GETTING STARTED
in the
COMPUTERIZED MEDICAL OFFICE
Fundamentals and Practice

Second Edition

CINDY CORREA

*Former Educational Coordinator and Curricula Developer for
City University of New York at Queens College—Allied Health Program/CEP*

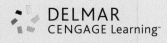

DELMAR
CENGAGE Learning™

Australia • Brazil • Japan • Korea • Mexico • Singapore • Spain • United Kingdom • United States

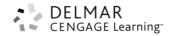
DELMAR
CENGAGE Learning

Getting Started in the Computerized Medical Office: Fundamentals and Practice, Second Edition
Cindy Correa

Vice President, Career and Professional Editorial: Dave Garza

Director of Learning Solutions: Matthew Kane

Senior Acquisitions Editor: Rhonda Dearborn

Managing Editor: Marah Bellegarde

Senior Product Manager: Sarah Prime

Editorial Assistant: Lauren Whalen

Vice President, Career and Professional Marketing: Jennifer Baker

Marketing Director: Wendy Mapstone

Senior Marketing Manager: Nancy Bradshaw

Marketing Coordinator: Erica Ropitzky

Production Director: Carolyn Miller

Senior Content Project Manager: Stacey Lamodi

Senior Art Director: Jack Pendleton

Senior Technology Product Manager: Mary Colleen Liburdi

Technology Project Manager: Erin Zeggert

Library of Congress Control Number: 2010920752

ISBN-13: 978-1-4354-3847-7
ISBN-10: 1-4354-3847-7

Delmar
5 Maxwell Drive
Clifton Park, NY 12065-2919
USA

Cengage Learning is a leading provider of customized learning solutions with office locations around the globe, including Singapore, the United Kingdom, Australia, Mexico, Brazil, and Japan. Locate your local office at:
international.cengage.com/region

Cengage Learning products are represented in Canada by Nelson Education, Ltd.

To learn more about Delmar, visit **www.cengage.com/delmar**
Purchase any of our products at your local college store or at our preferred online store **www.CengageBrain.com**

NOTICE TO THE READER

Publisher does not warrant or guarantee any of the products described herein or perform any independent analysis in connection with any of the product information contained herein. Publisher does not assume, and expressly disclaims, any obligation to obtain and include information other than that provided to it by the manufacturer. The reader is expressly warned to consider and adopt all safety precautions that might be indicated by the activities described herein and to avoid all potential hazards. By following the instructions contained herein, the reader willingly assumes all risks in connection with such instructions. The publisher makes no representations or warranties of any kind, including but not limited to, the warranties of fitness for particular purpose or merchantability, nor are any such representations implied with respect to the material set forth herein, and the publisher takes no responsibility with respect to such material. The publisher shall not be liable for any special, consequential, or exemplary damages resulting, in whole or part, from the readers' use of, or reliance upon, this material.

Printed in the United States of America
2 3 4 5 6 7 14 13 12 11

Dedication

*To the hard working educators, administrators, and directors
in technical career programs everywhere. Your efforts and dedication
make a difference in the lives of many.
Thank you.*

Contents

From the Author

When I began my journey as an educator in the early 1980s, mentored by a wonderful teacher and program administrator, I had no idea that she saw potential and would develop a love of teaching in me. She carefully directed me in curricula development, targeted lesson planning, and the art of presentation. In me, she had the raw materials. As my mentor, she provided the example to be followed, and put the finishing touches on my foundation for my future in education. Because of these early roots and personal instruction, many doors opened for me, allowing me to be creative with future courses and to demand the best from my students. As their successes became evident, this spurred me on to grow, change, and improve the time spent in the classroom with them. Through the years, many of my students have surpassed what they had hoped to do when they entered school, having had the support, knowledge, and tools to believe they could—and that they would—just as I did from my mentor.

This book is dedicated to everyone involved in the process of administrating and teaching in the technical schools and colleges. There are many challenges, but the ultimate goal we have for our students is for them to succeed in their chosen careers. I hope this book contributes to the success of your students, and that it provides another road to the destinations of solid employment, job satisfaction, and security. Students come to school seeking a change, a fresh start, and different personal goals. Most begin classes with excitement and enthusiasm and lots of hope for a better future. It is an honor for me to participate in this endeavor, and I commend you for your hard work and dedication in assisting your students in reaching their goals. I wish you the best in giving them their finishing touches and being their example, as together, we bring some of the best people—our students—into the medical field.

Cindy Correa

ABOUT THE AUTHOR

Cindy Correa has spent the majority of her time teaching in technical schools and colleges that offer medical career programs. Most recently, she was the Allied Health Educational Coordinator and senior instructor at City University of New York at Queens College. Cindy was responsible for the initial creation and curricula development of at least seven certificate programs of the Allied Health Program, and extended her expertise to satellite courses in outlying adult education programs. Her experience and understanding of the dynamics and challenges of teaching in technical schools, including computer lab courses, have helped create a book that facilitates the educational process for instructors and students. Her experience working in the private practice and administrative hospital environments includes oncology, cardiovascular surgery, pulmonology, and thoracic surgery.

Preface

Through the years, computers have revolutionized entire industries, changing and improving the way business is conducted. The field of medicine is an example of an industry that has benefited greatly from this technology in many areas. Diagnostic equipment and procedures have been enhanced through computer assistance. Therapeutic devices and instruments have been automated and improved, bringing a higher level of efficiency and accuracy to the medical office. Physicians are now prepared and trained to use innovative new ways of providing health care; examples would include telemedicine, computer-assisted equipment, and surgical robotics. Communications have expanded into the digital world, through e-mail, Web sites, and the Internet. Information is transferred and used via these channels, including dictation and medical transcription. Software has been developed to manage administrative office procedures, patient records, medical billing, coding, and multiple compliance issues, to name a few.

Students who enter the medical field will undoubtedly use software for one or more aspects of any position in the health care industry. By far, the most common software new graduates encounter is practice management software. Every medical administrative office manages operational, patient, and financial data. In addition, basic knowledge of medical insurance, especially managed care, is essential. Today's health care plans often require preauthorizations, referrals, and protocols directly related to providing services and receiving payment.

Further, different regions of the country have insurance carriers, plans, and guidelines specific to them. To make matters more difficult, there are hundreds of medical software titles used in the field. This presents a challenge to educators and schools to provide a well-rounded education, so that graduates are best equipped to succeed in their new careers.

Getting Started in the Computerized Medical Office: Fundamentals and Practice, Second Edition, was written to address these challenges in the classroom. This book offers a foundation to the health care learner that encompasses the entire reimbursement process and applies it to using practice management software. Starting with appointment scheduling, the material sequentially moves through patient registration, procedure posting, medical billing with paper claims and electronically, payment posting, secondary insurance billing, patient billing, and patient collections.

Easy-to-follow content and step-by-step directions make *Getting Started in the Computerized Medical Office: Fundamentals and Practice*, Second Edition, ideal for self-study learners and students in the classroom. Instructors can organize lectures and apply concepts learned from related course work to practical software use. This allows learners to work according to their individual abilities and pace. The content is flexible and easily adaptable to both entry-level and advanced curricula. The book can be used in stand-alone courses, as part of the computer/insurance billing component of a comprehensive program, or as a prerequisite to courses that actually use medical software. It accommodates schools that offer cyclic, open enrollment and classes to learners who possess different levels of computer skill.

Getting Started in the Computerized Medical Office: Fundamentals and Practice, Second Edition, offers a generic medical software with realistic simulations and training features, designed with career-training programs in mind.

ABOUT THE SOFTWARE: *MEDICAL OFFICE SIMULATION SOFTWARE (MOSS) 2.0*

Medical Office Simulation Software (MOSS) 2.0 is realistic in its look and functionality, containing elements that are representative of a broad cross section of popular practice management software on the market today. In MOSS, you will be oriented to the general functions of most practice management software (see Figure 1). There are eight basic components common to most practice management software:

- Appointment Scheduling
- Patient Registration
- Online Eligibility
- Procedure Posting
- Insurance Billing
- Claims Tracking
- Posting Payments

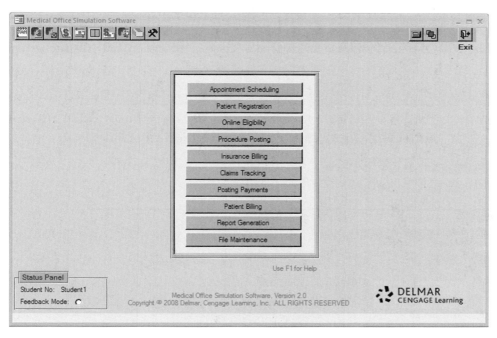

FIGURE 1
The Main Menu screen of MOSS. *Delmar/Cengage Learning.*

- Patient Billing
- Report Generation
- File Maintenance

MOSS 2.0 is available as a single-user version or as a classroom-led network version. As part of the network version, a classroom management Instructor's Console is available to provide comprehensive monitoring of individual students or entire classes.

Features have been built into the software that never before have been available in the classroom. They include a simulation of insurance verification/eligibility done online, and electronic submission of insurance claims. Figures 2 and 3 contain screen shots illustrating these features. Not only does the software simulate these procedures, but it also produces a report of the submission similar to those returned by insurance companies and clearinghouses. Furthermore, after simulating submission, the software treats the claims as "billed" for reports, secondary billing, and patient billing. The learner can then continue working further in the reimbursement process realistically.

Other educational features include Feedback Mode and Balloon Help Mode. Feedback mode will alert the user when essential fields have not been completed before allowing data to be saved, as shown in Figure 4. Balloon Help offers explanations, clarification, or reminders for certain fields, as shown in Figure 5. When using the single-user version, the user can easily turn these functions on or off in the File Maintenance area of the software. When using the network version, the instructor controls the application of these features, and may turn them on or off as required.

It is not uncommon for busy computer labs to experience printer and hardware problems. Should this occur, alternate methods of using reports are often available, including on-screen viewing and saving options. These features permit instructors to progress with the day's lesson plan, despite potential equipment problems unrelated to the software.

Because the software was designed for use by students, the ability to make "on-the-fly" corrections, deletions of data, or even entire patient records, can be done without disrupting the database or report output. This also makes MOSS ideal for learners engaged in distance education and self-study programs,

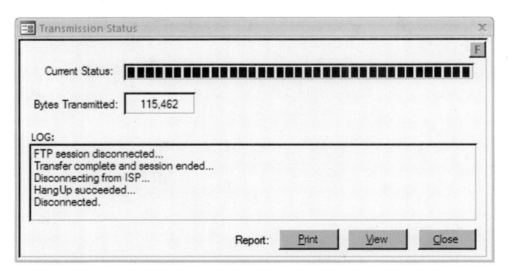

FIGURE 2

Electronic submission of insurance claims using MOSS. *Delmar/Cengage Learning.*

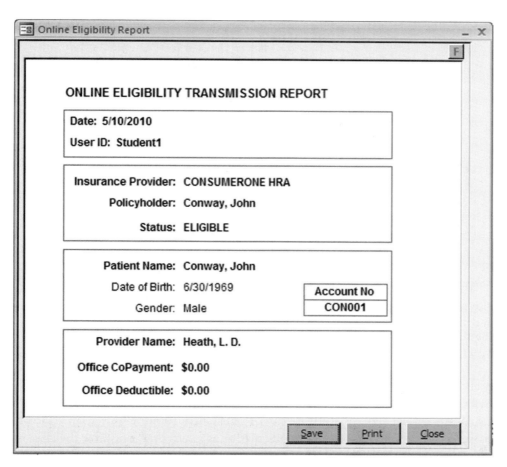

FIGURE 3

Online Eligibility report displayed by MOSS after using the simulator for this function.
Delmar/Cengage Learning.

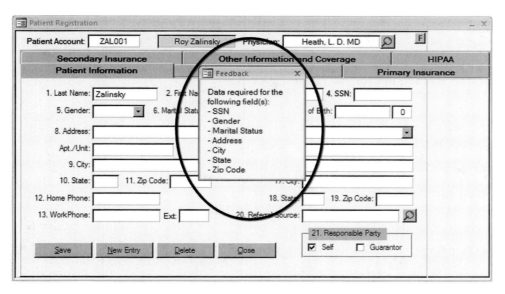

FIGURE 4

In feedback mode, a pop-up alerts the user that certain fields have not been completed.
Delmar/Cengage Learning.

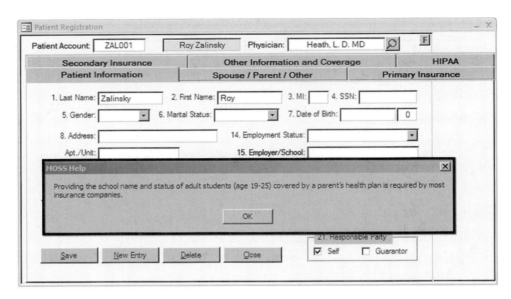

FIGURE 5

In balloon help mode, users can get additional information for certain fields within the software. *Delmar/Cengage Learning.*

since making corrections and being able to start again for individual exercises are possible. To facilitate learning, individual tasks or entire patient records can be deleted, so that learners can redo difficult tasks or make corrections. Also, if needed, the software can be reinstalled from the CD, allowing learners to restart the book and exercises over and over for more practice, or as a refresher long after the class is over.

The step-by-step directions and explanations in the text greatly assist classroom and self-study learners alike. This book is an asset to any program that wishes to offer in-classroom and distance education training, allowing both to use the same materials and curriculum.

NEW TO MOSS 2.0

- ✦ Claims-tracking module to simulate receiving electronic remittance advice reports from insurance carriers
- ✦ Separate fee schedules for each insurance type
- ✦ CMS–1500 claim forms populate data based on insurance type selected
- ✦ Several reports added, including prebilling report, monthly report, and individual patient ledger report
- ✦ Improved patient search functionality

NEW TO THE NETWORK VERSION

- ✦ Completely redesigned and streamlined Instructor's Console for more intuitive usability
- ✦ New Data Comparison reporting; improved student and class usage reporting
- ✦ Established security levels for students, instructors, administrators, and superadministrator
- ✦ Rebuilt infrastructure to accommodate more concurrent users

ORGANIZATION OF UNITS

Getting Started in the Computerized Medical Office: Fundamentals and Practice, Second Edition, consists of 11 units that walk the student through the theory and computer application of the entire management and reimbursement process of a private group practice. In order to accommodate the vast array of curricula and educational programs available, two units have been provided that either can be used or excluded accordingly. These are Unit 1, *Introduction to Computers,* and Unit 4, *Fundamentals of Medical Insurance.* These units can be safely removed from the lesson plan without affecting future exercises, report output, or the sequence of other units. However, all other units must be completed in sequence in order for the material and exercises to flow logically with the software.

UNIT 1—INTRODUCTION TO COMPUTERS

Unit 1 can be used for programs that wish to include an introduction as part of the medical software course. It is ideal for those who have little or no computer experience. It also can be used as a review for learners who have already taken an introductory computer course, or those who have learned to use computers only through hands-on experience. This unit clarifies many terms and misunderstandings regarding hardware, software, and technologies available today. A short introduction to Windows® and exercises to reinforce skills required to use MOSS are included.

UNIT 2—MEDICAL PRACTICE MANAGEMENT SOFTWARE

Unit 2 must be completed, and covers the components of practice management software and their function. Included is a general introduction to the Health Insurance Portability and Accountability Act (HIPAA) and relevant information, as applicable, to software use. Unit 2 introduces the software that accompanies the book, including logon procedures and instructions for navigating the software. Figure 6 illustrates an example of the HIPAA screen within the patient registration area. This screen is used with exercises to introduce learners to the procedures for notifying patients of privacy practices.

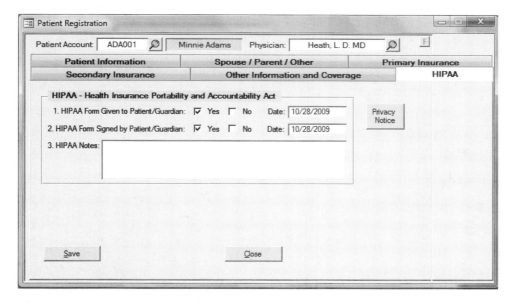

FIGURE 6
The HIPAA tab in the patient registration screen. *Delmar/Cengage Learning.*

UNIT 3—BASIC MANAGEMENT CONCEPTS FOR MEDICAL ADMINISTRATIVE STAFF

Unit 3 must be completed, and provides an understanding of the medical front and back offices and the staff members for each area. Basic principles of appointment scheduling for patients are covered, then applied using the software. Figure 7 shows an example of the Appointment Scheduling window included with MOSS. The flow of the office and information is discussed, including routines for preparing for patient visits, the check-in and check-out processes, and the reimbursement process.

UNIT 4—FUNDAMENTALS OF MEDICAL INSURANCE

Unit 4 can be used for programs that wish to include an introduction to medical insurance as part of the medical software course. It is ideal for learners who have not yet taken medical insurance courses (such as happens with open-enrollment schools), or as a review for learners who have already taken medical billing as a prerequisite. It is highly recommended that instructors and curriculum developers include this unit in their lesson plans. Many concepts are explained and reinforced, preparing learners for the situations and insurance plans encountered in the exercises of units that follow. The content of this unit sequentially occurs at Unit 4; however, if the unit is excluded, the instructor can safely begin Unit 5 without affecting the software database or report output.

UNIT 5—PATIENT REGISTRATION AND DATA ENTRY

Unit 5 must be completed, and begins the patient registration process. New patients are added to the software database. Complete demographics, guarantor, and insurance information are input, and some patients will have the simulated online insurance eligibility performed. Additionally, new patients who receive services outside the office, such as at hospitals and nursing homes, will be added to the database. Discussion of obtaining registration information for new patients outside the office is covered. Figure 8 shows an example of the comprehensive registration window. Registration includes patient demographics, guarantor information, and primary and secondary insurance information, all accessible in one area.

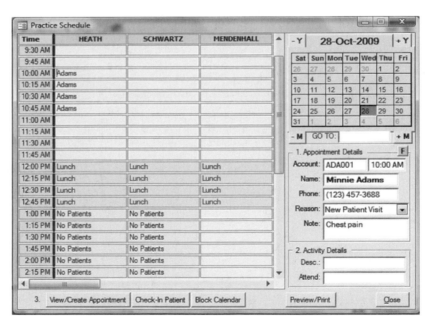

FIGURE 7

The Appointment Scheduling screen. *Delmar/Cengage Learning.*

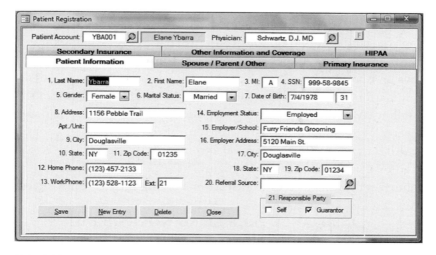

FIGURE 8

The patient information tabs in the Patient Registration screen.
Delmar/Cengage Learning.

UNIT 6—PROCEDURE POSTING ROUTINES

Unit 6 must be completed, and uses the software to apply procedural charges to patient accounts. Learners enter numerous case studies that include in-office, hospital, and nursing home procedures and services. As part of the patient check-out process, follow-up appointments are scheduled after the office visits are completed. An example of the Procedure Posting window is shown in Figure 9.

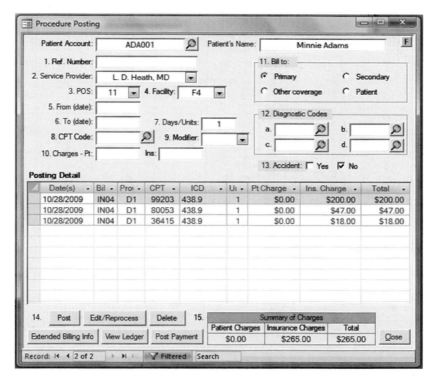

FIGURE 9

The Procedure Posting screen. *Delmar/Cengage Learning.*

UNIT 7—INSURANCE BILLING ROUTINES

Unit 7 must be completed, and builds upon the procedure charges entered in Unit 6. Basic requirements for insurance claims submission are covered, followed by utilization of the software to perform medical billing. Learners have an opportunity to prepare paper claims, as well as to send-claims electronically, using the MOSS simulation of online claims submission (see Figure 2). New to the second edition is the Insurance Pre-Billing Worksheet, allowing user review of claims details before they are submitted. This useful worksheet allows student and instructor to review data input before claims are finalized, as shown in Figure 10. All claims, whether paper or electronic, display on a CMS–1500 for preview before electronic submission or printing, as shown in Figure 11. A Claims Submission Report is generated after claims are submitted, creating a record of electronic billing activity, illustrated in Figure 12.

INSURANCE PREBILLING WORKSHEET
Student1

Dates of Service	Diag Code	Proc Code	POS	Units	Dr	As	Bill Amt	Receipts	Net
Medicare - Statewide Corp.									
Adams, Minnie									
10/28/2009	438.9	36415	11	1.00	D1	Y	$18.00	$0.00	$18.00
10/28/2009	438.9	80053	11	1.00	D1	Y	$47.00	$0.00	$47.00
10/28/2009	438.9	99203	11	1.00	D1	Y	$200.00	$0.00	$200.00
					Totals		$265.00	$0.00	$265.00
Blanc, Francois									
11/24/2009	401.9	99307	32	1.00	D1	Y	$68.00	$0.00	$68.00
					Totals		$68.00	$0.00	$68.00

FIGURE 10

A sample insurance pre-billing worksheet. *Delmar/Cengage Learning.*

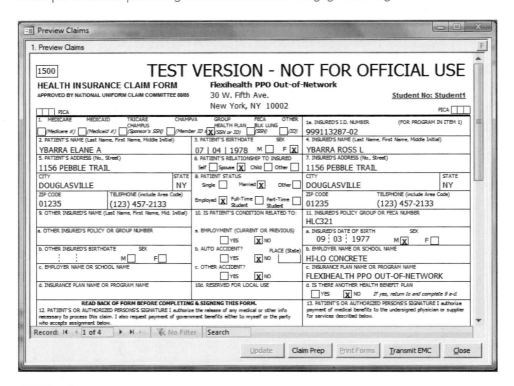

FIGURE 11

CMS–1500 forms are previewed on the screen prior to submission. *Delmar/Cengage Learning.*

Claims Submission Report
Student1

Medicare - Statewide Corp.

Patient Name
Minnie Adams

Account No ADA001	*DOS*	*Procedure*	*Charges*	*Result*
	10/28/2009	99203	$200.00	A
	10/28/2009	80053	$47.00	A
	10/28/2009	36415	$18.00	A
Patient Totals			$265.00	

FIGURE 12

A sample Claims Submission report generated after electronic submission.
Delmar/Cengage Learning.

UNIT 8—POSTING PAYMENTS AND SECONDARY INSURANCE BILLING

Unit 8 must be completed, and sequentially follows the insurance claims that were prepared and submitted in Unit 7. Learners use realistic examples of explanation of benefits or remittance advice notices to post payments from insurance companies and to patient accounts. Attention is given to patients who have deductible applications—co-insurance for balance billing to secondary plans or for patient billing. Figure 13 illustrates a sample Remittance Advice notice from a simulated insurance plan from the books students will use to post insurance payments. Figure 14 demonstrates the Payment Posting window in MOSS.

Explanation of Medical Benefits   **FlexiHealth PPO Plan**

Service Date	Type of Service	Charge(s) Submitted	Not Covered or Discount	Amount Covered	Patient Co-payment Co-insurance Deductible	Covered Balance	Plan Liability	See Note
Insured Name WORTHINGTON, CYNTHIA		Insured/Patient ID 999215992			Patient Name WORTHINGTON, CYNTHIA			
Provider Name: L.D. Heath, MD – In-Network Provider Reference Number: 987556								
10/30/2009	99213 Est. Pat/Level 3	$111.00	$28.60	$82.40	$20.00 co-pay	$62.40	$62.40	A
						Total Paid:	$62.40	
Insured Name YBARRA, ROSS		Insured/Patient ID 999113287			Patient Name YBARRA, ELANE			
Provider Name: D.J. Schwartz MD – Out-of-Network Provider Reference Number: 987557								
10/16/2009	99214 Est. Pat/Level 4	$180.00	$11.50	$168.50	$33.70 co-ins	$134.80	$134.80	B
10/16.2009	87081 Strep Screen	$16.00	$0.00	$16.00	$3.20 co-ins	$12.80	$12.80	B
11/06.2009	99215 Est. Pat/Level 5	$249.00	$33.20	$215.80	$43.16 co-ins	$172.64	$172.64	B
11/06.2009	81000 UA w/micro	$12.00	$0.00	$12.00	$2.40 co-ins	$9.60	$9.60	B
						Total Paid:	$329.84	
Insured Name TATE, JASON		Insured/Patient ID 999561133			Patient Name TATE, JASON			
Provider Name: L.D. Heath, MD – In-Network Provider Reference Number: 987558								
11/03/2009	99221 Hosp Admission	$145.00	$52.00	$93.00	$18.60 co-ins	$74.40	$74.40	A
11/04/2009	99231 Hosp Subsequent Care	$79.00	$26.00	$53.00	$10.60 co-ins	$42.40	$42.40	A
11/05/2009	99238 Hosp Discharge	$145.00	$86.80	$58.20	$11.64 co-ins	$46.56	$46.56	A
						Total Paid:	$163.36	

Notes on Benefit Determination:
A - Preferred provider discount. Patient is not required to pay this amount.
B – Patient is responsible for non-covered amounts for Out-of-Network providers.

FIGURE 13

A sample Remittance Advice used to post insurance payments.
Delmar/Cengage Learning.

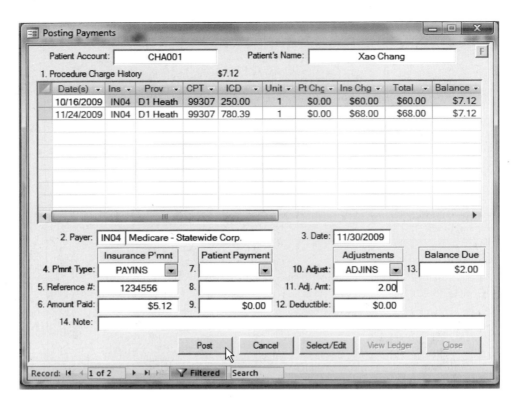

FIGURE 14

The Patient Posting screen. *Delmar/Cengage Learning.*

UNIT 9—PATIENT BILLING AND COLLECTIONS

Unit 9 must be completed. Discussing financials with patients is covered, including role-playing exercises learners can use with each other in class. The software is used to run reports to identify patients who require statements to collect balances due. Learners prepare statements, provide dunning messages, and print statements. Discussion of collections, both written and by telephone, is included. Exercises for writing collection letters and role-playing telephone collection techniques with patients are provided. Figure 15 illustrates the reports available for use with MOSS. Figure 16 is an example of the information contained in the Billing and Payment Report. Reports have been designed to reflect the learner's work, containing information directly related to the work done by the student. Both instructors and learners can review work for accuracy, pinpoint errors, or even use the results for grading purposes.

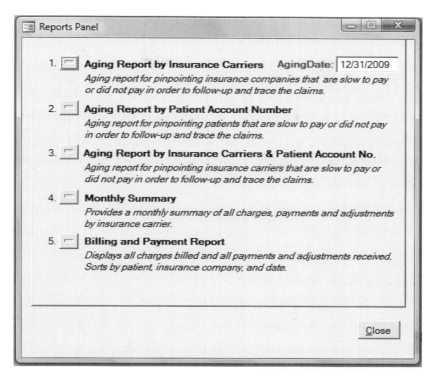

FIGURE 15

Reports available when using MOSS. *Delmar/Cengage Learning.*

Billing & Payments for Student1

Account / Insurance Provider	Date of Service	Submitted By	Total Claim	Patient Payment	Payment Code	Insurance Payment	Dis-count	Adjust. Code	Adjust. Amount	Deduct-ible	Balance Due
ADA001 Minnie Adams											
IN04 Medicare - Statewide Corp.	28-Oct-09	Electronic	$200.00	$21.40	PAYINS	$85.59	0	ADJINS	$93.01	$0.00	$0.00
IN04 Medicare - Statewide Corp.	28-Oct-09	Electronic	$47.00	$0.00	PAYINS	$14.77	0	ADJINS	$32.23	$0.00	$0.00
IN04 Medicare - Statewide Corp.	28-Oct-09	Electronic	$18.00	$0.00	PAYINS	$3.00	0	ADJINS	$15.00	$0.00	$0.00
								Minnie Adams Balances:		$0.00	$0.00
BEA001 Kimberly Beals											
IN03 Signal HMO	03-Nov-09	Electronic	$283.00	$10.00	PAYINS	$5.93	0	ADJINS	$267.07	$0.00	$0.00
IN03 Signal HMO	03-Nov-09	Electronic	$47.00	$0.00	PAYINS	$15.93	0	ADJINS	$31.07	$0.00	$0.00
IN03 Signal HMO	03-Nov-09	Electronic	$18.00	$0.00	PAYINS	$15.93	0	ADJINS	$2.07	$0.00	$0.00
								Kimberly Beals Balances:		$0.00	$0.00

FIGURE 16

A sample Billing and Payments report generated by MOSS. *Delmar/Cengage Learning.*

UNIT 10—POSTING SECONDARY INSURANCE PAYMENTS AND ELECTRONIC REMITTANCE ADVICE PAYMENTS

Unit 10 must be completed, and provides an opportunity to use the software to post payments from secondary insurance plans. A different set of explanation of benefits or remittance advice notices is used to read payment details and apply them to patient accounts. Figure 17 illustrates a Patient Ledger after the student has completed posting a payment from a secondary insurance plan.

New to the second edition, payments are posted from an HMO plan using an electronic Remittance Advice generated by the software, after direct deposit has been made to the provider's account. Figure 18 shows an example of the electronic RA for the HMO plan from the book.

PROVIDER PAYMENT ADVICE
Signal HMO
Student1

Patient Name   Kimberly Beals   (BEA001)

Claim ID	DOS	Procedure	Charges	Allowed Amount	Patient Responsibility	Rejected Amount	Paid to Provider	Remarks
1000351	11/3/2009	36415	$18.00	$15.93	$0.00	$0.00	$15.93	A
1000350	11/3/2009	80053	$47.00	$15.93	$0.00	$0.00	$15.93	A
1000349	11/3/2009	99204	$283.00	$15.93	$10.00	$0.00	$5.93	A
Patient Totals			$348.00	$47.79	$10.00	$0.00	$37.79	

FIGURE 17

A sample electronic Remittance Advice generated with the Claims Tracking feature. *Delmar/Cengage Learning.*

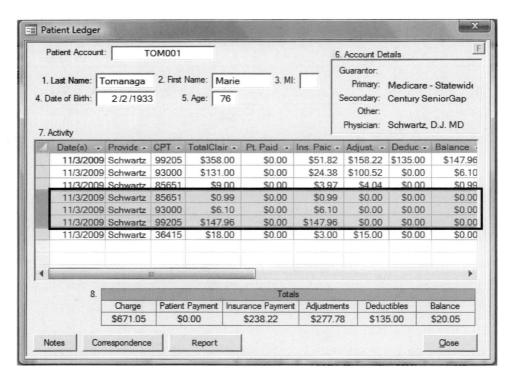

FIGURE 18

Patient Ledger screen. *Delmar/Cengage Learning.*

UNIT 11—INSURANCE CLAIMS FOLLOW-UP AND DISPUTE RESOLUTION

Unit 11 reviews tracking and follow-up of unpaid and problem claims from insurance companies. Various types of problem claims are discussed, as well as how to resolve them. Types of actions are covered, whether the action be rebilling a claim, providing documentation, or disputing a payment decision by submitting a formal review or appeal. Medicare's specific procedures are covered, as well as actions pertaining to private third-party payers.

FEATURES IN THE BOOK

- ◆ Objectives at the beginning of each unit clearly specify the content to be learned and the skills that will be mastered using the software, where applicable.

- ◆ Content within the book is grouped by subject for easy reading and instructor presentation, followed by immediate application of the concepts by using the software. Learners have an opportunity to study a topic in small segments, and then see it in action through software use. This also helps to start and end classes at logical points, and accommodates class sessions of varying lengths.

- ◆ Each exercise has its own objective, giving the instructor and the learner direction on the purpose of the task and the desired outcome upon its completion.

- ◆ Exercises include step-by-step directions supported by many screen shots, showing how the screen should look before and after processing data.

- ◆ Hints and special notes are interspersed throughout the exercises to remind students of important information, preventing common errors and thereby saving time.

- ◆ Each unit ends with the Final Notes section, summarizing the material just learned, and relating it to the topic in the next unit.

- ◆ Each unit provides a Check Your Knowledge review section to reinforce the topics learned.

NEW TO THE SECOND EDITION

- ◆ All exercises updated to correspond with new MOSS 2.0 features, functionality, buttons, and dates

- ◆ Source documents located in an appendix to allow for easier viewing and use of important forms and documents utilized in the exercises

- ◆ Bookmark provided to cover data entry field answers within the text in Units 5, 6, and 8 to check work and ensure accuracy

- ◆ Key Terms identified at the beginning of each chapter

- ◆ MOSS Notes that identify usability and troubleshooting tips

- ◆ Many more screen shots to check work

NEW TOPICS IN UNIT 1

+ Implications and impact of HIPAA and EHR
+ Dedicated and shared servers and firewalls
+ Blu-ray discs, flash memory, and Bluetooth technology
+ WiFi technology

NEW TOPICS IN UNIT 2

+ Implications of minicomputers and mobile phones as they relate to the medical office
+ The use of clearinghouses
+ The American Recovery and Reinvestment Act of 2009 (ARRA)
+ Using the backup and restore functions of MOSS, with new *Let's Try It!* activity
+ Resources for additional information

NEW TOPICS IN UNIT 3

+ Larger date range in MOSS, from January 1, 2008 to December 31, 2013
+ Revised appointment scheduling instructions based on changes in MOSS
+ Screen shots for each appointment scheduled, to check work
+ Implications of EHRs on appointment scheduling

NEW TOPICS IN UNIT 4

+ The Patient Protection and Affordable Care Act
+ Medicare Part D prescription drug program
+ Medicare Advantage Plans

NEW TOPICS IN UNIT 5

+ Data entry answers that can be covered by the Bookmark prior to entering information into MOSS

NEW TOPICS IN UNIT 6

+ Updated superbill
+ Data entry answers that can be covered by the Bookmark prior to entering information into MOSS
+ Updated fee schedules in MOSS

NEW TOPICS IN UNIT 7

+ Instructions in generating prebilling worksheets within MOSS prior to claims submission

NEW TOPICS IN UNIT 8

+ Electronic payment and statement systems (EPS)
+ Data entry answers that can be covered by the Bookmark prior to entering information into MOSS

NEW TOPICS IN UNIT 9

+ Bill pay system
+ Two new case study patients for *Let's Try It!* Writing Collection Letters

NEW TOPICS IN UNIT 10

+ Posting Secondary Insurance Payments and Electronic Remittance Advice Payments
+ Post payments based on an electronic Remittance Advice
+ Print an electronic Remittance Advice from MOSS
+ New *Let's Try It!* Posting Payments from an Electronic Payment Advice with five patient case studies

NEW UNIT 11

+ Insurance Claims Follow-up and Dispute Resolution
+ The Medicare appeals process, with two new forms
+ New *Let's Try It!* Prepare a Letter of Appeal

LEARNING PACKAGE

To provide students and instructors with complete support in the classroom, the following products are available:

+ **Workbook.** Written by the author of the text, the Workbook includes additional practice using MOSS, by providing more exercises, review questions, and critical thinking problems. A comprehensive final examination with answer key is included.

+ **Instructor's Manual.** Written by the author of the text, the Instructor's Manual includes lesson plans, answers to questions posed in the text and workbook, and tips for software use.

+ **Instructor Resources.** This CD-ROM includes instructor slides created in Microsoft PowerPoint and electronic Instructor's Manual files.

+ **Instructor Companion Site.** Includes MOSS 2.0 tutorials and documentation, back up files, network version compare report files, and Instructor Resources materials. Directions for accessing are found in the Instructor's Manual.

+ **Student Companion Site.** Includes MOSS 2.0 tutorials, documentation, and updates. Go to www.cengagebrain.com, enter "Correa" in the search bar and click Find. Click on this book's title to bring up the Product page, then click the Access Now button.

+ **WebTUTOR™ on WebCT or Blackboard.** These course cartridges include online Class Notes, additional Activities, Quizzes with automatic feedback and scoring, Flashcards, and Midterm and Final Exams.

TECHNICAL SUPPORT

For technical support related to Medical Office Simulation Software (MOSS) 2.0, please contact Delmar Technical Support, Monday–Friday from 8:30 a.m. to 6:30 p.m. EST:

+ Phone: 1-800-648-7450

+ Email: delmar.help@cengage.com

Acknowledgments

There are always many people involved in the writing of a book such as this. I thank each and every one for the effort put into this ongoing project.

Special thanks go to Elizabeth Hartman, Senior Systems Consultant for InHealth Record Systems, and everyone at InHealth who assists me with all of my writing projects. You continue to provide the very best for my books, from making updates and edits to providing custom forms and keeping this book current with the latest information. It is truly a pleasure working with you!

Many thanks to the many individuals at Delmar Cengage Learning who contributed to the creation of this book, providing the guidance and support for this ongoing project: Rhonda Dearborn, Senior Acquisitions Editor; Mary Colleen, Senior Technology Product Manager; Erin Zeggert, Technology Project Manager; Stacey Lamodi, Senior Content Project Manager; Jack Pendleton, Senior Art Director.

A special thanks to Sarah Prime, my Senior Product Manager, who is always patient, intuitive, and extraordinarily helpful with every facet of the book and software. The time and effort Sarah has spent in knowing MOSS inside and out, participating in the development of the software, giving her input, and being willing to hear my suggestions and implement them, is very much appreciated. The rigorous scrutiny she has given to my book has improved the overall quality of this work.

I wish to thank each one of the reviewers for their contributions to this and the previous edition of this book. Their suggestions, edits, and "extra set of eyes" have been so helpful. Instructors and field reps who shared information for improvements—many thanks. I even received a book marked with suggestions and comments, which provided so much insight as to how this book is used on a page-by-page basis. To those who provided these materials and more, helping to make an even better product, I am indebted. I do not have all the names or academic addresses, but they know who they are.

Finally, heartfelt thanks to those who are close to me on a daily basis. Whenever I am hard at work in a complex project, family and friends are so important. They are the very backbone of my success.

REVIEWERS

The publisher, as well as the author, would like to thank the following reviewers for their feedback and suggestions for improvement at each manuscript stage:

Cherika DeJesus, CMA (AAMA)
Medical Assistant Program Coordinator
Minnesota School of Business
Plymouth, MN

Linda Demain, MS, BS, LPN
Lead Instructor, Medical Assistant Program
Wichita Technical Institute
Wichita, KS

William Griz, PhD
Associate Professor
International College
Naples, FL

Patricia Hamilton
Medical Instructor
Pittsburgh Technical Institute
Oakdale, PA

Linda Henningsen, MS, RN
Nursing Administrator and Department Chair for Allied Health
Brown Mackie College
Salina, KS

Michelle Lenzi, M.Ed, CPC, CPC-H, CPC-I
Adjunct Professor
Hesser College
Manchester, NH

Alice Macomber, RN, RMA, RPT, AHI, CPI, BXO
Medical Assisting Program Coordinator
Keiser University
Fort Pierce, FL

Dawn Pessa
Remington College
Nashville, TN

Tiffany Rosta, CMA (AAMA)
Medical Instructor
Kaplan Career Institute
ICM School of Business and Medical Careers
Pittsburgh, PA

Janet J. Sorahan, BA, MS
Business Technology Instructor
Central Community College
Grand Island Campus
Grand Island, NE

Gayla Taylor
Instructor/Assistant Director of Education
PCI Health Training Center
Dallas, TX

Thomas J. Wesley, AS, BS, EMT
Medical Assistant Program Coordinator
Minnesota School of Business
Elk River, MN

How to Use this Book

Getting Started in the Computerized Medical Office: Fundamentals and Practice, Second Edition, offers a hands-on approach to learning office practice management software and computer skills, and includes targeted reading, practical applications, and pedagogy.

LET'S TRY IT!

Found in most units, the *Let's Try It!* exercises acclimate the user to practical applications of MOSS. Each exercise begins with an objective, and offers step-by-step instruction as the user goes through each activity. The exercises become more challenging as the user becomes more competent and confident with the software.

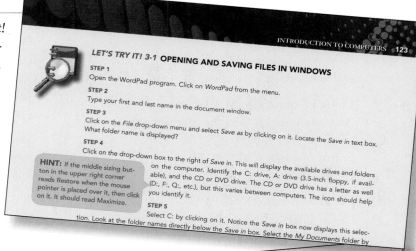

LET'S TRY IT! 3-1 OPENING AND SAVING FILES IN WINDOWS

STEP 1
Open the WordPad program. Click on *WordPad* from the menu.

STEP 2
Type your first and last name in the document window.

STEP 3
Click on the *File* drop-down menu and select *Save as* by clicking on it. Locate the *Save in* text box. What folder name is displayed?

STEP 4
Click on the drop-down box to the right of *Save in*. This will display the available drives and folders on the computer. Identify the C: drive, A: drive (3.5-inch floppy, if available), and the CD or DVD drive. The CD or DVD drive has a letter as well (D:, F:, Q:, etc.), but this varies between computers. The icon should help you identify it.

HINT: If the middle sizing button in the upper right corner reads Restore when the mouse pointer is placed over it, then click on it. It should read Maximize.

STEP 5
Select C: by clicking on it. Notice the *Save in* box now displays this selection. Look at the folder names directly below the *Save in* box. Select the *My Documents* folder by

SCREEN CAPTURES

Exercises include step-by-step directions supported by many screen captures of the actual software, showing how the screen should look before and after processing data.

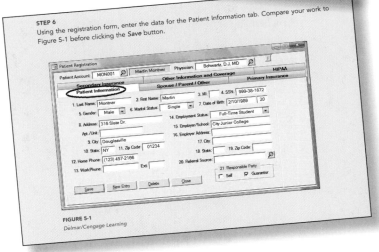

STEP 6
Using the registration form, enter the data for the Patient Information tab. Compare your work to Figure 5-1 before clicking the *Save* button.

FIGURE 5-1
Delmar/Cengage Learning

HINTS AND NOTES

Hints and Notes within the *Let's Try It!* exercises point out important information to help prevent common errors and save time.

HINT: Choose a password that is easy to remember, yet not something obvious that many people may know about you, such as a birth date.

STEP 4
Move your cursor into the Password field and delete the existing password. Enter a new password of your choice, making sure it is at least five characters in length.

STEP 5
Retype the new password in the next field to confirm it. Click *Save Record* (see Figure 2-8).

NOTE: If there is a typing error, a prompt will alert you to re-enter the password correctly.

FINAL NOTES

A Final Notes section concludes each chapter and emphasizes major discussion points, as well as relates the material to the next unit.

FINAL NOTES

It is important to have as broad-based a knowledge about computers and the use of their software as possible. Historically, many individuals resisted the advent of computerization and were left behind in terms of missed opportunities for advancement, higher income, or even upgrading skills until it was very late. Computer skills are no longer an option, but a necessity in today's work force.

Computers are now the standard tools in the medical office environment to perform daily tasks. Technology and new innovations that make health care professionals and their support staff more efficient are in use and will expand in the future. Mastering the information in this unit will provide you with a strong foundation of knowledge on which to build, and make you a more valuable staff member. This knowledge will facilitate on-the-job training during an externship or with your new employer. It will also position you for advancing your skills faster. Take advantage of all opportunities for learning new software, especially various practice management programs; the broader your skills set, the more doors will open to your future.

CHECK YOUR KNOWLEDGE

Each unit provides a Check Your Knowledge review section to reinforce the topics learned. Each of these sections includes a variety of types of questions that will appeal to many different learning styles, such as true/false, multiple choice, and short answer.

CHECK YOUR KNOWLEDGE

Select the correct answer for 1 through 4 from the following list.
a. Interconnected computers located in the same building
b. A computer that is not part of a network system
c. A computer operator
d. The process of interconnecting computers so that information can be exchanged between the machines

1. ____Networking
2. ____Stand-alone unit
3. ____User
4. ____LAN

In the blank, write *input, output,* or *both* for each of the following.
5. Mouse _____
6. Monitor _____
7. Digital camera _____
8. Printer _____
9. Software application _____
10. Speakers _____
11. Keyboard _____

Introduction to Computers

OBJECTIVES

Upon completion of this unit, the reader should be able to:

- **Identify types of computers common in medical environments**
- **Identify components of a personal computer**
- **Explain the data processing cycle and how it applies to computer tasks**
- **Differentiate between software and hardware**
- **Discuss common software used in the medical workplace and its function(s)**
- **Identify common hardware devices and their function(s)**
- **Demonstrate basic skills for using Microsoft® Windows**
- **Explain how to manage files in a Windows environment.**

The main difference between people who like using computers and those who do not is knowledge. In the beginning, we have a tendency to be afraid of computers—that they will break with the press of a wrong key or a stray click of the mouse. We panic as screens seem to disappear, then reappear. We worry about where our work has gone—lost, it seems—somewhere in the machine. At one time or another, everyone experiences this; with time and an understanding of how computers function, the fear begins to disappear. Everyone learns at a different pace. Remember to allow yourself the time needed, practice often, and be patient. The first step is tackling the basics. With knowledge of computer terminology and fundamental skills, your understanding will not only lay the foundation for learning more advanced work, but also it will help you enjoy using computers as the wonderful tools they really are.

KEY TERMS

Active window

Application window

Applications software

Central processing unit (CPU)

Command buttons

Data

Data processing

Dedicated server

Desktop

Dialog box

Digital camera

Digital files

Disk

Document window

Double click

Firewall

Floppy diskette

Hard copy

Hard drive

Hardware

Hot-swapped

Increment box

Input

Interface

TYPES OF COMPUTERS

While computers are manufactured with similar components, their use or purpose may be different from one another. Often, computers in an office are interconnected, or linked, so that information can be exchanged between them for many users. This is referred to as a **network**. Networking allows several users to share the same programs, files, and equipment—such as printers and an Internet connection. The most common type of network for computers that are located in the same building is referred to as a **local area network** or **LAN**. Networks can be hardwired, or wireless. When a computer is not part of a network, and all of its information is stored on and used from that computer only, it is called a **stand-alone unit**.

There are three main types of computers relevant to most medical environments:

1. **Mainframes.** These are powerful computers capable of supporting hundreds or thousands of users simultaneously. Government offices, schools, and large businesses, including medical environments, are good examples of where mainframes are used. Medical workers from various departments and outlying medical facilities can access patient information, records, and other pertinent data from these massive computers at the same time. In recent years, pressure to control costs has resulted in more use of mainframes in the hospital environment in areas such as billing and quality management. Mainframes are better equipped to secure patient records and data, helping to comply with stricter Health Insurance Portability and Accountability Act (HIPAA) regulations. The increased need to transfer patient records between facilities has created a demand for Electronic Health Records (EHRs), which require increased storage. This increased storage, best provided by the mainframe computer, also allows storage and viewing of huge image files, such as those from MRIs and CT scanning, allowing faster diagnostic results to reach providers faster.

2. **Servers.** A server is a computer that is accessible to other computers in a network, usually on a smaller scale than mainframes. Their job is to "serve" other computers connected to it by providing storage for data and access to files or programs. Servers often provide protection for the computers connected to them by providing a **firewall**. A firewall is software residing on a computer that is configured with rules that allow certain traffic, programs, and other network requests to move to and from the computers connected to the server. This helps protect from viruses, malicious attacks, or unauthorized access or use of certain areas or programs within the network.

   There are different types of servers with specific functions. These servers fall into two main categories: **dedicated servers** and **shared servers**. Dedicated servers perform only the specific tasks they were set up to do, such as hosting a website. Shared servers provide access to software, disk drives, and other areas to the users connected to them. Computers that are networked to the servers are often called **workstations** or **nodes**. As a medical staff member, you will probably use a workstation for much of your work on the computer. The information you use will be located and accessible on the server.

3. **Personal Computer.** The company IBM, International Business Machines, first coined the term PC, or *personal computer*, and introduced a desktop computer model in 1981. Although this was IBM's first entry into this market, other companies including Apple, Commodore, and Tandy had already introduced personal computers as far back as the mid-1970s.

   A personal computer is a machine that contains a **microprocessor**, also known as the **central processing unit** or **CPU**. This device contains the **silicon chip**, which is composed of electrical components that are responsible for all functions that run the computer. The CPU is often called the brain of a personal computer. Without it, the computer cannot run programs, perform calculations, or direct instructions to other parts of the computer. Figure 1-1 illustrates and identifies components of the personal desktop computer.

   While desktop computers continue to be the standard in any office environment, for those with the need to stay mobile, the laptop computer is the ideal solution. They come in all sizes, even small enough to fit in the palm of your hand. Since laptop computers first came to market around 1989, their capabilities have improved to the point where they now provide all of the computing power and features of a desktop computer. Laptops now come with long battery life, Internet connectivity, video cards, and high-quality stereo sound. While generally more expensive than the desktop computer, the modern laptop can do everything the desktop computer does.

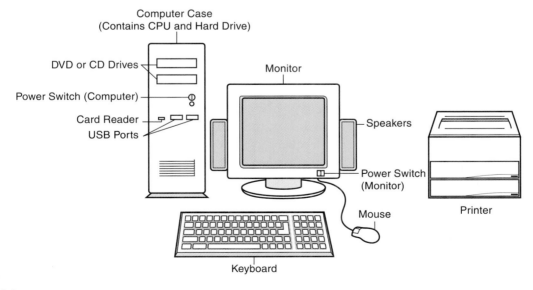

FIGURE 1-1

Components of a personal computer (PC). *Delmar/Cengage Learning*

THE DATA PROCESSING CYCLE

The **data processing** cycle of a computer usually includes three functions: input, processing, and output. Information, also known as **data**, needs to go into the computer. For example, if you are adding information on three new patients, it must be keyed or entered into the computer. This is referred to as data **input**. You are probably familiar with common input devices, such as the keyboard and mouse. A microphone is also an input device used to input sound in a format that can be played by the computer.

Other examples of input devices are **digital cameras** and **scanners**, which are used to convert pictures or text into digital files. **Digital files** is a term used to refer to any data in a format that can be recognized and used by the computer. Once data is input, the computer can then process the data. **Processing** occurs when the computer performs arithmetic and logical operations so that the data can be productively used or manipulated.

Digital cameras are popular in medical offices because pictures of patients, for identification, can be quickly and easily taken and immediately transferred to the computer. A camera is useful for storing photographs where tracking or comparisons are needed, such as with dermatology or plastic surgery cases. For example, a physician may want to document changes in a mole by keeping a photographic history over several months or years. Plastic surgeons typically take before and after photos, and can even alter photos using software to show a patient the approximate desired outcome of surgery.

In the area of medical records, scanning paper documents and then saving them on the computer as digital files make access and storage more convenient. Records can then be quickly viewed on the monitor instead of pulling out patient files and sifting through numerous papers. As previously mentioned, the increasing demand to convert to digital records, thus eliminating paper files and diagnostic films, has created a need for electronic health records, utilizing specialized programs for this purpose. The ease of use, faster access, simplification of routine tasks, and the overall positive impact on the environment by reducing paper use and waste material have made electronic records very desirable.

Processing requires the computer to use a **software program**. Software programs generate specific instructions the computer follows that cause it to function in a certain manner. For instance, once images are input from a digital camera to the computer, it is likely those images will need to be viewed. A software program, such as Adobe® Photoshop, can be used for this purpose. Manipulation means that the data can be altered or changed—for example, to resize the images or make improvements to their appearance. These files can then be stored in the computer for later use.

The last function in the data processing cycle is **output**, which refers to anything that comes out of a computer. Output can appear in many forms, the most common being information displayed on the monitor screen. Another example of a frequently used output is the printer. Printers produce **hard copies** of digital files. Hard copy is the term used to describe the paper documents produced by the printer. Speakers are output devices used to hear sound files, such as music, or any other sound that comes from the computer and its programs.

SOFTWARE

Many components of a computer system have been mentioned, such as the CPU, monitor, keyboard, mouse, and printer. In this section, common terminology associated with computers is discussed. Often, software and hardware concepts are misunderstood. The definitions that follow will demystify these concepts and help you understand computer systems in general.

As mentioned previously, software programs are instructions that are followed by the computer that cause it to function in a certain manner. Software has no physical characteristics, but rather, consists of ideas, concepts, and symbols. Software is divided into two categories: applications software and systems software.

APPLICATIONS SOFTWARE

Applications software allows the computer user to perform specific tasks or work. For example, word processors, spreadsheets, and database management programs are in the category of applications software. Medical practice management software is also applications software used by medical offices for many functions, including scheduling patient appointments, accounting tasks, and insurance billing. It is not uncommon for medical staff members to use additional software, alongside the practice management software, for completing necessary tasks associated with the office. The following list will familiarize you with the broad categories of applications software you might use in your place of employment.

- **Word processing programs** allow the use of text for producing documents such as correspondence, reports, medical notes, journal manuscripts, etc. Examples are Microsoft® Word and WordPerfect®.

- **Spreadsheet programs** allow information, namely numbers, to be used in rows and columns. Mathematical formulas can be applied to these numbers for various uses and results. Such uses might include payroll preparation and tracking sales figures. These formulas can range from simple addition to complex calculations. An example of a popular spreadsheet program is Microsoft® Excel.

- **Database management programs** enable information to be stored, modified, and retrieved in useful ways. Examples of database information include memberships, client lists, and inventory tracking, such as pharmaceuticals and medical supplies. Microsoft® Access is a popular database program.

There are many types of applications software. Sometimes, combinations of these programs are used within a large, single software program. Such is the case with medical practice management software, which is capable of using databases for patient information, practice and provider data, places of service, and other records. It can also use mathematical functions for financial purposes, such as maintaining patient accounts. A combination of these functions produces the reports needed for medical practice analysis and tracking specific information. In general, many programs can interface, or communicate, and function with each other within a primary software program in order to accomplish multiple tasks.

SYSTEMS SOFTWARE

Systems software refers to the **operating system (OS)** that enables the computer to communicate between its various components. This software is necessary in order for the applications software to run, and for any devices connected to the computer, such as printers and the keyboard, to work. Without the operating system, not only would software and devices not function, there would be no way for the user to communicate with the computer. Figure 1-2 shows various input and output sources and the operating system.

An example of an operating system is the popular Microsoft Windows program, which comes in various versions as updates are developed. These include the earlier Windows versions,

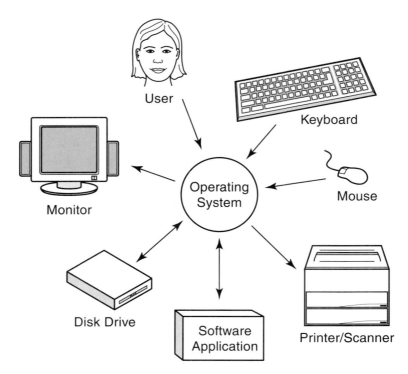

FIGURE 1-2

Input and output sources and the operating system. *Delmar/Cengage Learning*

called Windows®95 and Windows®98, and the more recent versions 2000, Me, NT®, XP, Vista, and Windows®7. There are a number of operating systems available for a vast array of uses, including popular names such as Linux, Unix®, and NetWare®, as well as the Apple Macintosh® operating systems, such as the MAC OS, and MAC OS X Snow Leopard.

HARDWARE

Unlike software, **hardware** refers to the physical parts of a computer. Often, the word **peripherals** is used to describe hardware devices connected to the computer. There are specific types of hardware and related terms that will be used for your work in the office and throughout this book. Following are short descriptions of the most common hardware components with which you should be familiar.

DRIVES

A drive is a machine, usually part of the computer system, that reads data from a disk or other storage media. In most cases, it can copy data to the disk as well. A **disk** is a round plate on which information, or data, can be recorded. A drive makes it possible for the data on these plates to be accessed and used by the computer. A common example of a disk is the *hard disk* that resides in the computer, which is discussed in the next section. A computer system can have several drives for different purposes; these are discussed further below. Note that the alternate spelling for disk is *disc*, although there are no real rules about their use.

Hard Disk Drive

The *hard disk drive* (HDD) is also referred to as the *resident drive*, *local drive*, or just *hard drive*. A **hard drive** is the disk that resides inside the computer and stores all software and files. Documents, software programs, presentations, games, and even the operating system itself, such as Windows, are stored on the hard drive. Because the computer can have more than one drive in it, letters are assigned to distinguish the various drives. The most common letter assigned to the hard drive is "C." It is commonly written as the letter followed by a colon—"C:"—and is also referred to as the *C: drive* (pronounced *see-drive*). Keep in mind that some computers may have more than one hard drive. Each drive has its own letter designation, such as the *F: drive*, *G: drive*, etc., which are assigned automatically by computers using Windows operating systems.

Floppy Diskette and Drive

A **floppy diskette** is a disk that stores data, similar to the hard drive, except it is portable and holds less information. Up until 2005, all computers came equipped with a floppy diskette, which was thin, 3.5 inches in size, and encased in a plastic cover. The diskette went into a slot in a drive located in the computer, usually at the front of the case. Data could be accessed and copied to and from the diskette as often as needed. This drive was usually identified by the letter "A" and is often written as "A:"— referred to as the *A: drive* (pronounced *ay-drive*). Again, depending on the installation, the floppy disk drive may have a different letter designation assigned to it. This drive is mentioned in this book because it was in common use up until fairly recently, and many computers are still around that have floppy drives in them. Some people are still using older operating systems and software that utilized floppy disks. However, it has been done away with in favor of more efficient drives and storage media, and is not found on today's modern computers.

CD-ROM and Drive

CD-ROM stands for Compact Disc-Read Only Memory. This means that the computer can use and transfer data from the compact disc (CD), but cannot erase or add any data to it. Thus, the terminology that the computer can read only, but not write or add data files to the CD, makes sense. Data CDs look like music CDs; however, they can hold graphics, videos, software programs, text, and sound files. One CD-ROM can hold 650–700 MB of data, or 74 to 80 minutes of music, respectively. CDs are used in the CD-ROM drive, also known as a CD player, located in the computer, usually in the front of the case. There are also external CD drives that can be connected to the computer. The drive is designated by a letter to identify it, such as "D:", although other letters might be used.

CD-R and CD Burners

Previously, we mentioned that a computer could not erase or add information to a CD-ROM. However, there are compact disc drives and special software that enable this to be done.

CD-R stands for Compact Disc-Recordable. This is a type of CD that permits data to be copied, or saved, onto it. Once the data is recorded onto the disc, the result is a CD-ROM, which can then be used in virtually any computer's CD-ROM drive in order to access and use the files. One drawback of the CD-R disc is that it can be recorded only once; data cannot later be added or erased from the disc once it has been *closed* or *finalized*. To close a CD means that it is prepared and finalized in order to be usable on most other computers. On modern computers, you can transfer files to and from a CD-R as long as it has not been closed. This allows the CD-R to be used in the same manner as an additional drive. Once you have completed copying files to the CD and you eject it from the CD player, the computer automatically closes the session on the CD, making it usable on most other computers with a

CD drive, but it is read-only (ROM). The information contained on the CD-ROM can be accessed as many times as needed, and can even be copied to the computer's hard drive, where permissible. There is also the CD-RW (rewritable), similar in just about all aspects to a CD-R, except that a CD-RW disc can be written to and erased many times.

Drives that can write (record) data onto a blank CD are typically called CD burners because data is burned onto the disc using a laser. Thus, the expression "burn a CD" means to copy, or write, data onto a CD-R or CD-RW disc. CD burners require special software for recording data, music, and other files onto the CDs. The Windows operating system includes built-in capabilities for burning data to CDs.

DVD and Drive

DVD stands for Digital Versatile Disk or Digital Video Disk. A DVD looks like a CD, but is based on different technology. Additionally, it holds much more data—roughly five to ten times more than a CD at 4.7 GB (gigabytes). This is why a DVD has the capacity to store a full-length movie. These discs are sometimes referred to as DVD-ROM and are also read-only, like their CD-ROM counterparts. A DVD drive plays not only DVDs, but also CD-ROMs and CD-R disks. Again, the drive is usually located in the front of the computer case.

Recordable DVDs are available in several formats. These function similar to the CD-R, and are also commonly referred to as DVD-R or DVD+R, DVD-RW, and DVD+RW. Although there were several compatibility issues when this technology first came out in the late 1990s, there have been improvements with the disks and players since that time. While special software is also required to burn to a DVD, the Windows operating system includes built-in capabilities for burning data to DVDs.

Blu-ray Discs (BD)

In 2006, the Blu-ray Discs (BD) were introduced. These discs were designed to function with high definition video, and eventually will probably replace the DVD. It derives its name from the blue-violet laser used to read the disc. Because of a vastly large storage capacity, Blu-ray discs can store and play back high definition video and digital audio, photos, and other digital content, such as computer data. These discs also come in ROM/R/RW formats.

A single-layer Blu-ray disc, which is about the size of a DVD, can hold up to 27 GB of data. That size can accommodate more than two hours of high definition video or roughly 13 hours of standard video. A double-layer Blu-ray disc stores up to 50 GB, which is enough to store approximately 4.5 hours of high definition video or more than 20 hours of standard video. As technology advances, and storage and playback demands continue to require more space, development of discs that hold much more are in the works. A Blu-ray disc player is required; however, these units will also play DVDs and Audio CDs.

RANDOM ACCESS MEMORY (RAM)

Random access memory (**RAM**) is the actual memory of the computer. It is often incorrectly referred to as storage and confused with the hard drive. There are several types of RAM; however, its basic function is to temporarily hold currently operating software programs and files while they are in use by the computer. The RAM feeds information to the processor as it is needed. Once you exit a program or turn off your computer, the information in the RAM is erased, since it is no longer being used. This is why it is important to remember to save your work often while you have software programs open.

Never exit a software program or the computer improperly, such as turning the machine off at the power switch, without closing programs. You might risk losing important data and hours of work, or cause software malfunctions. Furthermore, it is absolutely necessary to back up critical files at least weekly, if not more frequently, to prevent loss of data.

SERIAL, PARALLEL, AND USB PORT CONNECTIONS

Ports are the connectors on the computer that allow peripheral devices to be connected using special cables designed to fit into them. The **serial port** is a simple port and can be identified by its 9-pin socket. The **parallel port** is a 25-pin socket, which is most popular for plugging in the printer in older computers. It is rarely used for other purposes.

Because there are different ports with differing capabilities to connect peripheral devices, a universal port was developed in 1995 to help standardize peripheral connectivity. This port is called the **USB**, which stands for *universal serial bus*. Over the past few years, devices have been manufactured with USB cables and ports. The acceptance and versatility of USB has been so successful that it has quickly replaced serial and parallel ports in most modern computers. In fact, some computers come equipped only with USB ports, making it the only way peripherals can be connected to the computer. USB ports are especially attractive because devices can be **hot-swapped**, meaning one device can be disconnected and a different one plugged into the same slot with smooth transition from one to the other.

Most computers, both desktop and laptop, now come with several USB ports, in the front, back, and sides, so that several peripheral devices can be connected at one time. Special hubs can also be used, allowing one USB port to accept several devices by having several USB ports available on the hub to connect devices.

Flash Memory

As more digital devices became available and demand has increased, the need for storage of the output from these devices, such as images from digital cameras, has also increased. Flash memory refers to computer storage that can be electrically erased and reprogrammed, usually in the form of a small, portable memory card or stick that can be read in special card drives or in the USB port. This technology allows for general storage and transfer of data between computers and other digital products. A good example is the small memory cards that go inside a digital camera. When you take pictures, the images are stored on the card (often the approximate size of a postage stamp, and a little thicker than a credit card). When the images are ready to be viewed on the computer, the card can be put into a card reader and is accessed just like an additional drive (and is assigned a letter, such as F: or J:, etc.). Image files can then be viewed, copied, deleted, or opened on the computer. An external memory card reader can be connected to the computer, often via a USB port. Many of the modern computers and printers come equipped with built-in card readers right in the front panel, eliminating the need for an external card reader. These memory card readers contain several different sized minidrives to read the various sizes and types of cards that have been available since their introduction. Common ones in use today are the compact flash (CF), and more recently, the secure digital (SD) cards.

An example of a device popular with office workers, or anyone who uses more than one computer, is the **USB flash memory drive**, sometimes called a *jump drive, flash drive, pen drive,* or a *thumb drive*. These devices are about the size of a person's thumb, and come with various storage sizes. The flash memory drive plugs into the USB port and serves as additional storage, allowing files to be copied to and from the drive. It's a good tool for individuals who must take data from a home computer to a work computer or even exchange data between several computers. It is endlessly reusable, and most jump drives can be attached to a lanyard, so it can be worn around the neck or on the wrist, keeping the drive handy.

Bluetooth Technology

Bluetooth technology is a short-range wireless radio technology that allows electronic devices to connect to one another. It is capable of transmitting voice and data. Generally, Bluetooth has a range of up to 30 feet, and even over 100 feet in some newer devices.

In terms of data transmission, the purpose of Bluetooth wireless technology is to make connections between devices, in the same manner that cables and wires connect a computer to a keyboard, mouse, or printer. Bluetooth technology makes these same connections, except it does it without the cables and wires.

A common use of Bluetooth for voice transmission is the use of a wireless headset with a cell phone, so that you can answer and talk on the phone without any wires connecting the two devices.

Bluetooth is very secure, utilizing several layers of data encryption and user authentication protocols. Bluetooth devices use a combination of the personal identification number (PIN) and a Bluetooth address to identify other Bluetooth devices. Instead of transmitting over one frequency within a particular band, Bluetooth radios use fast frequency-hopping spread spectrum (FHSS), which allows only synchronized receivers to access the transmitted data. In this way, devices do not interfere with each other and communicate only with devices they are "paired" with. Because of its low cost and efficiency, it is likely that Bluetooth technology will be used for years to come.

DEVICES FOR INTERNET ACCESS

The **Internet** is a global network that connects millions of computers, enabling the exchange of data, news, and other information. When connections between computers are made on the Internet, the term "being **online**" is used. Currently there are many innovative uses for the Internet for medicine and medical practices, and new ideas are constantly being developed. Practice management applications are available for use through Web sites, including obtaining medical insurance verifications, referral authorizations, and status reports on payments. Some practices have online registration forms and questionnaires the patient can fill out and submit. Software at the medical office can be quickly updated with the latest data and upgrades by simply connecting to the company computers that provide these services. There are many choices for connecting to the Internet. The following list outlines some of the more common options likely to be encountered in medical offices.

1. **Modem.** The word *modem* is actually an acronym, which stands for <u>Mo</u>dulator-<u>Dem</u>odulator. A modem is a device that translates digital information from the computer into analog signals (audible tones) used by telephones, and vice versa. This allows computers to connect to each other and communicate over the phone wires. Because this type of access does not allow for normal use of the telephone line, offices will dedicate a line for modem use. Although modems are still a popular and relatively inexpensive method of accessing the Internet, they are slow and less effective for work purposes compared to other options, such as DSL or cable access.

2. **DSL.** The acronym DSL stands for *digital subscriber line*, a high-speed access to the Internet. It uses existing copper wires used for telephone service in the home or office without interfering with voice services. This means the telephone can be used at the same time the Internet is

accessed. A special modem is still necessary. Various forms of DSL technologies are available, but whether these options can be used often depends on how close the home or office is located to the central facility that provides the DSL service.

3. **Cable Modem.** A cable modem is another type of device that enables high-speed access to the Internet using cable television (CATV) wires instead of telephone lines. Cable modems translate radio frequency signals to and from the cable plant into usable information understood by all computers connected to the Internet. Cable Internet activity does not interfere with television service, and it allows for use of the telephone, since the phone wires are not used in any way.

4. **WiFi Technology.** WiFi, short for Wireless Fidelity, uses networking standards called 802.11, which come in several types. These types refer to the radio frequencies and speed with which data is moved. Common types are 802.11a, 802.11b, 802.11g and 802.11n, the latter being the newer standard with improved speed and range. This technology allows mobile users with laptop computers, personal digital assistant (PDA) devices, and smart phones to wirelessly connect to networks and, through that connection, reach both local and Internet resources for work, study, and recreational purposes. Wireless accessibility installed in certain areas of offices, colleges, libraries, and other locations are referred to as *wireless hotspots*. Computing devices must be equipped with wireless capability in order to access the Internet in this manner while in a hotspot.

In the near future, it will be commonplace for health insurance companies, practitioners, and patients to access each other easily for all types of business and communication. Patients will soon be able to videoconference effectively with their physicians, and many are now using e-mail to communicate with their health care professionals. It is easier and faster than ever to send medical records, X-rays, or scans as digital files to be viewed by health care professionals, both locally and anywhere in the world. Surgeons will perform computer-assisted surgery on patients located miles away, or in another country, using robotics. The possibilities are endless, and are quickly becoming reality, as devices and Internet access become faster and more efficient.

CONNECTING AND INSTALLING HARDWARE

You will use many types of hardware as you work with computers in the medical office. There may be times when the office purchases new peripherals, such as a scanner or an additional printer. You may be asked to connect and install these devices. It is important to remember that most hardware devices require software in order to be installed. It is often not sufficient to simply connect the device to the computer. Even though **plug-and-play (PnP)** hardware is popular, this simply means that the computer is able to automatically configure the hardware during installation using a generic driver. Software may still be required in order for the operating system to recognize and properly run the device. Because of this, after installing any device, remember to always save the software (the actual CDs or other media) that came with it in a safe location. These will come in handy if the device ever needs to be re-installed, or if additional files or programs are required at a future date. These files are often located on the software installation CD. Additionally, some software is now available as a downloadable execute (.exe) installation file. If software was purchased as a downloaded file, and did not come on a CD, be sure to store the execute file in a safe place, preferably copied to a CD in case of computer failure in the future. Any registration codes, keys, or other information needed to unlock the software for use should also be stored carefully with the execute file for downloaded software programs.

USING THE COMPUTER: A TOUR OF WINDOWS

As you have already learned, operating systems are programs that allow the computer to function. The operating system controls the information going to and from the various parts of the computer, and serves as the intermediary between software, hardware, and the user. Windows is currently the most widely used operating system for personal computers. In this section, a basic tour of Windows is covered to assist you in getting started with the software that accompanies this book. This knowledge will also be helpful when operating other software your employer may use on his or her computer system.

BOOTING THE COMPUTER

When the computer is turned on, the term *booting* the system is used. This simply refers to the computer using a special start-up program to load the operating system into memory. As the computer boots up, it may run a number of self-tests, configuration updates, and load programs. You may see several messages being displayed or simply a Windows screen as they are performed. You will not need to do anything during this process. When completed, this activity will either proceed to a logon screen, a password input screen, or directly to the Windows desktop screen. Since every computer lab, office system, and home computer is set up differently, make sure you follow the specific instructions of your school or facility for booting the computer and entering passwords (if used).

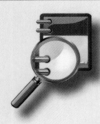

LET'S TRY IT! 1-1 BOOTING AND SHUTTING DOWN THE COMPUTER

Booting the Computer

STEP 1
Following the instructor's directions, turn on the computer using the power switch. If the monitor screen appears blank, turn on the monitor using the power switch. Do not repeatedly turn the computer on and off if there is no display on the monitor!

STEP 2
If the computer requires a password for you to gain access, use the information supplied by the instructor. Make a note of the information here for future reference:
User/Logon Name: _____
Password: _____

STEP 3
The computer will display a screen with several small pictures called *icons*. This area is known as the Windows *desktop* and is discussed in the next section. You have now properly booted up the computer and are ready to work.

Properly Shutting Down the Computer

STEP 1
When finished working with the computer, save all pertinent files and close all software programs.

STEP 2
Remove CDs, flash drives, and other removable media from the drives and put them away.

STEP 3

Take a moment now to label the CD from the back of your book, and any back up flash drives you may have, with your name, phone number, and instructor's name in case the CD discs are forgotten or lost. It is best to use a permanent marker on the labeled side of the CD; *do not* write on the unlabeled side—you will damage the CD.

TIP: Take special care of your CD and other computer media by never exposing them to extreme heat or handling them harshly. Protect the shiny, unlabeled side of the CD from scratches, smudges, and other damage.

JT: In Windows Vista, *Start* ears as a round icon in lower left corner with the dows logo in it.

STEP 4

Click on the *Start* button located on the far left bottom of the screen. Click on *Shut Down, Log Off,* or *Turn Off Computer,* following the instructor's directions. Wait until the entire system shuts down. If a message displays advising that the computer can be safely turned off, press the *power* switch to finish the process.

STEP 5

If you are working in a computer lab at a school, be courteous to the next class and remove your trash, papers, books, and supplies from the work area.

THE MICROSOFT WINDOWS DESKTOP

Recall when the computer was booted and loaded Windows. A screen with several small pictures, called *icons*, appeared. This area is called the **desktop**. The desktop is a graphical interface provided by Windows that allows users to manage resources visually. Icons represent software programs, files, and documents. See Figure 1-3 for examples of icons on the desktop.

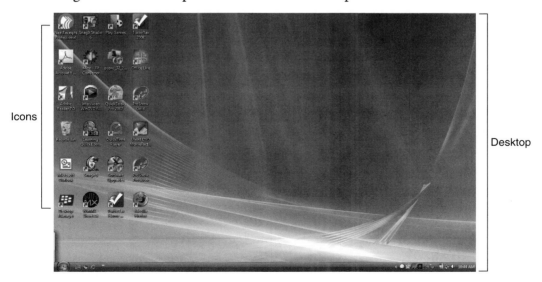

FIGURE 1-3

Icons on the Windows desktop. *Screen shot reprinted by permission from the Microsoft Corporation.*

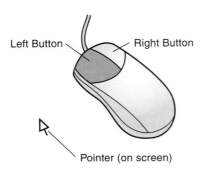

FIGURE 1-4

Two-button mouse and on-screen pointer. *Delmar/Cengage Learning*

Icons are actually shortcuts that will open the programs and files they represent when they are clicked on with the mouse. The mouse has two buttons, at a minimum, one on the left and one on the right. Some will have three buttons which may include a scroll wheel. The left mouse button is used to **single** or **double click** areas of the screen by using the **pointer**, usually depicted as an arrow displayed on the screen. By single or double clicking the left mouse button (where applicable), the computer will select, open, or execute a function. The right mouse button is used for special functions or displaying menu options (where available) in software programs. Refer to Figure 1-4 for an illustration of buttons on a mouse and the on-screen pointer.

APPLICATION AND DOCUMENT WINDOWS

Windows gets its name from the many window-like rectangular boxes that are displayed on the screen. There are basically two types of windows, the application window and the document window. The **application window** contains the actual software program. Whenever a document is created or opened within the program, it displays in its own window, called the **document window**. Thus, if you close the application window, you will also close any document windows that are open while using that program. Figure 1-5 shows an example of a document window opened inside of an application window.

To illustrate, suppose you are using the word processing program Word to write a letter. First, you must open the software program. When Word is opened, the application window is the one that displays the word processing program, ready for your use. Next, you open a new, blank document in which to write the letter. Another window opens inside, and as part of, the Word program. This is the document window in which you can begin to write the letter. When the letter is completed, you can give it a unique name and save it to the location of your choice—such as the hard drive or a flash drive.

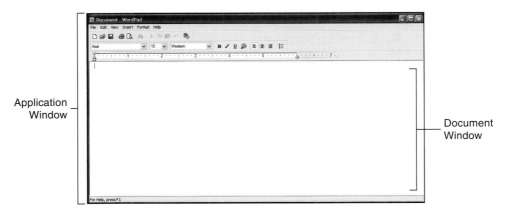

FIGURE 1-5

Software application and document windows. *Screen shot reprinted by permission from Microsoft Corporation.*

Next, the document window is closed, and the application window for the Word program can also be closed if there is no further work to be done.

USING WINDOWS

One of the most convenient features of Windows is that all application and document windows basically work the same way and have similar appearances. Here we will explore the features of a typical window. You will use these features when you work with just about any software program. Use Figure 1-6 as a reference for each component that is discussed in the following sections.

Title Bar

The **title bar** is along the top of a window and displays the name of the program or document on the left side. If several windows are open at the same time, the window that has a vivid-colored title bar (not dimmed or grayed) is called the **active window**. The active window is the one currently in use. To activate a different window, click on any area, including the title bar, of the desired window. This will cause the window to display in front of the other windows, which become inactive. As long as they are not completely closed, inactive windows remain available for use.

Maximize, Minimize, and Close Buttons

On the right side of the title bar are the sizing buttons. These buttons allow you to make the window larger or smaller, or to close it. A window can also be sized by using the mouse pointer on the screen. Point to the edges of the window border until the pointer changes into a double-headed arrow. When the double-headed arrow appears, do not move the mouse. Immediately hold down the left mouse button and, without letting it go, move the mouse in the direction that you would like to size the window. Whenever you hold down the left button and move the mouse, it is called **dragging** or **grabbing**. When you let go of the left mouse button so that the item that was dragged is left in its new location, it is referred to as **dropping**. You will commonly hear the phrase "drag and drop" when using software programs that use this technique.

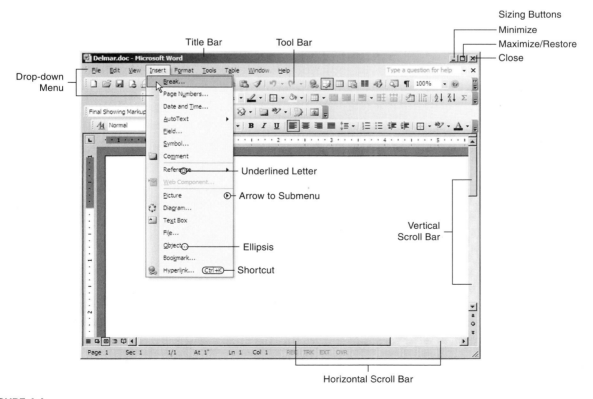

FIGURE 1-6

Components of a window. *Screen shot reprinted by permission from Microsoft Corporation.*

Drop-down (or Pull-down) Menus

Under the title bar are menu options for accessing the various functions and commands for the software in use. These drop-down menus typically read *File, Edit, Help,* etc. By single clicking on one of these options with the left mouse button, other menu options display on a drop down list. Move the pointer over the selections until the desired one is highlighted and single click the left mouse button to access it. If a menu selection is grayed out, it means that it is not available for use.

You may notice that there are symbols alongside some menu selections. It is useful to know the meaning of these symbols because this may assist you in using Windows more effectively. The most common ones are listed here.

- An *Ellipsis* is a group of three dots (...) that appears to the right of certain menu selections. This means there is a **dialog box** available for that selection. A dialog box is a window that either presents more information or allows the user to provide input. For example, if you are printing a letter, the dialog box for the printing command will allow you to input how many pages to print, to select color or grayscale, to collate, and to choose other options. Once the dialog box has been used, it closes and disappears from the screen. A dialog box that appears unintentionally can be canceled or simply closed by using the close button. More about dialog boxes is discussed later in this unit.

- *Arrows* and *arrowheads* that appear to the right or at the bottom of menu selections indicate that there are more selections, or a submenu is available. Normally, submenus are automatically displayed by placing the mouse pointer over the selection that has an arrow pointing to the right. Hold the pointer in place for a few moments (without moving it) to display the submenu. Arrows pointing down may need to be single clicked in order to display the remaining items.

> **HINT:** With some programs running in Windows Vista, the user must press the *Alt* key first so that the underlined letter in the menu options display. Otherwise, you may not see any underlined letters to use as a shortcut.

- *Underlined letters.* Menu options often contain an underlined letter. This indicates a shortcut feature that can be used with the keyboard instead of clicking on the selection with the mouse. For drop-down menu options, simply press and hold one of the *Alt* keys on the keyboard while pressing the underlined letter. To select items from the list of options that drop down, hold down the *Shift* key and press the underlined letter for that selection on the keyboard. To clear the drop-down menu from the screen, press the *Escape (Esc)* key at the top left of your keyboard.

- *Shortcut Keys,* sometimes called *hot keys,* are located to the right of some menu options. By using the shortcut keys indicated on the keyboard, menu options can be accessed directly without using the mouse. The keys to use are displayed to the right of the menu option. For example, *Ctrl+P* is next to the print option on the menu. This means that one of the *Control (Ctrl)* keys can be held down on the keyboard while the *P* key is pressed in order to immediately execute the print option.

- *Checkmarks* and *Black Circles.* In some cases, there might be a checkmark or a black circle to the left of some menu options. This indicates that the option is selected, or *on.* Often, software programs allow features to be turned on or off directly from their menus. Where applicable, clicking on the selection toggles the checkmark or circle to appear and disappear from the left side of the selection. Thus, the command is either *on* when the checkmark or circle is present or *off* when it is not.

◆ *Scroll bars*, located vertically on the right side of a window and horizontally along the bottom, are tools for scrolling text in a window up and down or left and right. Scroll bars have a small arrow box at either end of the bars. The slider bar, which is shaped like a box or rectangle, is located between these arrow boxes. There are two methods for scrolling. Either the arrow boxes can be clicked or you can hold down the left mouse button on the slider bar and drag it in the desired direction.

Toolbars

A **toolbar** is a collection of buttons that can be clicked to activate the most common commands of a software program. They are typically grouped by function, such as *formatting* or *drawing*. Toolbars, which can vary in each software program, are located under the drop-down menus along the top of the application window, and sometimes they will also open along the sides or the bottom of the application window. Available toolbars can be displayed in most programs by clicking on the *View* drop-down menu and clicking on *Toolbars*.

DIALOG BOXES

Dialog boxes are special windows that appear on the screen when more information or settings are required from the user before a command can be executed. It is important to know the components of dialog boxes, since just about every software program written for Windows uses them extensively. Refer to Figure 1-7 and Figure 1-8 as you review the following components of dialog boxes.

Command Buttons

Command buttons are used to execute a function when clicked. Some command buttons will open another dialog box so more choices can be made. Common command buttons in a dialog box are *Save*, *Open*, *Close*, *Cancel*, *OK*, and *Options*.

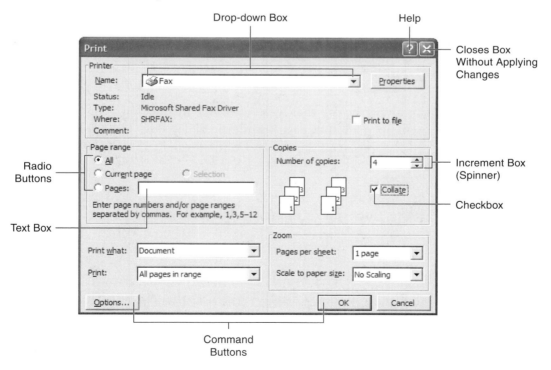

FIGURE 1-7

Example of a print dialog box. *Screen shot reprinted by permission from Microsoft Corporation.*

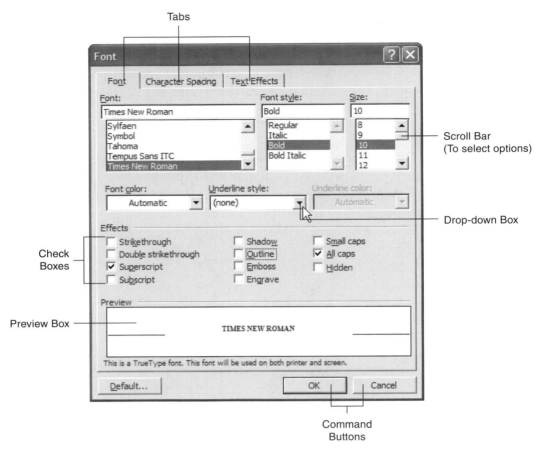

FIGURE 1-8

Example of a font formatting box. *Screen shot reprinted by permission from Microsoft Corporation.*

Tabs

Some dialog boxes have tabs along the top that look much like the tabs on a file folder. The tabs are labeled, and when clicked will open another page within the dialog box. These additional pages contain more command boxes or options. You can switch from one tab to another by clicking on the tabs without closing the dialog box.

Text Boxes

A text box provides an area to enter text or numbers. The information entered will customize the function to be executed.

Drop-Down Boxes

A drop-down box looks like a text box with a small, downward-pointing arrowhead on the right side. When this arrow is clicked, a list drops down displaying choices that can be clicked for selection.

Increment Boxes (or Spinners)

An increment box, also called a spinner, looks like a text box with a special button on the right that contains a small arrowhead pointing up and another one pointing down. These are typically found where choices involving size or quantity (number) are involved. Each click of the up arrow increases the size or quantity; the down arrow decreases the value. For instance, if you send a document to the printer and want five copies, use the increment box by clicking on the up arrow on the spinner until the number "5" is displayed; then click on print. If a margin of 1.5 inches needs to be reduced to 1 inch in a document, click the down arrow on the spinner until "1" is displayed in the margin box.

Check Boxes

Check boxes are located to the left of an available option and are used to select or deselect an option. By clicking in the box, a checkmark appears to turn the option *on*. By clicking on it again, the checkmark is removed, turning the option *off*. If a group of options with check boxes is available, it means more than one can be selected and applied at the same time.

Radio Buttons (or Option Buttons)

Radio and option buttons are two names for the same thing. These are round buttons located to the left of an available option. Click on these buttons with the mouse to select or deselect options. The option is *on* if a black dot appears in the button, and *off* if there is no dot. Unlike check boxes, if there are a group of options with radio buttons to the left of them, only one choice can be made.

THE TASKBAR

The *taskbar* is typically located at the bottom of the desktop, with the *Start* button on the far left and the time display on the far right. It usually stays on the screen at all times, even when software programs are open. It can be moved or even resized; take care when using the mouse in the taskbar to avoid unintentionally doing this, especially if the taskbar is *unlocked*. If you don't see the taskbar on your desktop, move the mouse pointer to the bottom edge of the lower screen to see if it pops up. If so, it means the taskbar autohide feature is turned on to hide the taskbar when it's not in use. If a double-headed arrow appears, you can drag the taskbar up slightly to bring it back into view. See Figure 1-9 for an illustration of the taskbar.

> **HINT:** In Windows Vista, *Start* appears as a round icon in the lower left corner with the Windows logo in it

The taskbar has many uses. By clicking on the *Start* button, the Start menu opens, allowing access to programs, files, help, and other important features. This is also where the command to properly shut down the computer is found. Always use the shut down command, when you are finished using your computer, by clicking on the Start button. Never shut down your computer by turning off the power to the computer unless you absolutely must. If your computer appears "frozen," or the mouse does not seem to be working, always consult with your instructor before pressing the power switch. There may be another way to solve the problem without losing your work or improperly restarting the computer.

In the center of the taskbar, there is one button for each program that the computer has open. If you open many programs or document windows, there could be many small boxes with name labels located here. Point at the boxes with the mouse (without clicking) and the name of the file and program will display in a pop-up box. Be sure not to open too many programs if they are not being used; this will deplete memory resources. Close all programs and files that are not currently needed and be careful not to open multiple sessions of the same software program. If you minimize an application window, it is not closed. Click on the box in the center of the taskbar to maximize the desired window.

Often, many small icons appear to the left of the time display. This area is called the *system tray*. These icons represent programs, special functions, volume adjustments, and online status, depending on what is installed on the computer.

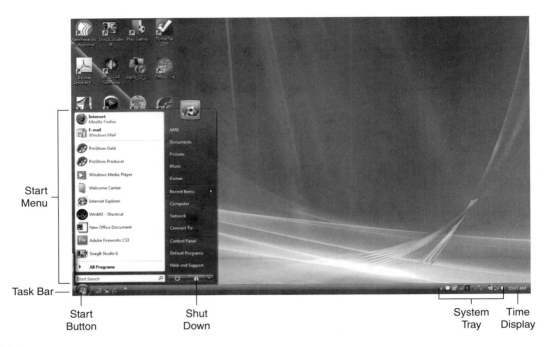

FIGURE 1-9

The Windows Vista taskbar. *Screen shot reprinted by permission from Microsoft Corporation.*

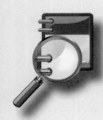

LET'S TRY IT! 1-2 LEARNING TO NAVIGATE WINDOWS

> **HINT:** Click on *Start, All Programs,* then *Accessories.* On the menu, click on *WordPad* to open the program.

STEP 1

Beginning on the desktop, follow directions from your instructor to open the WordPad program.

STEP 2

Locate the title bar along the top of the application window, where it reads *Document-WordPad.* The *Minimize, Restore,* and *Close* buttons are located to the far right of the windows title. Experiment with these buttons by left clicking them. Remember, when using the minimize button, click on the program from the center of the taskbar to bring it back into view.

STEP 3

Click on the drop-down menu *Format.* Notice the ellipses to the right of *Font,* indicating a dialog box for this feature. Click on *Font* to view that dialog box.

STEP 4

Experiment in the dialog box by clicking on the scroll bars for font types and sizes. Turn on effects by clicking the check boxes. Practice using drop-down boxes by viewing the color and script options. Click the *Cancel* command button to exit the dialog box.

STEP 5

Click on the drop-down menu *View.* Notice the check marks in front of the options. Click on each selection in the *View* menu and observe how the feature is turned on or off, causing each toolbar to be removed, then returned.

Click on the *Options* selection from the *View* menu. Notice the tabs along the top of the dialog box. Click on each one to view the page. Click on the *Write* tab. Notice the options with radio buttons and those with check boxes. Remember, radio buttons only allow one choice. Click on the buttons and check boxes to experiment. Click the *Cancel* command button when finished.

STEP 6

Click on *File* from the drop-down menus. Notice the shortcut keys on the right, such as Ctrl+N and Ctrl+S. To open a new file using the keyboard, *Ctrl+N* can be used. To try this, first, close the drop-down menu by pressing *Esc* on the keyboard. Next, hold down the *Ctrl* key on the keyboard while pressing the letter *N*. A *New file* window should appear on your screen. Cancel the window. Now, click on *File* from the drop-down menus; then click on *Print*. Notice the spinner next to where it reads *number of copies*. This increases or decreases the number of copies to print (if an option is grayed out, this feature is visible but not available for use). Click the *Cancel* command button when finished.

STEP 7

With the mouse, point at the various buttons on the toolbars without clicking (the pictures under the drop-down menus). Observe the pop-up captions, describing what each button is for. Locate the buttons for print, open, and save files.

STEP 8

NT: If the middle sizing
:on in the upper right cor-
reads "Restore" when the
se pointer is placed over it,
click on it. It should read
aximize."

Next, make sure the WordPad window is not maximized and is displayed on the desktop. To resize the window using *drag-and-drop*, point the mouse on any outer edge of the window. When a double-headed arrow appears, hold down the left mouse button and move the mouse in either of the directions indicated by the double-headed arrow. This is an example of dragging. When the window is resized to the size you want, let go of the mouse. This is an example of dropping.

Continue practicing this technique by pointing with the mouse at the lower right corner of the window. A diagonal double-headed arrow should appear. Drag and drop the window to size it diagonally. Next, make sure the window is sized fairly small in the middle of the screen. Point to the title bar and hold down the left mouse button. Without letting go, move the mouse and observe how the entire window moves on the screen. Drag and drop the window in this manner to various locations on the screen. This is an easy way to move windows on the desktop so the contents of more than one window can be viewed at the same time.

STEP 9

NT: Click in the blank area
ne middle of the WordPad
en with the mouse to make
cursor appear.

There should be a blinking vertical line in the document window area. This is called the cursor. Type your first name; then press *Enter* on the keyboard. This will move the cursor to the next line. Now type your last name and press *Enter* again. Click the mouse pointer to the left of the first letter of your first name. Next, hold down the left mouse button and move it to the right without letting go. Your name should be highlighted. Release the mouse button. This is called *selecting*. Next, point with the mouse to your first name (which is highlighted) and hold down the left mouse button. Drag the name down and to the right of your last name. The first and last names should switch places. Experiment until you have mastered selecting, dragging, and dropping.

continues

LEARNING TO NAVIGATE WINDOWS *continued*

STEP 10

Click on *File* from the drop-down menu. Click on *Exit* to close the WordPad program. A **prompt** will appear. Prompts are special windows that provide user messages. This prompt asks you if you want to save changes to your document. Since you are not saving this document, click on the *No* command button. The WordPad program will then close.

> **NOTE:** It is a good idea to practice these 10 steps until you have mastered the basic skills for navigating Windows.

HOW FILES ARE STORED

One of the most confusing and frustrating aspects of computer use for beginners is storing and retrieving files. The actual system is quite simple and, once properly explained, is relatively easy to understand.

The problem typically begins when a document is created or opened for use. Once the document is ready to be saved and you click on the *Save* command, a dialog box will display. Beginners who are unsure about what to do will often save the document without first looking *where* the document is being saved. Worse yet, many do not give the document a name. Consequently, when the file is needed again, it seems to have disappeared. Since there is no name for the file or knowledge of its location, the file is often difficult to find. Many people have retyped documents or re-entered work thinking their file has been forever lost, when it is actually stored somewhere on the hard drive.

Once you have an understanding of Windows Explorer, it will become easier to work with dialog boxes for opening and saving documents.

WINDOWS EXPLORER

Windows Explorer is the application used to browse a PC for files and folders. You can access this application by right clicking the *Start* button in the lower left corner of the taskbar. Choose *Explore* in the menu that pops up to open Windows Explorer.

In order to understand Windows Explorer better, visualize a filing cabinet with drawers, as shown in Figure 1-10. Each drawer in the cabinet represents a drive on the computer; the top drawer is the C: Hard Drive, the middle drawer is the D: DVD Drive, and the bottom drawer is the F: removable flash drive.

When each drawer of the cabinet is opened, folders are found inside. Folders typically are named, labeled, and stored in alphabetical order. When you look at the contents of a drive in Windows Explorer, you will also see a number of folders. The name of the folder is located to the right of each folder picture-icon. They also are listed alphabetically.

As you know, folders in a filing cabinet typically hold papers. This concept is similar with the computer. When a folder is clicked and opened, there are files inside, just like those papers. Like a real filing cabinet, these files can be very different from one another. Some pertain to various software programs and have different names to identify them. Others are reports, letters, data files, etc. Figure 1-11 illustrates files within Windows Explorer. By carefully comparing Figure 1-10 with Figure 1-11, the similarities between them, and their set up, become apparent.

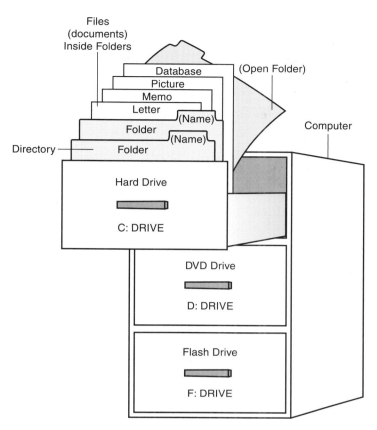

FIGURE 1-10

Windows Explorer is like a filing cabinet. *Delmar/Cengage Learning*

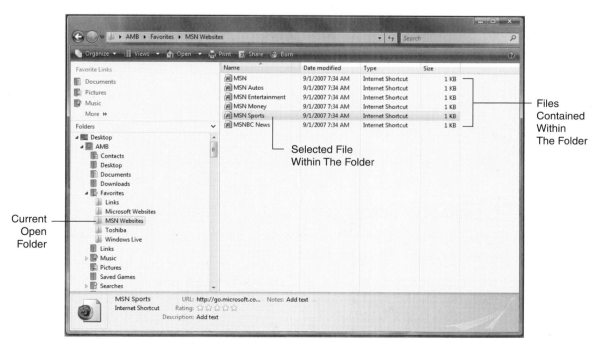

FIGURE 1-11

Folders and files displayed with Windows Explorer. *Screen shot reprinted by permission from Microsoft Corporation.*

Computers have a number of folders and files already on their hard drives. These are there as a result of software installations, devices being connected, and perhaps documents already created and stored by other people. You have the ability to save files to specific folders on the computer. Folders can be created, named, and grouped in order to make finding and using them easy. Files can be opened from or saved to the hard drive (C:), a flash drive or CD-R, or other drives capable of reading and writing files. Remember, each drive on the computer is like a different drawer of the filing cabinet—capable of holding folders and files. Therefore, each drive is another location where files can be saved.

Windows Explorer not only allows a user to browse the files on any given drive, but also maintain the content. Folders and files can be moved, copied, or deleted. As you gain more experience, it will become more apparent how to organize files and folders according to your own preferences and needs. When working on computers at school or work, be sure to use only the folders and files authorized for your use.

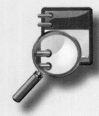

LET'S TRY IT! 1-3 **TAKING A LOOK AT WINDOWS EXPLORER**

STEP 1
With the mouse, point at the *Start* button on the lower left of the taskbar. Right click to display the submenu and click on *Explore*. This will open Windows Explorer on the screen.

STEP 2
Observe the two columns. In the left, drives and folders are listed. When a folder is clicked, the contents of that folder are displayed in the right pane. Notice that some folders have subfolders inside of them.

STEP 3
Looking again at the left pane, notice the small boxes with plus and minus signs. If you have Vista or a later version, you may have black and white arrowheads that point down and to the right. By clicking on these, the contents are expanded or collapsed for easy viewing of many folders and subfolders.

STEP 4
Close Windows Explorer by clicking on *File* and then *Close*, or simply clicking on the close button at the top right corner of the window.

OPEN AND SAVE DIALOG BOXES

Now that you understand how Windows Explorer works, the *Open* and *Save* dialog boxes for retrieving and storing files should be easy to understand.

Whenever you want to open a file, first you must select *File*, then *Open* from the pull-down menu. The *Open* dialog box displays and its drop-down box (along the top) will show the location field. You can open various folders in different locations on your hard drive in order to find the file you want. Refer to Figure 1-12. Once you find the file you need, double click to open it. Another way to open the file is to click once to select it and then click the *Open* command button.

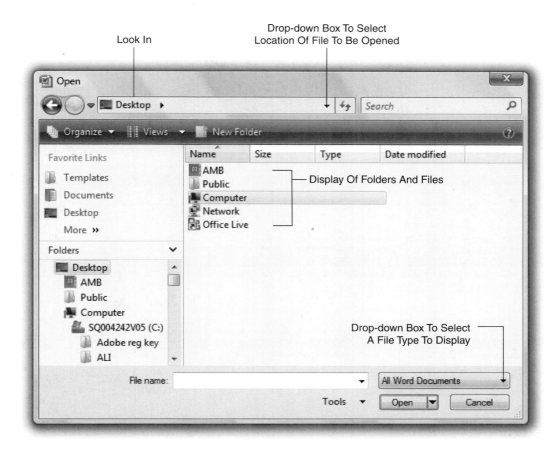

Look In

Drop-down Box To Select
Location Of File To Be Opened

Display Of Folders And Files

Drop-down Box To Select
A File Type To Display

FIGURE 1-12

The open dialog box. *Screen shot reprinted by permission from Microsoft Corporation.*

To save files, follow a similar process. Select *File* from the pull-down menu, then *Save As*. See Figure 1-13. Again, by dropping down the list, you can select the folder in the specific drive in which to save a file. Once the location has been selected, give the file a name by typing it in the text box that reads *File name*, near the bottom of the window.

These general steps can be followed in any software application; there are few differences to the basic function. By following these steps, you will be more likely to find your files on the computer. Because you are selecting the drive or folders the files are to be saved in, you know their location. When you name the files, you are more likely to recognize them when browsing for a lost file. You should be aware that some software programs will automatically assign a temporary name to a file if you don't select one. Others will prompt you for a name by displaying a reminder message. Be sure to investigate how the program you are working with handles naming files. As a last resort, you can always use the *Search* feature, found at the bottom of the Windows Start button at the lower left of the desktop screen. This will allow you to select basic and advanced searches for folders and files on the computer's various drives.

Before practicing saving documents, it is important to note two main differences between the commands *Save as* and *Save*. *Save as* is used to save files that have not been previously saved; these are new documents. Another common use for the *Save as* command is to change the name of an existing file so that there are multiple versions with different file names.

Save In

Drop-down Box To Select
Location To Save File To

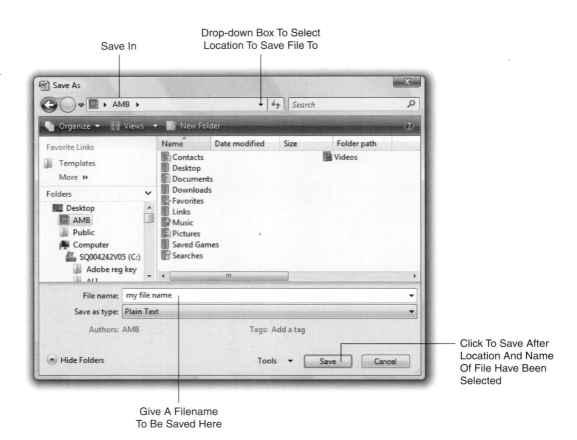

Click To Save After
Location And Name
Of File Have Been
Selected

Give A Filename
To Be Saved Here

FIGURE 1-13

The save dialog box. *Screen shot reprinted by permission from Microsoft Corporation.*

The *Save* command is used primarily to re-save files that were previously stored along with any edits or updates that were made. In other words, if a previously saved file is opened and edited, by using the *Save* command the revised document will *replace* the old document and use the same file name. Take care when using the *Save* command, because the old document generally cannot be recovered once it is re-saved with edits.

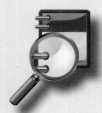

LET'S TRY IT! 1-4 OPENING AND SAVING FILES IN WINDOWS

HINT: Click on *Start, Programs,* and then *Accessories* to access this program.

STEP 1

Open the WordPad program. Click on *WordPad* from the menu.

STEP 2

Type your first and last name in the document window.

STEP 3

Click on the *File* drop-down menu and select *Save as* by clicking on it. Locate the *Save in* field. What folder or location name is displayed?

STEP 4

Using the *Folder* pane on the left side (click on the *Browse Folders* button, *if needed*), select *Desktop* by clicking on it. In the *File Name* field, enter your last name in the box to give the file a name so you are able to identify and find it. Click on the *Save* command button. Close the WordPad program.

STEP 5

Re-open the WordPad program. This time, click on *File* and then *Open* from the drop-down menus. Using the vertical scroll bars in the *Folders* pane at the lower left of the window, locate *Desktop* and click on it. Using the scroll bars on the right side of the window, scroll and look for the file with your last name. Double click on it to open the file in WordPad.

STEP 6

Click on *File* in the drop down menus, then *Exit* to close the WordPad program.

NOTE: It is a good idea to practice these six steps until you have mastered the basic skills for opening and saving files in Windows.

FINAL NOTES

It is important to have as broad-based a knowledge about computers and the use of their software as possible. Historically, many individuals resisted the advent of computerization and were left behind in terms of missed opportunities for advancement, higher income, or even upgrading skills until it was very late. Computer skills are no longer an option, but a necessity in today's work force.

Computers are now the standard tools in the medical office environment to perform daily tasks. Technology and new innovations that make health care professionals and their support staff more efficient are in use and will expand in the future. Mastering the information in this unit will provide you with a strong foundation of knowledge on which to build, and make you a more valuable staff member. This knowledge will facilitate on-the-job training during an externship or with your new employer. It will also position you for advancing your skills faster. Take advantage of all opportunities for learning new software, especially various practice management programs; the broader your skills set, the more doors will open to your future.

Select the correct answer for 1 through 4 from the following list.

  a. Interconnected computers located in the same building

  b. A computer that is not part of a network system

  c. A computer operator

  d. The process of interconnecting computers so that information can be exchanged between the machines

  1. _____ Networking

  2. _____ Stand-alone unit

  3. _____ User

  4. _____ LAN

In the blank, write *input, output,* **or** *both* **for each of the following.**

  5. _____ Mouse

  6. _____ Monitor

  7. _____ Digital camera

  8. _____ Printer

  9. _____ Software application

  10. _____ Speakers

  11. _____ Keyboard

Select the correct answer for 12 through 17 from the following list.

  a. A digital versatile disc that is capable of storing more than a CD, up to 4.7 GB

  b. A high storage capacity disc that can accommodate high-definition video

  c. A compact disc that can have files accessed from but not copied onto it

  d. A drive that enables files to be copied onto recordable discs

  e. A drive that plugs into the USB port and serves as additional storage, allowing files to be copied to and from the drive

  f. A compact disc that can have files accessed from and recorded (copied) onto it

  12. _____ CD-ROM

  13. _____ CD-R

  14. _____ DVD

  15. _____ CD or DVD burner

  16. _____ Blu-Ray Disc

  17. _____ Flash Memory Drive

  18. It is safe to shut down the computer while programs are open by turning it off at the power switch.

    a. True

    b. False

19. To safeguard them best, critical files on the computer should be backed up at least once a month.
    a. True
    b. False

20. Printers, monitors, keyboards, and scanners are examples of peripherals.
    a. True
    b. False

21. Without the operating system software, a computer would not function.
    a. True
    b. False

22. A special drive and software is needed in order to record information onto a CD-R disc.
    a. True
    b. False

23. DSL and cable modem access to the Internet is considered slow and ties up the telephone lines when used.
    a. True
    b. False

24. The terminology *booting the computer* refers to starting up the computer for use.
    a. True
    b. False

25. Software is a physical part of the computer.
    a. True
    b. False

26. The *brain* of the computer is considered to be the
    a. hardware.
    b. CPU.
    c. software.
    d. data.

27. Word processing, database, and practice management programs are examples of
    a. applications software.
    b. systems (OS) software.
    c. software found only in medical offices.
    d. all of the above.

28. Of the following choices, which is capable of storing the most data?

    a. DVD

    b. CD

    c. Blu-Ray

    d. Flash memory

    e. All hold the about the same amount of data.

29. The computer's memory, which feeds information to the processor while programs are in use, is called the

    a. RAM.

    b. hard drive.

    c. CPU.

    d. none of the above.

30. When connections are made between computers over the Internet for exchanging data, it is called

    a. a LAN.

    b. connecting peripherals.

    c. being online.

    d. none of the above.

31. A universal connecting port that enables hot-swapping of peripheral devices is known as the

    a. parallel port.

    b. USB port.

    c. serial port.

    d. all of the above.

32. Large facilities, such as hospitals, that require hundreds of users to access data simultaneously, are likely to be equipped with

    a. mainframes.

    b. Internet access.

    c. stand-alone computer units.

    d. LAN network.

    e. none of the above.

33. All software programs, files, data, and the operating system are located on the computer's

    a. resident hard drive.

    b. CD drive.

    c. monitor.

    d. USB drive.

34. The monitor, device cards, keyboard, printer, CPU, cables, and mouse are examples of

    a. software.

    b. input devices.

    c. hardware.

    d. operating systems.

    e. none of the above.

35. A message or alert that appears in a window with a reminder or request for input is referred to as the

    a. prompt.

    b. dialog box.

    c. text box.

    d. none of the above.

36. Explain why turning off the computer by using the power switch might be harmful to the system.

    _____

    _____

    _____

37. Four medical assistants work at their own computer workstations, which are networked to a server. Explain the function of a server.

    _____

    _____

    _____

38. How are digital cameras and scanners being used in some medical offices? Can you think of some additional or innovative uses for these devices in a medical office?

    _____

    _____

    _____

39. Can you think of any problems or issues regarding digital records, files, and transfer of files that contain patient information? What ideas or suggestions do you have for addressing those problems or issues?

    _____

    _____

    _____

40. How will your knowledge of computers, their components, and software help you with your career in health care?

_____

_____

_____

41. Explain the differences between these Internet access options: Modem, DSL, Cable, and WiFi.

_____

_____

_____

Medical Practice Management Software

OBJECTIVES

Upon completion of this unit, the reader should be able to:

- **Discuss the eight basic components of a medical practice management software application and their functions**

- **Explain the advantages and disadvantages of computerization in the medical office**

- **Understand the Health Insurance Portability and Accountability Act (HIPAA) regarding privacy of electronic records**

- **Demonstrate the logon procedure and navigation of *Medical Office Simulation Software* (MOSS)**

- **Demonstrate proper input of data using MOSS**

In the past, as with most businesses, the administrative procedures of running a medical office were done on paper using manual systems. Because there are so many components to a well-organized practice, coupled with hundreds, if not thousands, of patients, the manual process is quite monumental. Changes in the health care industry, including the many managed care plans, reimbursement methods, and varying rules for authorizing procedures and referrals, complicate the process even further.

The advent of computers, and the development of practice management software that addresses the many needs of the medical office, has improved the way everyday tasks are performed. Record keeping, medical insurance billing, appointment scheduling, and tracking referrals can be done easily with comprehensive software. In addition to using computers in the office, the ability to network and use the

KEY TERMS

Adjustment

Ancillary

Appointment scheduling system

Business Associate Agreement

Clearinghouse

Co-insurance

Co-payment

Covered entities

CPT-4

Deductible

Demographic information

Dunning message

Exclusions

Fee schedule

File maintenance system

Guarantor

Health Insurance Portability and Accountability Act (HIPAA)

ICD-9

Inpatient

Insurance billing system

Managed care

Internet and handheld digital devices that function as minicomputers (called personal digital assistants [PDAs], such as the Palm®) has simplified how work is done. Some modern mobile phones, often called *smartphones*, combine the attributes of cell phones and PDAs, such as the Blackberry® or iPhone®. New applications and software are continuously being developed for these devices that enable health care professionals to work efficiently and quickly. It is now possible for physicians visiting patients in the hospital to enter patient data and billing information using hand-held devices and to send it to the billers before arriving at the parking lot at the end of their workday. In addition, the capability to monitor patients' vital signs, to receive alerts, and to communicate with nurses, office staff, and transcriptionists, plus a multitude of other functions, is now available and under development.

The use of innovative technologies has also contributed to faster and easier methods of taking care of several key office functions. These include verification of a patient's eligibility for insurance benefits, approving referrals to specialists, and obtaining authorizations for medical procedures.

In this book, you will be exposed to the general functions of most practice management software. There are many different types of software on the market, some more powerful in their features than others. Programmers who develop and create the software may include features that are "extras" or exclusive to that software, making the software easier to use or more customized to the needs of an office. For this reason, it is impossible in a classroom setting to learn how to use every available piece of practice management software. However, most medical software has common components that perform similar functions. Once you have learned these common functions, it is easy to transfer your knowledge and skills to just about any other software designed for the same purpose.

KEY TERMS (*cont.*)

Participating physician

Patient billing system

Patient registration system

Posting payments system

Primary

Procedure posting system

Protected health information (PHI)

Reference sheet

Registration form

Report generation system

Source documents

Statement

Superbill

COMPONENTS OF A PRACTICE MANAGEMENT SOFTWARE APPLICATION

There are eight basic components common to most practice management software. While the use and look may be a little different from program to program, the output, or result, is usually about the same. Each of these components is explained in the following sections. A description of the tasks performed by each component is included.

APPOINTMENT SCHEDULING

Most practice management software programs come available with an **appointment scheduling system**. This system handles most of the tasks associated with patient visits. Scheduling of services performed outside the office, such as hospital rounds by the doctor, may be an available feature. Depending on the software, the appointment scheduling system can be very sophisticated or somewhat basic. Some offices still prefer to use traditional appointment books and logs, even if there is a computer system in the office. Whether an electronic or manual system is used, it is important to learn the fundamentals of appointment scheduling, especially as they apply to specific specialties and the needs of the individual office.

At a minimum, the appointment scheduling system should be able not only to make appointments, but also to cancel, reschedule, and search for appointments. It is especially useful if the system can sort appointments by time or type of visit, so that a **reference sheet** can be printed and distributed to staff members. A reference sheet shows all patients scheduled on a given day. It is provided to the physician, front desk, medical billers, office manager, and other staff as a guide at the start of the work day. See Figure 2-1 for an example of a reference sheet. The appointment scheduling system can be a useful tool for organizing this information, not only with patients' names and appointment times, but also by providing type of visit, symptoms, doctor to be seen, and special rooms or testing that will be required.

Schedule For Thursday, October 22, 20xx   **Student No:** Student 1

Time	Health	Reason	Schwartz	Reason	Mendenhall	Reason
9:00 AM	Meeting					
9:15 AM	Meeting					
9:30 AM	Meeting					
9:45 AM	Meeting					
10:00 AM	Meeting		Harold Englema	Heartburn, hypertension		
10:15 AM	Meeting		Harold Englema	Heartburn, hypertension		
10:30 AM			Harold Englema	Heartburn, hypertension		
10:45 AM			Harold Englema	Heartburn, hypertension		
11:00 AM	Derek Wallace	Follow-up UTI	Naomi Yamagat	Shortness of breath and		
11:15 AM			Naomi Yamagat	Shortness of breath and		
11:30 AM						
11:45 AM						
12:00 AM	Lunch		Lunch		Lunch	
12:15 AM	Lunch		Lunch		Lunch	
12:30 AM	Lunch		Lunch		Lunch	
12:45 AM	Lunch		Lunch		Lunch	
1:00 AM	Nancy Herbert	Follow-up COPD, needs				
1:15 AM	Nancy Herbert	Follow-up COPD, needs				
1:30 AM	Nancy Herbert	Follow-up COPD, needs				
1:45 AM	Alan Shuman	COPD				
2:00 AM	Alan Shuman	COPD				
2:15 AM						
2:30 AM						
2:45 AM						
3:00 AM			Emery Camille	Ear pain and sore throat		
3:15 AM						
3:30 AM	Deanna Hartsfe	Recheck cholesterol and	Martin Monter	Severe sore throat		
3:45 AM	Deanna Hartsfe	Recheck cholesterol and	Martin Monter	Severe sore throat		
4:00 AM			Martin Monter	Severe sore throat		
4:15 AM						
4:30 AM			Aimee Bradley	Sore throat and fever		
4:45 AM			Aimee Bradley	Sore throat and fever		
5:00 AM			Tina Rizzo	Allergies, sneezing and c		
5:15 AM			Tina Rizzo	Allergies, sneezing and c		
5:30 AM						
5:45 AM						

FIGURE 2-1

Sample of a reference sheet. *Delmar/Cengage Learning*

PATIENT REGISTRATION

The **patient registration system** allows the user to input information about each patient in the practice. As new patients arrive at the office, a **registration form**, also called a patient information data sheet, is completed. The person (or guardian of the person) to be treated by the physician fills out the form. Refer to Figure 2-2 for an example of a patient registration form.

The registration form contains what is typically referred to as demographic and medical insurance information. **Demographic information** basically includes the patient's address, phone number, date of birth (DOB), gender, marital status, employer or school, etc. The person responsible for paying medical expenses is often included on the registration form and is referred to as the **guarantor**. The guarantor is usually the patient. However, there are situations where that is not the case. For instance, parents typically are financially responsible for services rendered to their children, and are therefore the guarantors. The insurance information on the registration form includes the name of the health plan that covers the patient, identification numbers, names of the policyholders or dependents, and other relevant data.

In addition to creating the initial record using the software program, the patient registration system also allows for updating the record should any changes occur. Data that tends to change frequently includes addresses, phone numbers, employers, marital status, e-mail addresses, and insurance coverage.

The information in the patient registration system is extremely important and should always be entered carefully and checked for accuracy. Updating information, whenever there is a change, is of utmost importance because this becomes part of the database that the software uses to perform other functions within the program. For example, when payments are applied to patient accounts, or insurance claims are prepared, portions of the demographic information are used by the software. A software program can only be as effective and as accurate as the users who input and maintain the information it contains.

FILE MAINTENANCE

The **file maintenance system** is a utility area of the program that contains common information used by various systems within the software. It is also an area where the setup of the software system can be adjusted or customized for the needs of the practice.

Practice management software requires some initial data before it is operational. This data is specific to the medical office that will be using the software. Such items include the name, address, and phone number of the practice and any **ancillary** offices. Ancillary offices are additional office locations that are part of the same practice or one business entity. For example, four offices are located throughout a city. Ten physicians are working together out of those four offices as one professional corporation, or practice, called ABC Medical Associates. Each location is an ancillary office of the practice. In most cases, the computer system is networked, allowing staff members from each location to access information, appointment schedulers, and other functions relevant to daily operations. As computer technology and networking have become more practical, physicians' offices, hospitals, pharmacies, and diagnostic centers are often part of a system where an interchange of patient data and other information can be centrally accessed.

The file maintenance system contains information about each physician of the practice, referring physicians, and other professional health care providers. Information such as insurance provider and tax identification numbers, Drug Enforcement Administration (DEA) numbers, specialty numbers, and other pertinent data is also included.

Welcome To Our Office
PLEASE PRINT

NEW PATIENT INFORMATION

DATE _____

LAST NAME	FIRST NAME	MI	SSN		GENDER	MARITAL STATUS	DATE OF BIRTH

ADDRESS	APT/UNIT	CITY	STATE	ZIP	HOME PH ( )	WORK PH ( ) EXT

EMPLOYER/SCHOOL	EMPLOYER ADDRESS	CITY	STATE	ZIP

REFERRING PHYSICIAN (LAST NAME, FIRST NAME)	ADDRESS	CITY	STATE	ZIP	PHONE

GUARANTOR – Person responsible for payment: ☐ self   ☐ spouse/other   ☐ parent   ☐ legal guardian If not "self", please complete the following:

LAST NAME	FIRST NAME	MI	SSN		GENDER	DATE OF BIRTH

ADDRESS (IF DIFFERENT FROM PATIENT)	CITY	STATE	ZIP	HOME PH ( )	ALT. PHONE

EMPLOYER NAME	EMPLOYER ADDRESS	CITY	STATE	ZIP	WORK PHONE EXT

OTHER RESPONSIBLE PARTY:

LAST NAME	FIRST NAME	MI	SSN		GENDER	DATE OF BIRTH	

ADDRESS (IF DIFFERENT FROM PATIENT)	CITY	STATE	ZIP	HOME PH ( )	ALT. PHONE

EMPLOYER NAME	EMPLOYER ADDRESS	CITY STATE	ZIP	WORK PHONE EXT

INSURANCE – PRIMARY

PLAN NAME	PATIENT RELATIONSHIP TO INSURED: ☐ self ☐ spouse ☐ child ☐ other

POLICYHOLDER INFORMATION

LAST NAME	FIRST NAME	MI	DATE OF BIRTH	ID#	POLICY #	GROUP #

EMPLOYER NAME	PCP NAME, IF APPLICABLE:

INSURANCE – SECONDARY

PLAN NAME	PATIENT RELATIONSHIP TO INSURED: ☐ self ☐ spouse ☐ child ☐ other

POLICYHOLDER INFORMATION

LAST NAME	FIRST NAME	MI	DATE OF BIRTH	ID#	POLICY #	GROUP #

EMPLOYER NAME	PCP NAME, IF APPLICABLE:

ACCIDENT? ☐ YES ☐ NO IF YES, DATE OF INJURY	OCCUR AT WORK? ☐ YES ☐ NO	AUTO INVOLVED: ☐ YES ☐ NO	STATE

NAME OF ATTORNEY	PHONE NUMBER EXT.		

ALL PROFESSIONAL SERVICES RENDERED ARE CHARGED TO THE PATIENT. NECESSARY FORMS WILL BE COMPLETED TO HELP EXPEDITE INSURANCE CARRIER PAYMENTS. HOWEVER, THE PATIENT IS RESPONSIBLE FOR ALL FEES, REGARDLESS OF INSURANCE COVERAGE. IT IS ALSO CUSTOMARY TO PAY FOR SERVICES WHEN RENDERED UNLESS OTHER ARRANGEMENTS HAVE BEEN MADE IN ADVANCE WITH OUR OFFICE BOOKKEEPER.

INSURANCE AUTHORIZATION AND ASSIGNMENT

Name of Policy Holder _____ HIC Number _____
I request that payment of authorized Medicare/Other Insurance company benefits be made either to me or on my behalf to _____
for any services furnished me by that party who accepts assignment/physician. Regulations pertaining to Medicare assignment of benefits apply.
I authorize any holder of medical or other information about me to release to the Social Security Administration and CMS or its intermediaries or carriers any information needed for this or a related Medicare claim/other Insurance Company claim. I permit a copy of this authorization to be used in place of the original, and request payment of medical insurance benefits either to myself or to the party who accepts assignment. I understand it is mandatory to notify the health care provider of any other party who may be responsible for paying for my treatment. (Section 1128B of the Social Security Act and 31 U.S.C. 3801-3812 provides penalties for withholding this information.) Acknowledgment of Receipt of Privacy Notice - I have been presented with a copy of this provider's Notice of Privacy Policies, detailing how my information may be used and disclosed as permitted under federal and state law. I understand the contents of the notice, and, subject to the following restriction(s) concerning my personal medical information, I agree to the disclosures named in the Notice;_____

Signature _____   Date_____

FIGURE 2-2

Sample of a patient registration sheet. *Used with permission. InHealth Record Systems, Inc., 5076 Winters Chapel Road, Atlanta, GA 30360, 800-477-7374, http://www.inhealthrecords.com.*

The names and addresses of places where services are rendered, such as hospitals and nursing homes, also need to be input into the practice's file maintenance system. Insurance companies, and the identification numbers for providers used for preparing claims on paper or electronically, are also entered. The various codes that identify procedures performed for patients, called Current Procedural Terminology, or **CPT-4** codes, are maintained in the file maintenance area. A set of codes called International Classification of Diseases codes, or **ICD-9**, are also maintained in file maintenance. ICD-9 codes are used to identify patient diagnoses.

There is an extensive amount of information, used for a variety of purposes, that can be entered into the file maintenance system. Very often, because you will begin employment in an office that has already set up the file maintenance system with the required data, you will not need to enter this initial information. However, you can expect that new information will need to be added on occasion. For example, a patient may come to the office, having been referred by a physician who is not in the computer's records. The physician will need to be entered as a new referral source. In addition, changes and deletions will occasionally need to be made to records, such as when certain CPT-4 codes and ICD-9 codes are updated or replaced annually. For these reasons, it is important to learn how to use the file maintenance system of any practice management software.

PROCEDURE POSTING

When a patient receives services, whether in the office, hospital, nursing home, or other facility, the fees must be applied to the patient's account. This process is handled by the **procedure posting system** of the software. In this system, not only will fees for services be applied, but also other information relevant to the encounter between patient and physician. This includes the date(s) of service (DOS) and the place of service (POS). When posting procedures, the CPT-4 codes must have appropriate ICD-9 codes to support, or qualify, performing those procedures. This is especially important for claims sent to insurance companies. Claims will be denied payment if an appropriate match is not made.

In an obvious example, an insurance carrier will deny payment if a procedure code for a chest X-ray is billed with a diagnostic code for migraine headaches. It is clear that these do not match. However, because of medical terminology, circumstances unique to a case, or certain coding rules, mismatches may be subtle and not as easy to catch.

How does one know which codes to use? The physician determines the procedures and diagnoses for each patient by providing documentation used as a reference by the medical office staff. This documentation is referred to as **source documents**. Source documents include the notes written in the patient's record and special forms called **superbills**. Other common names for a superbill are *encounter form*, *charge ticket*, and *visit/fee slip*. Different offices may refer to this document by any of these names; however, for the purposes of this book, the term superbill is used throughout.

Superbills contain all of the information insurance companies require in order to consider a claim for payment. This information includes the patient's name, the date of service, itemized services with CPT-4 codes, and the diagnoses with ICD-9 codes. The superbill also identifies the practice and physician who renders the service. The physician usually signs the superbill before it is returned to the administrative staff.

The information contained on the superbill is needed by medical administrative staff in order to post procedure charges to patient accounts using medical practice management software. See Figure 2-3 for an example of a superbill.

PLEASE RETURN THIS FORM TO RECEPTIONIST

NAME _____

PLACE OF SERVICE:
( ) OFFICE
( ) NEW YORK COUNTY HOSPITAL
( ) COMMUNITY GENERAL HOSPITAL
( ) RETIREMENT INN NURSING HOME
( ) _____

DATE OF SERVICE _____

A. OFFICE VISITS - New Patient

Code	History	Exam	Dec.	Time	
99201	Prob. Foc.	Prob. Foc.	Straight	10 min.	____
99202	Ex. Prob. Foc.	Ex. Prob. Foc.	Straight	20 min.	____
99203	Detail	Detail	Low	30 min.	____
99204	Comp.	Comp.	Mod.	45 min.	____
99205	Comp.	Comp.	High	60 min.	____

B. OFFICE VISIT - Established Patient

Code	History	Exam	Dec.	Time	
99211	Minimal	Minimal	Minimal	5 min.	____
99212	Prob. Foc.	Prob. Foc.	Straight	10min.	____
99213	Ex. Prob. Foc.	Ex. Prob. Foc.	Low	15 min.	____
99214	Detail	Detail	Mod.	25 min.	____
99215	Comp.	Comp.	High	40 min.	____

C. HOSPITAL CARE

Dx Units

1.	Initial Hospital Care (30 min)	____ ____	99221	____
2.	Subsequent Care	____ ____	99231	____
3.	Critical Care (30-74 min)	____ ____	99291	____
4.	each additional 30 min.	____ ____	99292	____
5.	Discharge Services	____ ____	99238	____
6.	Emergency Room	____ ____	99282	____

D. NURSING HOME CARE

Dx Units

Initial Care - New Pt.
1.	Expanded	____	99322
2.	Detailed	____	99323

Subsequent Care - Estab. Pt.
3.	Problem Focused	____	99307
4.	Expanded	____	99308
5.	Detailed	____	99309
5.	Comprehensive	____	99310

E. PROCEDURES

1.	Arthrocentesis, Small Jt.	____	20600
2.	Colonoscopy	____	45378
3.	EKG w/interpretation	____	93000
4.	X-Ray Chest, PA/LAT	____	71020

F. LAB

1.	Blood Sugar	____	82947	____
2.	CBC w/differential	____	85031	____
3.	Cholesterol	____	82465	____
4.	Comprehensive Metabolic Panel	____	80053	____
5.	ESR	____	85651	____
6.	Hematocrit	____	85014	____
7.	Mono Screen	____	86308	____
8.	Pap Smear	____	88150	____
9.	Potassium	____	84132	____
10.	Preg. Test, Quantitative	____	84702	____
11.	Routine Venipuncture	____	36415	____

F. Cont'd

Dx Units

12.	Strep Screen	____	87081	____
13.	UA, Routine w/Micro	____	81000	____
14.	UA, Routine w/o Micro	____	81002	____
15.	Uric Acid	____	84550	____
16.	VDRL	____	86592	____
17.	Wet Prep	____	82710	____
18.	_____	____	____	____

G. INJECTIONS

1.	Influenza Virus Vaccine	____	90658	____
2.	Pneumococcal Vaccine	____	90772	____
3.	Tetanus Toxoids	____	90703	____
4.	Therapeutic Subcut/IM	____	90732	____
5.	Vaccine Administration	____	90471	____
6.	Vaccine - each additional	____	90472	____

H. MISCELLANEOUS

1. _____ ____ ____
2. _____ ____ ____

AMOUNT PAID $ _____

Mark diagnosis with
(1=Primary, 2=Secondary, 3=Tertiary)

DIAGNOSIS NOT LISTED BELOW _____

DIAGNOSIS	ICD-9-CM	1, 2, 3
Abdominal Pain	789.0	____
Allergic Rhinitis, Unspec.	477.9	____
Angina Pectoris, Unspec.	413.9	____
Anemia, Iron Deficiency, Unspec.	280.9	____
Anemia, NOS	285.9	____
Anemia, Pernicious	281.0	____
Asthma w/ Exacerbation	493.92	____
Asthmatic Bronchitis, Unspec.	493.90	____
Atrial Fibrillation	427.31	____
Atypical Chest Pain, Unspec.	786.59	____
Bronchiolitis, due to RSV	466.11	____
Bronchitis, Acute	466.0	____
Bronchitis, NOS	490	____
Cardiac Arrest	427.5	____
Cardiopulmonary Disease, Chronic, Unspec.	416.9	____
Cellulitis, NOS	682.9	____
Congestive Heart Failure, Unspec.	428.0	____
Contact Dermatitis NOS	692.9	____
COPD NOS	496	____
CVA, Acute, NOS	434.91	____
CVA, Old or Healed	438.9	____
Degenerative Arthritis (Specify Site)	715.9	____

DIAGNOSIS	ICD-9-CM	1, 2, 3
Dehydration	276.51	____
Depression, NOS	311	____
Diabetes Mellitus, Type II Controlled	250.00	____
Diabetes Mellitus, Type II Controlled	250.02	____
Drug Reaction, NOS	995.29	____
Dysuria	788.1	____
Eczema, NOS	692.2	____
Edema	782.3	____
Fever, Unknown Origin	780.6	____
Gastritis, Acute w/o Hemorrhage	535.00	____
Gastroenteritis, NOS	558.9	____
Gastroesophageal Reflux	530.81	____
Hepatitis A, Infectious	070.1	____
Hypercholesterolemia, Pure	272.0	____
Hypertension, Unspec.	401.9	____
Hypoglycemia NOS	251.2	____
Hypokalemia	276.8	____
Impetigo	684	____
Lymphadenitis, Unspec.	289.3	____
Mononucleosis	075	____
Myocardial Infarction, Acute, NOS	410.9	____
Organic Brain Syndrome	310.9	____
Otitis Externa, Acute NOS	380.10	____

DIAGNOSIS	ICD-9-CM	1, 2, 3
Otitis Media, Acute NOS	382.9	____
Peptic Ulcer Disease	536.9	____
Peripheral Vascular Disease NOS	443.9	____
Pharyngitis, Acute	462	____
Pneumonia, Organism Unspec.	486	____
Prostatitis, NOS	601.9	____
PVC	427.69	____
Rash, Non Specific	782.1	____
Seizure Disorder NOS	780.39	____
Serous Otitis Media, Chronic, Unspec.	381.10	____
Sinusitis, Acute NOS	461.9	____
Tonsillitis, Acute	463.	____
Upper Respiratory Infection, Acute NOS	465.9	____
Urinary Tract Infection, Unspec.	599.0	____
Urticaria, Unspec.	708.9	____
Vertigo, NOS	780.4	____
Viral Infection NOS	079.99	____
Weakness, Generalized	780.79	____
Weight Loss, Abnormal	783.21	____

ABN: I UNDERSTAND THAT MEDICARE PROBABLY WILL NOT COVER THE SERVICES LISTED BELOW

A. _____ B. _____ C. _____

Patient Signature _____

Date _____

Doctor's Signature _____

RETURN: _____ Days _____ Weeks _____ Months

REF# 122949 SB (05.07.09)   TO REORDER CALL INHEALTH RECORD SYSTEMS 800-477-7374

DOUGLASVILLE MEDICINE ASSOCIATES
5076 BRAND BLVD., SUITE 401
DOUGLASVILLE, NY 01234
PHONE No. (123) 456-7890
L.D. HEATH, M.D.   D.J. SCHWARTZ, M.D.
NPI# 9995010111   NPI# 9995020212
EIN# 00-1234560

FIGURE 2-3

Sample of a superbill. *Used with permission. InHealth Record Systems, Inc., 5076 Winters Chapel Road, Atlanta, GA 30360, 800-477-7374, http://www.inhealthrecords.com.*

Although the physician provides the information on source documents for coding purposes, those involved with billing should be trained in coding principles. This will assist with making good coding choices in addition to spotting errors, omissions, and inconsistencies that could cause a claim to have payment reduced or denied altogether.

When procedures are input into the procedure posting system, the software assigns the fee to be charged according to the **fee schedule** for the patient's insurance. Typically, medical practices have at least two fee schedules; most have several. In fact, many practice management software programs can accommodate up to 99 fee schedules! A fee schedule is much like a price list. There is a corresponding price, or fee, for each CPT-4 procedure code.

The advent of managed care and the various types of models and plans available have contributed much toward changing the way procedures and payments are accounted for. **Managed care** is a broad term describing organizations that combine the delivery of health care and reimbursement for services in order to control costs and manage access to health care. Although not exclusive to managed care plans, most require that the patient use participating plan physicians within a network to obtain the best coverage and incur the lowest expense.

A **participating physician** agrees to provide medical services to specific patient populations and negotiates for reimbursement under a contract. This sometimes involves a certain fee schedule that must be adhered to under the provisions of the contract, and the physician may have charge limits. Because fee schedules can be different from insurance company to insurance company under these agreements, multiple fee schedules must be used.

To illustrate, assume a physician participates as a provider for six different managed care plans. He is also a Medicare provider and has patients with other private insurance. Additionally, he accepts patients without insurance, offering a discount to those who pay cash. For this physician, the software has been set up with eight fee schedules. There is one for each managed care plan and one for Medicare. There is a standard fee schedule for all patients with insurance coverage who do not fall into any of the previous categories. It is clear to see how practice management software simplifies tracking eight different sets of fees according to insurance coverage. It would be cumbersome, indeed, to find each of the fees in a manual system!

Another important function of the procedure posting system is the compilation of information required by the insurance billing system in order to create claims. Once the fees, CPT, and ICD codes, along with service dates and place of service information have been input, the claim to the insurance company can be completed.

INSURANCE BILLING

The **insurance billing system** is designed to prepare claims that are sent to insurance companies in order to receive payment for services rendered by medical providers. The insurance billing system gathers patient information, procedures and diagnosis information with the corresponding codes, and place of service codes, and then uses the appropriate fee schedule to produce the claims.

Claims can be submitted to insurance companies either by mailing paper claim forms or sending them electronically. Because of the variety of health insurance plans and secondary billing, it is still typical for most medical offices to use both methods. It is customary for claims to first go through a **clearinghouse** before reaching insurance payers. A clearinghouse is a service that facilitates the movement of electronic claims from the medical office to the insurance companies. During this process, the claims are edited and validated to ensure they are error free. Then, they are reformatted to the specifications of the insurance payer and submitted electronically. Some of the better clearinghouses offer additional premium services that are beneficial to medical practices. These can include eligibility verification of benefits, claim status reports, online access to edit and correct claims on-the-fly, analysis of rejected claims, electronic claims tracking for paper claims, and patient invoicing services.

POSTING PAYMENTS

Practice management software plays an important role in simplifying and tracking the insurance billing process. There are several steps involved in preparing claims. The software assists in sorting information and directing how and when claims are sent, especially for patients who have more than one insurance coverage. As discussed previously, once a patient has received services, and fees are applied to the account, the software will use the insurance information that was entered on the patient to prepare claims. Once the claim is sent to the insurance company and a payment returns, it will be applied to the patient's account. This is accomplished with the posting payments system. Not only will the payment be posted, but also any adjustments that may be necessary. Adjustments are amounts that are taken away from (or added to) the balance of an account. Adjustments are often used to reflect contract agreements, credits, refunds, discounts, bad debt, corrections to erroneous entries, and other accounting situations. When amounts are removed from a balance, the adjustment is sometimes referred to as a *write-off*.

The following example illustrates a write-off.

A physician has a contractual agreement with an insurance plan to accept only what the insurance pays as payment-in-full for services. The balance left for that fee, called the adjustment (or write-off), must then be subtracted from the patient account once the insurance payment is posted.

Physician's fee for a given service:	$60.00
Insurance company paid:	($52.00)
Amount adjusted, or the write-off:	($8.00)
Patient balance due:	$0.00

Remember, since the physician's contract with the insurance plan states that the insurance payment will be accepted by him or her as payment-in-full, the $8.00 balance will be subtracted from the patient's account. This is why the patient does not owe anything.

For patients who have more than one insurance coverage, once payment from the first, or primary, insurance company is received and any appropriate adjustments have been posted, the software can generate a claim to the second insurance company. For those patients who have both a primary and secondary insurance, known as *dual coverage*, the secondary insurance is customarily billed for any remaining amount once the primary insurance has paid its portion. If there is no secondary plan, the bill can be sent directly to the patient in order to collect the remaining amount.

PATIENT BILLING

As claims are sent to insurance companies and payments are received and posted, the patient billing system uses this information to generate statements. It is customary for patients to receive a bill, or statement, each month from the practice if there is a balance due. The source of payments that have been applied and adjustments to the balance due are shown on the patient statement. This provides the patient with an ongoing picture of the financial standing of his or her account and the status of insurance billing activity. If any money is due from the patient, the statement should indicate this. An envelope should be included with the statement to make it easy to mail a payment to the medical office.

There are other instances when patients need to make payments to the practice. These include payments toward services that are not covered by the insurance plan, annual deductibles, and co-insurance amounts. If this money is not collected at the time a patient is in the office for service, a statement will need to be sent to collect it.

Services not covered by a health insurance plan are called exclusions. These will need to be paid by the patient out of his or her own pocket. In other cases, a patient's health insurance plan may cover a service but deny payment due to a particular reason. The denial could be due to a medical service seen as unnecessary, the frequency of service required, or some other reason. A number of plans require that the physician disclose to the patient which services will not be approved, and why, before they are rendered. It is important to know when, and for which plans, these requirements apply. If the medical office inadvertently collects money without following proper procedures of disclosure, the physician may have corrective action taken against him or her and could even be fined.

Some health plans have an annual deductible. The deductible is an out-of-pocket expense the patient must pay before the insurance company will pay for covered services. Typically, the deductible due starts over at the beginning of every year on January 1. For example, a patient who has a $2000 annual deductible will need to pay that amount every year, out-of-pocket, toward medical services. This could mean several office visits, diagnostic procedures, etc., until eventually a total of $2000, or one procedure that is at least $2000 or more, is reached. When the $2000 has been reached, the insurance company will start to pay toward services according to their policy. On January 1 of the next year, the patient will again have to pay $2000 toward medical services until the deductible has been met.

Some insurance plans pay a percentage of an approved amount of the fees after the deductible has been paid. A typical percentage is 80/20, where 80% is the amount paid by the insurance company and 20% is the patient's share. This 20% is generally referred to as the co-insurance. If the patient has dual coverage, the 20% co-insurance will be billed to the secondary insurance. As mentioned previously, if there is no secondary insurance, then a statement will be sent to the patient requesting payment of the remaining balance.

Most medical offices customarily send statements monthly to all patients who have a balance due on their accounts. It is helpful to include a dunning message on the statement. A dunning message is a short collections note that appears on the bill; most patient billing systems include this feature. These notes vary, and can be used to indicate to the patient the exact amount to be paid. For instance, if a patient has a balance of $250, but $200 has been billed to the insurance company and $50 is now due for co-insurance, a note clarifying this encourages the patient to pay his or her portion. Dunning messages can also read "60 days overdue, please send your payment today!" or "Do not send payment, your insurance company has been billed." Follow the office policy of your employer for including dunning messages when preparing statements with the patient billing system.

Despite the fact statements are sent monthly, it is best to collect money due for exclusions, deductibles, and co-insurance amounts at the time a patient is in the office to see the doctor. This helps maintain good reimbursement flow and encourages patients to come prepared to make payments. Remember to always follow the policy of your employer regarding the collection of money.

A managed care plan that requires a fixed payment at each office visit is called a **co-payment**. Typical co-payments can range from $10 at every visit to $35 or more. Many insurance plans have different co-payments depending on the service rendered. For instance, a patient may have to pay $30 each time he or she visits the office, but a visit at the emergency room may require a $100 co-payment. If the patient will be staying at the hospital more than 24 hours, known as an **inpatient**, the same plan may have a $200 co-payment for admission. Each patient's insurance coverage details will need to be carefully reviewed and verified. All patients (new to the practice and established patients) who change insurance plans should have their benefits eligibility checked and reimbursement issues verified.

Although it is standard practice to collect co-payments from patients with managed care plans at the time of office services, sometimes patients will forget or be unable to pay. Every medical office has its own policies regarding collection of co-payments. Some will send a statement; others will reschedule the patient to be seen at another time. Be sure to follow and enforce these policies carefully in order to ensure the best possible reimbursement for services.

REPORT GENERATION (RUNNING REPORTS)

The purpose of the **report generation system** is to retrieve and organize the data from various parts of the practice management software program into useful information, or reports. These reports can be as simple as a list of diagnostic codes to as complex as analytical reports reflecting the practice's financial statistics.

Reports can be useful tools for tracking insurance payments, income by physician, or ancillary facilities. Many business and practice activities can be documented and reviewed for any number of purposes, using a comprehensive and flexible report generation system. Members of the medical office staff, including the physician and even the accountant, will utilize different types of reports. Aging of accounts, for collections or assignment to a collection agency, can be reviewed quickly. Reports can yield results for decision making regarding equipment or services, and for statistical purposes. It is likely that you will generate reports at the end of each day—as needed for your purposes, and to be distributed to others.

ADVANTAGES AND DISADVANTAGES OF COMPUTERS IN THE MEDICAL OFFICE

Computer use is now the standard more than the exception in most medical practices and other health care provider offices. Technology has moved quickly in a short amount of time. New software, improvements in equipment, and amazing innovations make computer use exciting and promising in the field of medicine. However, the computer should not be mistaken for the solution to all problems, nor can the computer be treated as something capable of having reasoning powers. The computer is a useful tool, a machine; but, the skills of the user are still necessary, especially for recognizing errors and malfunctions. The user must be knowledgeable of office procedures and how software functions so it can be used correctly, and to ensure that the information is accurate, especially for reports.

ADVANTAGES OF COMPUTER USE

Up to this point, there have been many advantages mentioned for using computers for the purpose of managing a medical practice. An overview of the most pertinent points is covered in this section.

Working Efficiently

Unlike manual systems, where information must be looked up and referenced constantly, computers have the ability to search, sort, and retrieve information with unmatched speed. Databases are used with ease for multiple tasks, making repetitive jobs, especially in large volume, efficient and precise.

Computers are unlikely to replace medical office staff. However, they do make specific work less time-consuming, actually increasing staff productivity. This may even free specialized staff to concentrate on higher priority tasks. Medical billers have already recognized a faster turnaround time for receiving insurance payments. This has much to do with software that edits insurance claims for errors, coding discrepancies, and omissions. Programs with managed care modules track when referrals have been used up or are about to expire.

Physicians can upload information to and download information from the computer and PDAs to view and use information on patients who are receiving services at hospitals and other facilities. A health care professional talking into a recording device to create medical documents is called *dictation*. A transcriptionist is a specially trained professional who listens to the dictation and types the medical documents using proper formatting. Dictation can now be transferred from these handheld digital devices or be made available directly to computer servers where medical transcriptionists at various locations can retrieve and transcribe documents. The fact that cassette tapes, now becoming antiquated, no longer need to be physically delivered to the transcriptionist, and that digital voice recordings can be transferred directly to computers, of themselves, increase efficiency.

Easy Accessibility

With networking, wireless capabilities, larger storage, and faster Internet service, data of all types, from medical record documentation to detailed images, has become widely available. In the office, essential information regarding patient registration, insurance coverage, and other details is accessible to many staff members when needed, without having to pull out files for nonclinical tasks.

On a larger scale, communication between patients and health care professionals increased and expanded in ways never imagined just a decade ago. It is now estimated that more than 80% of homes in the United States have a computer and Internet access. As more people become computer savvy, the use of Web sites, e-mail, digital files, and other technology is creating a more involved and highly informed medical consumer. In the near future, health insurance companies will need to start considering how to reimburse health care professionals for services rendered to patients, using non-traditional methods.

Speed and Cost Reduction

The convenience of displaying information quickly on the computer monitor, instead of manually looking for it and then having to return it to its place, adds up to saved time. The same applies to gathering data and compiling it for statistics and reports. Additionally, when specific tasks have been set up to be done by the software program, the computer can be left to accomplish large amounts of repetitive work and processing.

Computerization saves time and money in the long run. For example, only essential information needs to be printed on paper. If the software produces receipts, statements, and various forms, these can be generated on demand. This eliminates having to order large quantities of custom, preprinted supplies that may become outdated with time and take up storage space. In many instances, the increasing use of digital information has done away with the need to use paper at all. Data can be stored easily and transferred where and when it is needed, using computers.

Software that is used properly, and to its full potential, will perform the mundane, daily business tasks that keep the practice running smoothly. Overall, this type of efficiency translates to better organized office procedures, decreased collections, and increased reimbursement.

DISADVANTAGES OF COMPUTER USE

Unfortunately, there are several disadvantages to computerization of the medical office. However, these necessary difficulties are usually overcome. In the end, these disadvantages do not outweigh the many benefits of a good practice management software program.

System Failures and Problems

Regardless of how expensive or high quality the software and equipment is, certainly there will be occasional system glitches. Whether problems arise because of errors made by users, or issues with the software, anytime a computer goes down, the operation of the medical office may very well come to a standstill. Alternative manual methods of performing office procedures will need to be implemented until problems with the computer are resolved.

At times, malfunctions with the software's programming, called *bugs*, will interfere with use of the computer. There is always potential for complete hardware failure, because computers are machines and subject to mechanical breakdowns. If the hard drive fails, the term for this unfortunate event is a system *crash*. Because of this risk, backing up of all pertinent data needs to be performed diligently and regularly in order to protect the digital records of the practice from being permanently lost. Reliable backup software and a regular schedule for using it are essential in any medical practice. In addition, it is wise to invest in high quality support from software and equipment vendors. Should any of these aforementioned failures occur, having made good choices and investments regarding technical support will prove invaluable.

Patient Confidentiality

A serious consideration when using computers is maintaining confidentiality of patient information. At present, the problem of finding complete and foolproof methods of safeguarding data from inappropriate use is a disadvantage. However, it is a problem that is under constant scrutiny. Because the United States government has encouraged electronic data use, guidelines and laws have been proposed and revised for safeguarding digital data related to health information. Some laws, such as those relating to HIPAA (discussed in the next section), started to be enforced in 2001 and were implemented in stages through 2004.

HEALTH INSURANCE PORTABILITY AND ACCOUNTABILITY ACT (HIPAA)

Since 1996, health care providers have been required to modify their office procedures to protect patient health information. The latest bill providing the guidelines for these regulations is the **Health Insurance Portability and Accountability Act**, also known as **HIPAA** (pronounced hip' ah).

The *portability* part of the law ensures that persons have an opportunity to keep their health insurance when they leave an employer, despite pre-existing medical conditions, including pregnancy. However, the major focus of HIPAA lies with the security and privacy of health information.

Every entity, including medical practices that transmit or store electronic data and records, must comply with HIPAA regulations. There are three components to these regulations:

1. **Transactions and Code Sets.** In an effort to standardize how health information is electronically stored and transmitted, these regulations affect the following transactions:

   + Insurance claim submissions
   + Insurance claim payments and remittance advice
   + Obtaining status of insurance claims
   + Patient eligibility for a health plan
   + Certification and referral authorizations
   + Enrollment information for a health plan
   + Information regarding health plan premium payments
   + Coordination of benefits (COB) for dual coverage situations.

   Additionally, the rules require that providers and health plans both use specific code sets, including CPT-4 and ICD-9, eliminating all local codes and bringing uniformity to the system.

2. **Security Rules.** In February 2003, the final mandatory rules were released regarding what must be done to safeguard electronic information from unauthorized disclosure. These rules encompass the storage, transmission, and access to health information. Reasonable requirements must be used properly to identify the user of health information before it is given out. In addition, the use of electronic signatures is authorized as a means of assuring user identification. Electronic signature is a technique for signing electronic documents that provides a means for proving the document has not been inappropriately tampered with.

3. **Privacy Rules.** Privacy rules apply to health information that can be individually identified in any form: orally, on paper, or electronically. This information is referred to as **protected health information (PHI)**. Because PHI is routinely used by hospitals, physicians, health care plans, clearinghouses, and others, the privacy rules apply to these entities. Collectively, under the HIPAA privacy rules, these users are referred to as **covered entities**. A *covered entity*, as defined by the Centers for Medicare & Medicaid Services (CMS), is a health plan, health care clearing-house (such as billing services), or a physician or hospital that transmits health information in electronic form.

The privacy rules component of HIPAA is probably the most recognizable by both health care workers and patients since April 2003, when they went into effect. This is due to the immediate and obvious changes that were put in place simultaneously by all medical providers. One of the changes involved something as commonplace as patient sign-in sheets.

In the past, many offices had patients sign a list, called the *sign-in sheet*, to identify who had arrived at the office for a visit. Depending on the office, sign-in sheets often included what is now protected health information. Such information as symptoms, diagnoses, type of appointment, and of course, the patient's name and other information could be seen by anyone else signing the list. If the sign-in sheet was in proximity, even visitors to the office for other business could easily view this information. Today, as a result of HIPAA, individual data cards, or specially designed sign-in sheets that have removable strips, immediately remove patient information from unauthorized access to others. See Figure 2-4 for an example of a modified sign-in sheet.

1. Please sign your name below
2. Remove strip from sheet
3. Hand the strip to receptionist

NAME: _____ ARRIVAL TIME: _____

APPOINTMENT WITH: _____ ADDRESS CHANGE? ☐

PHYSICIAN/OTHER: _____ INSURANCE CHANGE? ☐

NAME: _____ ARRIVAL TIME: _____

APPOINTMENT WITH: _____ ADDRESS CHANGE? ☐

PHYSICIAN/OTHER: _____ INSURANCE CHANGE? ☐

NAME: _____ ARRIVAL TIME: _____

APPOINTMENT WITH: _____ ADDRESS CHANGE? ☐

PHYSICIAN/OTHER: _____ INSURANCE CHANGE? ☐

NAME: _____ ARRIVAL TIME: _____

APPOINTMENT WITH: _____ ADDRESS CHANGE? ☐

PHYSICIAN/OTHER: _____ INSURANCE CHANGE? ☐

NAME: _____ ARRIVAL TIME: _____

APPOINTMENT WITH: _____ ADDRESS CHANGE? ☐

PHYSICIAN/OTHER: _____ INSURANCE CHANGE? ☐

NAME: _____ ARRIVAL TIME: _____

APPOINTMENT WITH: _____ ADDRESS CHANGE? ☐

PHYSICIAN/OTHER: _____ INSURANCE CHANGE? ☐

NAME: _____ ARRIVAL TIME: _____

APPOINTMENT WITH: _____ ADDRESS CHANGE? ☐

PHYSICIAN/OTHER: _____ INSURANCE CHANGE? ☐

NAME: _____ ARRIVAL TIME: _____

APPOINTMENT WITH: _____ ADDRESS CHANGE? ☐

PHYSICIAN/OTHER: _____ INSURANCE CHANGE? ☐

NAME: _____ ARRIVAL TIME: _____

APPOINTMENT WITH: _____ ADDRESS CHANGE? ☐

PHYSICIAN/OTHER: _____ INSURANCE CHANGE? ☐

NAME: _____ ARRIVAL TIME: _____

APPOINTMENT WITH: _____ ADDRESS CHANGE? ☐

PHYSICIAN/OTHER: _____ INSURANCE CHANGE? ☐

Inhealth Record Systems (800)477-7374, in Atlanta (770)396-4994   Form # PCS3

FIGURE 2-4

Sample of a modified patient sign-in sheet for HIPAA compliance. *Used with permission. InHealth Record Systems, Inc., 5076 Winters Chapel Road, Atlanta, GA 30360, 800-477-7374, http://www.inhealthrecords.com.*

The following list contains aspects of the privacy rules you should be familiar with. You will most likely encounter them in the medical workplace and have some responsibility for these during the course of your duties.

- Covered entities must make an effort to provide patients with a written privacy notice and practices. The notice must also explain the patient's privacy rights and, by signing for the notice, the patient acknowledges receipt of these rights. If the patient refuses to sign, a written explanation must be completed. Figure 2-5 shows an example of an authorization for the use and disclosure of PHI that the patient might sign in a medical office. An example of a complete privacy notice can be viewed directly from the software included with this book under the HIPAA tab of the registration screen.

- Covered entities must designate a person, known as the *privacy officer*, to be responsible for developing and implementing privacy policies and procedures. An existing staff member (such as an office manager) may be assigned to fulfill this role. Additionally, staff members must all be made aware of, and trained in, the privacy rules, policies, and procedures of the covered entity.

- Covered entities can share PHI with business associates only with written assurance from the associate that the information will be appropriately safeguarded. This assurance is usually in the form of a contract, known as a **Business Associate Agreement**. The agreement includes a number of areas regarding not only the safeguarding of PHI, but also establishing the way this information can be used by the associate, how it may be disclosed, and how to report unauthorized disclosures. It also outlines the terms by which the agreement can be terminated and the return or destruction of the PHI, if feasible, upon termination.

  The American Recovery and Reinvestment Act of 2009 (ARRA), signed by President Barack Obama on February 17, 2009, and better known as the Stimulus Bill, has expanded the scope of HIPAA privacy and security regulations. Instead of the regulations applying only to covered entities, the ARRA requires not only written agreements with business associates, but also now subjects business associates to direct federal regulation, including civil and criminal penalties for violating HIPAA standards.

- Patients have the right to review their PHI and obtain copies. Covered entities are permitted to charge a reasonable fee for providing copies. If patients find inaccuracies in their PHI, they have the right to request corrections. If a covered entity denies this request, the denial must be provided in a written statement.

- Covered entities must disclose only the minimal amount of PHI necessary to meet the purpose of the disclosure. In addition, policies must be in place that limit the information to be disclosed. It is important to note that these limitations are not applicable to health care providers for PHI related to treatment.

Whenever in doubt about patient information, and the possibility of disclosing information, always consult with the proper authority in your office. The penalties for accidental disclosure of PHI and consistent misuses are high.

Sample only, this is not intended as legal advice.

Douglasville Medicine Associates
5076 Brand Blvd., Suite 401
Douglasville, NY 01234

Effective: April 14, 2003

I authorize Douglasville Medicine Associates or its re-insurers and consumer reporting agencies, or any of its authorized representatives, to obtain, use, and/or disclose certain information about me as indicated below.

Douglasville Medicine Associates may obtain and maintain Protected Health Information (PHI) about me to perform specific functions. This authorization describes the type of information that is collected and my rights regarding how that information can be used.

Protected Health Information (PHI) includes individually identifiable health information that is created or received by my provider, my health plan or insurer, a data clearinghouse, a health authority, employer, school or university. PHI can be maintained or transmitted in any form or medium. It relates to the past, present, or future:

- Condition of my physical or mental health;
- Health care provided to me; or
- Payment for the health care provided to me.

PHI does not include summary health information or information that has been de-identified according to the standards for de-identification provided for in the HIPAA Privacy Rule.

This information may be obtained from a number of sources including, but not limited to, applications for health plan coverage, questionnaires, health care providers, claims for payment filed by myself or health care providers, referrals made by health care providers, and my medical records. Other sources of PHI include group health plan administrators, insurance carriers, the Medical Information Bureau, employers, and other business partners such as pharmacy benefit managers, third-party administrators, consultants, agents or brokers. PHI may be obtained over the telephone, by mail, or E-mail.

PHI may be used by Douglasville Medicine Associates employees, business associates, vendors and others as may be necessary to perform activities such as determination of benefit level usage, new benefit programs, and a variety of managed care programs, including but not limited to prescription drug management, disease management and health care risk assessment.

Douglasville Medicine Associates is committed to the privacy of your PHI and has required all business associates and vendors to agree in writing to those same protections. Despite these efforts, we are required by law to advise you that your information may at some point fall outside of these protections, be re-disclosed and would no longer be protected.

I understand I have a right to inspect and copy my own PHI to be used or disclosed.

I understand that I have a right to revoke this authorization at any time and my request must be in writing. Please refer to the [name of covered entity] Privacy Notice for additional information on how to revoke this authorization. I am aware that my PHI already used and disclosed will not be affected by my revocation.

I agree this authorization will be valid for twenty-four (24) months from the date signed or until coverage under this plan has terminated and all benefits have been determined.

_____   _____
Signature   Date

_____
Name

_____   _____
Name of Personal Representative   Relationship to Patient

FIGURE 2-5

Sample privacy notice for patient authorization to use and disclose protected health information (PHI). *Used with permission.* *InHealth Record Systems, Inc., 5076 Winters Chapel Road, Atlanta, GA 30360, 800-477-7374, http://www.inhealthrecords.com.*

USING *MEDICAL OFFICE SIMULATION SOFTWARE (MOSS)* VERSION 2.0

Medical Office Simulation Software (MOSS) version 2.0 comes in a single-user version and a network version. If you are working in a classroom computer laboratory, check with your instructor before proceeding with logon. Refer to the following instructions for the software version you are using.

LOG IN TO THE SINGLE-USER VERSION OF MOSS

When using the software from the back of the book as a single-user, the logon name and password will be auto-populated in the required fields.

> **TIP:** Note that logon names and passwords are case sensitive, so pay special attention to using capital and lowercase letters where needed.

The default logon name is "Student1," and the password, which is also "Student1," will appear as asterisks in the field. Simply click the *OK* command button to continue to the Main Menu screen.

Next, if you are using a single-user version, after logging in, skip to *Let's Try It! 2-2, Navigating Medical Office Simulation Software* on page 54, to continue.

LOGON PROCEDURE FOR MOSS NETWORK VERSION

If you are using the network version, begin the logon procedure by following the steps in the next section, *Let's Try It! 2-1, Logon Procedure for MOSS Network Version.*

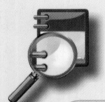

LET'S TRY IT! 2-1 LOGON PROCEDURE FOR MOSS NETWORK VERSION

Objective: The reader will log on to the network version and change the user password.

> **TIP:** Click on *Start*, then *Programs*, then click on the software title to open. If a desktop icon is available, you can also open the software by double clicking on it.

STEP 1
Start MOSS by following your instructor's directions.

STEP 2
A logon dialog box will open. The login level should be set to Student. If it is not, use the drop-down menu to select Student (see Figure 2-6).

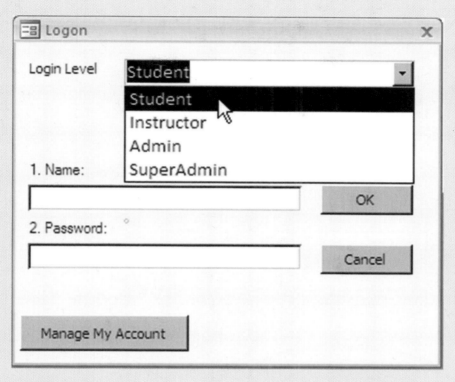

FIGURE 2-6

Delmar/Cengage Learning

NT: Note that logon names d passwords are case sensi- e, so pay special attention using capital and lowercase ers where needed.

STEP 3

Your instructor will provide you with your logon name and password. Using this information, enter the logon name in Field 1 and the password in Field 2 of the logon dialog box. Click on the *Manage My Account* button. See Figure 2-7.

continues

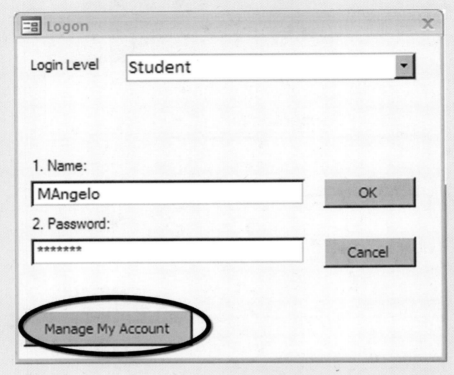

FIGURE 2-7

Delmar/Cengage Learning

HINT: Choose a password that is easy to remember, yet not something obvious that many people may know about you, such as a birth date.

STEP 4

Move your cursor into the Password field and delete the existing password. Enter a new password of your choice, making sure it is at least five characters in length.

STEP 5

Retype the new password in the next field to confirm it. Click *Save Record* (see Figure 2-8).

NOTE: If there is a typing error, a prompt will alert you to re-enter the password correctly.

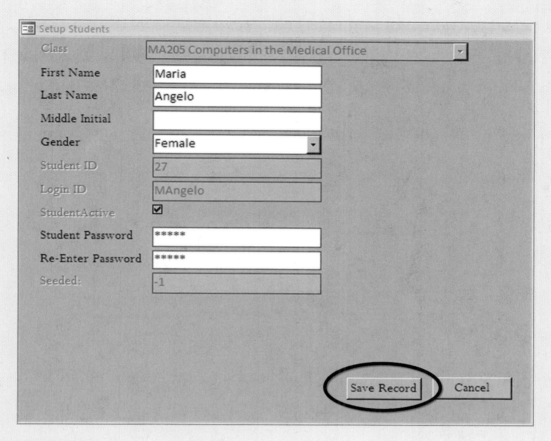

FIGURE 2-8

Delmar/Cengage Learning

STEP 6

The original logon dialog box should now be displayed on your screen. Move your cursor into Field 2, Password, and type the new password you just created. Click the *OK* button to enter the program. See Figure 2-9.

NT: You will select *Manage Account* to change your sword or other information; will choose *OK* to directly in to the program.

STEP 7

When logging in to MOSS Network in the future, you will simply enter your logon name and password and then click the *OK* button.

continues

LOGON PROCEDURE FOR MOSS NETWORK VERSION *continued*

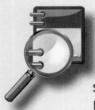

FIGURE 2-9

Delmar/Cengage Learning

LET'S TRY IT! 2-2 NAVIGATING MOSS

Objective: The reader will be oriented to the menus, navigation features, and screens of MOSS.

STEP 1

MOSS features a main screen with a Main Menu consisting of buttons that can be clicked to access specific areas. Refer to Figure 2-10.

STEP 2

In addition to the Main Menu at the center of the screen, there are alternate ways to access areas of the software. Along the top left, just below the software title bar, are the pull-down menus. Click on *File* and note the available menu selections. Without clicking, move the mouse pointer to the right until the next pull-down menu displays. Many of these selections are the same as the Main Menu choices at the center of the screen. Others, such as Lists, offer shortcuts that save time getting to certain functions of the software. See Figure 2-11 for an example of pull-down menus.

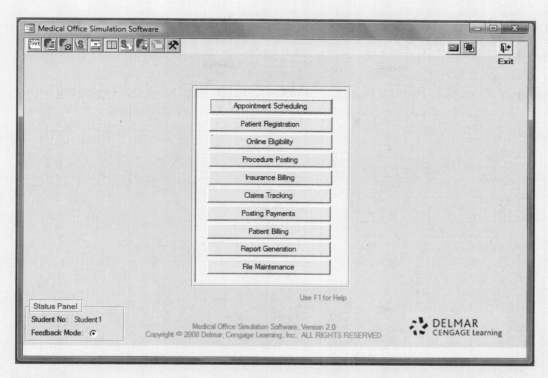

FIGURE 2-10

Delmar/Cengage Learning

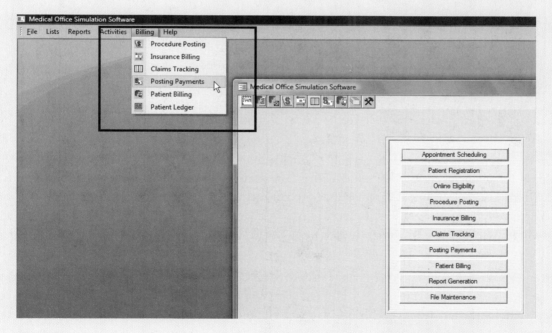

FIGURE 2-11

Delmar/Cengage Learning

continues

NAVIGATING MOSS *continued*

STEP 3

Another useful tool for navigating the software is the icon toolbar. The toolbar consists of small pictures that serve as buttons to quickly access areas of the software. See Figure 2-12. Place the mouse pointer over the first icon in the toolbar, without clicking. A caption will appear after a few seconds indicating what the button is used to access. View the captions for all of the icons in the toolbar.

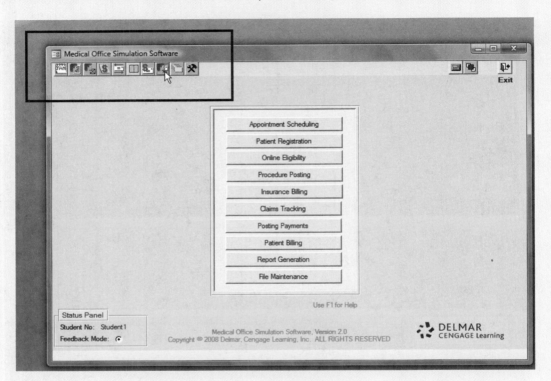

FIGURE 2-12

Delmar/Cengage Learning

STEP 4

On the right side of the main screen are utility icons. The first opens a calculator when clicked, handy for financial tasks. The middle icon has a caption that reads Restore Loaded Forms. This will maximize all forms or windows that are not immediately visible. If you cannot find a window you were working with, click this icon to restore any minimized windows for viewing. The last icon, labeled Exit, will close MOSS and return you to the Windows desktop. See Figure 2-13.

STEP 5

From the Main Menu, click on *Patient Registration*. This displays the patient selection dialog box. See Figure 2-14. This dialog box is used extensively throughout the software to select patient accounts for various tasks. The option buttons along the top allow searching for a patient either by name, social security number, or account number. When the desired patient is shown on the list, double-click on the patient's last name to make the selection. You can also click once in the space to the left of the patient name, and then click on the *Select* command button at the bottom. Try this a few times, using the *Close* button at the bottom right of any screen that opens. The *Close* button returns you to the patient selection dialog box.

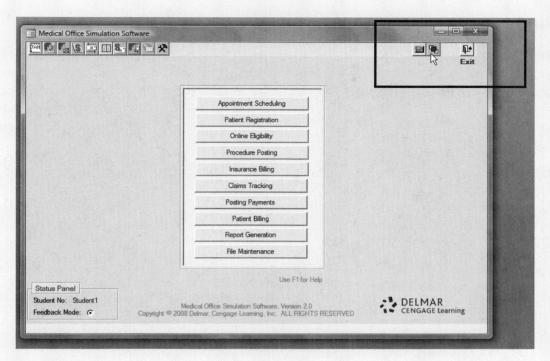

FIGURE 2-13

Delmar/Cengage Learning

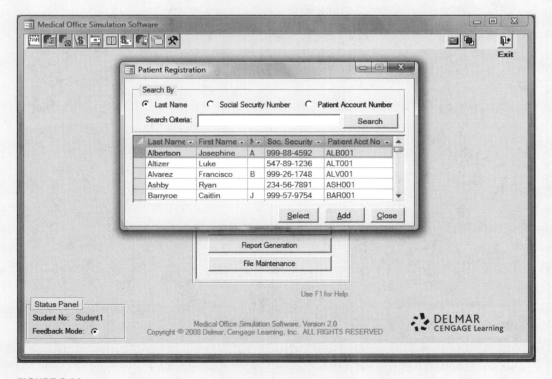

FIGURE 2-14

Delmar/Cengage Learning

continues

NAVIGATING MOSS *continued*

STEP 6

Along the bottom of the patient selection dialog box there is an *Add* button. Whenever the *Add* button is available, new data can be entered in the software database. What type of data can be entered with the *Add* button can differ depending on what area of the software you are working in. In the Patient Registration area, the *Add* command button will allow input of demographic and insurance data for new patients.

STEP 7

You should still be at the patient selection dialog box for Patient Registration. If not, click on *Patient Registration* from the Main Menu. Using one of the selection methods you just learned (Step 5), select Eugene Sykes from the patient list. The Patient Registration dialog box for this patient should display. See Figure 2-15.

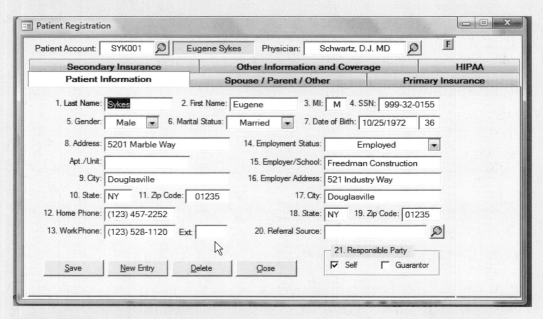

FIGURE 2-15

Delmar/Cengage Learning

STEP 8

Notice the tabs along the top, labeled "Patient Information," "Primary Insurance," "HIPAA," etc. By clicking on these tabs, more information regarding patient Sykes can be viewed. Practice clicking on each tab and take note of the information contained on each screen. Do not click on the *Save* or *Delete* buttons as you explore these tabs.

STEP 9

Click on the tab labeled Primary Insurance. Click on the search icon to the right of Field 1, *Insurance Plan* (it looks like a magnifying glass). See Figure 2-16.

This will display the insurance plans in the software database. Notice the familiar *Select* and *Add* command buttons along the bottom. There is an *Edit* button in this area to make corrections to the data if needed. See Figure 2-17. Click on the *Close* button to exit the Insurance Selection dialog box.

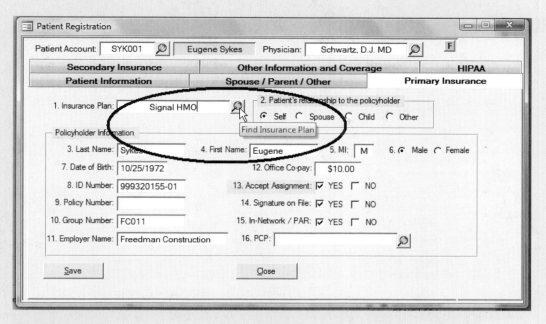

FIGURE 2-16

Delmar/Cengage Learning

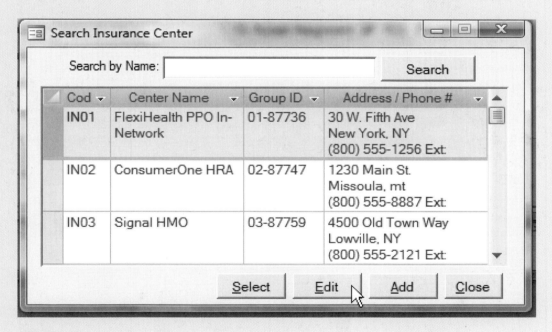

FIGURE 2-17

Delmar/Cengage Learning

STEP 10

You are now ready to close the Patient Registration screen. Click on the *Close* button. If a prompt appears that reads "Do you want to save changes?", click on the *No* button to exit. If the Patient Selection dialog box is open, you may close it. This will return you to the Main Menu.

USING HELP CAPTIONS AND FEEDBACK FEATURES

MOSS features a help file that offers two options: feedback mode and balloon help captions. Feedback mode will alert the user when essential fields have not been completed before allowing data to be saved. A window displaying the fields that require information to be input will appear, as shown in Figure 2-18.

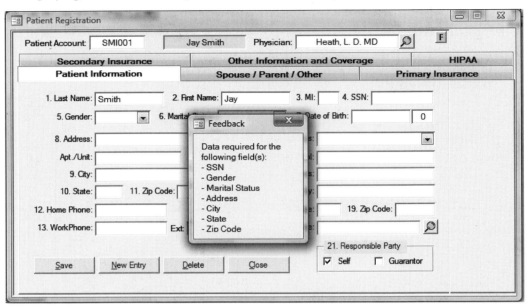

FIGURE 2-18

Delmar/Cengage Learning

Balloon help offers explanations, clarification, or reminders for certain fields. To utilize this feature, the F1 key is pressed after selecting the field for which information is desired. Not all fields have bubble captions; however, there are many throughout the software that can assist with difficult concepts. Figure 2-19 illustrates a bubble help caption for Field 20, Referral Source of the Patient Information tab of the registration screen.

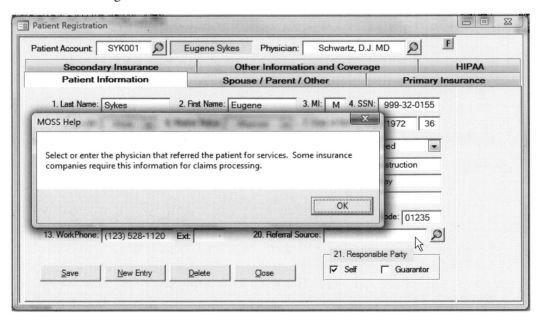

FIGURE 2-19

Delmar/Cengage Learning

Also, when clicking in fields that have additional help, information displays in the lower left MOSS screen with a tip or explanation about the data required. See Figure 2-20.

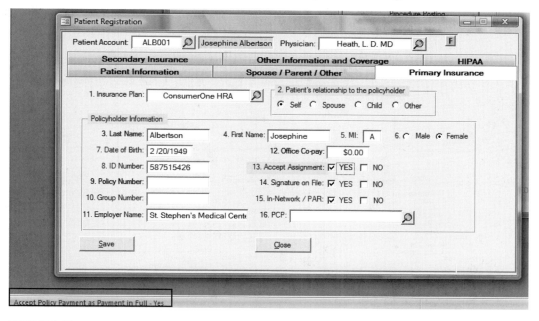

FIGURE 2-20

Delmar/Cengage Learning

MOSS NOTE: When using the network version in a classroom or computer lab, your instructor will turn the feedback and bubble help settings on or off as required. In the single-user version, these features can be selected by going to the Help tab of the File Maintenance area. Figure 2-21 illustrates the File Maintenance screen where these settings can be found. Clicking in the box in front of the desired feature will select it by placing a checkmark in the box. Be sure to close the software, and then reopen it in order for the selected features to activate.

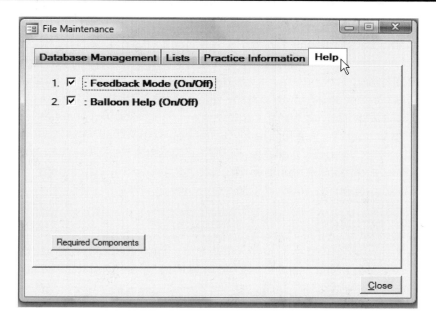

FIGURE 2-21

Delmar/Cengage Learning

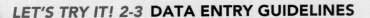

LET'S TRY IT! 2-3 DATA ENTRY GUIDELINES

Objective: The reader will become familiar with the guidelines for proper data entry using MOSS.

STEP 1

Starting from the Main Menu, click on *Patient Registration*. From the bottom of the patient selection dialog box, click on *Add*. This will display a blank patient registration screen, as shown on Figure 2-22.

FIGURE 2-22

Delmar/Cengage Learning

STEP 2

Click on Field 1, Last Name, and then type the word Practice. Use the Tab key to advance to Field 2. Type the first name Patty. Use the Tab key to advance to Field 4, SSN, or Social Security Number. All fields for social security numbers, telephone numbers, and dates will automatically format for you. Type the following SSN number in Field 4: 555231468. Advance by pressing the Tab key to Field 5. The SSN number should now display with dashes in place.

You may have also noticed that the software assigned a patient account number for Patty, displayed at the top left corner. See Figure 2-23. The software will allow the user to enter an account number, or will assign the next available. MOSS utilizes the first three letters of the patient's last name followed by a sequential number. Be sure to follow the instructions in your book before assigning account numbers to patients in the exercises.

STEP 3

With the cursor in Field 5, Gender, type the letter "f". This will display Female. You can then advance by pressing the Tab key. At Field 6, Marital Status, drop down the box to display the choices available. Select *Married* by clicking on it. Advance to the next field by pressing the Tab key.

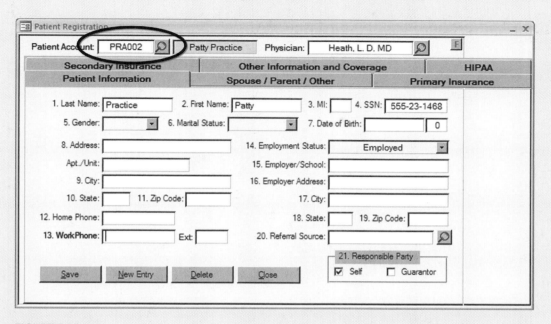

FIGURE 2-23

Delmar/Cengage Learning

STEP 4

Field 7 is a date field for the date of birth. It is important to remember that any date field throughout the software will accept only the eight-digit format. You do not have to include dashes or slashes between the numbers, the software will automatically format the date for you. Patty Practice's date of birth is 10/20/1974. In Field 7, type only the numbers 10201974, then press the Tab key. Notice that the software also provides the current age of the patient. Press the Tab key and advance to Field 12.

MOSS NOTE: MOSS calculates each patient's age based on today's date. Depending on when you work on your exercises, the age displayed on your screen for a patient may vary from the screen shots in the book.

STEP 5

Field 12 is for the patient's home phone number. Again, the software will automatically format the number; it is not necessary to type dashes or parentheses. Patty's phone number is (123) 987-6623. In Field 12, type only the numbers 1239876623; then press the Tab key. The home phone number should display in proper format.

STEP 6

Click on *Save*. If the Feedback mode is on, a window will display the missing information necessary to save this screen. Use the *Close* button at the top right corner of the Feedback window to close it, shown in Figure 2-24.

continues

DATA ENTRY GUIDELINES *continued*

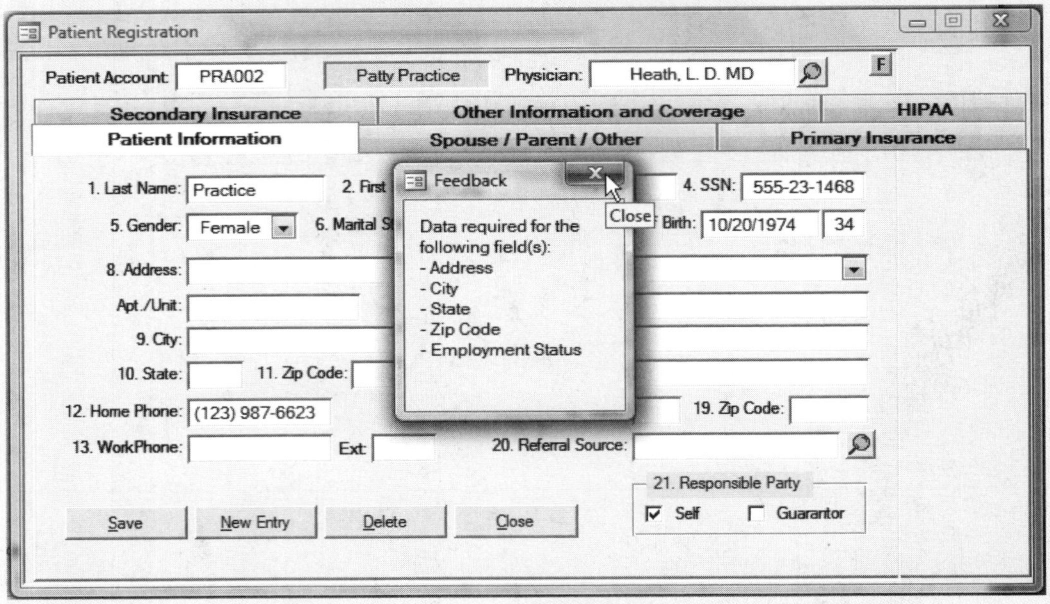

FIGURE 2-24

Delmar/Cengage Learning

STEP 7

Go back to Fields 8 through 11 and enter the following information:

123 Main St., Douglasville, NY 01234

Click on the *Save* button. If the Feedback window appears, it will indicate that employment status is required.

STEP 8

Close the Feedback window and go to Field 14, Employment Status. Use the drop-down box to select *Employed* from the list. Click the *Close* button, then *Yes* at the Save prompt. See Figure 2-25 for an example of the correct message when the record has been saved.

STEP 9

Click on the *Close* button. To verify that the patient is in the database, use the Patient Selection dialog box, which should still be on the screen. Use any of the previously discussed methods to find Patty Practice in the patient list. See Figure 2-26 to check your screen. Click on the *Select* button to open her account.

STEP 10

Next, click on the *Primary Insurance* tab. At Field 1, click on the *Search* button to view insurance health plans in the database. Select "FlexiHealth PPO In-Network" from the list by double clicking on it, or click on the plan name, then use the *Select* button.

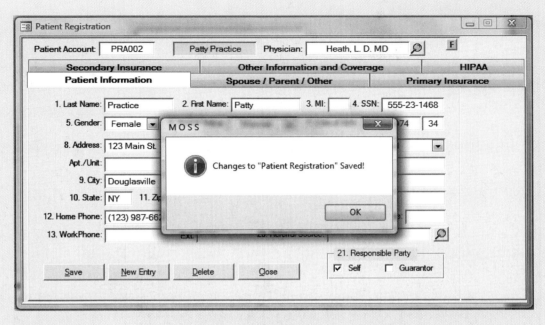

FIGURE 2-25

Delmar/Cengage Learning

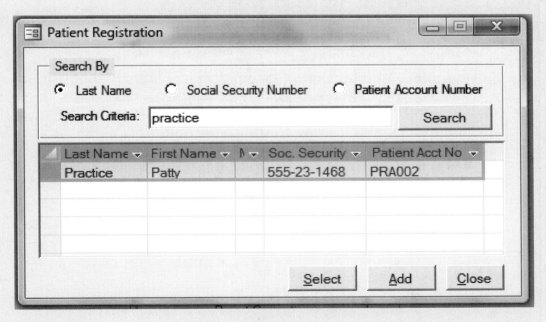

FIGURE 2-26

Delmar/Cengage Learning

continues

DATA ENTRY GUIDELINES *continued*

STEP 11

In Field 2, click in the radio button in front of *Self* to select this option. This will automatically fill in patient information previously input. Click in Field 8 and enter the following ID number: 555231468.

STEP 12

Next, tab to Field 10 and enter the following group number for her insurance plan: BY456.

STEP 13

Tab to Field 12 and enter 20.00 as the plan co-payment.

STEP 14

Patty's physician is Dr. Heath and he accepts assignment for this plan. Click *Yes* in Field 13 and also in Field 15, since Dr. Heath is also a network physician for this PPO.

STEP 15

Click the *Save* button. A confirmation that the changes to the primary insurance have been saved should appear. Click on *OK*, then check your screen with Figure 2-27. When finished, click *Close* and return to the Main Menu screen.

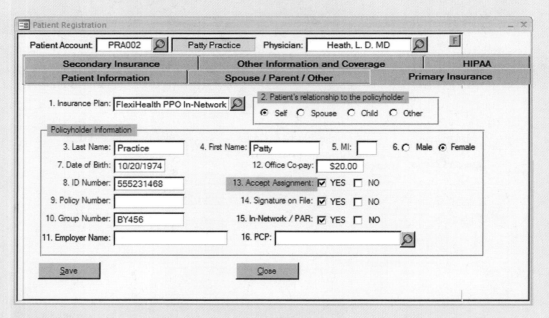

FIGURE 2-27

Delmar/Cengage Learning

It is advisable to use the Patty Practice account for testing or practicing certain tasks to try them out first. While learning to use this software, it is helpful to have a patient account strictly for practice purposes that can be easily deleted without affecting your other work.

USING THE BACK UP AND RESTORE FUNCTIONS OF MOSS

MOSS NOTE: The backup and restore functions are available only in the single-user version of MOSS. If you are using the network version in a classroom or computer lab, you may move to the next section. In the network version, the network administrator or instructor follows a different routine to back up your database.

Backing up your MOSS database is akin to saving a document or other file on your computer. In the single-user version, you can back up (save) your progress at any time using the backup function. The restore function allows you to return to a previous point in the program. For instance, if you realize you have made a mistake and cannot correct it, you could restore a previous backup file and start the exercise over again. In the single-user version, these functions can be accessed by going to the File Maintenance area. These functions have been improved to make it easier to create and restore your MOSS database. They have been changed so that readers can more easily select where backup files are saved, including to portable storage devices such as flash drives.

If you are using the single-user version of MOSS, follow the steps in the next section, *Let's Try It! 2-4*, Back Up and Restore Your MOSS Database, to create and restore backup database files.

MOSS NOTE: It is advisable to create a backup file of your MOSS database daily; at a minimum, after you complete each unit. For longer units (such as Unit 5 and Unit 6), it may be advisable to create backup files at several places within the unit.

LET'S TRY IT! 2-4 BACK UP AND RESTORE YOUR MOSS DATABASE

Objective: The reader will learn how to back up and restore the MOSS database using the single-user version of MOSS.

TO BACK UP (SAVE) YOUR MOSS DATABASE

STEP 1
Starting from the Main Menu, click on *File Maintenance*.

STEP 2
In the "Database Management" tab, click on the button next to *2. Backup Database*. See Figure 2-28.

continues

BACK UP AND RESTORE YOUR MOSS DATABASE *continued*

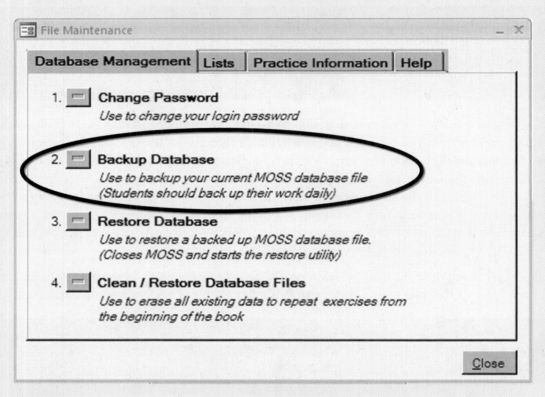

FIGURE 2-28

Delmar/Cengage Learning

STEP 3

You will receive a prompt: "Would you like to back up your current MOSS database?" Click *Yes*.

STEP 4

HINT: It is advisable to save your backup file on a portable storage device such as a flash drive.

The program will open a File Save dialog box. Browse to select the location to where you would like to save the backup file.

MOSS will automatically generate a file name based on the date and time you are creating the file. You may choose to rename the file; *however, if you rename the file, it is critical to keep the file extension (.mde) at the end of the file name*. See Figure 2-29.

STEP 5

Click *Save*. Click *OK* through the prompt indicating the backup was successful. Close the File Maintenance window and return to the Main Menu.

TO RESTORE A BACKUP FILE

STEP 1

Starting from the Main Menu, click on *File Maintenance*.

STEP 2

In the Database Management tab, click on the button next to *3. Restore Database*. See Figure 2-30.

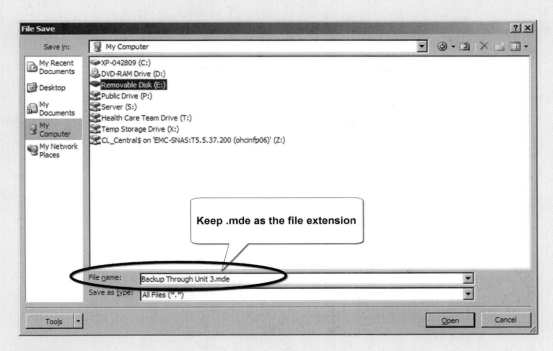

FIGURE 2-29

Delmar/Cengage Learning

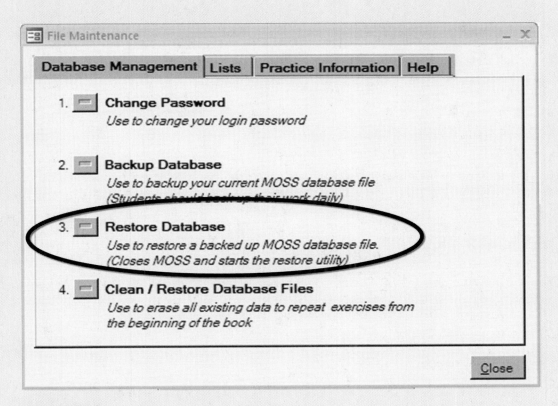

FIGURE 2-30

Delmar/Cengage Learning

continues

BACK UP AND RESTORE YOUR MOSS DATABASE *continued*

STEP 3

Click *Yes* through one prompt.

STEP 4

A MOSS Restore dialog box will open. Click on the button *Restore MOSS from Backup*. See Figure 2-31.

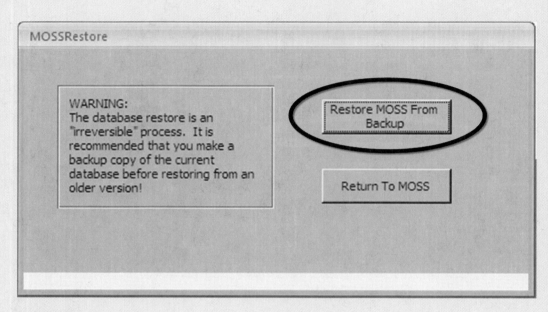

FIGURE 2-31

Delmar/Cengage Learning

STEP 5

Click *Yes* through one prompt.

STEP 6

Browse to find the location where you have saved the backup file you would like to restore (see Figure 2-32). Double click on the file name. (You can also highlight the file name and click *OK*.)

STEP 7

Click *Yes* through one prompt.

STEP 8

You are now on the MOSS Restore dialog box screen. Click on the button *Return to MOSS* (Figure 2-33).

STEP 9

Log in to MOSS. (You are logging into the new database you just restored.) You are now back on the Main Menu screen.

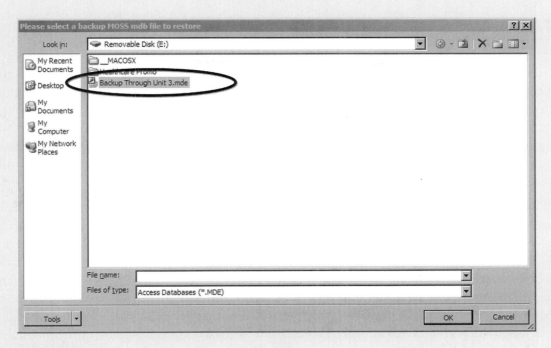

FIGURE 2-32

Delmar/Cengage Learning

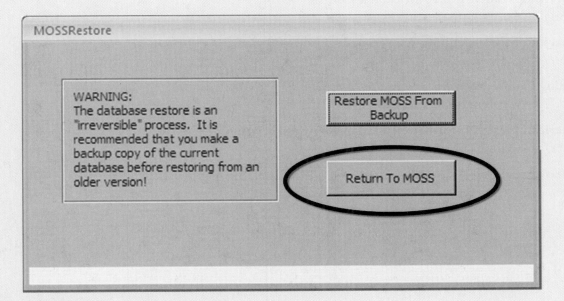

FIGURE 2-33

Delmar/Cengage Learning

FINAL NOTES

After completion of this unit, you will have a foundation of knowledge regarding the general components of practice management software and confidentiality issues, including HIPAA. With this general understanding, you will be familiar with the basic framework common to almost all practice management software. You are now ready to start learning and applying specific tasks, using the software that comes with this book. Upon completion of the activities found in the forthcoming units, you will be able to browse any medical practice management software and recognize the system components and know their function. This will greatly increase your ability to learn many different software titles that may be in use at various offices.

Because there are many changes that take place with guidelines for electronic billing and information management, including HIPAA, staying apprised of laws and regulations is a necessary part of this career. Become active with organizations that conduct seminars, such as the local chapter of the American Association of Medical Assistants or the American Medical Technologists. Attend workshops of interest to medical support staff sponsored by health insurance companies. Stay current with articles, publications, and web sites that report on issues concerning HIPAA, health insurance, reimbursement, and other areas of health care. There are several resources available at the end of this unit that can assist you with locating information related to software and computing for the medical office.

RESOURCES

American Academy of Professional Coders
http://www.aapc.com

American Medical Billing Association
http://www.ambanet.net/AMBA.htm

Coding Conferences
http://www.codingconferences.com/

American Health Information Management Association
http://www.ahima.org

American Coding Association
http://www.theamericancodingassociation.com

Select the correct answer for 1 through 5 from the following list.

    a. A system used to input demographic and insurance information about each patient in the practice.

    b. A system used as a utility to maintain common information or customize features of the program.

    c. A system used to apply fees for services to a patient account.

    d. A system used to retrieve and organize data from various parts of the software program into useful information.

    e. A system that prepares claims to be sent to the insurance companies.

    f. A system used to apply payments from various sources to a patient account.

    g. A system that generates statements to be sent monthly for balances due on patient accounts.

    h. A system that allows scheduling of patient appointments to be recorded.

1. ____Patient Billing System
2. ____Posting Payments System
3. ____File Maintenance System
4. ____Procedure Posting System
5. ____Report Generation System

Select the correct system used with practice management software in 6 through 13 to perform the following duties.

    a. A new patient is on the telephone and would like to know if the doctor can see her next Wednesday for a consultation.

    b. A patient has come to the front desk to check out after a visit and hands you the superbill. You need to apply the fees to the patient's account.

    c. The doctor wants to know how many routine prenatal patients the Physician's Assistant has seen in the office over the past three months.

    d. There are 43 payment checks from different sources in today's mail that need to be applied to patient accounts.

    e. Monthly statements need to be mailed out by the end of this week. The statements need to be prepared and printed.

    f. A new patient brings his patient information and insurance card(s) to the front desk. The patient needs to be added to the computer's records.

    g. The doctor has purchased new laboratory equipment to perform certain tests for patients during their visits. Fifteen CPT codes and fees not previously in the system need to be added for the tests that will now be billed by the office.

    h. Claims need to be prepared and submitted electronically to the respective insurance companies for payment.

6. ____Procedure Posting
7. ____File Maintenance
8. ____Posting Payments

9. ___Insurance Billing

10. ___Report Generation

11. ___Appointment Scheduling

12. ___Patient Registration

13. ___Patient Billing

14. There are no medical offices that still file insurance claims via paper.
    a. True
    b. False

15. Adjustments are amounts taken away or added to an account balance to reflect various accounting situations.
    a. True
    b. False

16. In general, a patient must pay the insurance deductible out-of-pocket every year.
    a. True
    b. False

17. "Please call the office to make payment arrangements for your past due amount," is an example of a dunning message.
    a. True
    b. False

18. Computers in the medical office have improved the way everyday tasks are performed.
    a. True
    b. False

19. When one practice management software is learned, the skills can be applied to learn other similar programs.
    a. True
    b. False

20. One advantage of computers is they will always correct the errors made by the users.
    a. True
    b. False

21. The registration form contains
    a. the patient demographics.
    b. the guarantor information.
    c. insurance information.
    d. a and c only.
    e. all of the above.

22. Multiple locations belonging to a medical practice are commonly referred to as
    a. incorporations.
    b. ancillary offices.
    c. network offices.
    d. none of the above.

23. Of the following, which is *not* an advantage of computerization of the medical office?
    a. Increased efficiency for staff members
    b. Easy accessibility to information
    c. Forms that can be generated on demand
    d. Vulnerability to *bugs* and system *crashes*

24. Codes that identify the procedures performed for a patient are called
    a. CPT.
    b. ICD.
    c. DOS.
    d. POS.

25. Codes that identify the date of service are called
    a. CPT.
    b. ICD.
    c. DOS.
    d. POS.

26. Codes that describe where procedures were performed are called
    a. CPT.
    b. ICD.
    c. DOS.
    d. POS.

27. Codes that describe the patient diagnoses are called
    a. CPT.
    b. ICD.
    c. DOS.
    d. POS.

28. Before practice management software can be used, initial data must be entered. This includes
    a. provider information.
    b. insurance companies.
    c. practice information.
    d. CPT and ICD codes.
    e. all of the above.

29. Physicians will determine the procedures for and diagnoses of the patient by providing

    a. information on superbills or encounter forms.

    b. making notes in the patient record.

    c. ICD and CPT codes on the patient registration form.

    d. all of the above.

    e. a and b only.

30. Multiple fee schedules are common in medical offices due to

    a. patients being able to afford only what their income allows.

    b. physicians participating with several different insurance companies that have different reimbursement agreements.

    c. the vast array of procedures that can be performed on a patient.

    d. none of the above.

31. A patient who has a primary and secondary insurance plan is said to have

    a. too much insurance.

    b. double insurance.

    c. dual insurance.

    d. none of the above; a patient can have only one insurance.

32. Services that are not covered by an insurance plan are referred to as

    a. procedures billed with incorrect CPT codes.

    b. adjustments.

    c. bad debt.

    d. exclusions.

33. A fixed payment to be made by the patient at each visit to the medical office is called

    a. a co-payment.

    b. a co-insurance amount.

    c. the deductible.

    d. none of the above.

34. A clearinghouse concerns itself with

    a. validating and editing claims sent to insurance companies.

    b. encoding software so that no one tampers with electronic files.

    c. clearing a patient's check before applying it to the account.

    d. none of the above.

35. List the advantages of computerization of the medical office.

    _____

    _____

    _____

36. List the disadvantages of computerization of the medical office.

_____

_____

_____

37. What does the acronym HIPAA stand for?

_____

_____

_____

38. Explain the "portability" part of HIPAA.

_____

_____

_____

39. What is a covered entity under HIPAA?

_____

_____

_____

40. List the three main components of HIPAA regulations.

_____

_____

_____

41. Explain the responsibilities of the privacy officer, as required by HIPAA.

_____

_____

_____

42. List and explain the five important aspects of HIPAA's privacy rules.

_____

_____

_____

43. What type of information do the privacy rules of HIPAA apply to?

_____

_____

_____

Basic Management Concepts for Medical Administrative Staff

OBJECTIVES

Upon completion of this unit, the reader should be able to:

- **Explain the responsibilities of the back and front office of a physician practice**

- **Explain basic principles of appointment scheduling**

- **Demonstrate basic appointment scheduling tasks using** *Medical Office Simulation Software* **(MOSS)**

- **Discuss the flow of information in a physician practice**

- **List the steps for collecting information and preparing patient files**

- **List the steps for the patient check-in and check-out process in a physician practice**

- **Explain the reimbursement process starting at patient check-in through claims submission and patient billing.**

Medical office management software is designed to do precisely that: manage a medical office. Whether scheduling appointments, accounting for services and payments, or medical billing, the software will handle many complex and multifaceted tasks. Because the software is a tool to help medical staff in many areas of practice management, it is important to have a basic understanding of how a medical office functions.

KEY TERMS

Appointment reminder card

Back office

Cancellation

Consultation

Electronic health records (EHR)

Established patient

Explanation of Benefits (EOB)

Flagging

Front office

Insurance card

Insurance verification

New patient

No-show

Office hours

Patient hours

Primary care physician (PCP)

Progress notes

Recall postcards

Referral

Tickler files

THE BACK OFFICE AND THE FRONT OFFICE

Typically, a medical office has two main areas: the back office and the front office. The **back office** is also referred to as the clinical area, or that part of the office where health care professionals examine patients. Diagnostic testing and medical procedures are performed in the back office according to type of medical specialty and equipment availability.

Medical staff members working in the back office alongside the physicians may include clinical medical assistants, nurses, and laboratory and X-ray technicians. Specialized professional health care providers, such as Nurse Practitioners and Physician Assistants (PA) also work primarily in the clinical back office. While these individuals work closely with the staff of the front office, and may even share responsibilities from both areas, their main focus is centered on direct patient care.

The **front office**, also referred to as the administrative area, is the hub of the medical facility. The front office and its staff are very important in terms of proper management of the medical office as a whole. At the reception area, patients are greeted as they arrive to visit the physician. Registration and other pertinent paperwork, including insurance matters, are attended to. If patients need to make a payment, the front office staff collects it. Follow-up appointments to see the physician are scheduled by the front-office staff, too. The administrative aspects of the front office are not limited to answering telephones and greeting patients. In reality, all activity related to proper insurance billing, reimbursement for services, and maintenance of patient records stems from the front office. The medical facility's image, as well as its patient and professional relations, depend strongly on the administrative medical staff.

Typical staff members of the administrative front office may include receptionists, medical secretaries, administrative medical assistants, medical transcriptionists, medical insurance billers, and office managers. Not all administrative staff are necessarily physically located in the front office area. In fact, some administrative staff have personal work stations or offices separate from the patient reception area, or may even be located in an ancillary office. However, the administrative functions and staff of a medical facility are often collectively referred to as front office staff.

BASIC PRINCIPLES OF APPOINTMENT SCHEDULING

The front office staff is usually the first contact for patients requesting appointments to see the doctor. In fact, scheduling appointments is one of the first opportunities the administrative staff has for collecting patient information. In order to best understand this important task, let us explore some terminology and techniques common with appointment scheduling.

ESTABLISHED AND NEW PATIENTS

On a continuing basis, appointments are scheduled for patients to see the physician for a variety of medical problems and procedures. Appointments are usually scheduled for patients who receive services in the medical office, but the physician also treats patients in other types of facilities, such as hospitals and nursing homes. Whether in the physician's office or an outside facility, services are provided to both established patients and new patients. Obtaining and preparing information for each type of patient is somewhat different, and will be discussed later in this unit.

An **established patient** is an individual who has received professional services from his or her physician, or another physician of the same specialty from the same group practice, within the past three years. Services may have been rendered either in the medical office or an outside facility. For example, a physician may treat a new patient in the hospital after he or she has been admitted through the emergency room. If the patient visits the physician for follow-up at the medical office after being discharged, the patient is no longer new, but established. The patient may be new in terms of visiting the office; however, the physician has previously rendered services (at the hospital) and is familiar with the patient's medical case.

New patients are those individuals who have not received services from the physician, or an associate physician of the same group within the same specialty, within the past three years. Most new patients have never been to the office or received services. Technically, however, if an established patient has not received services from the physician in more than three years, the patient is considered new and services can be billed as a new patient. Care should be taken when accepting patients who state they are new to the medical office. It is a good habit to check the medical software patient database, or the paper files, for every new patient, to make sure the individual is not already in the system. Instances occur where a patient has forgotten he or she has been to the office before, especially if it has been several years since his or her last visit. Some patients received services from the physician in the hospital or another facility, but did not need to return to the medical office for follow-up. There may be a patient record and medical billing activity on file, even if the patient has never physically visited the medical office. Checking all new patients against the existing records eliminates double entries and duplicate files.

INFORMATION DETAILS FOR APPOINTMENT SCHEDULING

When scheduling appointments, it is important to listen carefully to the patient. During the initial conversation, you can learn much about the patient's reason for contacting the office for an appointment. It may be necessary to ask further questions, as some patients will call simply to say they need an appointment, and will not offer information as to their symptoms or problem. It is useful to know whether the patient is new or established, the reason for their appointment, if there are serious symptoms, and if a particular physician has referred the patient. Based on this information, decisions must be made regarding whether a patient needs a routine appointment, immediate medical attention in the office, or should be referred to an emergency room. Depending on the nature of the medical problem, some patients can be scheduled in the coming days, weeks, or months. If you are uncertain about the urgency of a patient's medical condition, consult the physician or office manager to assist in deciding when the patient should be scheduled.

The following list contains important details to be aware of when handling appointment calls from patients.

1. **Distinguish between consultations and referrals.** The distinction between a consultation and a referral is not always well understood. In general, a referring physician requests a consultation. A consultation involves the consulting physician rendering an opinion and advice regarding a patient's diagnosis and treatment. Sometimes, requests for consultations can be made for the purpose of a second opinion. The consultant customarily provides a report to the physician who requested the consultation. The report contains the findings, recommendations, and results of any further testing that may have been done. The patient's regular physician usually sees the patient in follow-up after the consultation.

    Referrals occur when a patient is actually transferred to another physician for partial or complete care for a specific medical problem.

Medical office staff must take care with the term *referral*, which is also widely used by most managed-care plans. A referral in the context of managed care is an authorization for the patient to see a specialist or receive special services, such as diagnostic testing or surgery, or even a consultation.

To clarify the difference between a consultation and a referral, study the following example. A patient is experiencing chest pain and visits her regular physician, Dr. Jones, who is an internist. After examining the patient and obtaining diagnostic test results, Dr. Jones determines that the patient is showing signs and symptoms of coronary artery disease (hardening of the vessels of the heart). He *refers* the patient to Dr. Smith, a cardiologist. In this case, the patient has been transferred to the cardiologist for partial or complete care of the patient's coronary artery disease. However, after more testing, the cardiologist finds that the patient's vessels are in advanced stages of disease and are almost completely blocked. Dr. Smith believes that the patient will require bypass surgery of three vessels. As such, he requests a *consultation* from Dr. Brown, a cardiovascular surgeon. Dr. Brown is being asked for his opinion, and to evaluate the patient for possible surgery. Dr. Brown determines that the patient does require surgery, and sends his evaluation and recommendations in a report to Dr. Smith, the cardiologist. The patient has surgery, performed by Dr. Brown. After her recovery, the patient is discharged to the care of her cardiologist, Dr. Smith, who will monitor her as needed for coronary artery disease. She will continue to see Dr. Jones, her internist, for other medical problems.

2. **Inquire about insurance coverage.** Ask the patient before scheduling an appointment what type of insurance coverage he or she has. It is important to confirm that the insurance plan is one accepted by the medical office. Additionally, if authorization is required in the form of a referral from the patient's primary care physician, this is the time to ask if that referral has been made.

A **Primary Care Physician (PCP)**, common with some types of managed-care plans, is often called the "gatekeeper." The PCP decides when the patient can see a specialist or receive special services and procedures. Most PCPs practice general medicine, and include family medicine physicians and internists. The PCP must authorize the patient to receive care through a referral in order for the covered services to be paid by the insurance plan. Examples of physician specialists include cardiologists, oncologists, surgeons, and neurologists—basically, any provider who has a specialty field and is not the patient's PCP. The typical exceptions are gynecological and obstetrical services, and some other services for women, such as mammography. Most managed-care plans permit women to seek these services without a PCP referral. Examples of other services that may require referrals are rehabilitative medicine (such as physical therapy), hospital admissions, surgical procedures, and diagnostic testing—especially those considered to be of high cost.

Keep in mind that many specialists and diagnostic facilities will not make appointments for patients unless referral procedures have been completed as required by insurance companies. These procedures may differ from plan to plan.

3. **Ask the patient about existing test results.** Where applicable, ask patients if they have had testing and where it was performed. Some patients have films, scans, and other diagnostic records in their possession. Others will need to pick them up. It is a good idea to remind patients to bring pertinent diagnostic records for their visit(s). For instance, a patient who has had a stress test, or other cardiac tests, should bring results or films to the office of a consulting cardiovascular surgeon for evaluation. Having these test results available for review will be useful to the physician, and will avoid wasting time during the appointment by having results faxed or otherwise tracked down.

4. **Obtain basic information from the patient.** When adding the patient to the appointment schedule, ask for the patient's complete name and daytime telephone number. The daytime telephone number is useful for contacting the patient in case appointments need to be rescheduled by the medical office due to an emergency or delay. This is most likely to happen during regular business hours and a patient will need to be contacted during the day.

Follow the office policy for any additional patient information required by the practice. Some practices require more complete insurance information so that verification can be done in advance of the visit. Others require extensive medical histories or patient questionnaires. You may be asked to advise new patients to come a few minutes early for their initial appointments in order to fill out forms. Other offices will have you mail forms and other paperwork to patients so they can be completed at home prior to their initial visit. If this is the case, obtain the mailing address for the patient. Some medical practices and hospitals now offer online patient registration, where data can be entered securely by the patient at the website.

FACTORS THAT AFFECT APPOINTMENT SCHEDULING

Patients will be scheduled not only according to whether they are new or established, but also based on their medical condition, equipment that may have to be used, and the amount of time required. As discussed previously, information details obtained at the time of appointment scheduling will help you evaluate when to make a patient appointment and how much time to allot. Each office will train you regarding how much time to schedule according to procedure type or services to be rendered, how many examination rooms there are, and how many staff members are available to assist the physician.

In order to illustrate how these factors affect appointment scheduling, it is useful to compare two types of medical offices.

Office A is a small group with two physicians. The office has three examination rooms and one clinical medical assistant for both physicians. Because of the small office space, only one physician can see patients during a block of time. All blood drawing, minor procedures, and tests—such as electrocardiograms (EKGs)—must be done in the examination rooms, because there is no separate procedure area.

Office B is a larger group with six physicians. The office has ten examination rooms, three clinical medical assistants, and one physician assistant who handles routine office visits. Additionally, a laboratory technician has a separate area in which to draw blood and collect other specimens from patients. If needed, all six physicians can see their own patients during the same time block.

From these two examples, it is clear to see that rooms, staff, and equipment have a direct impact on when patients are scheduled. Furthermore, the personal preferences, medical specialty, and habits of physicians must be taken into account. Some physicians need more or less time for consultations and certain procedures, depending on each doctor's requirements, working routines, or the level of complexity of the medical examination.

Other factors that may affect scheduling of patients are the routines of a physician's busy work week. Many have responsibilities outside the office, such as meetings at hospitals, surgery in the operating room, patient rounds, and other functions. Some of these will consistently take place at certain times and days of the week. These times must be blocked from the scheduling calendar, as obviously, the physician will not be in the office to treat patients during these events.

Finally, other considerations when scheduling appointments lie with the patients themselves. The elderly, patients who are fasting for blood tests, after school hours for children, and working patients with irregular hours are examples of individuals who may require particular time slots for appointments. It is impossible to meet every patient's needs. However, an effort should be made to accommodate patients with special scheduling requirements.

SITUATIONS THAT COMPLICATE APPOINTMENT SCHEDULING

Regardless how hard the front desk staff tries to keep the appointment schedule running smoothly, inevitably, things happen that complicate the day. The following situations are common in most medical offices. Some actions to be taken, should they occur, are offered here.

1. **The walk-in patient.** The definition of a walk-in patient is a person who comes to the office without an appointment. This patient is usually established, but did not call ahead or attempt to schedule an appointment, and simply shows up. Usually, these patients are either very ill or have a medical problem that requires urgent attention. At times, a person accompanying another patient who does have an appointment, such as a spouse, will request to also be seen by the physician during the same visit. Obviously, while this may appear convenient to the patient, it can be a detriment to the office schedule. In either case, the office staff will need to make a decision, based on the office policy and time availability, as to whether the patient can be seen. In some cases, especially if the schedule is already very heavy, the doctor may need to be consulted so that a decision can be made.

2. **The work-in patient.** A patient who calls the day before or on the same day an appointment is needed, is called a work-in patient. Again, the patient is usually very ill or requires immediate service, and must therefore be fit into the schedule, or "worked in." These patients may have high temperatures, a minor (but deep) cut, a bad flu, or any number of ailments that are not serious enough for the emergency room, but require urgent medical attention.

   There are times when patients do not have an immediate need for an appointment, and simply have a habit of calling at the last minute. It is important to develop a good sense of what is an urgent situation, and what is not, so that the physician's time is best used, especially on very busy days.

   Typically, work-in patients are established, but it is not unusual for new patients to be worked into the schedule. This is especially true if another physician personally requests immediate or urgent services. These patients are customarily worked into the schedule as a professional courtesy. When, check with the physician or office manager for further direction or advice regarding patients with immediate needs.

3. **Emergencies and unforeseen delays at the office.** There are times emergencies and unforeseen delays occur that will necessitate rescheduling appointments in a certain time block. For instance, the physician may have an unexpected family emergency and cannot come in for patient visits. There may be a need to travel for an urgent matter and arrangements must be made immediately. A surgeon may have a patient who experiences complications during surgery, extending the time in the operating room beyond what was expected, and causing her to be late returning to the office. Whatever the circumstances, patients who were scheduled for appointments need to be contacted as soon as possible and rescheduled. It is not necessary to give patients any details; only that an emergency has occurred and the appointment cannot be honored. If the cancellation of visits occurred just before patients were scheduled to arrive, start by calling the earliest appointments first in an attempt to intercept patients before they leave their home, office, etc. Apologize for the inconvenience, and promptly offer to reschedule the appointment. Another

physician will customarily cover, or fill in, for a colleague when needed. This may be a physician from the same group practice or another medical office. If required, patients needing prompt medical care can be rescheduled to visit the covering physician.

APPOINTMENT SCHEDULING TOOLS

Now that the basic principles of appointment scheduling have been reviewed, the tools for recording and tracking appointments can be discussed. Medical office staff need to document appointments when they are scheduled. Offices that use a manual system should use an appointment book appropriate for the medical practice environment. Offices that use practice management software usually have an appointment scheduling component as part of the software. Even if an office doesn't use practice management software, there are several stand-alone software packages that handle only appointment scheduling tasks.

For both manual and software appointment scheduling systems for medical offices, a day is commonly divided into lines that represent 15-minute intervals. If required, other time intervals are available. If a patient appointment requires more than 15 minutes, additional lines are blocked off for the time needed. For instance, if a patient requires 30 minutes, two lines are blocked for the patient appointment. If one hour is needed, 4 lines are blocked. See Figure 3-1 for an example of blocking a manual appointment scheduling page from a sample medical office.

Software used for appointment scheduling will typically display calendar pages with lines representing 15 minutes as well. Using software for scheduling is convenient and offers capabilities such as searching, cancelling, and rescheduling patients with ease and speed. See Figure 3-2 for an example of the appointment scheduling system screen for *Medical Office Simulation Software* (MOSS).

> **MOSS NOTE:** The calendar display may show Sunday through Saturday, or Saturday through Sunday, depending on your computer system installation.

As mentioned previously, if the physician has meetings or other responsibilities outside the office, these times should be clearly blocked and made unavailable for scheduling patients. In this manner, the only open lines on the scheduling system are those slots available for patients.

Another tool used in relation to appointment books and software scheduling is the reference sheet. This document was mentioned in Unit 2 and is typically prepared the day before or the same morning that patients visit the office. It is a list of all patient names with appointment times in chronological order. A reference sheet also shows each patient's reason for his or her visit and other details as required by the office. The list is distributed to all staff members and helps track patients receiving services in the office on that day. Refer to Figure 2-1 on page 35.

When patients finish with their appointments, some will need to return for follow-up visits. Medical offices usually provide an **appointment reminder card** to patients, or the software creates a reminder slip. The reminder card is the size of a standard business card and contains information for the next appointment, including day, date, and time. The front desk staff member who schedules the next appointment for the patient fills out the reminder card and gives it to the patient. See Figure 3-3 for an illustration of a reminder card.

Some patients require follow-up in the distant future—for example, returning for annual pap smears. It is not always convenient to schedule appointments that far in advance. **Tickler files** or **recall postcards** are reminder systems designed to monitor distant follow-up appointments and provide a

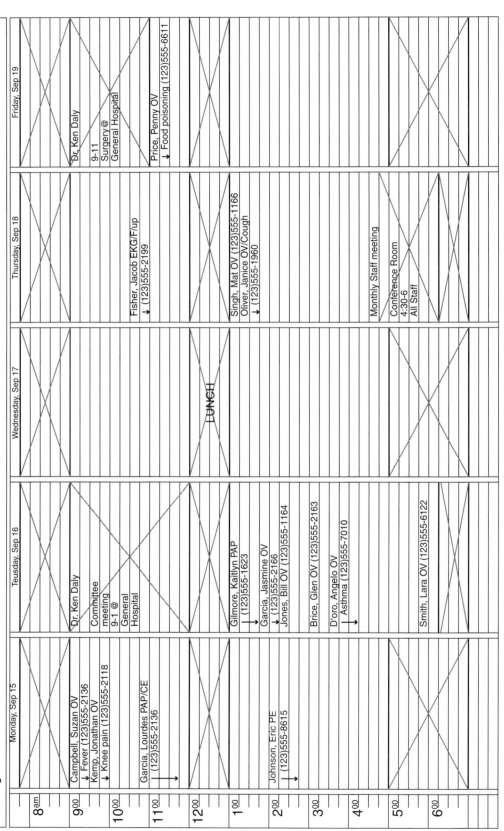

West Side Medical Associates
123 Main St., Suite 600
Anytown, XY 00235

Kenneth Daly, M.D.

Internal Medicine

September 15 – September 19

FIGURE 3-1

Sample of a blocked schedule from a medical appointment book. *Delmar/Cengage Learning*

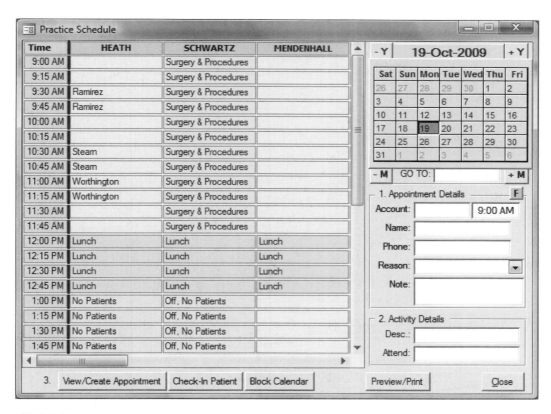

FIGURE 3-2

The appointment scheduling screen in MOSS. *Delmar/Cengage Learning*

---

has an appointment with

Dr. D.J. Schwartz

5076 Brand Blvd, Suite 401, Douglasville, NY 01234

Tel. (123) 456-7890

☐ MON.   ☐ TUES.   ☐ WED.   ☐ THURS.   ☐ FRI.   ☐ SAT.

A.M.

_____ AT _____ P.M.

FIGURE 3-3

Sample appointment card. *Delmar/Cengage Learning*

mailer that can be sent to patients approximately one to two months before an appointment should be scheduled. These reminder systems can be manual, using postcards that patients address to themselves. The postcards are then stored in file boxes under the month they are to be mailed. Practice management and scheduling software often have features to prepare reminder notices to be sent to patients as well.

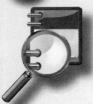

LET'S TRY IT! 3-1 NAVIGATING THE APPOINTMENT SCHEDULER

Objective: The reader will be oriented to the appointment scheduler and its features. For the purpose of this educational software, dates for simulated exercises are limited from January 1, 2008 to December 31, 2013.

HINT: Click on *Start,* then *Programs*, then click on the software title to open it. If a desktop icon is available, you can also open the software by clicking on it.

STEP 1

Start MOSS and use your logon information to begin using the software.

STEP 2

Click on *File Maintenance* on the *Main Menu*. Click on the *Practice Information* tab. Click on the button in front of *Practice Settings* to open the dialog box. See Figure 3-4.

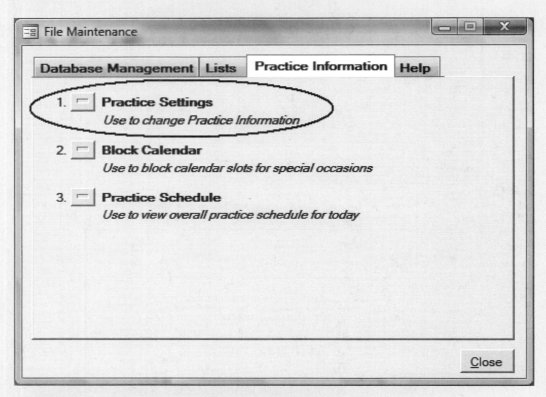

FIGURE 3-4

Delmar/Cengage Learning

STEP 3

At the bottom of the dialog box, Field 12, there are practice hours that can be set. This should read "start time: 09:00 a.m." and "stop time: 06:00 p.m." Lunch is scheduled from 12:00 p.m. to 1:00 p.m. daily. Time slots should remain at 15-minute intervals. If this data is correct, do not make changes. If not, enter or correct as required. See Figure 3-5.

STEP 4

When finished, click on *Save,* then *OK,* and click *Close* on both remaining dialog boxes to return to the Main Menu.

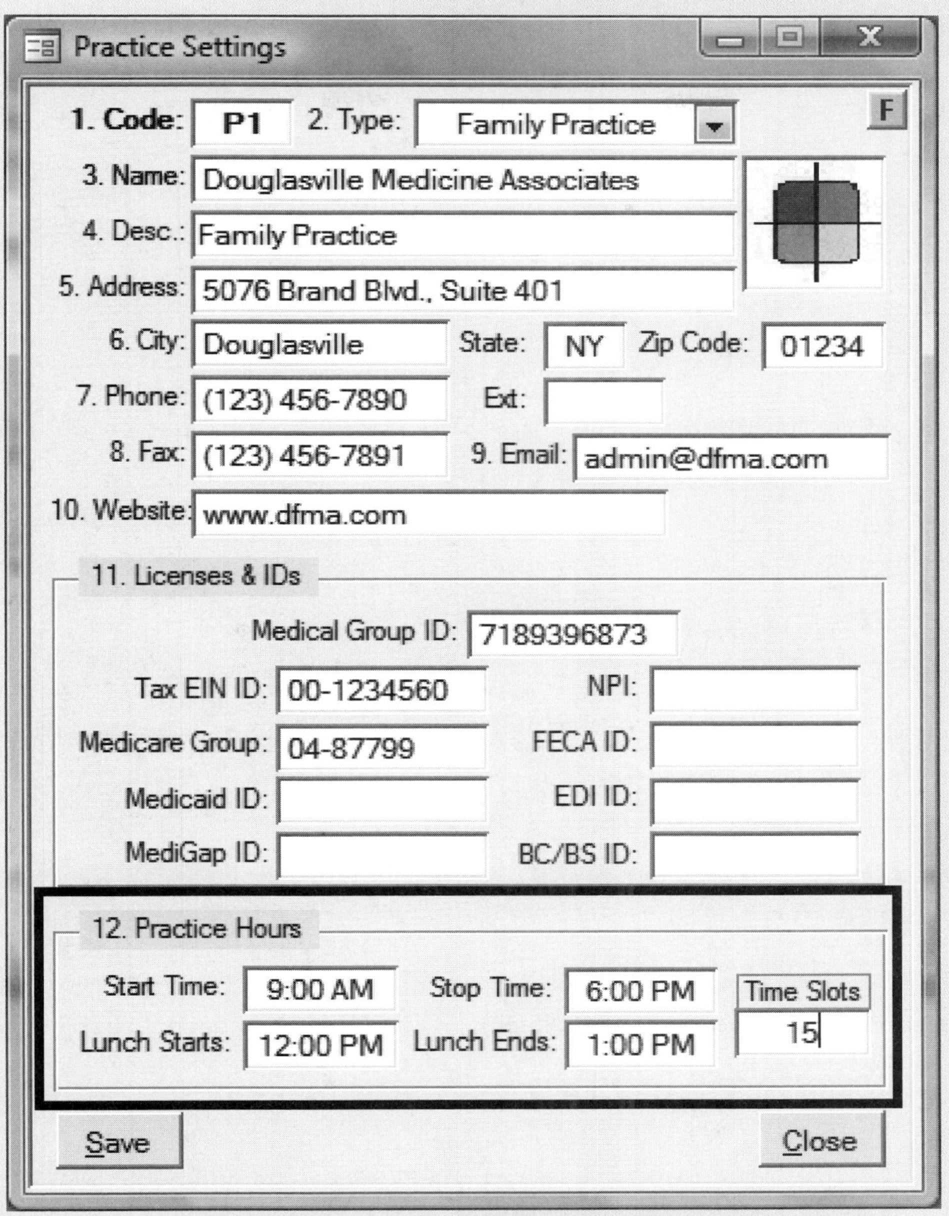

Practice Settings

1. Code: **P1**   2. Type: Family Practice ▼   F

3. Name: Douglasville Medicine Associates

4. Desc.: Family Practice

5. Address: 5076 Brand Blvd., Suite 401

6. City: Douglasville   State: NY   Zip Code: 01234

7. Phone: (123) 456-7890   Ext:

8. Fax: (123) 456-7891   9. Email: admin@dfma.com

10. Website: www.dfma.com

11. Licenses & IDs

Medical Group ID: 7189396873

Tax EIN ID: 00-1234560   NPI:

Medicare Group: 04-87799   FECA ID:

Medicaid ID: EDI ID:

MediGap ID: BC/BS ID:

12. Practice Hours

Start Time: 9:00 AM   Stop Time: 6:00 PM   Time Slots
Lunch Starts: 12:00 PM   Lunch Ends: 1:00 PM   15

Save   Close

FIGURE 3-5

Delmar/Cengage Learning

STEP 5

Verify that the appointment scheduling screen now displays these times by clicking on *Appointment Scheduling* on the Main Menu. Using the calendar on the upper right side of the scheduler, click on October 02, 2009. The start time should display 09:00 a.m.; the lunch hour is blocked from 12:00 p.m. to 01:00 p.m. By scrolling down to the end of the day, 05:45 p.m. should display as the stop time. All dates from October 02, 2009 forward should display these time settings. See Figure 3-6 to check your screen.

HINT: Use the Y+/Y− and M+/M− buttons to move through the calendar.

continues

NAVIGATING THE APPOINTMENT SCHEDULER *continued*

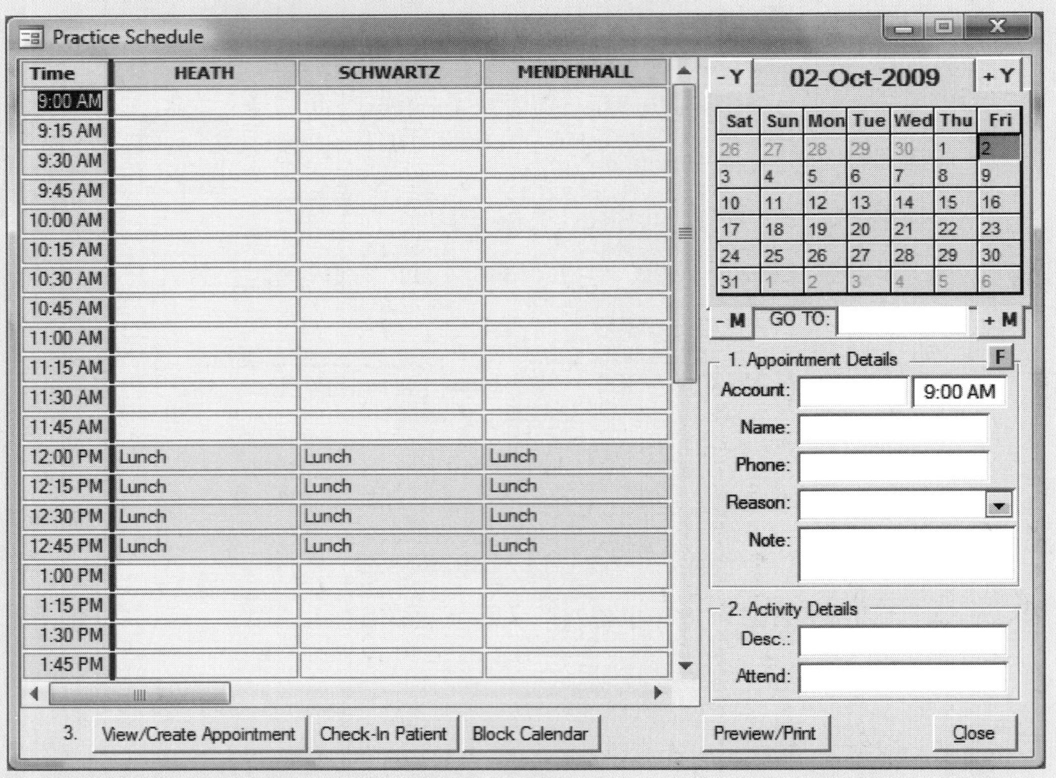

FIGURE 3-6

Delmar/Cengage Learning

> **NOTE:** It appears that lunch ends at 12:45 p.m.; however, the first patient appointment available is in fact 1:00 p.m.

STEP 6

Click on October 5, 2009 on the calendar to display that date. Observe the blocks that are already in place for Drs. Heath and Schwartz. Each physician has one column per day for scheduling patient appointments. Time slots that are unavailable for patients are blocked out in gray with a message indicating the reason for the block. See Figure 3-7. For more information, single click on one of the *Surgery & Procedures* slots in Dr. Schwartz's column, and then click on the *Block Calendar* button down below. A window with complete information on this event will display, as shown in Figure 3-8.

STEP 7

Although the office is closed on Saturday and Sunday, these days are not blocked, because it is understood that no patients will be scheduled on these days. Click on each day, Monday through Friday, October 5 through October 9, and observe the time slots already blocked for each physician. Compare this to the Practice Information shown in Figure 3-9.

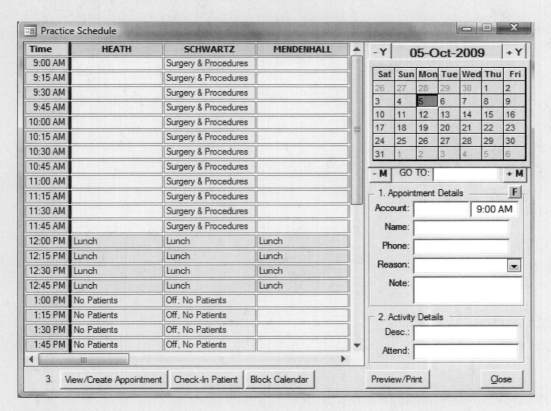

FIGURE 3-7

Delmar/Cengage Learning

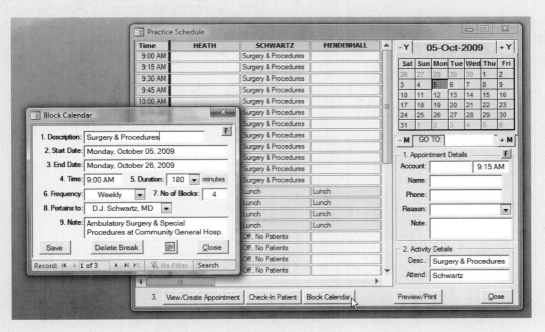

FIGURE 3-8

Delmar/Cengage Learning

continues

NAVIGATING THE APPOINTMENT SCHEDULER *continued*

Douglasville Family Practice
Medicine Associates
5076 Brand Blvd., Suite 401
Douglasville, NY 01234
(123) 456-7890

Physicians	**Office Staff**	
L.D. Heath, M.D.	K. Betran, CMA	Full-time office manager
D.J. Schwartz, M.D.	S. Dowdy, RMA	Full-time back-office medical assistant
	P. Khan, CPC	Part-time medical biller
	_____	Full-time front-office medical assistant
	(your name)	

Office Hours (closed all legal holidays)

9:00 am – 6:00 pm Monday through Friday
12:00 pm – 1:00 pm Lunch

Patient Hours (By appointment only)

Dr. Heath	Monday, Wednesday, Friday	9:00 am – 12:00 pm
	Tuesday	1:00 pm – 6:00 pm
	Thursday	10:30 am – 12 pm & 1:00 pm – 6:00 pm
Dr. Schwartz	Wednesday	9:00 am – 12:00 pm
	Tuesday, Thursday	9:00 am – 6:00 pm
	Friday	10:30 am – 12:00 pm

Professional Commitments

Dr. Heath	**Tuesday** Nursing home rounds	9:00 am – 12:00 pm
	Thursday Family Practice Chairman/weekly meeting NY County Hospital	9:00 am – 10:30 am
Dr. Schwartz	**Monday** Ambulatory Surgery and Special Procedures Community General Hospital (Off rest of day, 1:00 pm – 6 pm)	9:00 am – 12:00 pm
	Friday Phone calls/paperwork catch-up Volunteer, physician services Allcity Medical Clinic	9:00 am – 10:30 am 1:00 pm – 6:00 pm

FIGURE 3-9

Practice Information for Douglasville Family Practice Medicine Associates. *Delmar/Cengage Learning*

STEP 8

Next, click on October 19, 2009 on the calendar to display the schedule for that date. Observe that Dr. Heath has patients scheduled on that morning. Each slot represents 15 minutes of time. In this example, patients Ramirez, Stearn, and Worthington each have two slots, or 30-minute visits. See Figure 3-10.

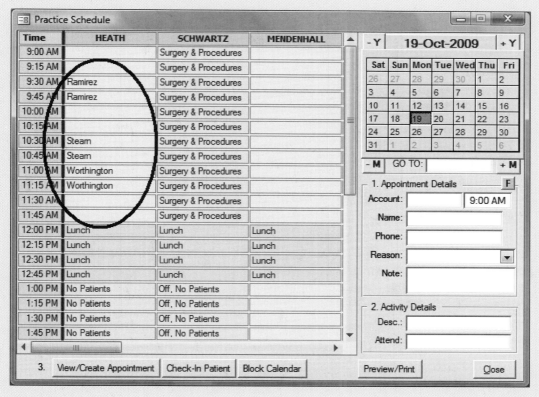

FIGURE 3-10

Delmar/Cengage Learning

STEP 9

When more information is required regarding an appointment, single click on the patient's name. Try this now with patient Ramirez. On the right of the screen, under Appointment Details, Field 1, more information regarding this appointment is provided. See Figure 3-11.

continues

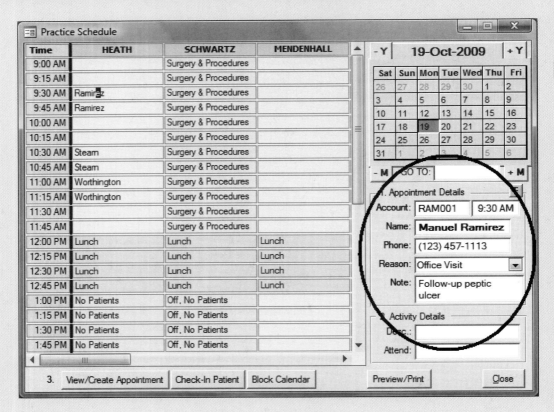

FIGURE 3-11

Delmar/Cengage Learning

Next, double click on patient Ramirez's name to display the Appointment Form window, which contains more information about the appointment. See Figure 3-12. When finished, click on the *Close* button to close the Appointment Form window.

STEP 10

Practice viewing other months by clicking on the −M and +M buttons below the calendar, then click on various days to view them. When finished, click on the *Close* button until you return to the Main Menu.

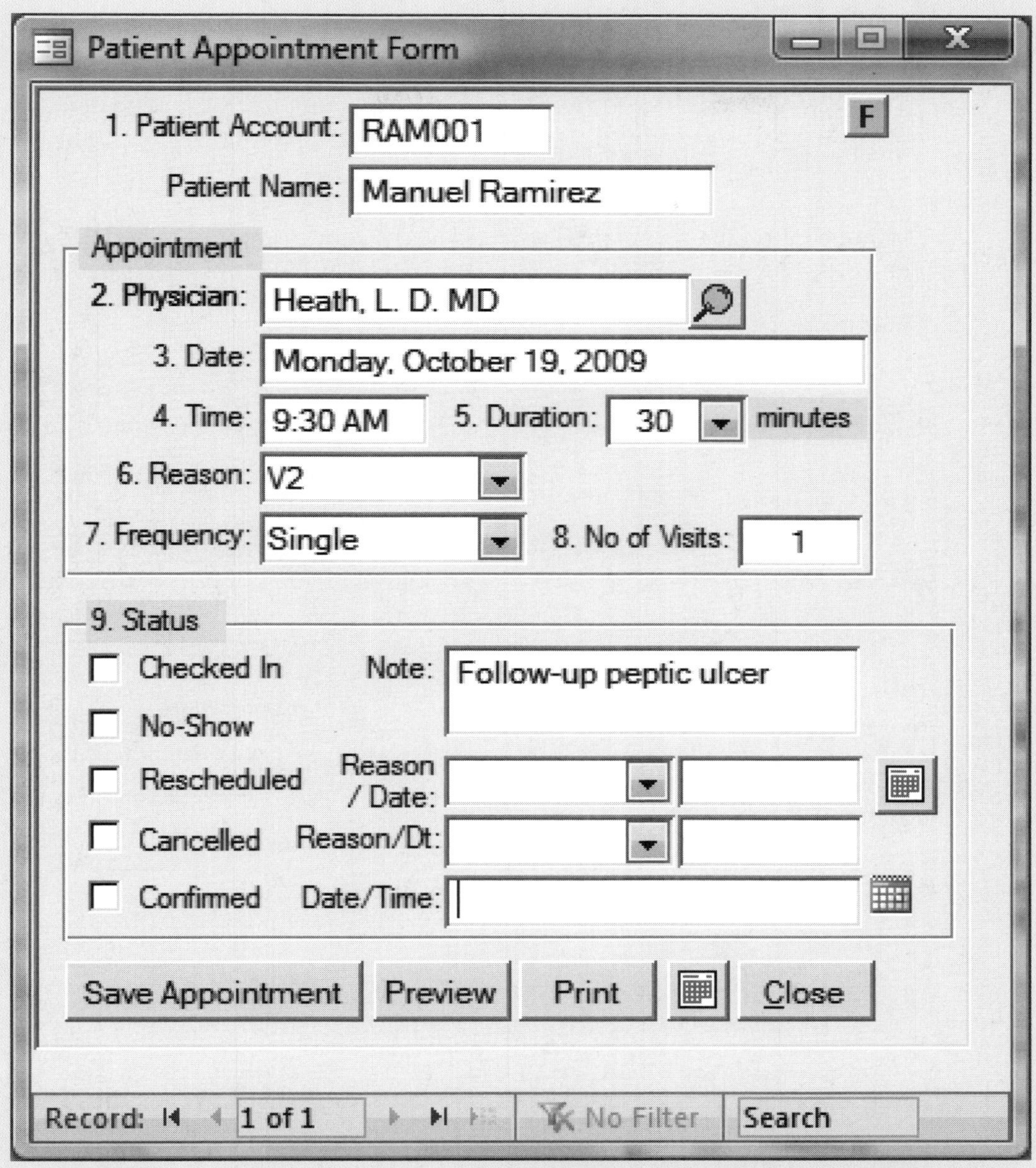

Patient Appointment Form

1. Patient Account: RAM001   [F]

Patient Name: Manuel Ramirez

Appointment

2. Physician: Heath, L. D. MD

3. Date: Monday, October 19, 2009

4. Time: 9:30 AM   5. Duration: 30 minutes

6. Reason: V2

7. Frequency: Single   8. No of Visits: 1

9. Status

☐ Checked In   Note: Follow-up peptic ulcer

☐ No-Show

☐ Rescheduled   Reason / Date:

☐ Cancelled   Reason/Dt:

☐ Confirmed   Date/Time:

Save Appointment   Preview   Print   Close

Record: 1 of 1   No Filter   Search

FIGURE 3-12

Delmar/Cengage Learning

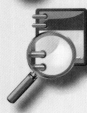

LET'S TRY IT! 3-2 SCHEDULING APPOINTMENTS FOR ESTABLISHED PATIENTS

Objective: Schedule appointments as indicated in the following exercise for established patients. These patients have demographic and insurance information in the software database.

STEP 1

On the Main Menu, click on the *Appointment Scheduling* button. When the scheduler opens, click on *10/21/2009* to display the schedule for that date, including patient hours, for Dr. Schwartz. See Figure 3-13.

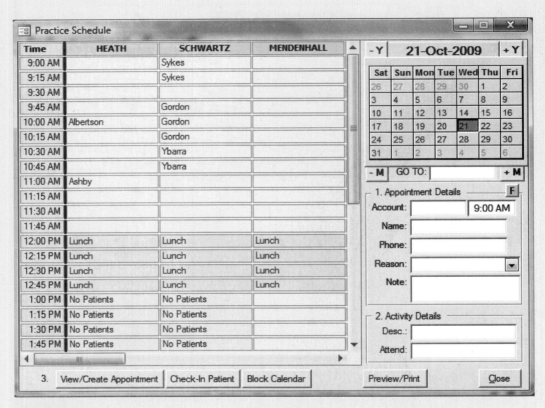

FIGURE 3-13

Delmar/Cengage Learning

STEP 2

The following patient calls the office and requires an appointment with Dr. Schwartz on 10/21/2009 at 11:00 a.m.:

    Richard Manaly   **30 minutes**   **Office visit**
    Reason: Follow-up Diabetes

STEP 3

On the scheduler for October 21, single click on the *11:00 a.m. slot* in the column for Dr. Schwartz.

STEP 4

Next, click on the *View/Create Appointment* button in the lower left corner. Locate Richard Manaly in the patient selection box for appointment scheduling, then single click on his name. See Figure 3-14. Notice the buttons along the bottom: *Add New Patient, Select,* and *Add.* Click on *Add,* since an established patient is being added to the calendar.

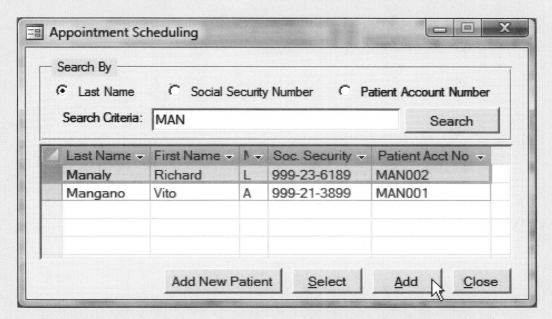

FIGURE 3-14

Delmar/Cengage Learning

STEP 5

An appointment window that shows October 21, 2009 at 11:00 a.m. is displayed. Check your screen with Figure 3-15.

continues

SCHEDULING APPOINTMENTS FOR ESTABLISHED PATIENTS *continued*

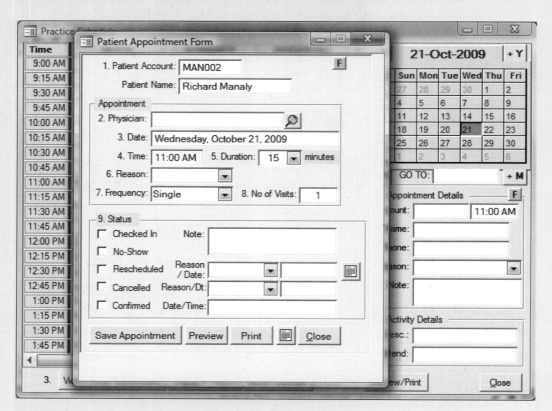

FIGURE 3-15

Delmar/Cengage Learning

Click on the search icon (magnifying glass) in Field 2, *Physician*, and select Dr. Schwartz by double clicking his name. This ensures that the patient is placed in that doctor's column. In Duration, Field 5, drop down the box and select 30 minutes. At Field 6, Reason, drop down the selections and click on *Office Visit*. Click in the box at Field 9, *Note*, and enter the reason for visit: "Follow-up diabetes." Check your work with Figure 3-16.

STEP 6

Click on the *Save Appointment* button. A prompt indicates that the appointment has been posted. Click *OK*, and then close the Appointment Form window (not the scheduler in the background).

STEP 7

Check your appointment schedule for Richard Manaly with Figure 3-17. Because the visit is for 30 minutes, there are two time slots with Manaly's name (15 minutes each). To view details for this appointment, single click on the name Manaly, then refer to Field 1 on the Scheduling screen.

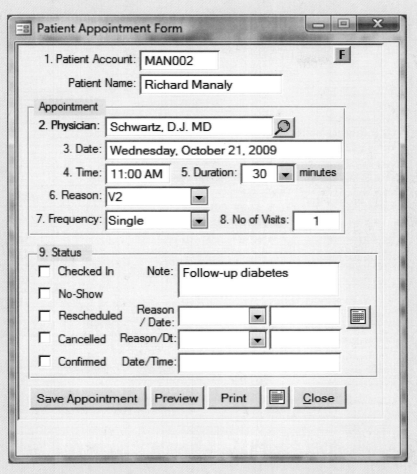

Patient Appointment Form   **F**

1. Patient Account: MAN002

   Patient Name: Richard Manaly

Appointment

2. Physician: Schwartz, D.J. MD

3. Date: Wednesday, October 21, 2009

4. Time: 11:00 AM   5. Duration: 30 minutes

6. Reason: V2

7. Frequency: Single   8. No of Visits: 1

9. Status

☐ Checked In   Note: Follow-up diabetes

☐ No-Show

☐ Rescheduled   Reason / Date:

☐ Cancelled   Reason/Dt:

☐ Confirmed   Date/Time:

Save Appointment   Preview   Print   Close

FIGURE 3-16

Delmar/Cengage Learning

HINT: Don't forget to select the physician and correct amount of time for each appointment.

STEP 8

Using the procedures just learned for scheduling appointments, add the following established patients as indicated.

A.   John Conway   30 minutes   Office visit
     Reason note: Abdominal pain, fever
     Doctor: Heath   Date: 10/23/2009   Time: 11:00 a.m.
     Check your work with Figure 3-18.

B.   Paula Shektar   30 minutes   Office visit
     Reason note: Congestive Heart Failure (CHF)
     Doctor: Schwartz   Date: 10/23/2009   Time: 10:30 a.m.
     Check your work with Figure 3-19.

continues

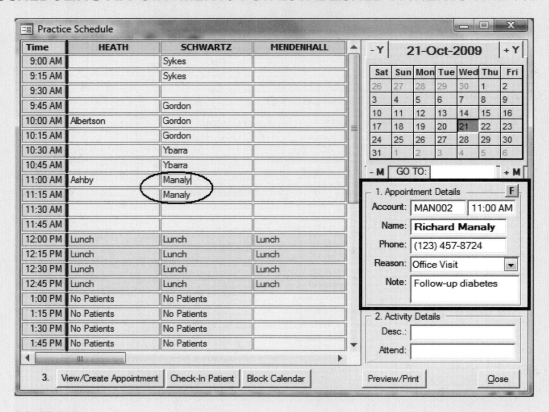

FIGURE 3-17

Delmar/Cengage Learning

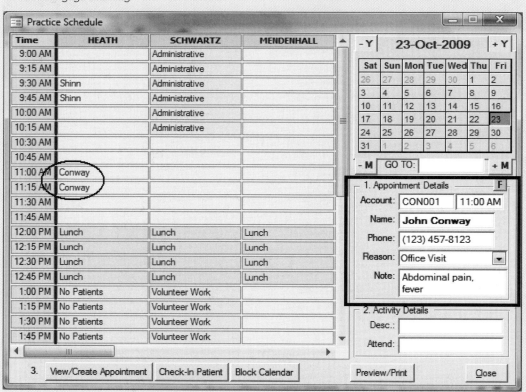

FIGURE 3–18

Delmar/Cengage Learning

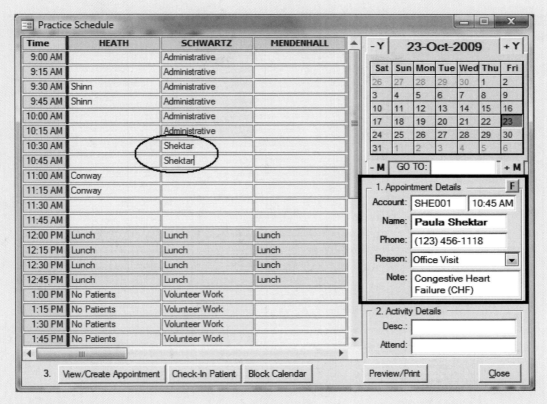

FIGURE 3–19

Delmar/Cengage Learning

C.   Robert Shinn   15 minutes   Walk-in visit
     Reason note: Ear ache
     Doctor: Heath   Date: 10/30/2009   Time: 09:00 a.m.
     Check your work with Figure 3-20.

D.   Manual Ramirez   15 minutes   Office visit
     Reason note: Cholesterol check/patient fasting
     Doctor: Heath   Date: 11/16/2009   Time: 09:30 a.m.
     Check your work with Figure 3-21.

E.   Cynthia Worthington   15 minutes   Office visit
     Reason note: Rash post antibiotic therapy
     Doctor: Heath   Date: 10/30/2009   Time: 09:30 a.m.
     Check your work with Figure 3-22.

continues

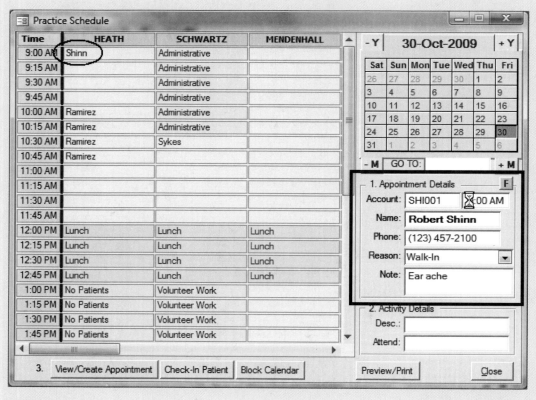

FIGURE 3-20

Delmar/Cengage Learning

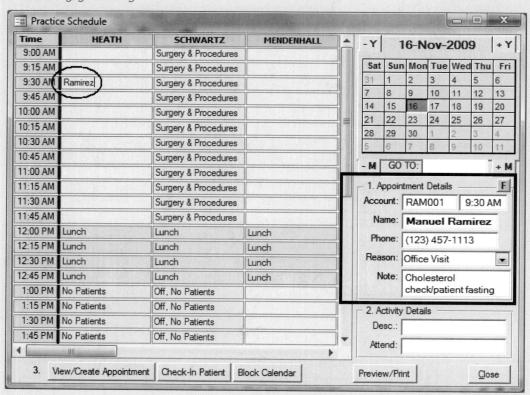

FIGURE 3-21

Delmar/Cengage Learning

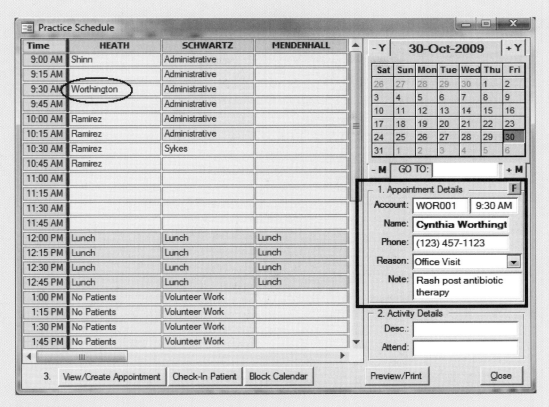

FIGURE 3-22

Delmar/Cengage Learning

F. Patty Practice   45 minutes   Office visit
    Reason note: Practice for cancellation
    Doctor: Heath   Date: 10/28/2009   Time: 10:00 a.m.
    Check your work with Figure 3-23.

STEP 9

Correcting errors. If you make an error and need to remove an appointment from the schedule, the action must be documented with a reason code. Go to October 28, 2009 and double click on Patty Practice at 10:00 a.m. In the Appointment Form window, click to place a checkmark in front of Cancelled, then use the drop-down box in the Reason field to select *Erroneous Entry* from the list. Use the date 10/22/2009 as the cancellation date. See Figure 3-24. Next, click on the *Save Appointment* button. A prompt alerts you that the information has been posted; click *OK*. The appointment should now be gone from the 10/28/2009 column for Dr. Heath. However, the cancelled visit is documented by being included with the patient's appointment history.

continues

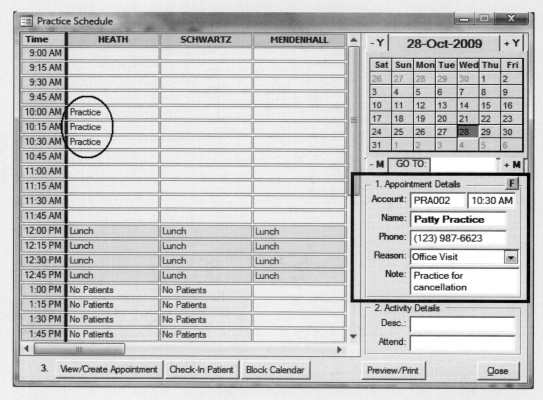

FIGURE 3-23

Delmar/Cengage Learning

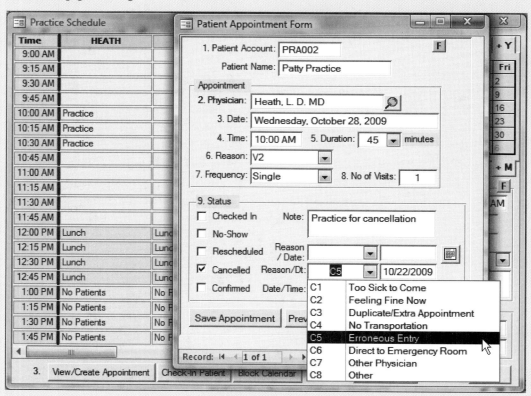

FIGURE 3-24

Delmar/Cengage Learning

STEP 10

Click on the *Close* button to close the Appointment Form window, and then close the Practice Scheduler and return to the Main Menu.

LET'S TRY IT! 3-3 SCHEDULING APPOINTMENTS FOR NEW PATIENTS

Objective: The following exercise includes new patients who have called the office to schedule appointments. Remember that new patients should be searched in the database to be certain they are not already in the system. Each patient has been screened via telephone for name, daytime telephone number, insurance coverage, referring physician, and reason for visit. Because he or she does not have demographic information listed in the software database, an account must be created and basic information entered. The remainder of the required information and copies of the insurance cards should be obtained at the time of the office visit, when the patient completes his or her registration form.

MOSS NOTE: For these exercises, turn the feedback mode off; if it is on, then shut down and restart the software program.

STEP 1

On the Main Menu, click on the *Appointment Scheduling* button. When the scheduler opens, click on *10/22/2009* to display the schedule for that date.

STEP 2

Martin Montner, a new patient and college student, requires a 45-minute appointment at 3:30 p.m. with Dr. Schwartz.

Daytime telephone:	Home—(123) 457-2166
Insurance:	Signal HMO
Felicia Anderson is Martin's mother. She is the guarantor and insurance policyholder.	
Reason for visit:	Severe sore throat
Referring physician:	None

STEP 3

On the scheduler for 10/22/2009, double click on the *3:30 p.m. slot* in the column for Dr. Schwartz. When the appointment patient selection window appears, search for Martin Montner to make certain he is not already in the database. If he is not, click on the *Add New Patient* button, as shown in Figure 3-25. This will open the patient registration window.

continues

SCHEDULING APPOINTMENTS FOR NEW PATIENTS *continued*

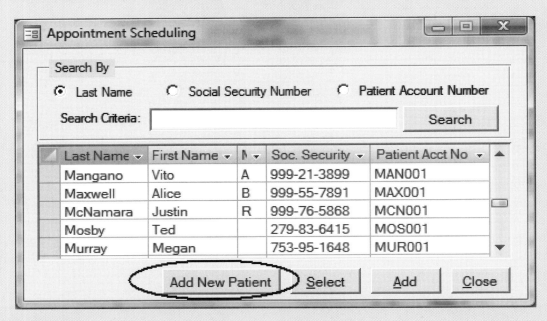

FIGURE 3-25

Delmar/Cengage Learning

STEP 4

Look along the top of the screen and locate the Physician field. Dr. Heath is the default physician; however, Martin will be visiting Dr. Schwartz. Click the search icon (magnifying glass) and select *Dr. Schwartz* by double clicking on his name.

STEP 5

On the Patient Information tab, enter the patient's first and last name and home telephone number (in Field 12) and click to select *Guarantor* in Field 21—his mother will be entered elsewhere. Notice that the software has automatically assigned a patient account number. Check your work with Figure 3-26. Next, click on the *Save* button.

STEP 6

Click on the *Spouse/Parent/Other* tab. In Field 1, click on the radio button for *Parent.* In Field 2, click on the *Yes* radio button for Guarantor. Enter the name of the patient's mother, Felicia Anderson, and click the button for *Female.* Check your work with Figure 3-27. Click on *Save* when finished.

STEP 7

Click on the *Primary Insurance* tab. At Field 1, click on the search icon (magnifying glass) and select Signal HMO as the primary insurance. In Field 2, click on the radio button for *Child,* since the patient is on his mother's policy. Check your work with Figure 3-28. Click on *Save.* Remember, the rest of the information will be obtained from the registration form when the patient comes for his first visit. This preliminary information was obtained at the time the patient made an appointment in order to start an account. Click on the *Close* button.

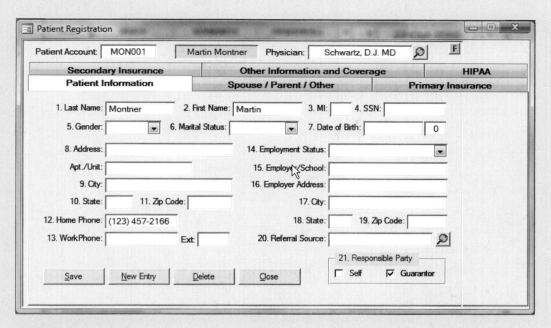

FIGURE 3-26

Delmar/Cengage Learning

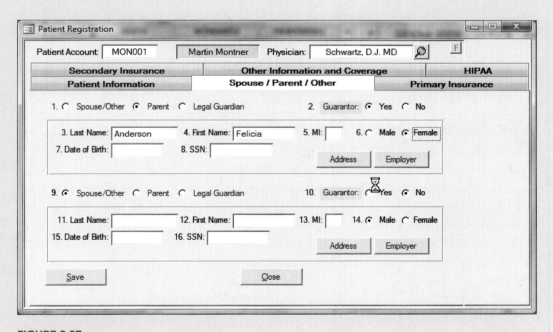

FIGURE 3-27

Delmar/Cengage Learning

continues

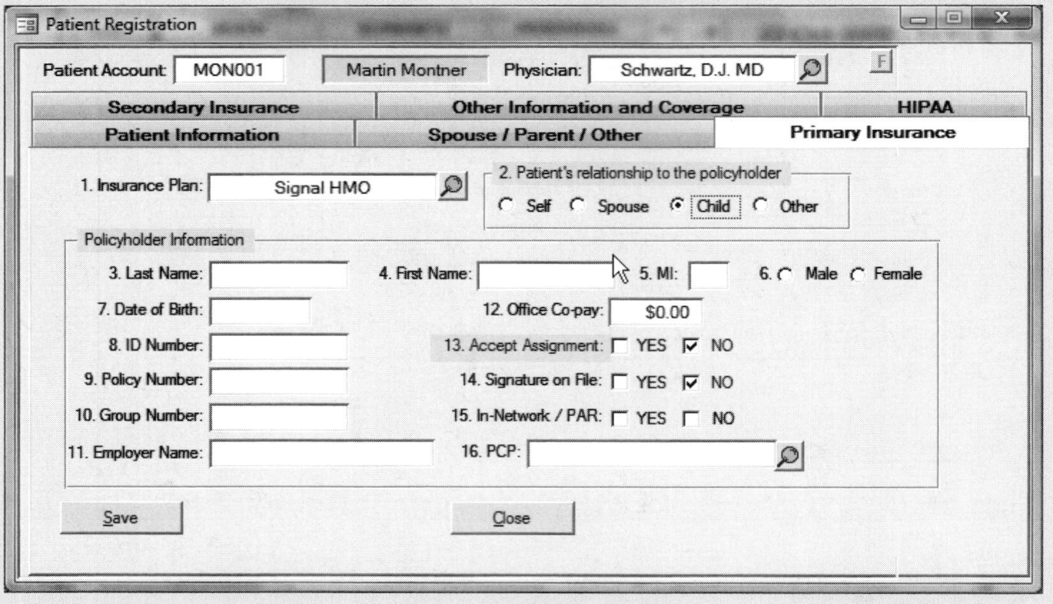

FIGURE 3-28

Delmar/Cengage Learning

STEP 8

Return to the Appointment Scheduler for 10/22/2009 and single click on the *3:30 p.m. slot* for Dr. Schwartz. Use the *View/Create Appointment* button to open the patient selection screen. Martin Montner should now be on the list. Locate the patient, single click on his *name* and click on *Add*, since the patient is being added to the calendar.

STEP 9

The Appointment Form window you previously learned to use should display. Enter the patient's physician, Dr. Schwartz, 45 minutes for visit duration, and select *New Patient Visit* for Field 6. Enter "severe sore throat" in the note box. Make certain that Field 4 shows a 3:30 p.m. appointment. Check your screen with Figure 3-29. Click on the *Save Appointment* button; then close the Appointment Form window. You should now have three slots at 3:30 p.m. showing patient Montner in the column for Dr. Schwartz. Single click on the name *Montner* and view the appointment details in Field 1. See Figure 3-30.

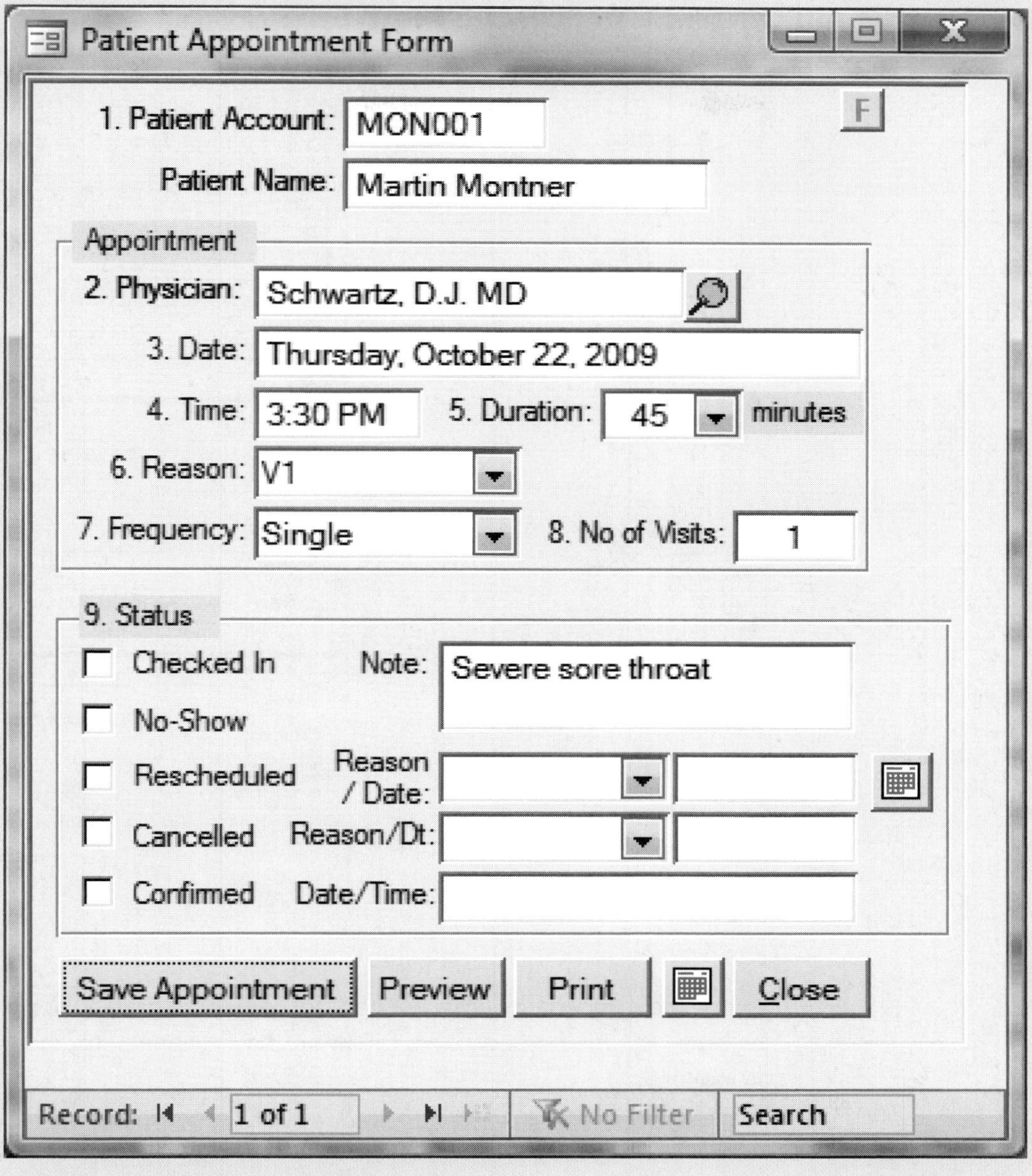

Patient Appointment Form

1. Patient Account: MON001

Patient Name: Martin Montner

F

Appointment

2. Physician: Schwartz, D.J. MD

3. Date: Thursday, October 22, 2009

4. Time: 3:30 PM   5. Duration: 45 minutes

6. Reason: V1

7. Frequency: Single   8. No of Visits: 1

9. Status

☐ Checked In   Note: Severe sore throat

☐ No-Show

☐ Rescheduled   Reason / Date:

☐ Cancelled   Reason/Dt:

☐ Confirmed   Date/Time:

Save Appointment   Preview   Print   Close

Record: 1 of 1   No Filter   Search

FIGURE 3-29

Delmar/Cengage Learning

continues

SCHEDULING APPOINTMENTS FOR NEW PATIENTS *continued*

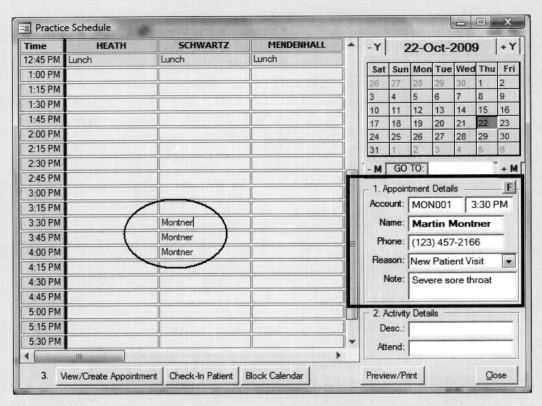

FIGURE 3-30

Delmar/Cengage Learning

HINT: Do not forget to search for each patient in the database before entering their information. When scheduling appointments, select the correct physician and amount of time for each visit.

HINT: There is a selection for self-pay in the primary insurance tab, Field 1.

STEP 10

Using the procedures just learned for scheduling new appointments in *Let's Try It! 3-3*, add the following new patients to the schedule as indicated.

A.   Name: Rodney Zuhl

       Doctor: Schwartz

       Daytime telephone: Home—(123) 457-4448

       Insurance: Self-Pay (No Insurance)

       Duration of visit: 45 minutes

       Date and time: 10/30/2009; 11:15 a.m.

       Reason for visit: Difficult urination

Check your work with Figure 3-31 and Figure 3-32.

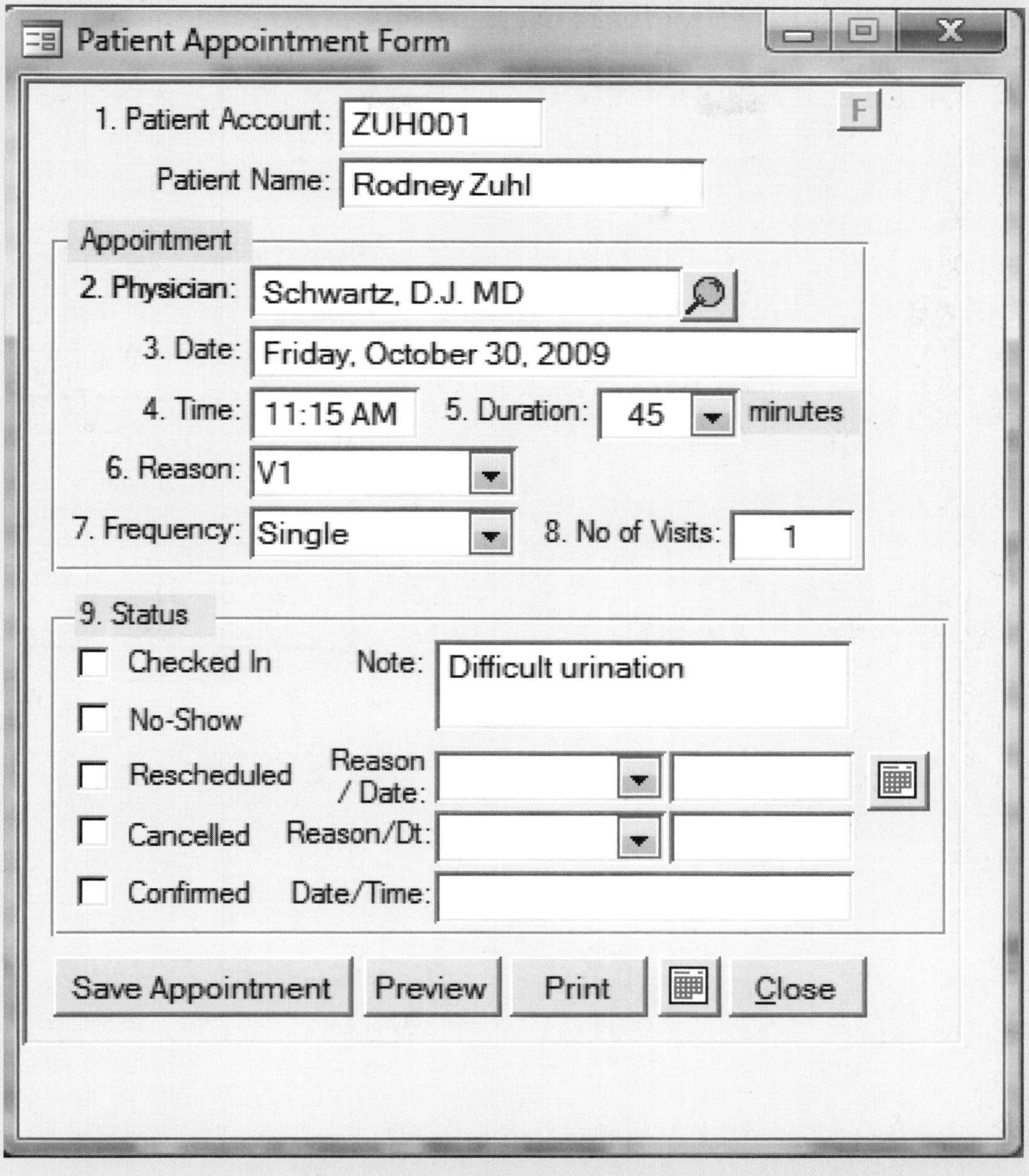

Patient Appointment Form

1. Patient Account: ZUH001

Patient Name: Rodney Zuhl

F

Appointment

2. Physician: Schwartz, D.J. MD

3. Date: Friday, October 30, 2009

4. Time: 11:15 AM   5. Duration: 45 ▼ minutes

6. Reason: V1 ▼

7. Frequency: Single ▼   8. No of Visits: 1

9. Status

☐ Checked In   Note: Difficult urination

☐ No-Show

☐ Rescheduled   Reason / Date: ▼

☐ Cancelled   Reason/Dt: ▼

☐ Confirmed   Date/Time:

Save Appointment   Preview   Print   Close

FIGURE 3-31

Delmar/Cengage Learning

continues

SCHEDULING APPOINTMENTS FOR NEW PATIENTS *continued*

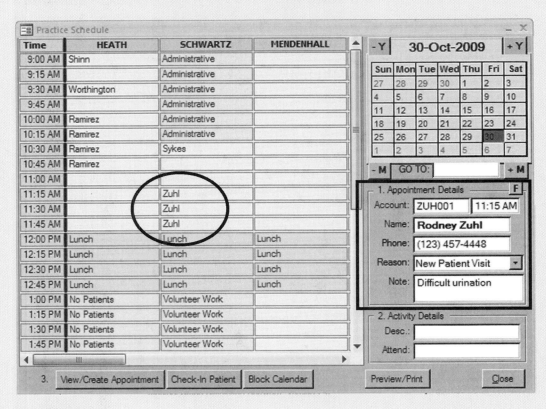

FIGURE 3-32

Delmar/Cengage Learning

B. Name: Melissa Corbett, born 6/16/1997

Duration of visit: 30 minutes

Doctor: Heath

Daytime telephone: Home—(123) 457-2133

Insurance: FlexiHealth PPO In-Network.

Guarantor and policyholder: Patient's father, Daniel Corbett

Duration of visit: 30 minutes

Date and time: 10/29/2009; 02:30 p.m.

Reason for visit: Possible flu

Check your work with Figure 3-33 and Figure 3-34.

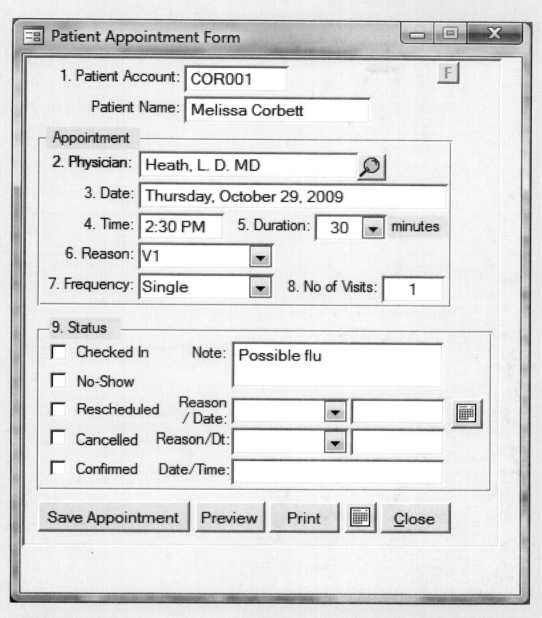

FIGURE 3-33
Delmar/Cengage Learning

continues

SCHEDULING APPOINTMENTS FOR NEW PATIENTS *continued*

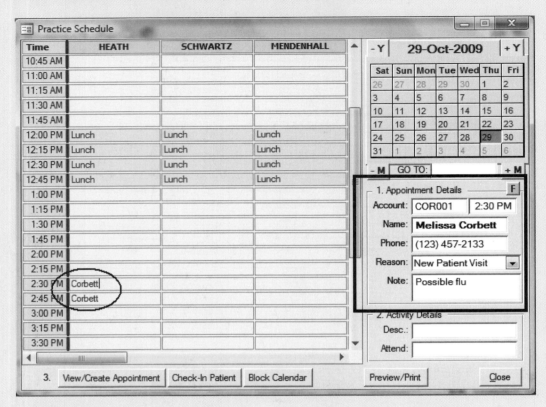

FIGURE 3-34

Delmar/Cengage Learning

C. Name: Kabin Pradhan

   Doctor: Schwartz

   Daytime telephone: Work—(123) 528-9772

   Insurance: ConsumerOne HRA

   Duration of visit: 30 minutes

   Date and time: 10/29/2009; 09:00 a.m.

   Reason for visit: Heartburn, indigestion

   Referring physician: None

Check your work with Figure 3-35 and Figure 3-36.

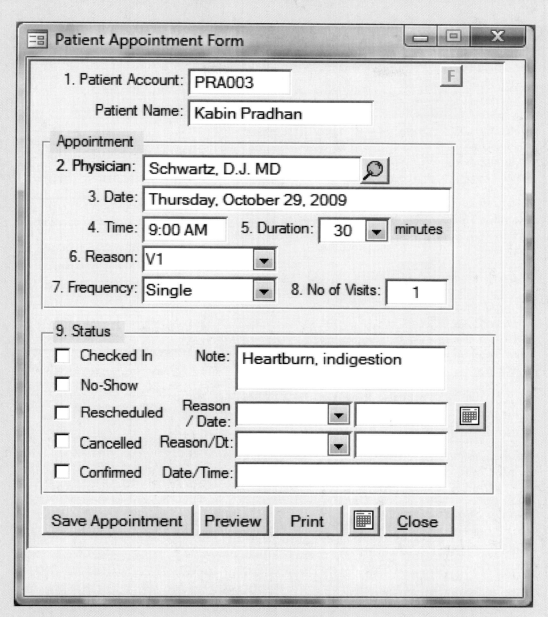

FIGURE 3-35

Delmar/Cengage Learning

continues

SCHEDULING APPOINTMENTS FOR NEW PATIENTS *continued*

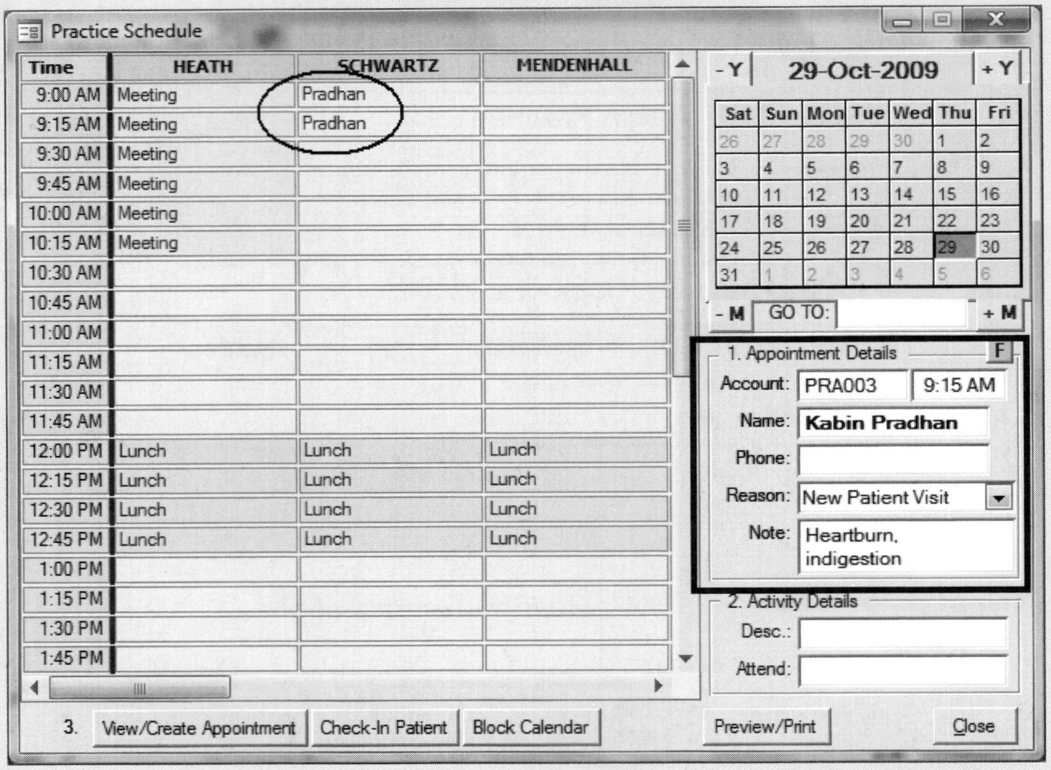

FIGURE 3-36
Delmar/Cengage Learning

D. Name: Ricky Villanova

Doctor: Schwartz

Daytime telephone: Work—(123) 457-6122

Insurance: Signal HMO

Duration of visit: 45 minutes

Date and time: 10/27/2009; 03:30 p.m.

Reason for visit: Thirst/frequent urination

Check your work with Figure 3-37 and Figure 3-38.

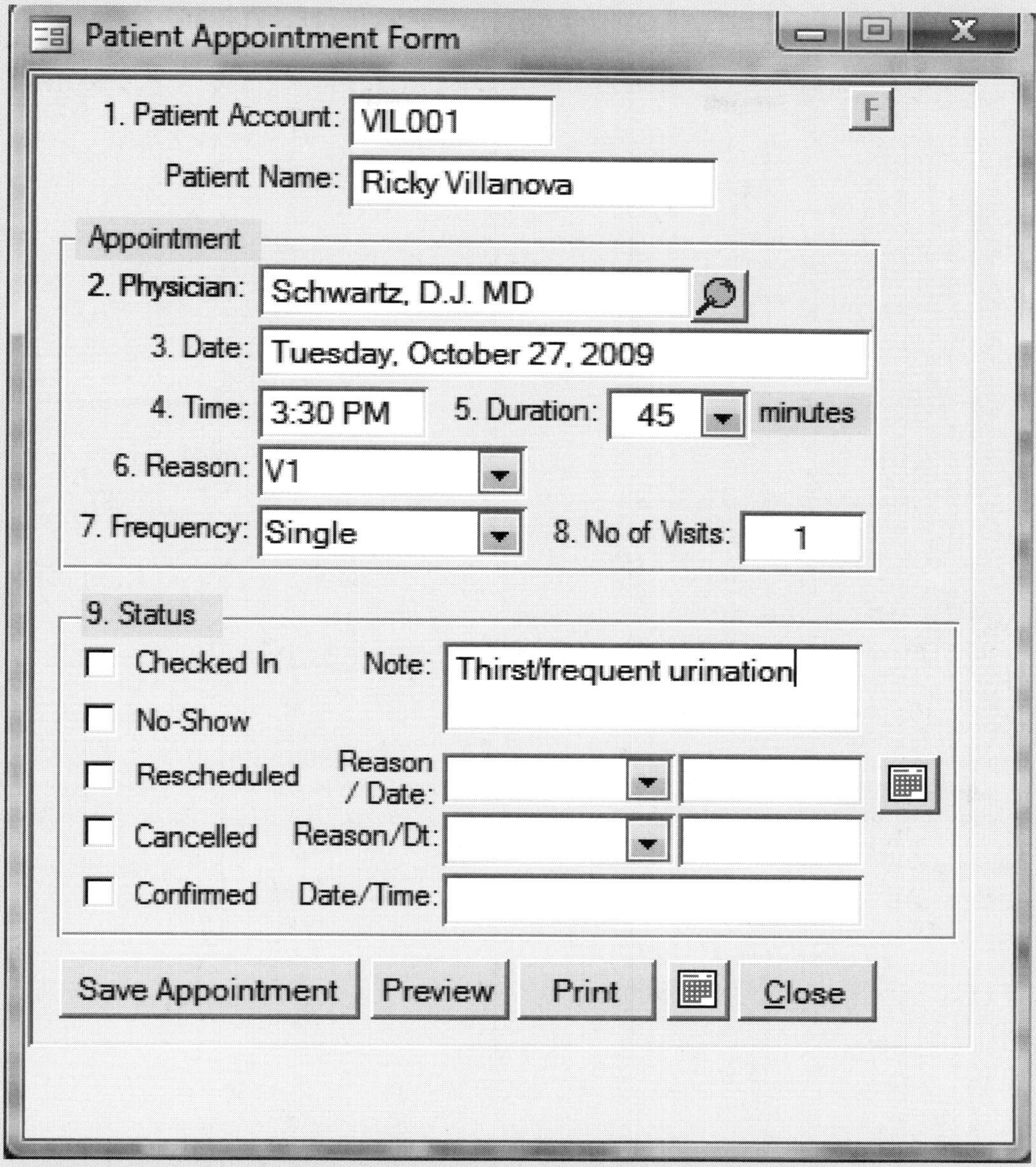

FIGURE 3-37

Delmar/Cengage Learning.

continues

SCHEDULING APPOINTMENTS FOR NEW PATIENTS *continued*

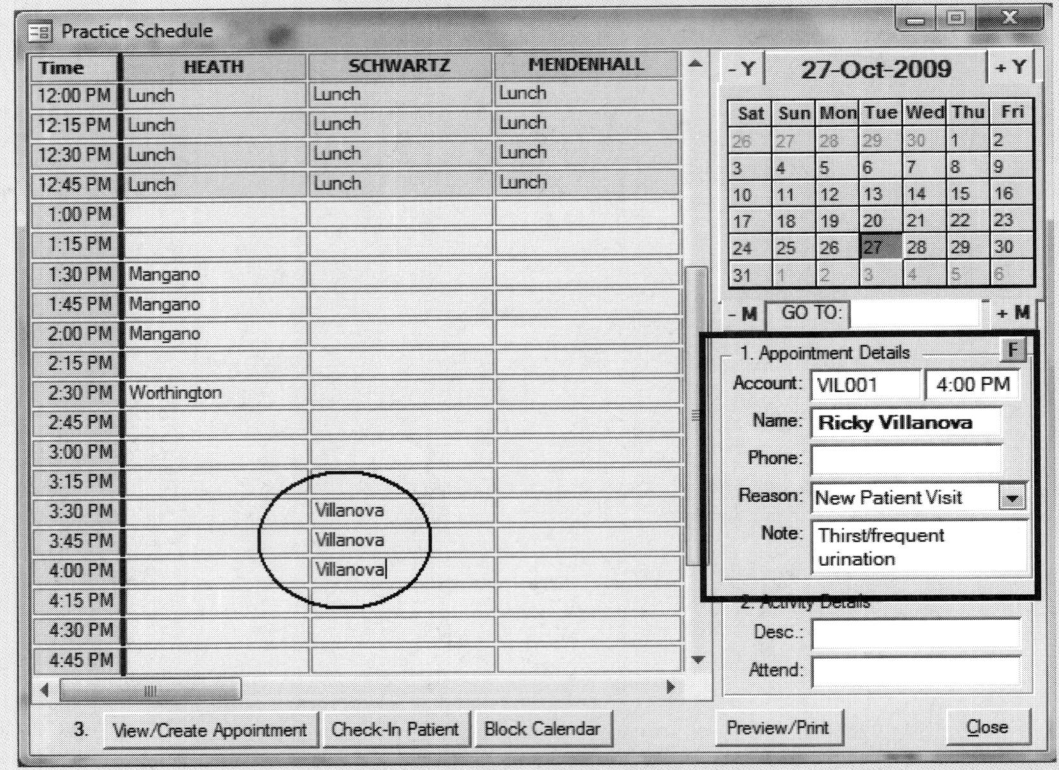

FIGURE 3-38
Delmar/Cengage Learning

E. Name: Minnie Adams

    Doctor: Heath

    Daytime telephone: Home—(123) 457-3688

    Insurance: Medicare, Statewide Corp.

    Duration of visit: 60 minutes

    Date and time: 10/28/2009; 10:00 a.m.

    Reason for visit: Chest pain

    Referring physician: None

Check your work with Figure 3-39 and Figure 3-40.

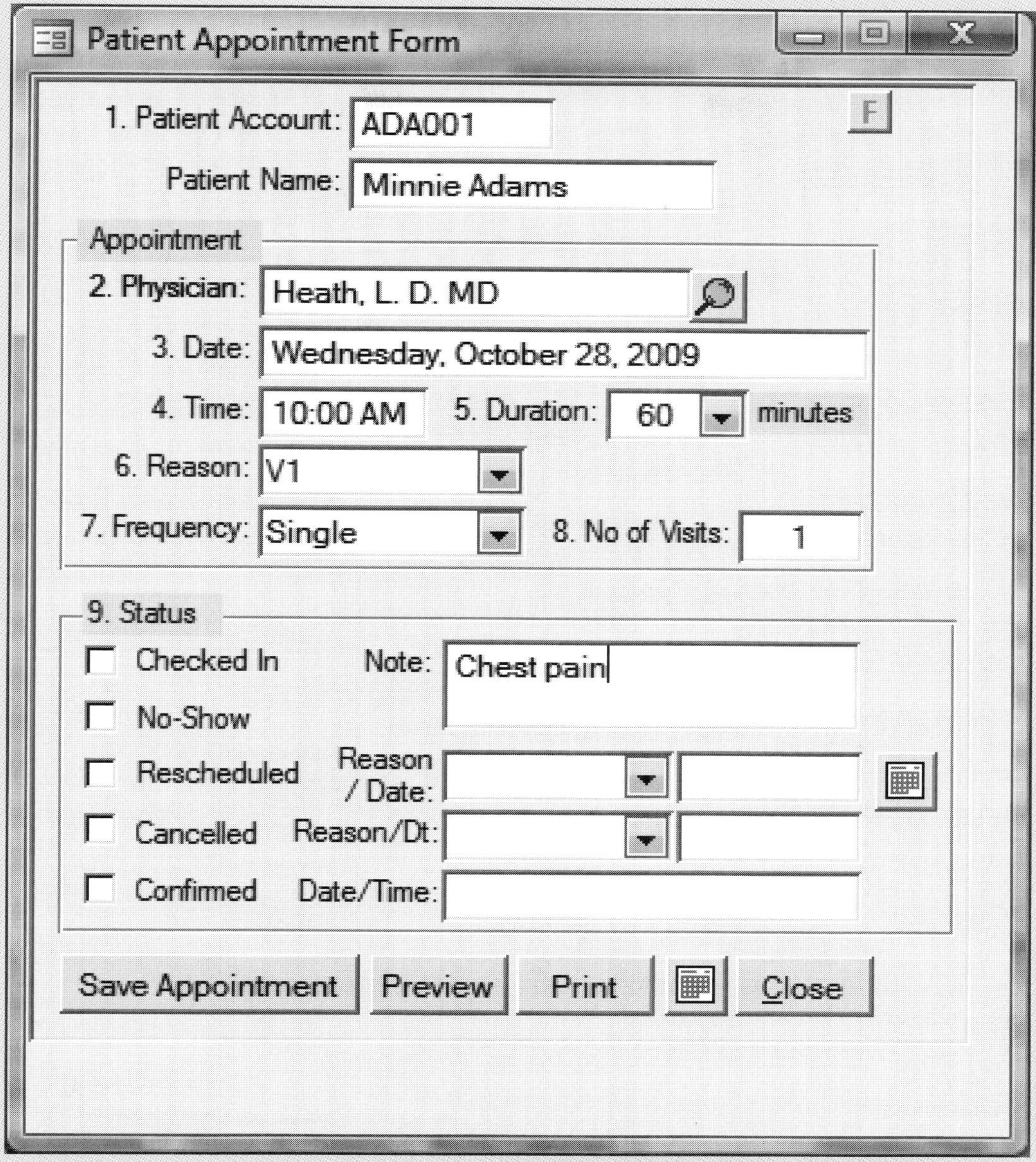

FIGURE 3-39

Delmar/Cengage Learning

continues

SCHEDULING APPOINTMENTS FOR NEW PATIENTS *continued*

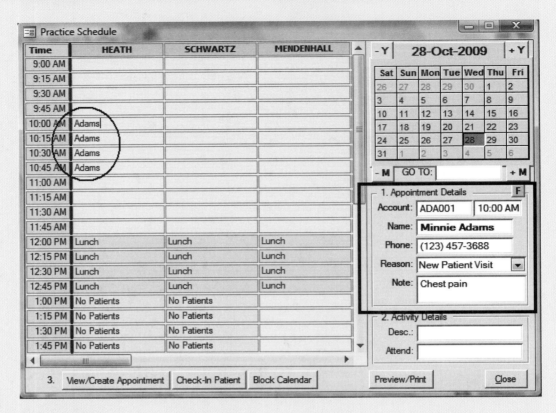

FIGURE 3-40

Delmar/Cengage Learning

STEP 11

Check your work and make corrections as needed. For each scheduled patient, click on the *Patient Registration* button on the Main Menu. Open each patient's record and check each one for the following:

A.   Correct doctor has been selected for the patient

B.   Daytime telephone number has been entered

C.   Correct guarantor has been selected (if applicable)

D.   Correct insurance has been selected for the patient

E.   Check the appointment scheduler to be certain each appointment and all details were entered correctly.

STEP 12

Click on the *Close* button and return to the Main Menu.

LET'S TRY IT! 3-4 SEARCHING AND RESCHEDULING PATIENT APPOINTMENTS

Objective: Search for and reschedule patient appointments as indicated. As previously discussed, the physicians or patients may need to reschedule appointments already on the schedule, such as cancellations, and rescheduled appointments. These should be documented for legal purposes. The following exercise guides the reader through the steps for rescheduling appointments to a new date.

Patient Manuel Ramirez has called the office to say he has an appointment in November, but does not remember the date. The reader will look up the appointment, and then reschedule it for a more convenient time.

STEP 1

On the Main Menu, click on the *Appointment Scheduling* button. When the scheduler opens, click on the *View/Create Appointment* button. This will open the Appointment Patient Selection window.

STEP 2

Locate Manuel Ramirez and single click on his *name*. Next, click on the *Select* button. This opens the Appointment Entry window and enables the user to search by viewing all appointments on record for this patient.

STEP 3

Along the bottom of the window is a label that reads "Record." To the right is a selection bar. If there is more than one appointment record to view, the number "1 of __" displays in the field. The far right indicates how many records. Click on the arrow as shown in Figure 3-41 to view each record until the appointment for November is displayed.

STEP 4

Patient Ramirez should have an appointment on record for November 16, 2009 at 09:30 a.m. for a cholesterol check. The visit was scheduled for 15 minutes with Dr. Heath. The patient is to come fasting (for blood tests that will be ordered). The patient informs you that his appointment will need to be rescheduled since the date is no longer convenient. With the November 16 appointment displayed, click on the *calendar icon* (between the Print and Close buttons) to be taken directly to that date. See the circled area on Figure 3-42.

STEP 5

On November 16, locate the Ramirez appointment. Double click on the patient's *name* to open the Appointment Form window.

STEP 6

Click in the *checkbox* in front of Rescheduled, and then use the drop-down box next to the Reason field to display the reason codes. Select *Needs Different Date* from the list, or R6.

continues

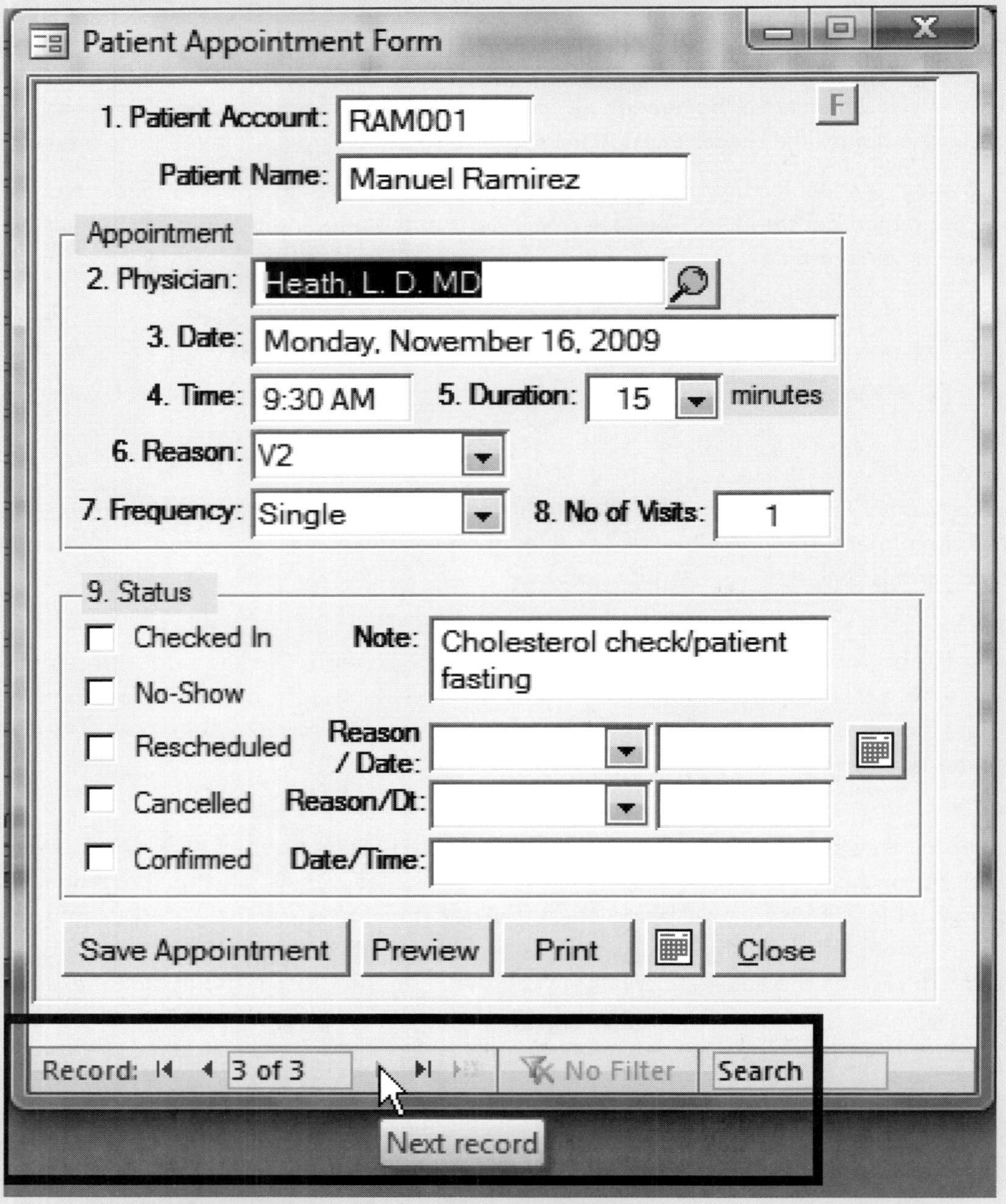

FIGURE 3-41

Delmar/Cengage Learning

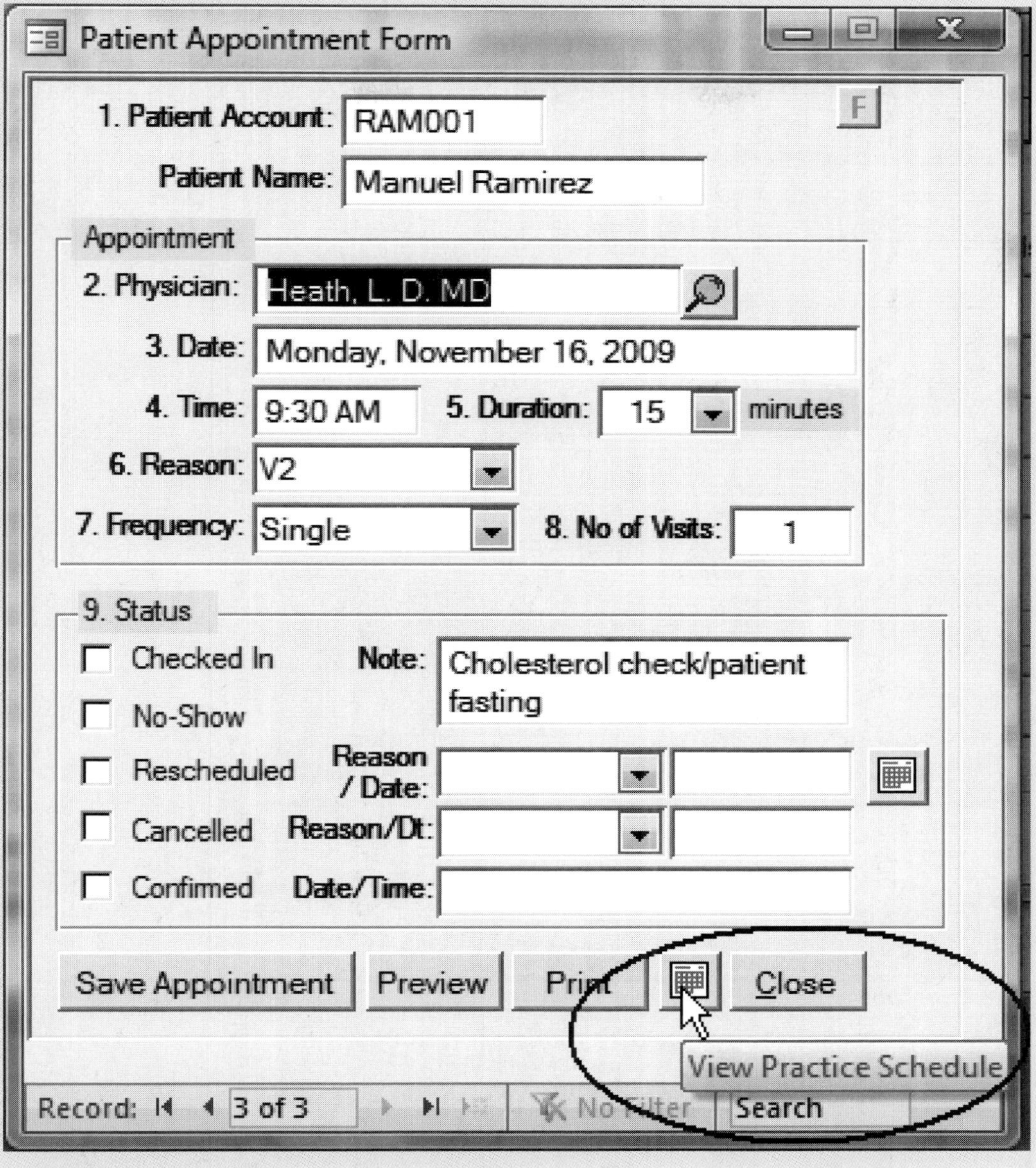

FIGURE 3-42

Delmar/Cengage Learning

continues

STEP 7

Next, click on the *calendar icon* on the far right, as shown in Figure 3-43. This opens a separate scheduler so that another date can be selected for the patient's appointment. Once you have opened the separate Practice Reschedule window, click to 11/18/2009.

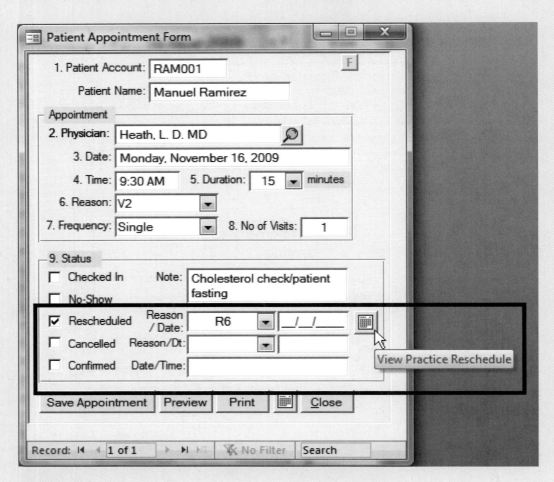

FIGURE 3-43

Delmar/Cengage Learning

STEP 8

Patient Ramirez would like to be rescheduled for 09:00 a.m. on 11/18/2009 with Dr. Heath. Double click in that time slot—it will appear that nothing has happened. Next, click on the *Close* button on the lower right corner. However, when the Appointment Form window displays, the new date will be in the proper field, as shown in Figure 3-44.

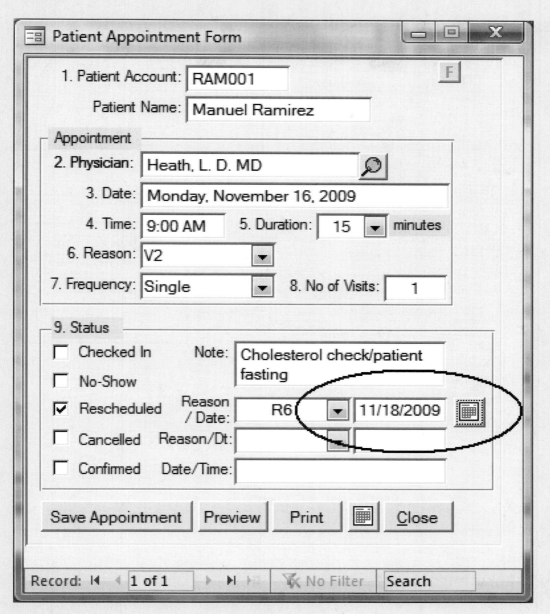

FIGURE 3–44

Delmar/Cengage Learning

STEP 9

Next, click on the *Save Appointment* button in order for the changes to take place on the Practice Schedule. Click *OK* through prompt, confirming the appointment has been moved, and then *Close* the Appointment Form window. The appointment that was previously shown on 11/16/2009 is cancelled and off that day's schedule, and now appears at 09:00 a.m. under Dr. Heath on 11/18/2009. See Figure 3-45.

continues

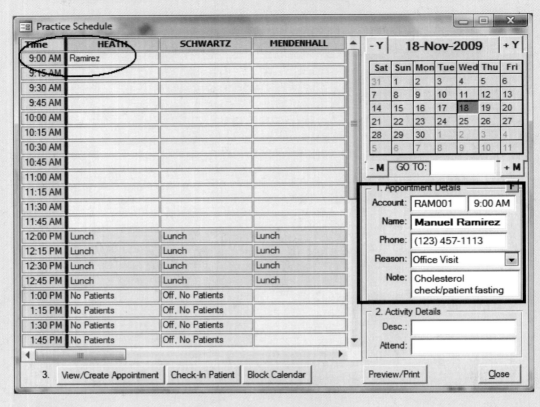

FIGURE 3–45

Delmar/Cengage Learning

HINT: Click on the *View/ Create Appointment* button, click on *patient name*, and then click on *Select* to find his appointment.

STEP 10

Following the procedures just learned for rescheduling an appointment, search for the appointment previously made for Kabin Pradhan.

STEP 11

Reschedule his appointment to November 3, 2009 at 09:00 a.m. with Dr. Schwartz. The reason is he needed a different date. Check your work with Figure 3-46. When finished, close the scheduler and return to the Main Menu.

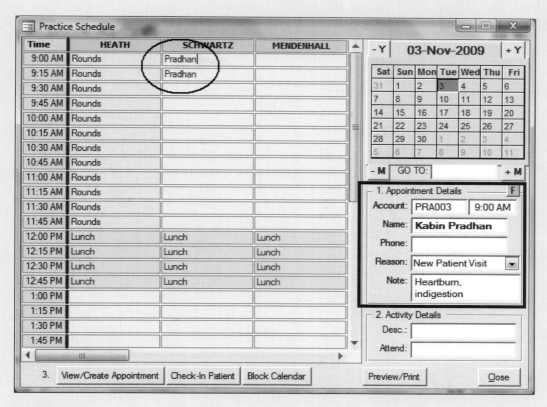

FIGURE 3–46

Delmar/Cengage Learning

LET'S TRY IT! 3-5 **REVIEW AND PRACTICE: SCHEDULING APPOINTMENTS**

Objective: Apply the skills you have learned for scheduling appointments to add established and new patients to the schedule.

STEP 1

> **HINT:** Established patients are already in the MOSS database.

Schedule Established Patients for Appointments. The following established patients have called the office to schedule appointments. Refer to the following information and schedule appointments using the procedures learned in this unit.

A. Eric Gordon   15 minutes   Office Visit
    Reason note: Diarrhea and stomach pain
    Doctor: Schwartz   Date: 11/5/2009   Time: 10:30 a.m.
    Check your work with Figure 3-47.

continues

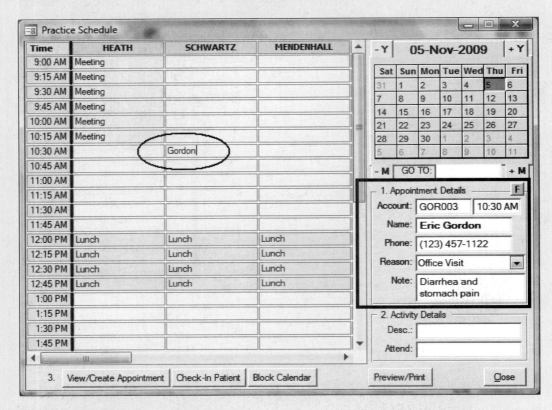

FIGURE 3–47

Delmar/Cengage Learning

B. Elane Ybarra   45 minutes   Office Visit
    Reason note: Painful urination/burning
    Doctor: Schwartz   Date: 11/6/2009   Time: 11:15 a.m.
    Check your work with Figure 3-48.

C. Vito Mangano   30 minutes   Office Visit
    Reason note: Follow-up anemia
    Doctor: Heath   Date: 11/9/2009   Time: 09:30 a.m.
    Check your work with Figure 3-49.

D. David James   15 minutes   Office Visit
    Reason note: Tender abdomen and fatigue
    Doctor: Heath   Date: 11/9/2009   Time: 11:15 a.m.
    Check your work with Figure 3-50.

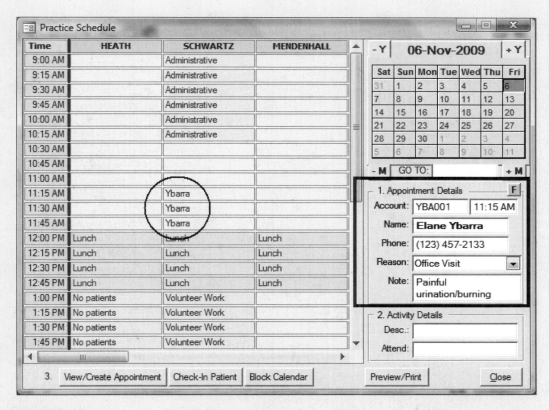

FIGURE 3–48

Delmar/Cengage Learning

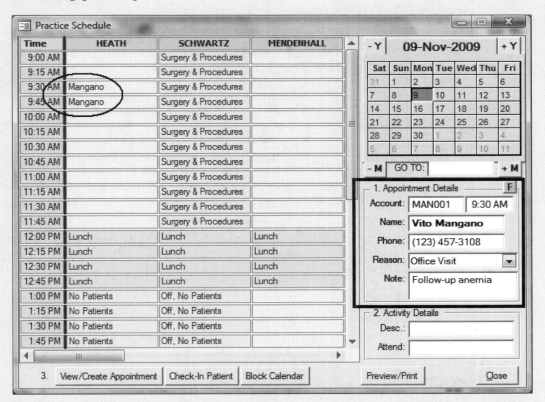

FIGURE 3–49

Delmar/Cengage Learning

continues

REVIEW AND PRACTICE: SCHEDULING APPOINTMENTS *continued*

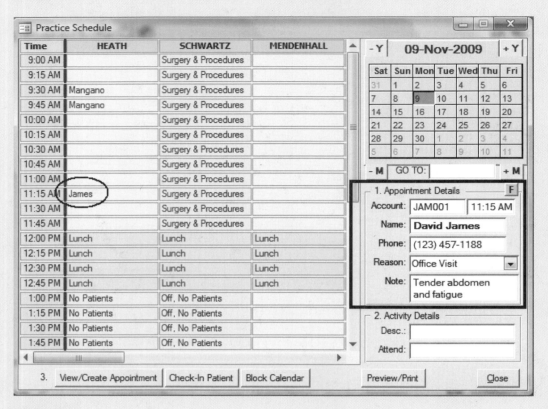

FIGURE 3–50

Delmar/Cengage Learning

E. Caroline Pratt   15 minutes   Office Visit
Reason note: Rash and itching
Doctor: Heath   Date: 11/18/2009   Time: 09:15 a.m.
Check your work with Figure 3-51.

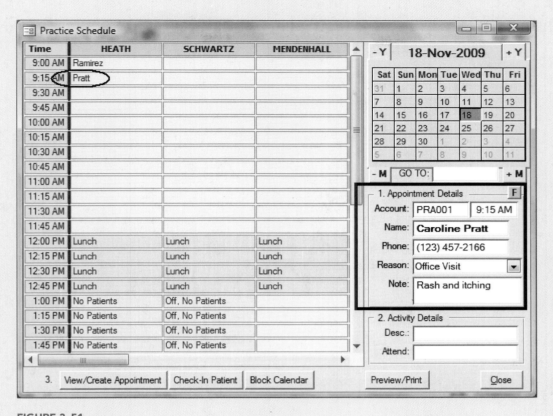

FIGURE 3–51

Delmar/Cengage Learning

STEP 2

Schedule New Patients for Appointments. The following new patients have called the office to schedule appointments. Each patient has been prescreened to be sure his or her insurance is accepted by the office. Use only the information given. The registration form completed at the time of the visit will provide any missing data.

HINT: Partial information will need to be used on the registration screen in order to create an account in the software.

MOSS NOTE: For these exercises, turn feedback mode off, if it is on; then shut down and restart the software program.

A. Name: Marie Tomanaga

Doctor: Schwartz

Daytime telephone: Home—(123) 457-2110

Insurance: Medicare, Statewide Corp.

Duration of visit: 60 minutes

Date and time: 11/03/2009; 10:00 a.m.

Reason for visit: Chest pain and hypertension

Check your work with Figure 3-52.

continues

REVIEW AND PRACTICE: SCHEDULING APPOINTMENTS *continued*

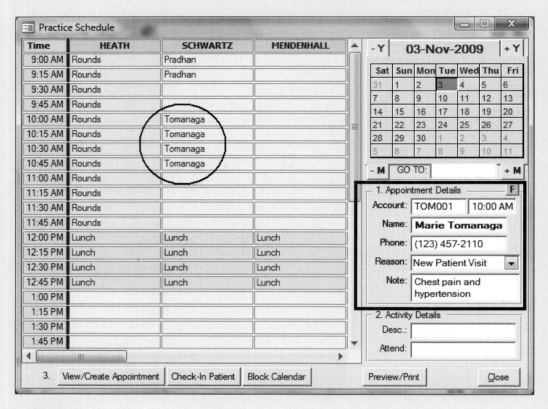

FIGURE 3–52

Delmar/Cengage Learning

B. Name: Kimberly Beals

   Doctor: Heath

   Daytime telephone: Work—(123) 528-1132

   Insurance: Signal HMO

   Duration of visit: 45 minutes

   Date and time: 11/03/2009; 03:00 p.m.

   Reason for visit: Unexplained weight loss

Check your work with Figure 3-53.

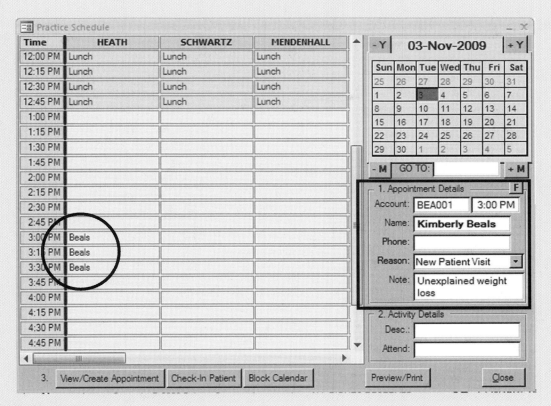

FIGURE 3–53

Delmar/Cengage Learning

C. Name: Linda Kinzler

    Doctor: Heath

    Daytime telephone: Home—(123) 457-5688

    Insurance: FlexiHealth PPO In-Network

    Duration of visit: 30 minutes

    Date and time: 11/09/2009; 10:15 a.m.

    Reason for visit: Flu shot, asthmatic

Check your work with Figure 3-54.

continues

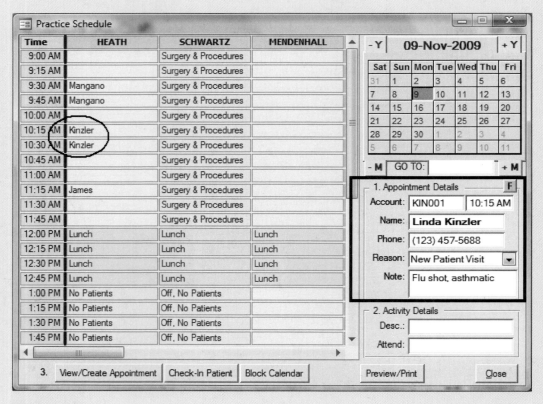

FIGURE 3–54

Delmar/Cengage Learning

FLOW OF THE OFFICE: THE INFORMATION CYCLE

Every medical practice has its own system and office policies when it comes to obtaining, processing, and preparing patient information. Fortunately, this process has many common procedures and terminology from office to office. These common aspects are discussed here, and will assist you in having a better understanding of the role of medical software in managing these tasks.

PREPARING FOR PATIENT VISITS: THE DAY BEFORE APPOINTMENTS

In medical offices that use hard copy patient files, the preparation of patient files begins a day or two before scheduled visits. It is best not to prepare files too far in advance, because patients may change their appointments. Additionally, too many patient files removed from the filing cabinet can create chaos and misplaced files, causing wasted time for staff members who may need to use them. The implementation of **Electronic Health Records (EHR)** Software is quickly replacing the paper patient file. It is not uncommon to see both physicians and clinical medical assistants using laptop computers with wireless access to an interoffice network and the Internet during patient visits. These laptop computers can be carried to each examination room, and all records easily accessed in digital format. Additionally, many offices have permanent desktop computers located in each examination or procedure room where patient records, including digital medical imaging, laboratory results, and other needed records can be instantly viewed and data input at the point of service. Orders for pharmacies, medical testing, specialist referrals, requests for insurance authorizations, and other requests can be easily processed via these computers using the electronic health records software.

In general, where paper patient records are used, all files of established patients with appointments will be pulled out and files for new patients will be assembled. This means getting together a folder, fasteners, initial documents, labels, and other needed items. It is a good idea not to create files completely for new patients until they actually arrive at the office, because cancellations or no-shows may occur. Even if electronic health records software is used in the medical office, preparing for the day's patient visits is still necessary, according to each patient's reason for visit and anticipated needs.

No matter how well an office prepares for patient visits, there will inevitably be patients that do not or cannot make their appointments. A **cancellation** is a patient who had an appointment, but called the office to either reschedule or opted not to visit the office. A **no-show** is a patient with a scheduled appointment who simply does not show up, and did not call the office to advise he or she would not be coming. In the case of both cancellation and no-show patients, be sure to document the reason on both the medical software and in the patient's file (or electronic health record) as a legal precaution. Additionally, no-show patients should be contacted to find out why, and to be rescheduled. The physician should also be apprised of any patients who fail to keep appointments. This is especially important for patients with medical conditions that require monitoring or follow-up.

PREPARING FILES FOR ESTABLISHED PATIENTS

When all established patients coming in for office visits are identified, each one is checked for a number of items, as shown in the following list.

1. **Date patient was last seen by the physician.** This can be easily done using medical software, checking the electronic health record, or by checking the date of the last notes written by the physician in the file. If more than six months have passed since the last visit, the file is flagged as a reminder to ask the patient if the address, phone number, marital status, employer, or insurance information has changed. **Flagging** a file means marking the file, or placing a note on it indicating special action is required. Any information that has changed will need to be updated in the paper record and computer database files.

   Instead of asking patients if any of their information has changed, some offices make it a standard practice to have all patients complete a new registration form once a year. Furthermore, copies (or scans) of insurance cards are made annually. In some offices, a copy or scan of the insurance card is made at each and every office visit. This is the best way to keep up with today's frequent changes in patient information and insurance coverage.

2. **The patient account is checked to verify if any balances are due.** Again, medical software makes this a quick and easy task. If the patient has an old balance, a forgotten co-payment, or any other amount due, the ideal time to collect it is at the time of an office visit. Some offices have the biller or collector place a note on the front of the file to alert the reception staff that additional money needs to be collected from the patient.

3. **All filing of loose documents (reports, test results, letters, etc.) is completed.** Most offices have stacks of documents waiting to be filed in patient records, whether hard copies for paper files or scans that need to be completed for the electronic record. Patients who have appointments should have all documents filed and ready before their office visits. Staff members who prepare patient files should read the notes written by the physician during the patient's last visit, to make sure all results of diagnostic tests that were ordered have been returned and filed in the patient's record. If any results have not been received in the office, tracking and obtaining them is necessary. It is likely the physician will need to refer to test results, consult details from other physicians, and review other important information when following up with a patient during the office visit.

4. **The progress note page is checked to make sure there is enough room for the clinical staff to write notes.** **Progress notes** are the handwritten or typed notes provided by the physician to document the details of the patient visit for the hard copy patient file. If there is not enough room left to write complete notes, a new page is inserted and the heading is filled out with the patient's name and other information, as needed. If a transcriptionist types the notes, these are typically provided on a sticky label that will be placed on the progress note sheet. For offices that use electronic health records, notes will be entered directly into the software and saved for viewing at any time. This information is stored as part of the patient's database on the computer.

5. **When the patient arrives for a visit, a blank superbill, also called an encounter form, is prepared.** During each patient visit, the clinical staff will document the procedures performed and the patient's diagnoses on the superbill. The superbill shows the date of service, place of service, signature of the physician, and an itemized list of services rendered.

   Superbills are returned to the front office at the end of each patient's visit. The information will be input into the medical software as required for accounting and medical billing purposes. The superbill also indicates when the physician would like to see the patient again, so that a follow-up appointment can be scheduled by the front office.

6. **Patients are contacted to confirm their upcoming office visits.** Many offices like to reduce no-shows by calling patients a day or two before their appointments as a reminder. A staff member may be assigned this task, or there are systems now available that function through a computer that can automatically dial the patient's phone number and leave prerecorded reminders. Another option is to have the system generate an e-mail reminder to the patient.

   For offices that are too busy to routinely call patients, it is highly recommended to at least call every new patient. Established patients with appointments expected to last 30 to 45 minutes or longer should also be reminded. It is not unusual for new patients to forget appointments. New patients sometimes misplace the office phone number or address, and some even forget the physician's name! Patients scheduled for complicated or lengthy visits who no-show not only waste the physician's time, but also take a valuable appointment slot away from other patients. Reminder calls are the best way to reduce these problems.

PATIENT HOURS: THE CHECK-IN AND CHECK-OUT PROCESS

The term **patient hours** refers to those times during the workday that are dedicated to patient visits in the clinical back office. A medical facility also has **office hours**, but there is an important distinction between the two. For instance, a facility may have office hours of Monday through Friday from 8:30 a.m. to 6:00 p.m. However, patient hours are Monday, Tuesday, and Friday from 9:00 a.m. to 12:30 p.m., and Wednesday afternoons, 2:00 p.m. to 6:00 p.m.

When patients are not visiting the office, the clinical and administrative staff occupies this time with completing the array of tasks to be done. These are the times medical billing, accounting, sending out patient statements, insurance follow-up, preparing patient files, and filing can be attended to. Equipment maintenance and office upkeep, as well as stocking supplies, is also done. These ongoing office management responsibilities are completed best when patients are not in the office.

Some of the most important tasks concerning patient information and office cash flow take place during patient hours. Without diligent attention to details by the staff located in the patient reception area, the rest of the administrative staff cannot perform their job efficiently or effectively. The following sections illustrate the responsibilities of the front-office staff at the patient reception area during patient check-in and check-out.

Checking in Patients

1. **As new patients arrive and check in at the office, each is given a registration form to fill out.** When the form is returned, each item must be reviewed for accuracy and completeness. If the patient has health insurance, photocopies (or scans) of the front and back of the insurance card(s) are taken and placed in the patient file. The **insurance card** is issued by the insurance company and contains information about the policyholder, identification numbers, important addresses, and phone numbers, among other data. This is the best opportunity to ask patients to clarify dual insurance issues, identify the policyholder, dependents, and the guarantor.

   Some medical offices have the reception area staff perform **insurance verification**, especially for eligibility. This involves contacting the insurance company, either by telephone or by using online resources on the computer, in order to verify that the patient is indeed eligible to receive benefits.

   Some medical offices have adopted the policy of collecting co-payments at the time of check-in, before services are rendered.

2. **Information is updated as needed for established patients when they check in.** If an established patient has a new insurance plan, due to a change of employment or plan availability, the same procedure as previously described for new patients is followed. Obtain photocopies (or scans) of the new insurance cards, including any needed signatures and forms, and perform insurance verification.

   Keep in mind that it is more common than ever before for employers to change the choices for health insurance plans available to employees. It is not unusual for plans to be changed yearly. It is especially important to be alert for this in the first three months of the year, when most new plans become effective.

3. **Referrals for managed-care patients are checked to be sure services are authorized.** As discussed previously, some managed-care health plans require PCP referrals before certain services can be rendered to a patient. It is the responsibility of the administrative staff to ensure managed-care patients arrive for visits with the appropriate referral, when required. This is usually accomplished at the time appointments are scheduled by reminding patients if and when referrals are required. This demands a good amount of tracking and follow up.

   Keep in mind that these referrals often have expiration dates or limits to how many times the patient can see the specialist. These details must also be carefully monitored; otherwise, a patient might receive unauthorized services, causing the physician to be denied payment. Practice management software, with managed-care modules, may offer tools to monitor referrals, expiration dates, and remaining visits, making the tracking of this information much more efficient.

These days, it is not unusual for referral authorizations to be completely handled by the referring and receiving medical offices. However, some degree of patient responsibility is involved in the process. Many medical offices have adopted policies that specify if a patient arrives for a visit without the proper referral, the appointment will be rescheduled. Some offices even charge the patient for the visit at the standard fee, if the patient insists on receiving services from the doctor without proper PCP referral.

Checking Out Patients

1. **Collecting payments.** If the patient's co-payment was not already collected upon arrival, it will be collected at check-out. All other payments, as applicable, will also be collected when the patient returns to the reception area after visiting the physician. It is most practical to take a direct approach when asking for payment. Statements such as "You have an old balance of $125.00. Will you be paying with a check or credit card?" are much more effective than, "Will you be making a payment today?"

2. **Further tests or referrals have been ordered.** If there are orders from the physician to schedule appointments for diagnostic tests outside the office, or to initiate referrals or consults to other physicians, follow the office policy. Some physicians prefer that the medical staff schedule outside tests for the patient; others will have the patient call directly to make his or her own appointment(s). Generally, the medical staff handles all surgery arrangements and hospital admissions.

3. **Follow-up visit to the office is scheduled.** At check out, the superbill indicates if and when the physician requires a follow-up visit to the office. If the doctor forgot to include that information, ask the patient whether he or she was told when he or she would be seen again. Progress notes written by the physician in the patient file can also be checked. Most physicians will indicate in their notes when the patient is to be seen again. The follow-up appointment can then be scheduled for the patient, and a reminder card given.

4. **Any final information, if required, is taken care of before the patient leaves the office.** Each patient has a different situation. If additional forms, prescription samples, or explanatory brochures for tests or medical conditions need to be given to the patient, these are provided before he or she leaves.

THE REIMBURSEMENT PROCESS

After patients receive services from the physician, the reimbursement process begins, starting with medical billing. The first step is completion of the superbill, or encounter form, by the clinical staff. As discussed previously, superbills show the patient's name, date of service, place of service, itemized procedures with CPT codes, and diagnoses with ICD codes. The fees are sometimes entered on the superbill for each itemized procedure, or selected by the medical software from a fee schedule. The physician usually signs the superbill to confirm services were rendered. Insurance companies require these pieces of information for billing purposes.

Next, the medical biller prepares and submits insurance claims in order to receive payment, using the information contained on the superbill. Any special forms, signatures, copies of insurance cards, or other information that was obtained by the front desk staff, are used to prepare the insurance claims. This is the reason the staff at the reception area plays an important role in how efficiently and accurately medical billers can perform their part of the job.

Ideally, for each claim sent to the insurance company, a payment returns. An **Explanation of Benefits (EOB)** accompanies payments received from an insurance company. If the medical office receives payment from the insurance company electronically, the explanation of benefits is referred to as an Electronic Remittance File, a document that shows the dates of service for a particular patient, which codes were considered for payment, and the physician or facility that rendered the services. If a payment was made, the explanation indicates the amount of the payment and provides information regarding any portion of the fees that were not allowed or not paid, including reason notes.

The medical biller, or other designated staff member, uses the explanation of benefits (or electronic remittance file) to properly post payments to patient accounts. If there are any payment denials or inaccurate payments and services listed, these must be followed up and pursued. This process is discussed in more detail in a later unit.

After the medical office receives payment from the insurance company, there are two actions that then can be taken. If there are any remaining balances due, either the secondary insurance plan is billed, or the patient is sent a statement requesting payment.

The last step in the reimbursement process is collections for overdue accounts. As previously mentioned, this commonly involves taking action in the form of letters and telephone calls to the patient, including offering monthly payment arrangements. Assigning overdue accounts to a collections agency is always a last-resort option.

FINAL NOTES

Good office management and reimbursement begins with an understanding of the flow of information in a medical office. Starting from the time a patient schedules an appointment through the time the payment is received for services rendered, every member of the health care team plays an important role in proper reimbursement. Like the links of a chain, every person participates in and is responsible for a component that contributes to the image, organization, efficiency, and success of the medical office as a whole.

Medical offices are both places of business and places of human care and compassion. The proper balance between business and patient care is essential; one cannot exist without the other. The medical administrative staff ensures that the logistics of the business aspect of a medical office are properly carried out, so that physicians and other clinicians have the ways and means with which to provide patient care.

Currently, new laws are affecting management procedures. Health insurance issues continue to diversify and at times seem to complicate reimbursement. Small practices merge, form associations, or join larger organizations in order to survive. Through it all, developers of all types of medical software continually strive to provide tools that assist medical administrative staff to best perform their work and maximize reimbursement.

CHECK YOUR KNOWLEDGE

1. From the following list, check the items that are important to update if the patient has not been to the office in six months or more.

   ____ Social Security Number

   ____ Marital Status

   ____ Address

   ____ Phone Number

   ____ Salary Rate

   ____ Employer

   ____ Past Medical History

   ____ Insurance Information

2. Referrals for managed-care patients typically have expiration dates and a limit to the number of visits authorized.

   a. True

   b. False

3. As long as the employer does not change, it is unlikely that a patient's health insurance plan will change.

   a. True

   b. False

4. A patient's daytime telephone number is best for recording appointments in case rescheduling is required.

   a. True

   b. False

5. Progress notes are provided by the physician to document details of a patient visit.

   a. True

   b. False

6. The reason for a patient cancelling or no-showing an appointment should be documented for legal purposes.

   a. True

   b. False

7. The back office of a medical practice is the area where

   a. health care professionals examine and treat patients.

   b. patients are admitted to the hospital.

   c. administrative functions are performed.

   d. medical billing is done.

8. The walk-in patient is

    a. a person who requires medical service, but calls the same day or day before an appointment and must be fit into the schedule.

    b. a person who comes to the medical office seeking service without having first made an appointment.

    c. a person who has not received services from the physician within the past three years.

    d. none of the above.

9. A list of patient names with appointment times, reason for visit, and other details, that is distributed to medical office staff for patient hours, is called

    a. the appointment book or scheduler.

    b. appointment reminder card.

    c. the reference sheet.

    d. none of the above.

10. A patient will receive complete or partial care for a medical problem from a physician and has been transferred to receive this care. This is known as a

    a. referral.

    b. consultation.

    c. surgery.

    d. office visit.

11. A patient will need to return next year for a follow-up appointment to monitor a medical condition. A useful reminder system consisting of postcards or notices that can be mailed to the patient when the appointment is due is called

    a. a reference sheet.

    b. a progress note.

    c. a tickler file.

    d. flagging the file.

12. When patients present their insurance card at check-in, the administrative staff will

    a. store the card in the patient's file.

    b. verify the information on the card, then return it to the patient.

    c. copy or scan the front and back of the card for the patient file, then return the card to the patient.

    d. take no action; it is not necessary to do anything with the insurance card.

13. The gatekeeper for some types of managed-care plans is also referred to as the

    a. attending physician.

    b. primary care physician.

    c. specialist.

    d. none of the above.

14. The best time to collect money due from a patient is
    a. at the time of the office visit.
    b. when the patient is sent a statement to his home.
    c. when the patient is admitted to the hospital.
    d. when the money is at least 60 days overdue.

15. At patient check-out, information regarding when the patient is due back for a follow-up appointment can be found
    a. on the superbill, or encounter form.
    b. in the physician's progress notes.
    c. by asking the patient if he was told when to return.
    d. all of the above.

16. The EOB, or explanation of benefits, is a document that
    a. explains payment details made on health insurance claims.
    b. authorizes a patient to see a specialist.
    c. explains what insurance coverage and benefits the patient has.
    d. none of the above.

17. When patient files are pulled in preparation for patient hours, describe four major items each file should be checked for.

    _____

    _____

    _____

18. Explain the difference between an established patient and a new patient.

    _____

    _____

    _____

19. Describe at least three factors that may affect scheduling patients for appointments.

    _____

    _____

    _____

20. Explain why confirming patient appointments, especially for new patients and long visits for established patients, is a good practice for medical offices.

    _____

    _____

    _____

21. Describe steps to take when patient appointments must be rescheduled due to an emergency or a delay on the part of the medical office.

    _____

    _____

    _____

Fundamentals of Medical Insurance

OBJECTIVES

Upon completion of this unit, the reader should be able to:

- **Explain the basic principles of the The Patient Protection and Affordable Care Act (PPACA)**

- **Understand concepts common to most medical insurance plans**

- **Differentiate between group plans and individual plans**

- **Discuss the major types of medical insurance plans: indemnity, managed care, Medicare, Medicaid, and Health Reimbursement Arrangements (HRAs)**

- **Discuss Health Maintenance Organization (HMO) models and their basic format(s)**

- **Discuss the basic concept of Preferred Provider Organizations (PPOs) and Point of Service Plans (POSs)**

- **Identify the differences between Health Reimbursement Arrangements (HRAs), Medical Savings Accounts (MSAs), and Flexible Savings Accounts (FSAs)**

- **Understand the coverage details of the insurance plans used in the simulation exercises for *Medical Office Simulation Software* (MOSS).**

KEY TERMS

Accepting assignment

Centers for Medicare & Medicaid Services (CMS)

Closed panel HMO

Consumer Driven Health Care (CDHC)

Group model HMO

Group plan

Health Flexible Spending Accounts (FSAs)

Health Savings Accounts (HSAs)

Health Reimbursement Arrangement or Account (HRA)

Indemnity plans

Independent Practice Association (IPA)

Individual plans

In-network benefits

Limiting charge (Medicare)

Major medical

Managed care

Medicaid

Medical savings account (MSA)

All members of the health care delivery team, from physicians to clinical personnel to administrative support personnel, need to have an understanding of the reimbursement process. Whether providing patient care, managing the office, or securing payment, each staff member has a role for ensuring the best possible return for professional services rendered. Having basic knowledge of the fundamentals regarding medical insurance is essential for accomplishing this.

It is a fact that numerous medical plans are available today, differing not only in the details of coverage, but also in the requirements and procedures for obtaining reimbursement. A single insurance company may offer several medical insurance products, and the plans may differ within a region or from state to state. It is typical for providers to participate, and have specific contracts, with many plans. With time, staff members of the medical office become familiar with the plans popular within an area, and the usual requirements for each.

Keeping up with the latest updates and changes often presents a challenge. How does one keep up with the most current insurance protocols with patients having so many different medical insurance plans? This requires diligence on the part of the staff by reading newsletters and journals, attending seminars, and joining associations. Many resources are provided by insurance carriers or by private organizations specializing in medical reimbursement issues. Once updates and changes that affect the practice have been identified, provisions to put them into effect need to be initiated. These may include diagnostic or procedural coding changes along with use of new forms, documentation guidelines, and referral or authorization requirements, to name a few possibilities. Medical office staff need to be apprised and trained regarding all changes and updates. Steps are being taken, concurrent with the writing of this book, to standardize the claims submission and reimbursement process in the United States.

In the administrative medical environment, practice management software is a useful tool for automating updates and assisting with monitoring patient data. Software developers and vendors are concerned with keeping software compliant with federal requirements, especially where HIPAA is concerned. Many offer online updating for code changes, online eligibility for insurance verification, and even tracking of claims and their status. Developers are offering tools available at Web sites to perform these functions customized to the needs of each medical office. The introduction of computers in medical office management, combined with the widespread use of the Internet, has automated many facets of the reimbursement process, continually improving how the work is done.

KEY TERMS (cont.)

Medicare Advantage (MA) plans

Medicare Part A

Medicare Part B

Medicare Part C

Medigap

Open panel or network HMO

Patient Protection and Affordable Care Act (PPACA)

Premium

Staff model HMO

Title XIX

Usual, customary, and reasonable rate (UCR)

THE PATIENT PROTECTION AND AFFORDABLE CARE ACT

The idea of a universal health system and medical care for all eligible people in the United States has been the topic of heated discussion among politicians and citizens for many years. On March 23, 2010, The Patient Protection and Affordable Care Act (PPACA) was signed into law in the United States by President Barack Obama. This, along with the Health Care and Education Reconciliation Act of 2010 (HCERA), signed into law on March 30, 2010, represents the health care reform agenda of the Obama administration.

The law stems from the fact that people in the United States with health problems but without health insurance have long struggled to find affordable coverage. For those that have preexisting medical conditions, the current health care system has been difficult to navigate or to assist patients with the cost of treatment. Patients with preexisting medical conditions were often offered coverage at unaffordable premium prices, or were not insurable at all. It seems that health insurance should be available when one needs it the most, but this has not been the case in the personal stories of many patients. Part of the problem is that insurance is designed to protect against future events that may happen—not events that have already occurred in the past. From the perspective of the insurance companies, covering a preexisting condition is akin to a person applying for flood insurance after a home has already been damaged by water. Of course, from a compassionate and human perspective, the fact that a person has an illness and requires help with medical expenses is an entirely different situation. Because of the health care reform, this should no longer be an issue for those with pre-existing health problems in the near future.

The **Patient Protection and Affordable Care Act (PPACA)** includes a large number of health-related provisions that will be put into effect over the next several years, anticipated to be in full effect by 2018. These provisions include expanding Medicaid eligibility, providing incentives for businesses to provide health care benefits to their employees, additional support for medical research, and eliminating pre-existing condition exclusions, among others. These changes will not come without their share of growing pains and costs. A variety of new taxes, cuts to current services or coverage, and adjustments to the plan to accommodate future needs are certain to happen. Some of these taxes include new Medicare taxes for those in a higher income bracket, taxes on indoor tanning, additional fees on pharmaceutical companies and certain medical devices, as well as tax penalties imposed on those that do not obtain health insurance (unless exempt). There will be changes to the Medicare Advantage program, which will affect senior citizens and may cut some of the broader benefits seniors now enjoy, in favor of Original Medicare. However, improvements to the Medicare Part D drug program are also included in the plan, which will close the current gap in prescription drug coverage, known as the "donut hole".

At the time of the writing of this book, the health care system in the United States was on the brink of landmark changes not experienced since Medicare rolled out in 1966 under the Johnson administration. Everyone in the medical field in all occupations, whether administrative or in direct patient care, will need to keep a careful eye on the upcoming reforms that are to take place in the coming years. This will most likely bring changes to how medical billing, coding, and medical documentation are done, as well as other significant changes. Electronic health records are expected to become mandatory in an effort to streamline information and create a more efficient method for using medical information and cutting costs overall.

GENERAL INFORMATION ABOUT MEDICAL INSURANCE

While there are many differences between medical insurance plans, there is still some common ground between most plans. The following list outlines general concepts about medical insurance that are important not only for medical staff to be aware of, but also for patients to understand.

1. **The insured and payer relationship.** Many patients present their medical insurance card at an office somewhat like a credit card, as if those services will be "charged" to it. They expect services to be billed to the insurance carrier without having to be much involved after that. Medical services are rendered when needed and payments follow later, the greater part usually from the insurance company. The assumption is made that everything will be taken care of. While it is proper for the patient to expect that the medical office will bill for services accurately and correctly, there are times when assistance from the patient is helpful when problems arise and reimbursement is difficult.

   Patients need to understand that the medical plan is actually a contract between the insured (patient) and the insurance carrier. The medical insurance contract is a promise, by the insurance company, to pay for expenses related to health care in exchange for payment of a **premium**. A premium is the amount the insured pays to assure coverage under a health insurance plan. Premiums may be paid in one lump sum, or, often, with a quarterly or monthly payment plan. In cases where groups of people have coverage through an employer, the contract is between the employer, the insurance carrier, and the insured. While the physician or medical facility may also have a contract to provide services to policyholders of a particular plan, it is still the patient's responsibility to utilize the medical plan only within its coverage guidelines.

As such, it makes sense that patients should understand their coverage, limitations, and exclusions, as well as financial responsibility. Medical office staff often spend a good amount of time educating patients about their deductibles, co-payments, non-covered services, and other insurance matters. However, it is not always possible to know every detail of coverage for every plan. It is a good idea to take a stance with patients that encourages active participation in knowing their coverage and assisting the medical office with reimbursement issues whenever necessary. Well-informed patients who understand what is expected of them are less likely to become collections problems later on.

2. **Method of payment is not consistent.** Not all medical insurance plans pay the same for services. Insurance payments vary according to the type of plan and the method used to determine payments. Some plans pay contracted rates; others, predetermined fee schedules. There are fee schedules that are based on average fees by specialty and geographic location. To illustrate, if four patients have four different plans and all receive the same service, it is likely that the physician will be reimbursed four different amounts according to the method used by each plan. Here again, the importance of practice management software for simplifying the task of applying payments to patient accounts becomes clear.

3. **Most policies have limitations or exclusions; therefore, not all services are covered.** If a medical plan limits the number or types of service, or does not cover them at all, called exclusions, the patient will most likely be responsible for payment. It is ideal for the patient to know about limitations and exclusions ahead of time, so that reimbursement can be discussed. This increases patient cooperation and helps avoid collections activity. As a medical staff member, you should be aware that some plans require disclosure to the patient of those procedures that are known to be not covered, or are expected to be denied payment for a particular reason. It is important to follow documentation criteria for plans that require disclosure, because the patient may not be responsible for payment if the provider fails to follow proper protocol before rendering services.

GROUP AND INDIVIDUAL PLANS

Most medical insurance plans are either individual or group plans. By far, the group plan is the more common type. When a single medical plan provides coverage for a group of people, such as employees or members of an organization, it is referred to as a **group plan**. The major difference between a group plan and the individual plan is that all eligible members of the group are covered regardless of age, health conditions, or medical history. Premiums are generally calculated according to the overall age, job risks, and size of the group, and therefore tend to reflect a lower premium compared to individual plans. Generally, a small group has less than 20 participants; a large group, more than 100. The law now requires that large groups be offered at least one managed care plan in their benefits choices. Details of coverage are often negotiated between the employer and the insurance company.

Medical insurance plans that are purchased directly by the policyholder from insurance companies or through agents are called **individual plans.** These are rather difficult to obtain, because one must be in very good health to qualify. In addition, the plans may have very high premiums. Insurance rates may go up according to changes in health status, or coverage can even be dropped. Limited coverage, or no coverage for certain services, is also a problem, and may include exclusion of maternity, prescription drug, and mental health services. Furthermore, individual plans may have higher deductibles and co-insurance amounts due from the patient. These are all factors that should be kept in mind when providing services to patients who have individual insurance plans, as status and coverage can change at any time.

COMMON TYPES OF MEDICAL INSURANCE PLANS

While there are many medical insurance products available that differ in coverage details from each other, for the purpose of this book, four main categories of medical insurance are discussed: indemnity plans, managed care plans, Medicare, and Medicaid. A more recent concept in health plans, known as Health Reimbursement Arrangements or Accounts (HRAs) will also be discussed. These plans are currently being offered by several large employers as part of their menu of choices for medical benefits.

INDEMNITY PLANS

Indemnity plans, sometimes called traditional or commercial insurance, were, at one time, the most common type of plans. In simple terms, this type of insurance gives patients the most choices. Patients have no restrictions on which doctors they can see, referrals are not required, and authorization for large procedures or expensive tests are rarely needed. The insurance company does not control or direct the patient's medical care; this is left to the patient's discretion and the decisions made by physicians. Additionally, patients are expected to pay fees in their entirety at the time of service, and send claims to the insurance company themselves in order to be reimbursed. As a result, indemnity plans are also referred to as fee-for-service plans. Often, there is an annual deductible and co-insurance involved, which tends to have a more expensive out-of-pocket cost to the patient than other types of medical plans. Premiums also tend to be significantly higher.

Since the advent of managed care, indemnity plans have dropped off as a viable option for medical coverage, mainly because they are higher cost plans. Presently, while these plans still exist, they represent a small percentage of medical insurance products in common use. However, it is important to understand how indemnity plans work—especially deductibles, co-insurance, and other out-of-pocket patient expenses. As we will see later, many managed care plans have adopted components of the indemnity plan model for out-of-network services and even some in-network services. In addition, the traditional Medicare plan, available since 1966 and known as *original* Medicare, is very much based on an indemnity plan model. There are many Medicare beneficiaries still using Original Medicare.

REIMBURSEMENT AND INDEMNITY PLANS

Indemnity plans use a system for tracking data related to procedure fees charged and payments accepted by physicians. The system also considers geographic location and other relevant factors. Once calculated, the results are referred to as the **usual, customary, and reasonable rate (UCR)** for the each procedure. The indemnity medical plan uses the UCR rate as the basis on which to make payment to the provider. Most indemnity plans pay a percentage of the approved, or allowed, amount for each procedure billed. The following example is typical for indemnity plans.

Dr. Heath performs a procedure for a patient. The standard fee is $150.00, and the patient pays Dr. Heath $150.00 at the time of service. The patient then sends a claim to his insurance company to be reimbursed. The claim is for $150.00. The insurance company determines that the UCR for this procedure is $125.00, and approves it at that rate. The patient's medical plan pays 80 percent of the approved amount, or 80 percent of $125.00. The patient receives a check for $100.00.

What happened to the other $50.00? The patient's plan pays only 80 percent of the approved amount. The other 20 percent is the co-insurance and comes out of the patient's pocket. In this example, the co-insurance is $25.00. The difference between the approved amount ($125.00) and the physician's fee ($150.00) also comes out of the patient's pocket. In this case, the non-approved portion of the fee was $25.00. Because most physicians do not have contractual obligations with indemnity plans and rarely offer discounts, they are entitled to full payment of their fee. Thus, the patient paid a $25.00 co-insurance and the $25.00 non-approved amount, or a total of $50.00. This example is shown line by line for clarification:

Physician standard fee:	$150.00
Insurance UCR/approved:	$125.00
Patient pays non-approved difference:	$ 25.00
Insurance pays 80% of $125.00:	$100.00
Patient pays 20% co-insurance:	$ 25.00

At times, the patient will have a deductible that has not been met. This decreases the payment from the insurance company and increases the patient's out-of-pocket costs. If you recall from Unit 2, a deductible is an out-of-pocket expense the patient must pay before the insurance company will pay for covered services. Let us look at the same example, but this time, the patient has a $100.00 deductible that has not been met.

Physician standard fee:	$150.00
Insurance UCR/approved:	$125.00
Amount applied to deductible:	$100.00 (deductible is now met)
Amount covered:	$ 25.00
Insurance pays 80% of $25.00:	$ 20.00
Patient pays 20% co-insurance:	$ 5.00
Patient pays the deductible applied ($100.00), the non-approved amount ($25.00), and the co-payment ($5.00) to physician. Total:	$130.00

Although fee-for-service indemnity plans served the American people well prior to the late 1970s, escalating health care costs started to increase insurance premiums to formidable levels. Advances in technology, increased lawsuits, and performing unnecessary medical procedures were some of the reasons for these increasing costs. This forced employers and the government to find alternative solutions and contain costs, leading to the managed care options that have become popular in the past three decades. The concept of patients sharing in their medical expenses by paying a deductible and a percentage of costs continues to be incorporated into current managed care and alternative coverage plans, often with interesting variations.

MANAGED CARE PLANS

Few people realize that the advent of the managed care idea in the United States began in the 1800s in California. With the arrival of large numbers of immigrants to San Francisco and Los Angeles, there was a need for health care and affordable ways to deliver it. At the time, many workers of the timber, aqueduct, railroad, and related industries were busy developing the West. The population was growing rapidly as people came in search of opportunity: gold, silver, land, and a better way of life. The needs for health care brought about the earliest prepaid health plan, offered by the French Mutual Benevolent Society in San Francisco in the mid-1800s. For an admission fee and monthly dues, or a lifetime membership fee, medical services could be sought from physicians at a participating hospital.

Unions, employers, ethnic societies, and other groups continued creating health care plans. Among them was the Ross-Loos Medical Group, generally accepted as the first health maintenance organization, started in 1929. Over the next 60 years, and into the 1980s, Ross-Loos underwent purchases and mergers that eventually became known as the CIGNA HealthPlans of California, part of the CIGNA Employee Benefits Division. The nation's first Blue Cross and Blue Shield programs would enter the scene in the 1930s, also originating in California. Soon after, the Kaiser Permanente Health Plan followed in 1946. Given that significant events took place in relation to health care coverage during the depression, and the introduction of Medicare and Medicaid in the 1960s, coupled with the health care reform issues leading into the 1990s, it is clear that the United States has always been in a state of change and innovation with its health care system.

What Is Managed Care?

Managed care is a system of health plans that attempts to control costs by limiting access to health care and focusing on preventative medicine. For example, with some plans, limiting access to health care is accomplished by requiring the patient to have routine care performed by a primary care physician (PCP), who also is the only one authorized to refer the patient to specialists, or approve certain tests and procedures.

With other types of managed care plans, PCPs are not used. However, access to health care is limited by encouraging patients to receive services from physicians who have a contract and participate with the health plan. By doing this, discounts or additional benefits may be available to the patient, making it more attractive to receive services from the participating providers.

Limiting access to care does not mean denying care or making less care available to patients. Rather, it is a means of funneling patients through a system that supervises when and by whom care will be provided. Choice, as compared to indemnity plans, is restricted to the degree outlined by the health plan. Consequently, following the proper procedures for obtaining care has a direct impact on reimbursement.

In addition to limiting access to health care, the concept of preventative medicine in managed care is also an effective way to control costs. While most indemnity plans of the past did not cover routine physicals, screening tests, and examinations, managed care plans encourage them. This is based on the philosophy that if patients are covered for annual physical examinations and preventative medical testing, they will be more apt to receive regular medical care. By doing so, medical problems can be detected earlier and perhaps treated with more success, rather than when severe symptoms or progression of disease have occurred. In other words, medical conditions can often be treated for less money in earlier stages; they become more expensive as they develop further.

Since managed care has become prevalent in recent years, you will work mostly with these plans in medical offices. To understand these health plans better, it is useful to become familiar with examples of coverage details. Additionally, you will need to learn about popular managed care models, as the medical facility you work at may be set up according to the type of contract the providers (physicians and hospitals) have with the health plans and payers. As a staff member screening and accepting new patients for a medical office, this becomes important, for there may be restrictions regarding the services patients can receive at a particular location according to the plans they have.

Managed Care Models

Although there are few basic managed care models, there are many diverse medical plans offered by insurance companies based on these models. Variations in coverage details and services are numerous; it would be unwise to generalize and assume all plans are the same if they are of a certain model. However, the guidelines that follow are helpful for understanding the basic definition, or setup, for each model. Each patient's plan will need to be verified on a case-by-case basis.

1. **Health Maintenance Organizations.** Health Maintenance Organizations (HMOs) are also known as Managed Care Organizations (MCOs). There are several standard models under the classification of HMO. The differences between these models are the contractual relationships that exist between the providers and the insurance plan(s). HMOs generally require the patient to have a PCP who provides routine medical care and authorizes the patient to see specialists, although some are "open access" HMOs that do not require a PCP. However, for such plans, the patient's out-of-pocket expenses could be higher.

   The standard models include the following:

   A. *Open Panel or Network HMO.* The **open panel** or **network HMO**, also called an **Independent Practice Association (IPA)**, includes physicians who provide services to enrollees of the plan in their own offices. Physicians are not employees of the HMO, but rather, have their own private practices. As such, they can contract with many different HMO plans, and also provide services to their own patients who are not members of any HMO plan. This model is the most common. Physicians can be reimbursed for their services either in a fee-for-service arrangement or with a predetermined fee schedule.

   B. *Closed Panel HMO.* The opposite of open panel HMOs are **closed panel HMOs**, also called **staff model HMOs**. These are plans that contract with physicians to provide services to their members, exclusively. Physicians are not allowed to see patients from other managed care plans. Physicians in this model type are actually employees of the HMO and receive a salary as reimbursement. In addition, the medical facilities and equipment are also owned by the HMO for use by its members. These facilities may include medical offices, pharmacies, diagnostic testing facilities (such as laboratory and radiology), and even hospitals.

   C. *Group Model HMO.* The **group model HMO** resembles the closed panel model. In the group model, instead of contracting with physicians to provide exclusive services in the HMO's facilities, the HMO has an exclusive contract with a medical group practice. Physicians of the medical group provide services to the members of the plan. The physicians, however, are employed by the group practice, not the HMO. These physicians are reimbursed for their services according to the arrangements they have made with the group practice: salary, fee-for-service, or other compensation.

From the HMO models discussed, it is clear to see that patients must receive services only from authorized providers. This is referred to as receiving **in-network benefits**. In the case of HMOs, receiving services out-of-network generally means there are no covered benefits, and the patient will pay out-of-pocket for those services.

The demand for more flexibility and choice brought about some variations in managed care plans. The variations relieved some of the restrictions, but the plans still had limitations. Others offered in-network and out-of-network options that left the decision up to the patient regarding which way to use the plan without losing all benefits. The following plans represent more flexible managed care options in common use today.

2. **Participating Provider Organizations.** Participating Provider Organizations (PPOs) are also called Preferred Provider Organizations. PPOs are physicians and facilities, such as hospitals, that have agreed to provide services to patients on a discounted fee schedule. In addition to the reimbursement the provider receives from the insurance company, the patient may have a co-payment and deductible to pay as well. In this model, the patient has a choice when selecting physicians, including specialists, without first consulting a PCP. Compared to HMOs, the out-of-pocket cost is higher for the patient. In order to receive the best benefit, selecting physicians that are in-network is required. Some PPO plans do allow the patient to receive services out-of-network; however, benefits may be greatly reduced, resulting in much higher out-of-pocket expenses for the patient.

3. **Point-of-Service Plans.** These plans are much like being covered by two or three types of plans. Point-of-Service plans (POSs) include an in-network component and an out-of-network component. The in-network component is typically set up like an HMO, requiring a PCP and referrals. It may also include a plan that works like a PPO, allowing choice of physicians who participate, without requiring a PCP. In both cases, the patient normally is responsible for a co-payment. The out-of-network component works like an indemnity plan, with choice of any physician outside of the POS plan; however, there are higher out-of-pocket costs to the patient through deductibles and co-insurance.

CONSUMER-DRIVEN HEALTH PLANS

In simple terms, **Consumer Driven Health Care (CDHC)** refers to high-deductible health insurance plans (HDHP) that are paired with targeted tax-advantage accounts that are used to pay for unreimbursed medical expenses. Examples of such targeted accounts include **Health Savings Accounts (HSAs)**, **Health Reimbursement Arrangements (HRAs)**, or similar type accounts that pay for routine health care expenses directly, while an High-Deductible Health Insurance Policy (HDHP) provides protection from catastrophic medical expenses, much as a major-medical plan does. **Major medical** covers expenses for catastrophic illness or accidents that go beyond what is covered by basic insurance or funds available in arrangement agreements. If the funds in the account run out, the insured pays for medical expenses, like a regular deductible, usually up to a predetermined limit. If the funds are not used, the balance is carried over to the next year and is cumulatively available in the future towards medical expenses.

These plans are attractive in that they offer the ability to see any doctor without requiring approval from a PCP. Procedures often do not require pre-authorization, and many other restrictions do not exist. However, the patient has the responsibility for overseeing how health care dollars are spent. The funds for medical costs are provided through contributions made by either the employer or the insured, depending on the plan.

In addition to the previously mentioned Health Savings Accounts (HSAs), and Health Reimbursement Arrangements/Accounts (HRAs), Consumer Driven Health Care (CDHC) plans may also include **Health Care Flexible Spending Accounts (FSAs)** and the **Archer Medical Savings**

Accounts (MSA), or, Archer MSA. The main focus of Consumer Driven Health Care (CDHC) plans is controlling costs by having the insured more actively participate with how and when available funds are used. Because many employers are now offering HRAs and people are seriously opting for them, you should be prepared for patients who have this plan by becoming familiar with its typical features. Very often, HRAs are confused with MSAs and FSAs. The following offers an overview of these accounts to help clarify important differences.

Health Reimbursement Arrangements (HRAs)

A HRA is an arrangement between an employer and the insured that provides funds for health care expenses. In the HRA model, employers contribute a set dollar amount for medical spending for each insured (employee). The insured uses the employer's money for qualified health care expenses, as needed, up to the specified limit. If the money is not used, or there is some left, it can be rolled over to the next year.

With some plans, various levels may exist. In the first level, the insured uses the employer's money. If the money is used up, the insured progresses to the next level and must pay for all expenses out-of-pocket, capped at a set amount. After that, the major-medical portion goes into effect to cover further medical costs. Typically, the major-medical portion is much like an indemnity plan and pays a percentage, such as 80 percent. The insured is responsible for the remaining co-insurance. The plan may also offer in-network physicians to the insured, which results in lower out-of-pocket co-insurance costs. In order to keep patients motivated to seek medical services, HRAs may cover preventative care at 100 percent without it counting against the money contributed by the employer.

Is there a deductible with HRA plans? Technically, there is. The deductible is considered to be the amount of money contributed by the employer, and any out-of-pocket amount paid by the insured, before access to benefits under the major-medical portion is available. For an illustration of a sample HRA plan, see Figure 4-1.

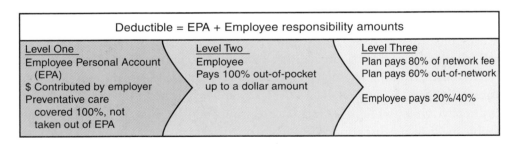

FIGURE 4-1

Example of an HRA plan. *Delmar/Cengage Learning*

Health Savings Accounts (HSAs)

Health Savings Accounts (HSAs) were established as part of the Medicare Prescription Drug, Improvement, and Modernization Act, which was signed into law by President George W. Bush on December 8, 2003. It was developed to replace the Medical Savings Account (MSAs). An HSA is a special savings account into which an employee can contribute a portion of pretax pay. The employee owns the HSA account and can take it with him or her when changing jobs. Money deposited, and any interest earned on the account, can be withdrawn and used to pay non-covered medical expenses, free of tax. Funds may be contributed to an HSA account by any person with a qualifying high-deductible insurance plan (HDIP). If the funds are not spent, they can be rolled over and accumulate for future use.

Medical Savings Accounts or Archer Medical Savings Accounts (MSAs or Archer MSA)

The Medical Savings Account (MSA) was a precursor to HSAs, which have basically replaced it. Existing MSAs were grandfathered. The MSA for the self-employed is now referred to as the *Archer MSA* by the IRS. Congressman Bill Archer of Texas sponsored the HIPAA amendment that created the accounts in 1996.

Like the HSA, the account holder of an MSA can make contributions to the account only if it is paired with a qualifying High Deductible Health Plan (HDIP) and no other coverage. Contributions made by the employer are tax exempt, and the contributions made by the account holder are tax deductible. Either the employer or the account owner can make deposits, but not both. The MSA was primarily for the self-employed or the employees of small businesses of less than 50 employees. Additionally, no matter who contributed money into the MSA, employer or employee, the employee owns the MSA funds and can take the money when employment ends.

Health Flexible Spending Accounts (FSAs)

Health Flexible Spending Accounts (FSAs) are another type of arrangement between employers and employees. Only employers can set up these accounts, and the employee typically contributes to it. FSAs provide a means for employees to put aside money for medical expenses that might not otherwise be reimbursed. This can include deductibles, co-insurance, dental, and vision care. Like the MSA, Health Flexible Spending Accounts (FSAs) are usually offered in combination with a medical plan, but this is not a requirement.

The main drawback with the FSA is that rollover of unused funds into the next year is not permitted, although a two-and-a-half month extension into the next year may now be permitted by the employer. In addition, a one-time roll-over of funds into an HSA is permitted. If the money is not used, the employee loses the funds. Also, the employer can keep the money that is not used, despite it being provided by the employee. Consult Figure 4-2 to study the differences between FSAs, HRAs, HSAs, and the Archer MSA.

MEDICARE AND MEDICAID

It is interesting to note that while there is much debate and speculation today about a national health care program that provides coverage for all, significant discussion actually started in 1937. At that time, Senator Robert Wagner introduced a bill to create the National Health Act of 1939. The bill closely resembled the future Medicare; however, it never made it out of committee. Even at that time, there was much argument and resistance to a socialized medicine program in the United States.

In 1945, President Harry S. Truman proposed a comprehensive, prepaid medical insurance plan for all people through the Social Security system. Two decades of debate on this subject ensued, resulting in amendments and bills along the way that would shape the major portions of Medicare and Medicaid by 1965. On July 1, 1966, only persons over age 65 were automatically covered for hospital insurance provisions under Medicare. Later, inclusion of additional coverage for medical services would follow. Originally, Medicare covered Americans age 65 and older, who at the time represented the largest segment of the uninsured in the United States. In 1972, it was expanded to include Americans with disabilities. Also in 1972, Congress passed legislation authorizing the End Stage Renal Disease (ESRD) program under Medicare.

It is important to remember that Medicare is an insurance program and not a health delivery system. Medicare pays for the cost of hospital or medical services, but does not employ or manage the

	Health Care Flexible Spending Accounts (FSA)	Health Reimbursement Accounts (HRA)	Health Savings Accounts (HSA)	Medical Savings Accounts (Archer MSA)
Eligibility	Employees whose employers offer this benefit. Former employees may be included. Employers are not restricted by size.	Employees whose employers offer this benefit. Former employees may be included. Employers are not restricted by size.	Individuals with qualifying insurance. Ineligible individuals may keep previously established accounts but cannot make contributions.	Individuals with qualifying health insurance who are employees of a small employer (50 or fewer workers) with a high deductible plan or self-employed. Ineligible individuals may keep previously established accounts but cannot make contributions.
Definition of Qualifying Health Insurance	No health insurance requirements.	No health insurance requirements, although HRAs are usually combined with high deductible health insurance.	Self-only deductible must be at least $1,150; the family deductible must be at least $2,300. Annual out-of-pocket expenses for covered benefits cannot exceed $5,800 for self-only coverage and $11,600 for family coverage. Deductible need not apply to preventative care.	Self-only deductible must be at least $2,000 but not over $3,000; the family deductible must be at least $4,000 but not over $6,050. Annual out-of-pocket expenses for covered benefits cannot exceed $4,000 and $7,350 respectively. Deductible need not apply to preventative care if absence of deductible is required by state law.
Contributions	By employer, employee, or both. Usually funded by employee through salary reduction agreement.	Only by employer.	By any person on behalf of an eligible individual.	By employer or account owner, but not both.
Annual Contribution Limits	None required, though employers usually impose a limit.	None required. Employers usually set their contributions below the annual deductible of the accompanying health insurance.	$3,000 for self-only coverage and $5,950 for family coverage. Account owners 55 years old or older and not in Medicare can contribute an additional $1,000 in 2009.	65% of the deductible for self-only coverage and 75% of the deductible for family coverage.
Qualifying Expenses	Most unreimbursed medical expenses, though employers may impose additional limitations. May not be used for long-term care or health insurance premiums.	Most unreimbursed medical expenses, though employers may impose additional limitations. May be used for long-term care and health insurance premiums, if the employer allows.	Most unreimbursed medical expenses. May be used for premiums for long-term care insurance, COBRA, health insurance for those receiving unemployment compensation under federal or state law, and health insurance (other than Medigap policies) for individuals who are 65 years of age and older.	Most unreimbursed medical expenses. May be used for premiums for long-term care insurance, COBRA, and health insurance for those receiving unemployment compensation under federal or state law.
Allowable Non-medical Withdrawals	None	None	Permitted, subject to income tax and 10% penalty except in cases of disability, death, or attaining age 65.	Permitted, subject to income tax and 15% penalty except in cases of disability, death, or attaining age 65.
Carryover of Unused Funds	Balances remaining at year's end (or up to 2½ months after year's end, if employer permits) are forfeited to employer. A limited, one-time rollover to an HAS is allowed.	Permitted, although some employers limit amount that can be rolled over. A limited, one-time rollover to an HAS is allowed.	Full amount may be carried over indefinitely.	Full amount may be carried over indefinitely.
Portability	Balances generally forfeited at termination, although COBRA extensions sometimes apply.	At discretion of employer, though subject to COBRA provisions.	Portable.	Portable.

FIGURE 4-2

providers (i.e., physicians and facilities) who administer care. Compare this to the Veterans Health Administration, which does pay for the cost of care and also provides the facilities and employs the physicians who deliver that care.

Those covered by Medicare are called beneficiaries, not policyholders. Until 1977, the Social Security Administration (SSA) administered the Medicare and Medicaid programs; then the Health Care Finance Administration (HCFA) was created to take over the task. In 2001, as a result of reforms that took place under President William J. Clinton, HCFA was renamed the **Centers for Medicare & Medicaid Services (CMS)**, which now serves the needs of Medicare and Medicaid beneficiaries.

IMPORTANT DETAILS ABOUT MEDICARE

Eligibility for Medicare is determined based on the following:

1. The beneficiary is 65 years or older and has worked for at least 10 years in Medicare-covered employment. United States citizenship or permanent legal residence for five continuous years is also required.

2. Social Security or Railroad Retirement Board disability benefits have been collected for at least 24 months.

3. The beneficiary is undergoing dialysis for permanent kidney failure or requires a kidney transplant (no waiting period required).

4. The beneficiary is diagnosed with Amyotrophic Lateral Sclerosis (ALS), also known as Lou Gehrig's disease (no waiting period required).

Medicare is divided into two parts: Part A and Part B. **Medicare Part A** covers inpatient hospital, skilled nursing facility, home health, and hospice care. **Medicare Part B** covers professional services that are reasonable and medically necessary. This includes physician services, laboratory and x-ray services, durable medical equipment (e.g., wheelchairs, walkers, hospital beds), ambulance services, outpatient hospital care, blood, and medical supplies. You may have also heard of Medicare Part C and Medicare Part D. Medicare Part C, or the Medicare Advantage (MA) plans, will be discussed later in this unit. Medicare Part D subsidizes the cost of prescription drugs for Medicare beneficiaries and was part of the Medicare Prescription Drug, Improvement, and Modernization Act of 2003 and took effect in January of 2006.

THE ORIGINAL MEDICARE PLAN—PART B

Original Medicare Part B works like a traditional fee-for-service indemnity plan. Under Part B for medical services, Medicare pays 80 percent of the approved charges and the beneficiary pays the other 20 percent. Currently, there is a $135.00 deductible that must be met every year. Patients with Original Medicare often purchase Medigap insurance. **Medigap** is coverage that helps pay for the deductible and co-insurance and other "gaps" in coverage in the Medicare plan. Medigap can be sold only in 12 standardized plans, referred to as plans A through L. The chart in Figure 4-3 shows the "gaps" covered by each Medigap plan. While the plans are standardized so that the same coverage is available regardless of which insurance carrier sells it, not every plan is available in all areas.

Once Medicare pays on a claim as the primary insurance, Medigap is billed as secondary and considers the remaining balance for payment. Instead of Medigap, some beneficiaries have employer group plans that are converted to supplemental policies to Medicare after retirement. When a Medicare beneficiary has Medicare only, the deductible and the co-insurance for all approved procedures must be

2009 Medicare Supplement Benefit	A	B	C	D	E	F*	G	H	I	J*	K	L
Medicare Part A Coinsurance and MediGap Coverage for Hospital Benefits	✓	✓	✓	✓	✓	✓	✓	✓	✓	✓	✓	✓
Medicare Part B Coinsurance or Co-payment	✓	✓	✓	✓	✓	✓	✓	✓	✓	✓	50%	75%
Blood (First Three Pints)	✓	✓	✓	✓	✓	✓	✓	✓	✓	✓	50%	75%
Hospice Care Coinsurance or Co-payment											50%	75%
Skilled Nursing Coinsurance			✓	✓	✓	✓	✓	✓	✓	✓	50%	75%
Medicare Part A Deductible		✓	✓	✓	✓	✓	✓	✓	✓	✓		
Medicare Part B Deductible			✓			✓				✓		
Medicare Part B Excess Charges						✓	80%		✓	✓		
Foreign Travel Emergency (Up to Plan Limits)			✓	✓	✓	✓	✓	✓	✓	✓		
At-Home Recovery (Up to Plan Limits)				✓			✓		✓	✓		
Preventive Care Coinsurance (Included in the Part B Coinsurance)	✓	✓	✓	✓	✓	✓	✓	✓	✓	✓	✓	✓
Preventive Care Not Covered by Medicare (Up to $120)					✓					✓		
2009 out-of-pocket limit:											$4,620**	$2,310**

*Medicare Supplement Plans F and J also have a high deductible option. **We don't recommend the high deductible plans.** If you select the high deductible plans you have to pay the first $2,000 (deductible in 2009) in MediGap-covered costs before the MediGap policy pays anything. You must also pay a separate deductible for foreign travel emergency ($250 per year).

**After you meet your out-of-pocket yearly limit and your $135 yearly Part B deductible, the plan pays 100% of covered services for the rest of the calendar year.

FIGURE 4-3

Medigap benefits offered with plans A through L. *Courtesy of the Centers for Medicare & Medicaid Services*

Financial Hardship Disclosure

Under Medicare law, physicians are required to collect any unpaid portion of the $135.00 annual Part B deductible and the 20 percent co-insurance from the Medicare beneficiary.

One condition that may permit the physician to waive the collection of these amounts is financial hardship. Based on discussions with you, the physician has determined that due to your financial hardship, you are unable to pay the unpaid portion of your deductible and/or the 20 percent co-insurance. Due to these circumstances, the physician waives your obligation for payment of the following services:

Service: _____ Charge: $ _____ Date: _____

Service: _____ Charge: $ _____ Date: _____

Service: _____ Charge: $ _____ Date: _____

Disclosure and Agreement:

"I understand that the physician is waiving the collection of the Medicare co-insurance and/or deductible amounts in my case due to financial hardship. I also understand that the physician can and will begin to attempt to collect charges should my financial situation improve."

Signature of Beneficiary: _____ Date: _____

Signature of Physician: _____ Date: _____

FIGURE 4-4

Medicare financial hardship exception form. *Courtesy of the Centers for Medicare & Medicaid Services*

collected. Medicare does not permit physicians to simply write off these amounts unless a true financial hardship exists. Even then, the hardship must be documented in the beneficiary's record in order to justify the write-off by using the Medicare Financial Hardship Exception Form, shown in Figure 4-4.

Assignment and the Original Medicare Plan

Medicare Part B uses a fee schedule to determine how much will be approved for services billed. Medicare informs physicians exactly how much will be approved. When the physician or supplier agrees to accept the approved amount as their full fee, this is called **accepting assignment**. Assignment only affects services provided under Medicare Part B.

Each year, physicians who provide services to Medicare beneficiaries must decide whether they will be participating providers. The medical administrative staff needs to be aware of the physician's participating status, because this affects information that must be submitted on the claim regarding assignment and how much the beneficiary pays out of pocket. There are three situations regarding physician participation in Medicare:

1. Physicians *can participate* with Medicare, meaning they sign a contract and are required to accept assignment for all Medicare patients. These physicians are usually referred to as PAR, or participating.

2. Physicians *can choose not to participate* with Medicare, but will still be subject to certain rules for reimbursement. These physicians are usually referred to as non-PAR, or non-participating. Non-PAR physicians can choose to accept assignment or not on a case-by-case basis. If they choose to accept assignment, Medicare will reduce the approved amount by 5 percent. Consider this a "penalty" for being a non-PAR physician, despite the fact that assignment has been accepted. If the physician does not accept assignment, there is a cap, called the **limiting charge (Medicare)**, on the amount that can be charged above Medicare's approved amount.

3. Physicians *can make private arrangements with the patient* and bypass Medicare. In other words, the physician can privately contract to provide services and be paid the agreed upon fee directly by the patient. Medicare will not be billed. Neither the physician nor the patient will be reimbursed by the Medicare plan.

The choice a physician makes in regard to participation and assignment has a direct impact on reimbursement. For the medical staff, it may be necessary to educate patients on the amounts they owe based on the choices made by the physician. It also impacts how payments and adjustments are posted to patient accounts. The examples that follow help illustrate these points.

Example A

Mrs. Jones, a Medicare patient, receives a service with a standard fee of $150.00. Her physician is PAR with Medicare and is required to accept assignment.

Standard fee:	$150.00
Medicare Approved:	$100.00
Medicare pays (80%):	$ 80.00
Patient co-insurance (20%):	$ 20.00

Because the physician accepts assignment, and is PAR with Medicare, the difference between the standard fee and the Medicare approved amount ($50.00) will be written off the account. The patient pays the co-insurance of $20.00. Total reimbursement to the physician is $80.00 from Medicare and $20.00 from the patient, which equals the total amount approved by Medicare: $100.00.

Example B

Mr. Smith, a Medicare patient, receives a service with a standard fee of $150.00. His physician is non-PAR with Medicare and accepts assignment.

Standard fee:	$150.00
Medicare Approved: (Reduced 5%)	$ 95.00
Medicare pays (80%):	$ 76.00
Patient co-insurance (20%):	$ 19.00

In this example, remember that even though the physician accepted assignment, the physician does not participate with Medicare. Because of this, the approved amount was reduced by 5 percent ($100.00 − 5% = $95.00). Medicare then pays 80 percent of $95.00 ($76.00). The patient is responsible only for the remaining 20 percent co-insurance ($19.00). In this situation, the total reimbursement to the physician is $95.00. The difference between the standard fee ($150.00) and the approved amount ($95.00) will be written off the account: $55.00.

Example C

Ms. White, a Medicare patient, receives a service with a standard fee of $150.00. Her physician is non-PAR with Medicare and does not accept assignment.

Standard fee:	$150.00
Limiting Charge (cap):	$109.25
Medicare Approved:	$ 95.00
(Reduced 5%)	
Medicare pays (80%):	$ 76.00
Patient co-insurance (20%):	$ 19.00

Because the physician did not accept assignment, and is non-PAR, he can collect up to 15 percent above Medicare's approved amount from the patient. This is the limiting charge; in this example a total of $109.25. The patient is responsible for paying the co-insurance ($19.00) and the difference between the limiting charge and the approved amount ($14.25) for a total of $33.25. Although the physician is entitled to receive the $76.00 payment, Medicare will send the payment directly to the patient for all unassigned claims. The physician will need to collect the $76.00 Medicare payment from the patient. The difference between the limiting charge and the standard fee is written off the account ($40.75).

It is clear to see that the patient in Example C paid more out-of-pocket than the patient in Example A for the same service. This was completely dependent on whether the physician accepted assignment or not. It is also clear that posting of the payment is affected by assignment choices. This is another excellent example of how practice management software can help keep track of fees and approved amounts, and simplify making adjustments for write-off amounts. In the case of Original Medicare, the approved amounts for procedures are made available to the office through a fee schedule, which is released annually. Fee schedules can be loaded into the database to correctly calculate fees and write offs based on whether the physician accepts assignment or not.

As a final note, there are situations where all physicians, regardless of participation, must accept assignment for Medicare patients. These include Medicare-covered laboratory services, ambulance services, and certain drugs or supplies.

MEDICARE ADVANTAGE (MA) PLANS

Medicare Advantage (MA) plans are part of the Medicare program and are sometimes referred to as **Medicare Part C**. Medicare Advantage (MA) plans are health plan options that are approved by Medicare, but are run by private companies. These plans must provide all of the coverage available with Original Medicare, and may even offer additional services not covered by Original Medicare. If a beneficiary chooses to use an Medicare Advantage (MA) plan, the rules of the plan must be followed, and the procedures for using Original Medicare do not apply. The beneficiary in no way loses his or her Original Medicare; in fact, he or she can go back to that coverage if desired. However, while enrolled in an Medicare Advantage (MA) plan, the rules of the chosen plan are in effect.

Nationally, there are currently one or more MA plan types available in most areas. MA plans can include choices of Health Management Organisation (HMO), Preferred Provider Organisation (PPO), Private Fee-for-Service (PFFS), or Medical Savings Accounts (MSA) plans, as well as Medicare Special Needs Plans (Medicare SNP). Some of the plans require referrals to see specialists, and typically have a network of physicians and facilities from which the patient must receive services in order to be covered. Such facilities include hospitals, diagnostic centers (such as for X-rays, scanning, and laboratories), physical and occupational therapy providers, etc.

In most cases, the premiums and cost of services, such as co-payments and deductibles, are lower than in Original Medicare. Costs to the patient can be significantly lower than having Original Medicare with a secondary Medigap policy. The plans provide Part A (hospital) and Part B (medical) coverage for medically necessary services. Often, there are extra benefits, and many include prescription drug coverage. Costs for prescription drug coverage can be lower than in the stand-alone Part D Medicare Prescription Drug plans. Medicare SNPs go a step further. They are Medicare Advantage (MA) plans that limit membership to people with specific diseases or conditions. Medicare SNPs customize beneficiary benefits, providers, and drug formularies (a list of covered drugs) to best meet the specific needs of those they serve.

If a patient enrolls in an Medicare Advantage (MA) plan, there is no need to have a supplemental Medigap policy. However, the beneficiary continues to pay the Medicare premium, and in addition, pays an extra premium for the Medicare Advantage (MA) plan. These plans often have a co-payment requirement for primary physician and specialist physician care, as well as for other services, such as emergency, hospital, and skilled nursing facility services. Typical co-payment amounts are $10.00 for a primary physician visit and $30.00 for a specialist visit. As with all patients covered by managed care plans, the payment of the co-pay is expected at the time of the office visit.

THE MEDICAID PROGRAM

The **Medicaid** Program is also known as **Title XIX**, or Title 19, of the Social Security Act. In California, this program is called Medi-Cal. Medicaid is a federal/state entitlement program that provides medical assistance for families and individuals with low incomes and limited resources. The federal government establishes general guidelines for the program; however, Medicaid requirements are established by each state. Eligibility for Medicaid depends on guidelines from the state where the person applying lives.

Within federally imposed limits and restrictions, each state determines the rate of payment and method of payment. Some states pay using a fee-for-service method; others employ prepaid methods, such as HMOs. Rates of payment vary widely among states. However, regardless of the method, each participating Medicaid provider must accept payment rates as payment-in-full for services rendered to recipients.

It is important to note that some states may have deductibles, co-payments, and other cost-share arrangements for some services covered under Medicaid. However, certain Medicaid recipients are exempt. These include children under the age of 18, pregnant women, and hospital or nursing home patients who spend most of their income on institutional care. Recent policy discussions in government are looking at ways to change Medicaid, including allowing states to increase the amounts low-income beneficiaries are charged, through ways such as premiums, deductibles, co-payments, and co-insurance. Supporters of these changes believe they will make Medicaid more like private health insurance, and encourage beneficiaries to participate in a larger share of their health costs.

Medicare beneficiaries may also have Medicaid if they meet low income criteria that qualify them for coverage. In some areas, patients with both Medicare and Medicaid coverage are referred to as "Medi-Medi," or "care-caid" beneficiaries. If the beneficiary qualifies for full Medicaid coverage, Medicaid may provide supplemental coverage for items such as prescription drugs, eyeglasses, and hearing aids, in addition to extending certain benefits available under Medicare.

Medicare is the first payer for persons who have coverage under both Medicare and Medicaid. This means that Medicare is billed first, and pays on approved services before Medicaid makes any payments. As a general rule, Medicaid is always the second payer if the patient is covered by another health plan, because Medicaid is considered the "payer of last resort."

INSURANCE PLANS USED FOR BOOK SIMULATIONS

Now that the fundamentals of common insurance plans have been reviewed, the following section introduces the simulated medical insurance plans used in this book. Exercises have been prepared using these insurance plans and are much like the ones discussed thus far in this unit. They are intended to resemble actual plans used by patients in medical offices today. By becoming familiar with these insurance plans, you will apply your knowledge to the software provided with this book in order to bill and send claims to insurance companies. Later, you will post payments and adjustments according to the requirements of each plan. By doing so, you will not only reinforce how common insurance plans work, but also how to handle the transactions using practice management software.

FLEXIHEALTH PPO PLAN

FlexiHealth is a PPO plan used in the book simulations. It offers in-network and out-of-network benefits. Study the benefits chart for the FlexiHealth PPO plan in Figure 4-5 to become familiar with coverage details.

FlexiHealth PPO Plan Benefits at a Glance		
Provision	**Benefits: In-Network**	**Benefits: Out-of-Network**

Deductible
  Individual
  Family
	
	$200/hospital care
	$400/hospital care
		
		$400
		$600

Office Visits	$20.00 co-payment	Pays 80% after deductible
Hospital Care	Pays 80% after deductible	Pays 50% after deductible
Hospital Pre-Authorization	Required	Required
Emergency Care	$50.00 co-payment, waived if admitted, pays 80% after deductible hospital care	$50.00 co-payment, waived if admitted, pays 50% after deductible hospital care

Mental Health
  Inpatient Facility
 	
  Outpatient Facility
	
	Pays 80% after deductible, up to 30 days combined in- and out-of-network
	
	$20 co-payment up to 60 visits per year, combined in- and out-of-network
		
		Pays 50% after deductible, up to 30 days combined in- and out-of-network
		
		Pays 50% after deductible up to 60 visits per year, combined in- and out-of-network

Specialist Office Visits	$30.00 co-payment	Pays 80% after deductible

FIGURE 4-5

Flexihealth PPO. *Delmar/Cengage Learning*

Dr. Heath is a participating physician with this plan. Patients who receive services from her are subject to the in-network benefits column. Dr. Schwartz does not participate with this plan; however, there are patients who receive services from him and are covered by FlexiHealth PPO. When they do see Dr. Schwartz, they are subject to the out-of-network benefits column. When reviewing the out-of-network column, notice that the coverage is set up much like an indemnity plan.

SIGNAL HMO PLAN

Both Dr. Heath and Dr. Schwartz participate with the Signal HMO plan. Patients must use in-network providers in order for services to be covered. Study the benefits chart for the Signal HMO plan in Figure 4-6 to become familiar with coverage details. Most services require a co-payment from the insured.

Signal HMO Plan Benefits at a Glance	
Provision	**Benefits: In-Network Only**

Deductible
  Individual
  Family
	N/A
	N/A

Office Visits (PCP) Specialists (Referred by PCP)	$10.00 co-payment $30.00 co-payment
Outpatient Surgery	$50.00 co-payment
Hospital Care	$100 co-payment per hospitalization
Hospital Pre-Authorization	Required (arranged by PCP)
Emergency Care	$50.00 co-payment, waived if admitted

Mental Health
  Inpatient Facility
 	
  Outpatient Facility
	No co-payment up to 45 days
	
	$20 co-payment up to 50 visits per year

Specialist Office Visit	$25.00 co-payment

FIGURE 4-6

Signal HMO. *Delmar/Cengage Learning*

MEDICARE

Since Douglasville Medicine Associates is a family practice, both physicians have many patients age 65 and older who are covered by Medicare. These patients may have Medicare as their only coverage; others will have Medicare and Medicaid. Patients may have a supplemental plan, such as a Medigap or a private plan from a previous employer.

Dr. Heath participates with Medicare and is required to take assignment on all Medicare patients. Dr. Schwartz does not participate and will inform the staff on a case-by-case basis which patients he will accept assignment on. If needed, review the sections regarding Medicare and assignment discussed earlier in this unit. Remember, the non-PAR physician's choice where assignment is concerned affects charges for services, out-of-pocket amounts due from beneficiaries, and payment-posting procedures.

CENTURY SENIORGAP PLAN

Patients of Douglasville Medicine Associates who have Medicare coverage and a Medigap supplement will have a plan called Century SeniorGap. This Medigap plan is available from a local insurance carrier in Douglasville and is a Plan C. Review the chart in Figure 4-3 under Plan C to see which additional benefits are covered by this supplemental policy.

CONSUMERONE HRA

Major employers in the Douglasville area offer an Health Reimbursement Arrangement (HRA) plan to its employees, called ConsumerONE. Both Dr. Heath and Dr. Schwartz have decided to participate as in-network providers for enrolled members. As part of their agreement, they have accepted the network fee schedule as payment-in-full for services. A standard claim form will be submitted to ConsumerONE by the medical office for the patient.

Study the chart in Figure 4-7 under the in-network benefits column. The employer contributes $1,000.00 every year to the Employee Personal Account (EPA). Since the medical office bills the HRA and receives payment directly, patients generally do not pay anything at the time of service. If any

ConsumerOne HRA Benefits at a Glance		
Provision	**In-Network**	**Out-of-Network**
LEVEL ONE Health care services determined to be medically appropriate by the carrier, according to patient diagnosis.	100% of charges up to the network fee schedule. Insured not responsible for amount above network fees. Funds available: $1,000 (Employer contribution to EPA–Employee Personal Account). Any money left in the EPA at year's end is rolled over into next year's EPA.	100% of the charges up to the network fee schedule. Insured responsible for the difference between network fee and provider's standard fee.
Preventative Care (Annual exams, annual flu and pneumoccal vaccinations, cholesterol, colonscopy and fecal blood, mammogram and PAP smear, and Well-Child Care services).	Covered 100%, not taken out of EPA.	Covered 100% at network fee schedule, insured responsible for difference between network fee and provider's standard fee.
LEVEL TWO If EPA account is exhausted, insured pays up to $500 maximum out of pocket for medical expenses.	Insured pays 100% of network fee schedule.	Insured pays 100% of provider's standard fee.
LEVEL THREE If Level One and Level Two are exhausted (preventative care not included), Indemnity coverage begins.	Pays 80% of network fee schedule, insured pays 20% co-insurance.	Pays 60% of network fee schedule, insured pays 40% co-insurance plus difference up to standard fee.

Both Drs. Heath and Schwartz are in-network providers for ConsumerONE HRA.

FIGURE 4-7

ConsumerONE HRA. *Delmar/Cengage Learning*

of this money is not used, it rolls over and becomes available in next year's EPA and another $1,000.00 is added by the employer. Accordingly, it is possible for the insured to accumulate money in the EPA towards health care costs.

If all of the money in the EPA is exhausted, the coverage progresses to Level Two. Notice that in Level Two, the insured is expected to pay $500.00 out-of-pocket toward services. This, in addition to the employer's contribution, is considered the deductible. If all of the money in the EPA is used, and the insured pays for the next $500.00 of services out-of-pocket, the deductible is now met. Coverage is then available as an indemnity plan in Level Three and pays 80 percent of the network fee schedule. The insured pays the 20 percent co-insurance portion. When using an in-network provider, the insured does not pay for amounts greater than the network fee schedule.

At first glance, the HRA plan appears to be complicated, but in reality it is innovative and relatively straightforward. Because there are three levels that affect reimbursement, one might wonder how the medical office knows which patients are at what level. After all, one patient may have few medical problems and a large EPA fund, and another can experience unexpected illness or injury and be in Level Three within a few weeks! The key is tracking the explanation of benefits from the HRA. If a payment is denied based on EPA funds being exhausted, notification of the insured going to Level Two or Level Three, as applicable, is made known to the medical office. The medical office sends an invoice to the insured for any balance due. The insured has access to information regarding how much money is left in the EPA, and at which level of coverage he or she is. This information is made available to the insured in the form of quarterly statements, online via the member Web site, or by contacting the health plan via telephone or mail. In addition, many of the consumer-driven programs will issue a special credit card to be used for medical expenses that draw from the funds available to the patient from their plan. Remember, the philosophy of an HRA plan is based on giving health care consumers control and responsibility over how their benefit dollars are spent.

FINAL NOTES

The majority of revenue generated at medical facilities comes from payments on medical insurance claims. The importance of accurate billing, good follow-up, and monitoring for proper payments cannot be overemphasized. Every member of the health care delivery team is responsible for some aspect of reimbursement. Physicians and other clinical staff must provide adequate documentation of services in order for accurate coding of procedures and diagnoses to take place. Administrative staff must be diligent in obtaining updated and accurate demographic and insurance information on patients. Billers and collectors must follow guidelines and laws for insurance billing, assuring claims are complete and accurate. Patients must be educated about their responsibilities, and how they can assist so that proper reimbursement can be secured for services they receive.

Having a good understanding of the basic types of medical insurance plans, their architecture, and related terminology provides a good foundation of knowledge. As you have learned, there are a vast number of health plans, yet most are based on the basic principles of examples discussed in this unit. This knowledge will not only help you with details in your work, but also in understanding how practice management software processes information related to various medical insurances.

In 1 through 7, select the correct definition for each type of medical insurance plan from the following list.

   a. A federal program that provides health insurance primarily for those age 65 and older, and persons with chronic disabilities, Amytrophic Lateral Sclerosis (ALS), or End Stage Renal Disease (ESRD) under the age of 65.

   b. Also known as traditional, commercial insurance or fee-for-service plans; a type of health insurance that places no restrictions on which doctors may be used; referrals are not required and most pay a percentage of medical expenses based on a UCR, after an annual deductible is paid by the patient.

   c. Physicians and facilities, such as hospitals, who have agreed to provide services to patients on a discounted fee schedule.

   d. A federal/state entitlement program that provides medical assistance for families and individuals with low incomes and limited resources.

   e. New health plan products that give medical consumers more choices and control over spending by having access to funds reserved for health care.

   f. A type of managed care plan that requires patients to have a gatekeeper, or PCP, in order for health care services to be coordinated and costs to be better controlled.

   g. A type of managed-care plan that includes an in-network and out-of-network component allowing patients to choose how benefits will be used. Broader coverage and less out-of-pocket expense is realized when using services with in-network providers.

1. ___ PPO
2. ___ POS
3. ___ HMO
4. ___ Indemnity plan
5. ___ Medicare
6. ___ Medicaid/Medi-Cal
7. ___ Consumer driven health plans

8. As a general rule, physicians who accept Medicaid patients must accept the payment rate as payment in full for services.

   a. True

   b. False

9. Medigap is an insurance plan that supplements Medicare and helps pay for gaps in coverage.

   a. True

   b. False

10. A Medicare physician who is PAR must accept assignment on all Medicare patients.

   a. True

   b. False

Study the following situation; then answer questions 11 and 12. The patient has an indemnity plan and the physician does not have a contract with the health plan.

Physician standard fee (billed to insurance):	$ 60.00
Insurance UCR/approved:	$ 52.00
Insurance paid 80%:	$ 41.60
Co-insurance:	$ 10.40

11. Based on the information given for this indemnity plan, what is the patient's out-of-pocket responsibility for this service?

    a. $ 8.00

    b. $18.40

    c. $10.40

12. Based on the information provided, what is the total of the non-approved amount?

    a. $ 8.00

    b. $18.40

    c. $10.40

Study the following situation; then answer questions 13 and 14. The patient has Medicare and the physician is PAR.

Standard fee:	$80.00
Medicare Approved:	$75.00
Medicare pays 80%:	$60.00
Co-insurance pays 20%:	$15.00

13. Based on the information provided for this Medicare PAR situation, what is the patient's out-of-pocket responsibility for this service?

    a. $ 5.00

    b. $20.00

    c. $15.00

14. What is the physician's adjustment (write-off) based on the information provided?

    a. $ 5.00

    b. $20.00

    c. $15.00

    d. No adjustment

Study the following situation; then answer questions 15 and 16. The patient has Medicare and the physician is non-PAR and will not be accepting assignment.

Standard fee:	$145.00
Limiting charge (cap):	$135.70
Medicare Approved:	$118.00
(Reduced 5%)	
Medicare pays 80%:	$ 94.40
Co-insurance pays 20%:	$ 23.60

15. What is the physician's adjustment (write-off) based on the information provided?

    a. $41.30

    b. $ 9.30

    c. $27.00

    d. $23.60

16. Based on this Medicare non-PAR situation, where the physician does not accept assignment, what is the patient's out-of-pocket responsibility for this service?

    a. $42.30

    b. $ 9.30

    c. $27.00

    d. $23.60

17. A Medicare physician who accepts assignment is agreeing to

    a. accept the Medicare payment as payment in full.

    b. accept what Medicare approves as the full fee for services.

    c. not charge patients for co-insurance amounts.

    d. not charge patients for the Medicare deductible.

    e. all of the above.

18. A health plan where the employer contributes funds every year for the use of employees towards health care expenses is called a

    a. Health Maintenance Organization plan.

    b. Health Reimbursement Arrangement plan.

    c. Preferred Provider Organization plan.

    d. Flexible Spending Account.

    e. traditional indemnity plan.

19. A single medical plan that provides coverage for a group of people, such as employees, is referred to as

    a. a group plan.

    b. Medicare.

    c. an individual plan.

    d. managed care plans.

    e. none of the above.

20. A system for tracking data related to procedure fees charged and payments accepted by physicians is called

    a. practice management software.

    b. Health Maintenance Organization.

    c. usual and customary rates.

    d. fee-for-service.

    e. none of the above.

21. Describe the differences between Original Medicare and Medicare Adavantage plans.

_____

_____

_____

22. List suggestions for ways of staying up-to-date concerning details related to health care plans, laws, and other pertinent changes related to medical insurance and coding.

_____

_____

_____

23. Explain why it is useful for patients to understand their coverage, limitations, and exclusions, as well as financial responsibilities, as they relate to medical insurance coverage.

_____

_____

_____

24. When comparing indemnity plans to HMOs, PPOs, and POS plans, which ones offer

    a. more flexibility in terms of access to health care? Explain your answer.

_____

_____

    b. lower out-of-pocket costs? Explain your answer.

_____

_____

25. Describe some of the advantages and disadvantages of Health Reimbursement Arrangements (HRAs).

_____

_____

_____

Patient Registration and Data Entry

OBJECTIVES

Upon completion of this unit, the reader should be able to:

- Identify key demographic information from a patient registration form and input data into *Medical Office Simulation Software* (MOSS)

- Review insurance cards for relevant health insurance coverage details and input data into the registration system

- Demonstrate registering new patients using MOSS

- Describe types of medical facilities where patients receive services outside of the physician's office

- Discuss how information is collected for new patients receiving services at facilities outside the physician's office

- Review hospital admission forms and the emergency room record; input information into the registration system.

KEY TERMS

Ambulatory surgical center

Attending physician

Face sheet

Health Insurance Claim number (HIC number)

Health unit coordinator

Hospital

Nursing home

Skilled nursing facility (SNF)

Social Services

Wards

Most people have experienced visiting a doctor for the first time. It is common knowledge that a new patient is required to provide information for the purpose of record keeping and insurance billing. Basic information is obtained, such as address, telephone, employment, and insurance information. If a person other than the patient is financially responsible for health care expenses, information regarding that individual, known as the guarantor, must also be obtained. New patients often expect to fill out several forms, present their insurance cards, and provide medical histories when seeing a new doctor.

You have already learned about the protocols regarding protected health information (PHI) under HIPAA. Protection and proper use of patient information is now law, and special care must be taken to ensure that HIPAA guidelines are followed. Whenever new patients are registered, they need to be advised of the office policies regarding PHI. The privacy notice is given to the patient, a signature of receipt is obtained, and documentation that these steps were completed is generated. Practice management software has been updated to accommodate necessary HIPAA guidelines, including the privacy notice. New software is being introduced that tracks and documents patient information to ensure that it is released properly, and to provide a record of how, when, and to whom information is provided. *Medical Office Simulation Software* (MOSS) provides a sample privacy notice that can be viewed and printed. It also provides an area for documentation in the patient registration system. This will be addressed further in the case studies in this unit.

In the sections that follow, the patient registration process at the front desk is reviewed, and then applied to MOSS.

THE PATIENT REGISTRATION PROCESS

In Unit 2, the patient registration system of practice management software was discussed. This component of the software allows the user to input information about each patient. The following list reviews the steps previously learned regarding registering new patients.

1. The patient is greeted upon arrival at the office.

2. A registration form is given to the patient and any required signatures are obtained.

3. The HIPAA privacy notice is given to the patient to sign after the policies of the office, in regard to PHI, have been explained.

4. A copy (or scan) of the front and back of the insurance card is made for the patient record.

5. Verification of insurance eligibility is done either online or via telephone to ensure the patient has coverage.

6. Assembly of the new patient chart is completed and all required forms and documents are inserted in the file (or data is input on the electronic health record).

7. A superbill is prepared and attached to the front of the patient file.

8. The clinical back-office staff use the superbill to document the procedures and diagnostic codes relevant to the visit.

THE REGISTRATION FORM

All demographic and insurance information on a patient is contained on the registration form. When the patient completes a registration form, it is important for the front desk medical assistant to look it over to ensure it is complete and accurate. The insurance information should be compared to the copies or scans of the insurance card that were made.

It is important to keep alert for clarifications that may be required from the patient. For example, a Medicare patient might have other primary coverage. Patients covered by two health plans also need to inform the physician's office which insurance is primary, and front-office staff should confirm the information. Discrepancies of any kind are best resolved at the time patients are in the office, rather than after they leave.

At times, an elderly patient who has difficulty writing may need assistance completing a registration form. Patients who have difficulty speaking English may need help as well. Preferably, they will be accompanied by a friend or family member who can translate, as needed.

The variety of situations that can exist in the lives of patients is vast. Often, these situations affect the business relationship the medical office has with the patient. Personal issues related to a patient's employment, marital status, and financial situation that affects his or her ability to pay are everyday challenges to be dealt with. Issues with health insurance coverage are also a large factor. Whether this centers on deductibles to be met, co-payments, exclusions, or preauthorization requirements for special procedures, each patient may have a unique issue. It is not uncommon for the medical office staff to participate in educating, guiding, or advising patients, as needed, when these situations have an impact on receiving and paying for medical care.

Because the diversity of patient situations is so great, the simulations and software exercises in this unit have been presented as case studies. Review of the registration forms and insurance cards, including details about the patient's personal situation, are included. Supplemental information that furthers your knowledge about insurance is integrated within the case studies.

LET'S TRY IT! 5-1 REGISTERING NEW OFFICE PATIENTS

Objective: In Unit 3, several new patients were scheduled for appointments with Doctors Heath and Schwartz. The reader will be guided through the registration process for each of those patients as a case study. If you have not yet completed the appointment scheduling exercises contained in the *Let's Try It!* sections of Unit 3, do that now before proceeding.

CASE STUDY 5–A: MONTNER, MARTIN

Today's Date: **October 22, 2009**

New patient: **Montner, Martin**

After being greeted by the office staff, patient Montner is given a registration form to fill out and copies of his insurance card are made. The privacy notice is given to the patient and he is asked to sign, acknowledging receipt. See Figure 2-5, Unit 2, for a sample of the form provided by Douglasville Medicine Associates. He is a full-time college student, and his mother, who is the guarantor and policyholder for the health plan, has accompanied him for his visit today. Martin is complaining of a severe sore throat.

Refer to the Source Documents Appendix at the end of this book. Martin Montner's registration form (Source Document 5-1) and Signal HMO insurance card copy (Source Document 5-2) will be needed for the following exercise.

SPECIAL NOTES REGARDING CASE STUDY 5-A

It is important to recognize that Martin Montner is an adult child and a dependent on a parent's health plan. This is a detail that the office staff should be aware of when reviewing patient information during registration.

Currently, health plans that offer coverage for family members have differing rules about dependent children. Some accept children only up to the age of 18. Others continue coverage for adult children age 19 and older (with an age cap) under specific circumstances.

Case Study 5-A Continues >>

Case Study 5-A Continued

Those circumstances usually require the adult child to be financially dependent on the policyholder, unmarried, and that he or she still lives at home. Even if the adult child is a college student at a boarding school, the child is usually still considered "at home." The new reform bill specifies that beginning on and after September 23, 2010, insurers must provide dependent coverage for adult children up to age 26 for all individual and group policies. Some states have enacted mandates that require coverage for even older children. The specifics of eligibility are still to be defined at the time of this writing.

The majority of health plans require student status as a condition for coverage. Again, different health plans have different requirements. Some cover a college student on part-time status, others only if the student attends full-time. The number of credit hours to be recognized as a part- or full-time student is determined by each health plan and is not the same for all insurances. The policyholder will be required to periodically prove the status of the dependent adult child by providing a form and transcripts from the college or technical school to their Employee Benefits Office.

STEP 1
Carefully review the information on the registration form (Source Document 5-1) and answer the following questions. *Cover the answers using the tear-off bookmark from the cover of your book. Check your work before entering data into MOSS to be sure you have correctly interpreted the source documents.*

A.	What is the patient's date of birth?	**2/10/1989**
B.	Is the patient employed?	**No, he is a student**
C.	What is the patient's marital status?	**Single**
D.	What is the name of the patient's school?	**City Junior College**
E.	How many insurance policies is the patient covered by?	**1**
F.	What is the name of the primary health plan?	**Signal HMO**
G.	What is the policy ID number? Group number?	**ID: 999162133-02** **Group Number: BTPW39**
H.	What is the name of the patient's mother?	**Felicia Anderson**
I.	Where does the patient's mother work?	**Big Top Paper Warehouse**
J.	Does the patient live with his mother?	**Yes**

STEP 2
Compare the insurance card (Source Document 5-2) to the information on the registration form, and then answer the following questions. Identify other information on the card that may be pertinent to a medical office.

A.	Does the information match what is on the form?	**Yes**
B.	Does the patient have a co-payment for office visits? If yes, how much is it?	**$10.00**
C.	Which services require preauthorization?	**Hospitalization**
D.	What is the phone number to call for preauthorization purposes	**800-123-8877**
E.	Who is the patient's PCP?	**Dr. Schwartz**

NT: Click on *Start*, then *grams*, then click on the *tware title* to open it. If a ktop icon is available, you also open the software by king on it.

STEP 3

Start MOSS and use your logon information to begin using the software.

STEP 4

Click on the *Appointment Scheduling* button to open the scheduler. Click on *October 22, 2009* and locate patient "Montner." Double click on his *name* to open the appointment form window. Click in front of *Checked In*. This documents the patient's arrival. Click on the *Close* button when finished, and then close out of the scheduler and return to the Main Menu of MOSS.

STEP 5

Next, on the Main Menu, click on the *Patient Registration* button. Search for Martin Montner using the method of your choice. Be sure to click on the *Select* button, or double click on the patient's *name*. Recall that registration was started at the time the patient made his appointment, so partial information is already in the database.

STEP 6

Using the registration form, enter the data for the Patient Information tab. Compare your work to Figure 5-1 before clicking the *Save* button.

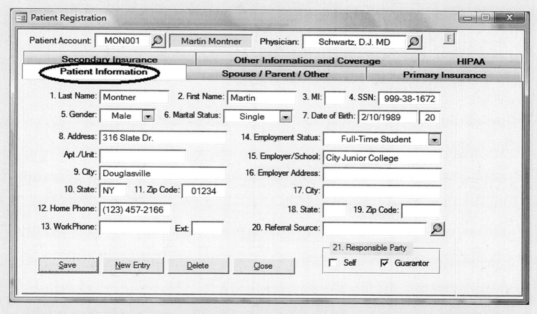

FIGURE 5-1

Delmar/Cengage Learning

MOSS NOTE: MOSS calculates each patient's age based on today's date. Depending on the date you work on your exercises, the age displayed on your screen for a patient may vary from the screen shots in the book.

Case Study 5-A Continues >>

STEP 7

Click on the *Spouse/Parent/Other* tab. Since the guarantor for this patient is his mother, complete the information for Felicia Anderson in Fields 1 through 7. Check your work with Figure 5-2, and then click the *Save* button. Next, click on the *Address* button. Since the patient and his mother live at the same address, click on the *Copy Pt Addr* button to autofill the fields, then close the window. Click on the *Employer* button and enter Felicia's work information. Check your work with Figure 5-3. Click *Close*, then the *Save* button when you are finished.

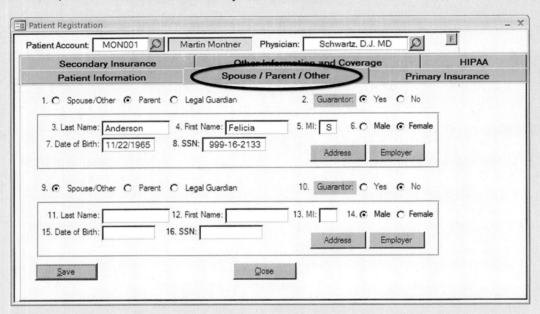

FIGURE 5-2

Delmar/Cengage Learning

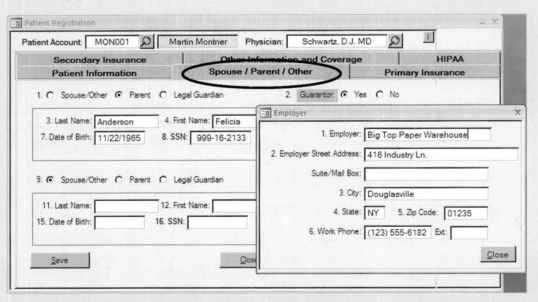

FIGURE 5-3

Delmar/Cengage Learning

STEP 8

Click on the *Primary Insurance* tab. Using the information on the registration form, complete the fields as needed. Include the following data:

A. $10.00 co-payment in Field 12.

NT: See Figure 4-6, Unit 4.

B. Recall that Dr. Schwartz participates with Signal HMO and accepts assignment. Click *Yes* in Fields 13 and 15.

NT: See bottom of registration form.

C. Signatures have been obtained from the insured, click on *Yes* in Field 14.

D. Leave Field 16 blank. This is used only when a patient has a PCP who has referred the patient to be seen by one of the physicians at Douglasville Medicine Associates. Check your work with Figure 5-4, then click the *Save* button when finished.

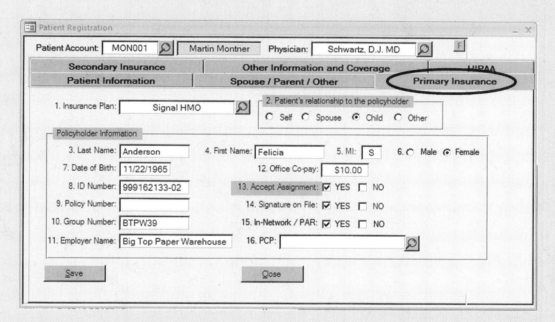

FIGURE 5-4

Delmar/Cengage Learning

STEP 9

Next, click on the *HIPAA* tab. The patient was given a privacy notice, which was signed. In Field 1, click on *Yes*, and then enter the date of signature, "10/22/2009." Check your work with Figure 5-5 before saving it. In order to view the privacy notice for Douglasville Medicine Associates, click on the *Privacy Notice* button. Print the notice so it can be reviewed later.

Case Study 5-A Continues >>

Case Study 5-A Continued

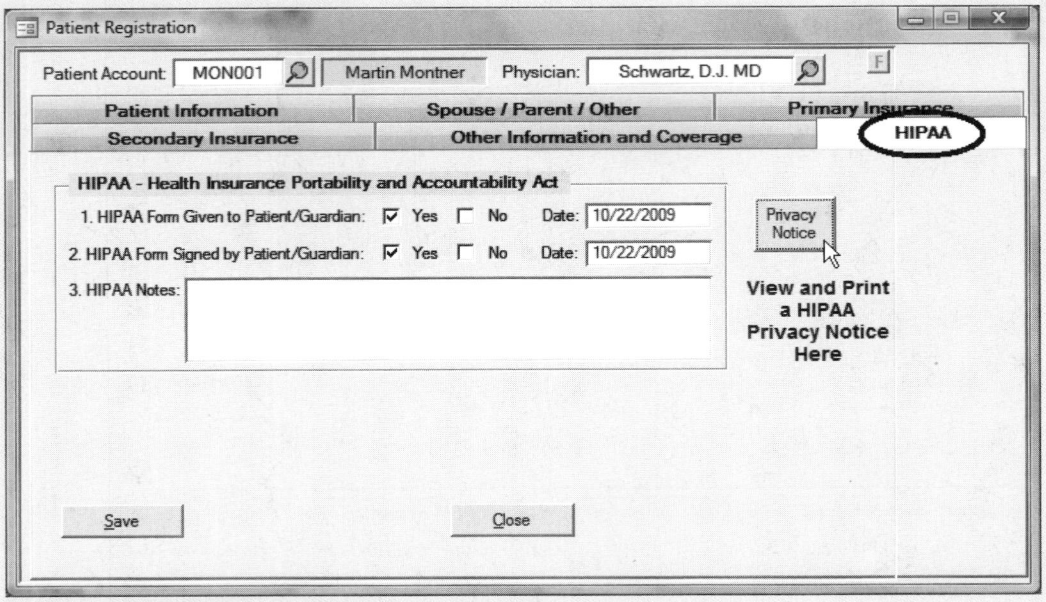

FIGURE 5-5
Delmar/Cengage Learning

STEP 10

Close the Patient Registration window. The medical office staff can clip a superbill to the front of the patient's file. The patient is now ready to visit the doctor.

VERIFYING INSURANCE ELIGIBILITY: CASE STUDY 5-A

Objective: Now that the registration of the patient has been completed, the Online Eligibility feature can be utilized to verify insurance coverage. When using MOSS, it is best to verify insurance after the patient registration data has been entered. The online eligibility feature will automatically fill the fields with required information, drawn from the data you have just entered. Follow the next steps to verify the health plan for Martin Montner.

HINT: You also can use the Activities drop-down menu as an alternative.

STEP 1

Starting at the Main Menu, click on the *Online Eligibility* button. Select patient Montner from the list using the method of your choice.

STEP 2

The online eligibility window opens. Check the window to be certain that the information displayed is correct by comparing it to Figure 5-6. If errors are found, close the window and go back to Patient Registration to make corrections as needed.

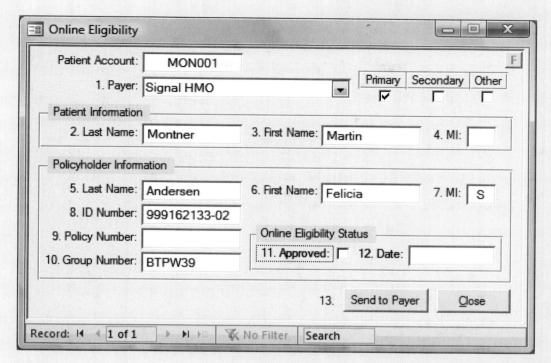

FIGURE 5-6

Delmar/Cengage Learning

MOSS NOTE: Some users have reported seeing a date of 12/31/1899 in Field 12 of the Online Eligibility screen. Go ahead and click the *Send to Payer* button. After the online eligibility is performed, the date of the report will then populate in that field.

STEP 3

If your information is correct, click on the *Send to Payer* button to begin the online verification process. A message displays indicating the session has disconnected and that the transfer was complete.

HINT: The User ID should be your own student number; the date will show today's date (the date you are completing this exercise).

STEP 4

Click on the *View* button to see the results. Check your work with Figure 5-7. Print the report for your records. Click the *Close* button when finished.

Case Study 5-A Continues >>

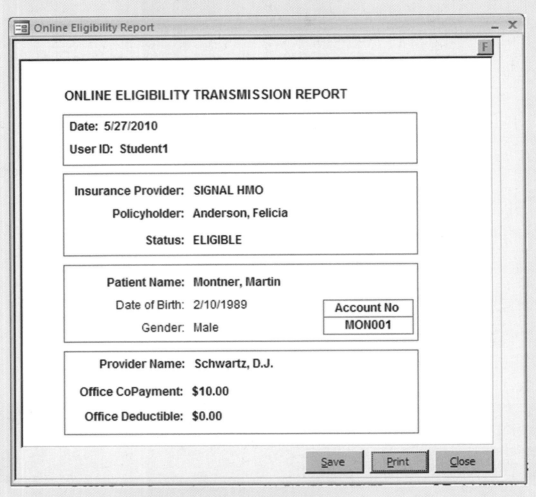

ONLINE ELIGIBILITY TRANSMISSION REPORT

Date: 5/27/2010
User ID: Student1

Insurance Provider: SIGNAL HMO
Policyholder: Anderson, Felicia
Status: ELIGIBLE

Patient Name: Montner, Martin
Date of Birth: 2/10/1989
Gender: Male

Account No
MON001

Provider Name: Schwartz, D.J.
Office CoPayment: $10.00
Office Deductible: $0.00

FIGURE 5-7
Delmar/Cengage Learning

CASE STUDY 5–B: ADAMS, MINNIE

Today's Date: October 28, 2009
New patient: Adams, Minnie

After being greeted by the office staff, patient Adams is given a registration form to fill out and copies or scans of her insurance card are made. The privacy notice is given to the patient and she is asked to sign, acknowledging receipt. Minnie is changing her doctor's office since Douglasville Medicine Associates is closer to her home. She has a history of an old cerebral vascular accident (CVA), which was minor and is healed.

Refer to the Source Documents Appendix at the end of this book. Minnie Adams' registration form (Source Document 5-3) and her Medicare Health Insurance Card copy (Source Document 5-4) will be needed for the following exercise.

SPECIAL NOTES REGARDING CASE STUDY 5-B

Minnie Adams has the original Medicare plan, which was discussed in Unit 4. She has a deductible due at the beginning of each year and is responsible for a 20% co-payment. Dr. Heath is a PAR physician and accepts what Medicare approves as the full charge for services.

The Medicare insurance card provides information useful to the office. See Source Document 5-4. The card shows the patient's Medicare number and whether the patient is entitled to hospital services (Part A), medical services (Part B), or both.

The patient's Medicare number is often referred to as the **Health Insurance Claim number,** or **HIC number** (pronounced *hick*). The HIC number has a suffix following it, consisting of an alpha letter (with or without numbers). Medicare beneficiaries who have Railroad Retirement benefits will have prefixes in front of their HIC number(s). There are in excess of 50 Medicare HIC suffixes; however, you will probably use only a handful of the most common ones in the medical office. The following list provides definitions of common suffixes:

- A Primary wage earner, age 65 or older (person who actually worked for the benefits)

- B Wife of wage earner, age 65 or older

- B1 Husband of wage earner, age 65 or older

- D Widow, age 65 or older

- D1 Widower, age 65 or older

Refer to the Medicare insurance card belonging to Minnie Adams. Which suffix is at the end of her HIC number? What does this tell you about her benefits?

STEP 1

Carefully review the information on the registration form (Source Document 5-3) and answer the following questions. *Cover the answers using the tear-off bookmark from the cover of your book. Check your work before entering data into MOSS.*

A.	What is the patient's date of birth?	**9/4/1928**
B.	Is the patient employed?	**No**
C.	What is the patient's marital status?	**Single**
D.	Was the patient referred by another physician? If yes, what is the physician's name?	**Samantha Green**
E.	How many insurance policies is the patient covered by?	**1**
F.	What is the name of the primary health plan?	**Medicare**
G.	What is the policy ID number?	**999571266A**

STEP 2

Compare the insurance card (Source Document 5-4) to the information on the registration form, then answer the following questions and think about other information on the card that may be pertinent to the medical office.

A.	Does the information match what is on the form?	**Yes**
B.	What types of coverage does the patient have under Medicare? (Part A, Part B, or both?)	**Part A and Part B**

Case Study 5-B Continues >>

Case Study 5-B Continued

HINT: Click on *Start*, then *Programs*, then click on the *software title* to open it. If a desktop icon is available, you can also open the software by clicking on it.

STEP 3

If MOSS is running, continue to the next step. Otherwise, start MOSS and use your logon information to begin using the software.

STEP 4

Click on the *Appointment Scheduling* button to open the scheduler. Click on *October 28, 2009* and locate patient Adams. Double click on her *name* to open the appointment form window. Click in front of *Checked In*. This documents the patient's arrival. Click on the *Close* button when finished, and then close out of the scheduler and return to the Main Menu of MOSS.

STEP 5

Next, on the Main Menu, click on the *Patient Registration* button. Search for Minnie Adams using the method of your choice. Be sure to click on the *Select* button or double click on the patient's *name*. Recall that registration was started at the time the patient made her appointment, so partial information is already in the database.

STEP 6

Using the registration form, enter the data for the Patient Registration tab. Compare your work to Figure 5-8 before clicking the *Save* button.

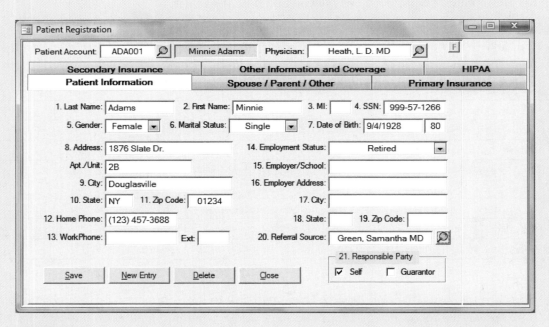

FIGURE 5-8

Delmar/Cengage Learning

STEP 7

Click on the *Primary Insurance* tab. Using the information on the registration form, complete the fields as needed. Include the following data:

A. Recall that Dr. Heath participates with Medicare and accepts assignment. Click *Yes* in Fields 13 and 15.

B. Signatures have been obtained from the patient; click on *Yes* in Field 14.

C. Leave Field 16 blank; this is used only when a patient has a PCP who has referred her to be seen by one of the physicians at Douglasville Medicine Associates.

Check your work with Figure 5-9, then click the *Save* button when finished.

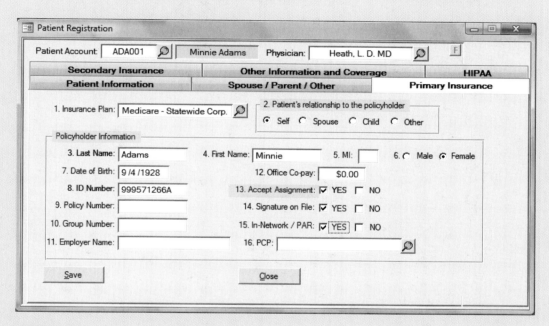

FIGURE 5-9

Delmar/Cengage Learning

Case Study 5-B Continues >>

STEP 8

Next, click on the *HIPAA* tab. The patient was given a privacy notice, which was signed. In Fields 1 and 2, click on *Yes,* then enter the date of receipt and signature, "10/28/2009." Check your work with Figure 5-10 before saving.

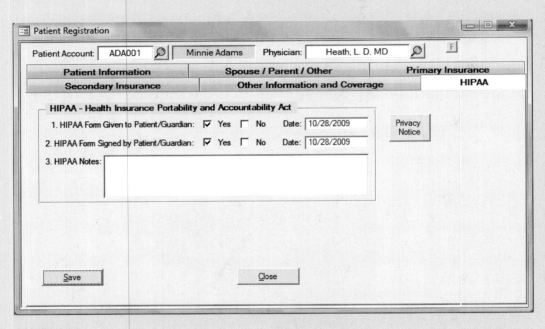

FIGURE 5-10

Delmar/Cengage Learning

STEP 9

Close the Patient Registration window. The medical office staff can clip a superbill to the front of the patient's file. The patient is now ready to visit the doctor.

VERIFYING INSURANCE ELIGIBILITY: CASE STUDY 5-B

Objective: Now that the registration of the patient has been completed, the Online Eligibility feature can be used to verify insurance coverage. Follow the next steps to verify the health plan for Minnie Adams.

STEP 1

HINT: You can also use the Activities drop-down menu as an alternative.

Starting at the Main Menu, click on the *Online Eligibility* button. Select patient "Adams" from the list using the method of your choice.

STEP 2

The online eligibility window opens. Check the window to be certain that the information displayed is correct by comparing it to Figure 5-11. If errors are found, close the windows and go back to Patient Registration to make corrections as needed.

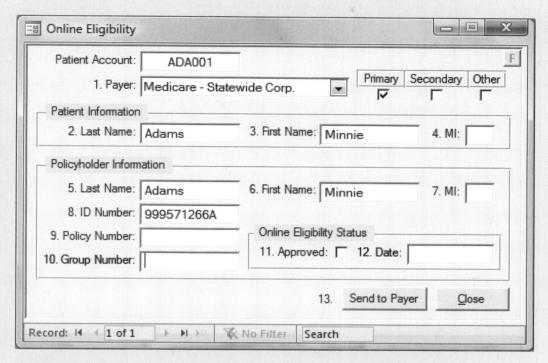

FIGURE 5-11

Delmar/Cengage Learning

STEP 3

Click on the *Send to Payer* button to begin the online verification process. A message displays indicating the session has disconnected and that the transfer was complete.

STEP 4

Click on the *View* button to see the results. Check your work with Figure 5-12. Print the report for your records. Click the *Close* button when finished.

MOSS NOTE: At the time MOSS was developed, the Medicare deductible was $110.00; this amount will appear on Online Eligibility Reports as the office deductible. At the time this book was written, the Medicare deductible had increased to $135.00.

Case Study 5-B Continues >>

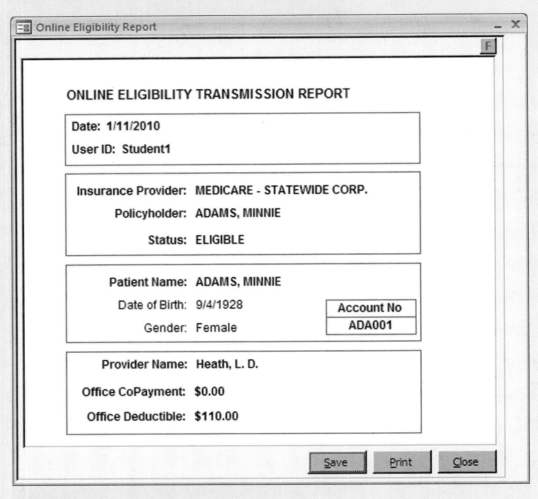

FIGURE 5-12

Delmar/Cengage Learning

CASE STUDY 5–C: CORBETT, MELISSA

Today's Date: **October 29, 2009**

New patient: **Corbett, Melissa**

After being greeted by the office staff, patient Corbett's father is given a registration form to fill out for Melissa, who is a young girl. She is a full-time student at her middle school. Copies of the insurance card are made. The privacy notice is given to the father and he is asked to sign, acknowledging receipt. Melissa is not feeling well and possibly has the flu.

Refer to the Source Documents Appendix at the end of this book. Melissa Corbett's registration form (Source Document 5-5) and FlexiHealth PPO Plan insurance card copy (Source Document 5-6) will be needed for the following exercise.

STEP 1

Carefully review the information on the registration form and answer the following questions. *Cover the answers using the tear-off bookmark from the cover of your book. Check your work before entering data into MOSS.*

A.	What is the patient's date of birth?	6/16/1997
B.	What is the name of the patient's school?	**Clear Lake Middle School**
C.	How many insurance policies is the patient covered by?	**1**
D.	Who is the policy holder of the health plan?	**Daniel Corbett**
E.	What is the name of the primary health plan?	**Flexihealth PPO In-Network**
F.	What is the policy ID number? Group number?	**ID: 999301255-04** **Group number: BH225**
G.	Who is the guarantor for the patient?	**Daniel Corbett**
H.	Where does the patient's father work?	**Banterfield Hobby**
I.	Does the patient live with her father?	**Yes**

STEP 2

Compare the insurance card to the information on the registration form, then answer the following questions and think about other information on the card that may be pertinent to the medical office.

A.	Does the information match what is on the form?	**Yes**
B.	Is there a co-payment for office visits? If yes, how much is it?	**$20.00**
C.	Which services require preauthorization?	**Surgery & hospitalization**
D.	What is the phone number to call for preauthorization purposes?	**800-123-3654**
E.	Does the patient require a PCP? Why or why not?	**No**

STEP 3

If MOSS is running, continue to the next step. Otherwise, start MOSS and use your logon information to begin using the software.

STEP 4

> **HINT:** Click on *Start,* then *Programs,* then click on the *software title* to open it. If a desktop icon is available, you can also open the software by clicking on it.

Click on the *Appointment Scheduling* button to open the scheduler. Click on *October 29, 2009* and locate patient Corbett. Double click on her *name* to open the appointment form window. Click in front of *Checked In.* This documents the patient's arrival. Click on the *Close* button when finished, and then close out of the scheduler and return to the Main Menu of MOSS.

STEP 5

Next, on the Main Menu, click on the *Patient Registration* button. Search for Melissa Corbett using the method of your choice. Be sure to click on the *Select* button, or double click on the patient's *name.* Recall that registration was started at the time an appointment was made for the patient, so partial information is already in the database.

Case Study 5-C Continues >>

Case Study 5-C Continued

STEP 6

Using the registration form (Source Document 5-5), enter the data for the Patient Information tab. Be sure that Field 21 indicates there is a guarantor. Check your work with Figure 5-13, and then click on the *Save* button.

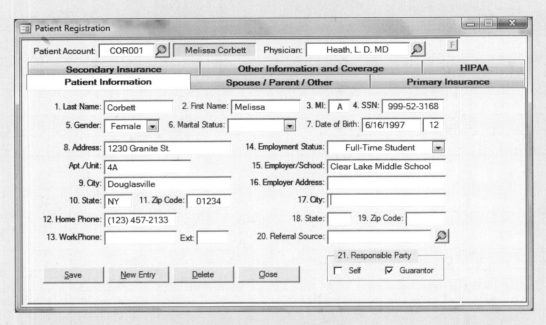

FIGURE 5-13

Delmar/Cengage Learning

STEP 7

Click on the *Spouse/Parent/Other* tab. Since the guarantor for this patient is her father, complete the information for Daniel Corbett in Fields 1 through 8. Click on the *Save* button. Next, click on the *Address* button. Since the patient and her father live at the same address, click on the *Copy Pt Addr* button to automatically fill the fields. Click on the *Employer* button and enter Daniel's work information.

Enter the mother's information starting at Field 9, as shown on the registration form for Other Responsible Party. Check your work with Figure 5-14 before clicking the *Save* button.

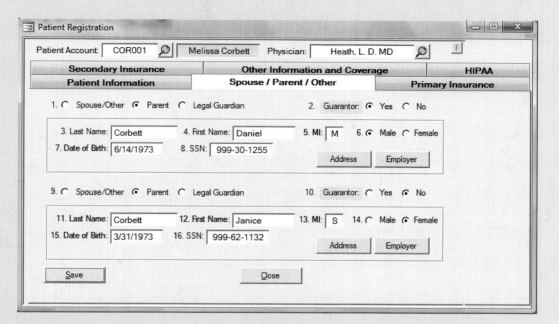

FIGURE 5-14

Delmar/Cengage Learning

STEP 8

Click on the *Primary Insurance* tab. Using the information on the registration form, complete the fields as needed. Include the following data:

A. $20.00 co-payment in Field 12.

B. Recall that Dr. Heath participates with FlexiHealth PPO and accepts assignment. Click on *Yes* in Fields 13 and 15.

C. Signatures have been obtained from the patient's father. Click on *Yes* in Field 14.

D. Leave Field 16 blank. This is used only when a patient has a PCP who has referred her to be seen by one of the physicians at Douglasville Medicine Associates.

Check your work with Figure 5-15, then click the *Save* button when finished.

NT: Refer to Figure 4-5,
t 4.

NT: See bottom of registra-
form.

Case Study 5-C Continues >>

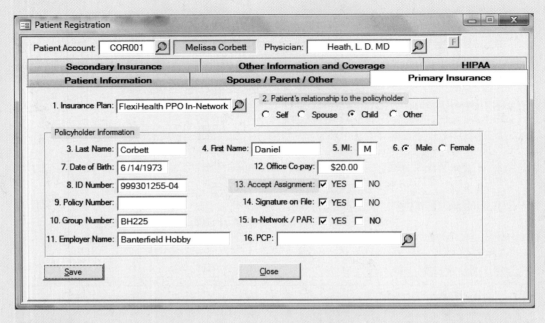

FIGURE 5-15

Delmar/Cengage Learning

STEP 9

Next, click on the *HIPAA* tab. The patient's father was given a privacy notice, which was signed. In Fields 1 and 2, click on *Yes*, then enter the date of signature, "10/29/2009." Check and save your entries. See Figure 5-16.

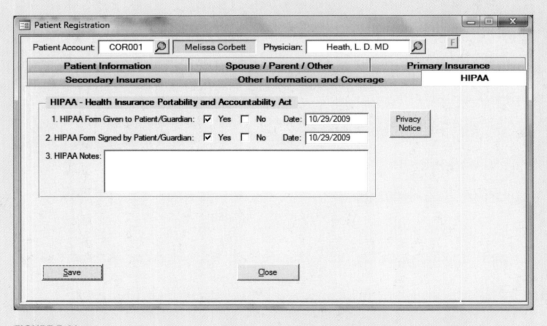

FIGURE 5-16

Delmar/Cengage Learning

STEP 10

Close the Patient Registration window. The medical office staff can clip a superbill to the front of the patient's file. The patient is now ready to visit the doctor.

VERIFYING INSURANCE ELIGIBILITY: CASE STUDY 5-C

Objective: Now that the patient registration has been completed, the Online Eligibility feature can be used to verify insurance coverage. Follow the listed steps to verify the health plan for Melissa Corbett.

NT: You also can use the tivities drop-down menu as alternative.

STEP 1

Starting at the Main Menu, click on the *Online Eligibility* button. Select patient Corbett from the list using the method of your choice.

STEP 2

The online eligibility window opens. Check the window against the registration form to be certain that the information displayed is correct. If errors are found, close the window and go back to Patient Registration to make corrections as needed. See Figure 5-17.

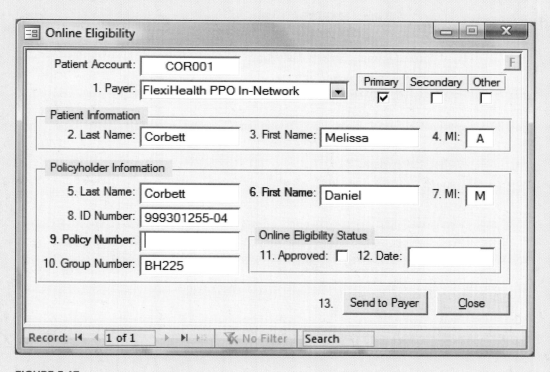

FIGURE 5-17

Delmar/Cengage Learning

STEP 3

Click on the *Send to Payer* button to begin the online verification process. A message displays indicating the session has disconnected and that the transfer was complete.

Case Study 5-C Continues >>

Case Study 5-C Continued

HINT: The User ID should be your own student number.

STEP 4
Click on the *View* button to see the results. Check your work with Figure 5-18. Print the report for your records. Click the *Close* button when finished.

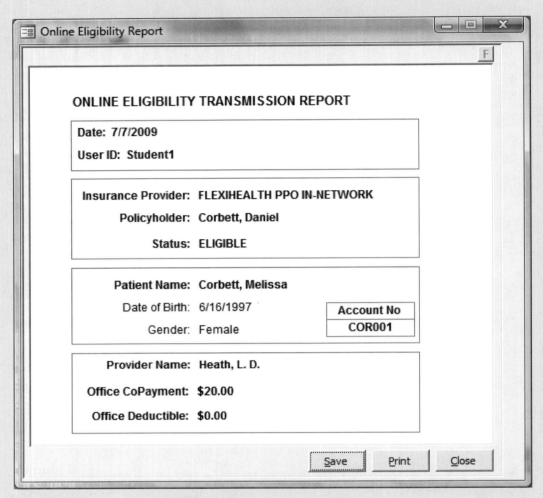

FIGURE 5-18
Delmar/Cengage Learning

CASE STUDY 5–D: ZUHL, RODNEY

Today's Date: October 30, 2009

New patient: Zuhl, Rodney

After being greeted by the office staff, patient Zuhl is given a registration form to fill out. Since Rodney does not have health insurance due to unemployment, there are no insurance cards to copy. The doctor has agreed to give him a hardship discount for paying cash. The privacy notice is given to the patient and he is asked to sign, acknowledging receipt. Rodney is complaining of difficulty in urinating.

Refer to the Source Documents Appendix at the end of this book. Rodney Zuhl's registration form (Source Document 5-7) will be needed for the following exercise.

STEP 1

Carefully review the information on the registration form and answer the following questions. *Cover the answers using the tear-off bookmark from the cover of your book. Check your work before entering data into MOSS.*

A.	What is the patient's date of birth?	12/21/1984
B.	Is the patient employed?	No
C.	What is the patient's marital status?	Single

STEP 2

If MOSS is running, continue to the next step. Otherwise, start MOSS and use your logon information to begin using the software.

NT: Click on *Start*, then grams, then click on the *ware title* to open. If a ktop icon is available, you also open the software by king on it.

STEP 3

Click on the *Appointment Scheduling* button to open the scheduler. Click on *October 30, 2009* and locate patient Zuhl. Double click on his *name* to open the appointment form window. Click in front of *Checked In*. This will document the patient's arrival. Click on the *Close* button when finished, and then close out of the scheduler and return to the Main Menu of MOSS.

STEP 4

Next, on the Main Menu, click on the *Patient Registration* button. Search for Rodney Zuhl using the method of your choice. Be sure to click on the *Select* button, or double click on the patient's *name*. Recall that registration was started at the time the patient made his appointment, so partial information is already in the database.

STEP 5

Using the registration form, enter the data for the Patient Information tab. Check your entries before clicking the *Save* button with Figure 5-19.

Patient Registration		
Patient Account: ZUH001	Rodney Zuhl Physician: Schwartz, D.J. MD	F

Secondary Insurance	Other Information and Coverage	HIPAA
Patient Information	Spouse / Parent / Other	Primary Insurance

1. Last Name: Zuhl   2. First Name: Rodney   3. MI: A   4. SSN: 999-61-9213

5. Gender: Male   6. Marital Status: Single   7. Date of Birth: 12/21/1984   24

8. Address: 62 Pebble Trail   14. Employment Status: Unemployed

Apt./Unit: 15   15. Employer/School:

9. City: Douglasville   16. Employer Address:

10. State: NY   11. Zip Code: 01234   17. City:

12. Home Phone: (123) 457-4448   18. State: 19. Zip Code:

13. WorkPhone: Ext: 20. Referral Source:

21. Responsible Party
☑ Self   ☐ Guarantor

Save   New Entry   Delete   Close

FIGURE 5-19

Delmar/Cengage Learning

Case Study 5-D Continues >>

STEP 6

Click on the Primary Insurance tab. Select *Self Pay* from the list in Field 1 and click on *Self* in Field 2. Check your entries before clicking the *Save* button.

STEP 7

Next, click on the *HIPAA* tab. The patient was given a privacy notice, which was signed. In Fields 1 and 2 click on *Yes,* then enter the date of receipt and signature, "10/30/2009." Check your entries before clicking the *Save* button.

STEP 8

Close the Patient Registration window and return to the Main Menu.

STEP 9

Because the physician has instructed the staff to give patient Zuhl a discount for cash payments, a note will be made on the record. Using the drop-down menus, click on *Billing*, then on *Patient Ledger*. See Figure 5-20.

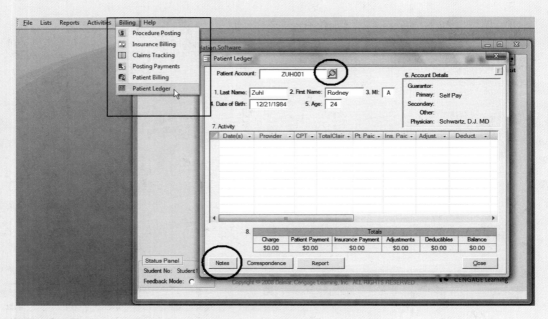

FIGURE 5-20

Delmar/Cengage Learning

STEP 10

Click on the *Search icon* (the magnifying glass), and find Rodney Zuhl. Click on the *View* button to open his ledger. Along the bottom of the screen, locate and click on the *Notes* button (shown in Figure 5-20).

STEP 11

At the Patient Notes window, click on the *Add* button to add a note. Then, click in the *box next to the asterisk (*)*. Type the following instruction:

"Patient receives 10% discount only when procedures are paid in full at time of service. No discount for services that are billed to patient or partial payments." See Figure 5-21.

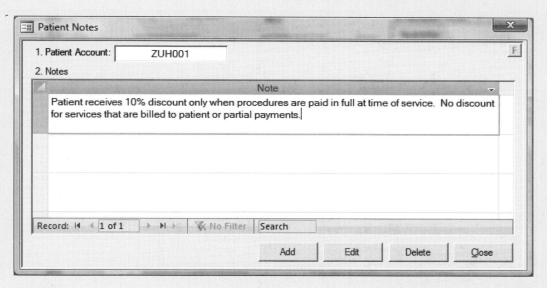

FIGURE 5-21

Delmar/Cengage Learning

STEP 12

When finished, click on the *Close* button for both the Patient Notes window and the Patient Ledger. This will return you to the Main Menu. The medical office staff can clip a superbill to the front of the patient's file. The patient is now ready to visit the doctor.

CASE STUDY 5–E: TOMANAGA, MARIE

Today's Date: **November 3, 2009**

New patient: **Tomanaga, Marie**

After being greeted by the office staff, patient Tomanaga is given a registration form to fill out and copies of her insurance card are made. The privacy notice is given to the patient and she is asked to sign, acknowledging receipt. She is complaining of occasional chest pain and has a history of high blood pressure.

Refer to the Source Documents Appendix at the end of this book. Marie Tomanaga's registration form (Source Document 5-8) and insurance cards for Medicare and Century SeniorGap (Source Document 5-9) will be needed for the following exercise.

Case Study 5-E Continues >>

Case Study 5-E Continued

STEP 1

Carefully review the information on the registration form (Source Document 5-8) and answer the following questions. *Cover the answers using the tear-off bookmark from the cover of your book. Check your work before entering data into MOSS.*

A.	What is the patient's date of birth?	2/2/1933
B.	Is the patient employed?	No
C.	What is the patient's marital status? If married, what is the spouse's name?	Walter Tomanaga
D.	Did another physician refer the patient? If yes, what is the physician's name?	No
E.	How many insurance policies is the patient covered by?	2
F.	What is the name of the primary health plan?	Medicare
G.	What is the name of the secondary health plan?	Century Senior Gap
H.	What is the policy ID number of the primary plan? Group number?	ID: 999213166A
I.	What is the policy ID number of the secondary plan? Medigap identification number?	ID: 999213166 Group number: MG612

STEP 2

Compare the insurance cards (Source Document 5-9) to the information on the registration form, and then answer the following questions.

A.	Does the information match what is on the form?	Yes
B.	What types of coverage does the patient have under Medicare? (Part A, Part B, or both?)	Both

> **HINT:** Click on *Start*, then *Programs*, then click on the *software title* to open it. If a desktop icon is available, you can also open the software by clicking on it.

STEP 3

If MOSS is running, continue to the next step. Otherwise, start MOSS and use your logon information to begin using the software.

STEP 4

Click on the *Appointment Scheduling* button to open the scheduler. Click on *November 3, 2009* and locate patient Tomanaga. Double click on her *name* to open the appointment form window. Click in front of *Checked In.* This documents the patient's arrival. Click on the *Close* button when finished, and then close out of the scheduler and return to the Main Menu of MOSS.

STEP 5

Next, on the Main Menu, click on the *Patient Registration* button. Search for Marie Tomanaga using the method of your choice. Be sure to click on the *Select* button, or double click on the patient's *name*. Recall that registration was started at the time the patient made her appointment, so partial information is already in the database.

STEP 6

Using the registration form, enter the data for the Patient Information tab. Check your entries before clicking on the *Save* button with Figure 5-22.

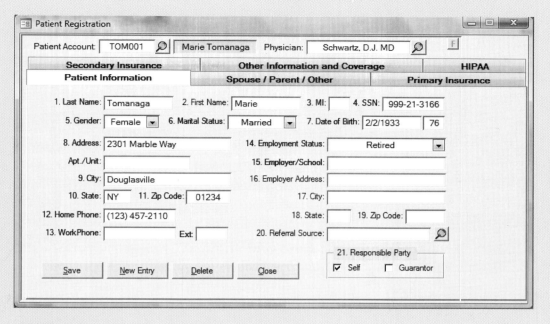

FIGURE 5-22

Delmar/Cengage Learning

STEP 7

Click on the *Spouse/Parent/Other* tab and enter information regarding the patient's husband, Walter. Do not forget to click on the *Address* button and complete the information there. Check your entries before clicking the *Save* button with Figure 5-23.

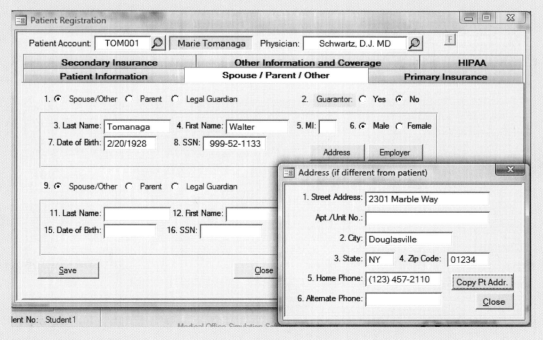

FIGURE 5-23

Delmar/Cengage Learning

Case Study 5-E Continues >>

Case Study 5-E Continued

STEP 8

Click on the *Primary Insurance* tab. Using the information on the registration form, complete the fields, as needed. Include the following data:

A. Recall that Dr. Schwartz does not participate with Medicare. However, since this patient has a Medigap policy as secondary insurance, he has chosen to accept assignment for both insurances. Click *Yes* in Field 13 and *No* in Field 15.

B. Signatures have been obtained from the patient. Click on *Yes* in Field 14.

C. Leave Field 16 blank. This is used only when a patient has a PCP who has referred him to be seen by one of the physicians at Douglasville Medicine Associates.

When finished, check your work with Figure 5-24 before clicking on the *Save* button.

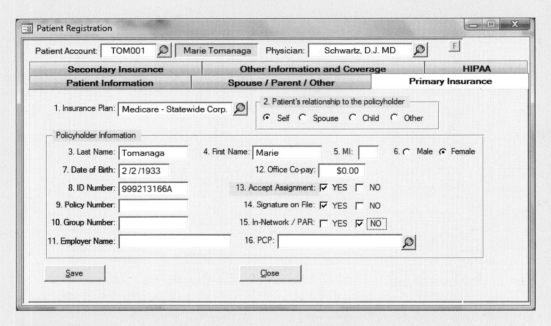

FIGURE 5-24

Delmar/Cengage Learning

STEP 9

Click on the *Secondary Insurance* tab. Using the information on the registration form, complete the fields as needed. Include the following data:

A. Select Century SeniorGap from the insurance list in Field 1.

B. Click in front of *Self* in Field 2 since the patient is the policyholder.

C. Place the ID number in Field 8 and the Medigap identifier number in the field for group number, Field 10.

D. The checkbox for Field 11 should be checked as a default indicating the secondary insurance is to be billed after the primary. If it is not, click the *checkbox* now.

E. Dr. Schwartz accepts assignment for the Medigap policy. Click on *Yes* for Field 14.

F. Signatures have been obtained from the patient. Click on *Yes* in Field 15.

G. Click on *No* for Field 16, since Dr. Schwartz is not a Medicare PAR physician.

Check your work with Figure 5-25 and then click the *Save* button when finished.

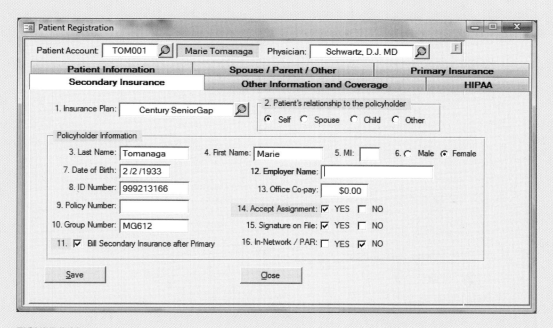

FIGURE 5-25

Delmar/Cengage Learning

STEP 10

Next, click on the *HIPAA* tab. The patient was given a privacy notice, which she signed. In Fields 1 and 2, click on *Yes,* then enter the date of receipt and signature, "11/3/2009." Click the *Save* button.

STEP 11

Close the Patient Registration window. The medical office staff can clip a superbill to the front of the patient's file. The patient is now ready to visit the doctor.

VERIFYING INSURANCE ELIGIBILITY: CASE STUDY 5-E

Objective: Now that the patient registration has been completed, the Online Eligibility feature can be used to verify insurance coverage. In the majority of medical offices, Medicare coverage is not typically verified if the patient holds a current and valid Medicare card. Follow the next steps to verify only the secondary health plan for Marie Tomanaga.

HINT: You also can use the Activities drop-down menu as an alternative.

STEP 1

Starting at the Main Menu, click on the *Online Eligibility* button. Select patient Tomanaga from the list using the method of your choice.

Case Study 5-E Continues >>

STEP 2

The online eligibility window opens. At the bottom of the online eligibility screen, click on the *record* button (lower left corner of window) to select and display the secondary insurance. Refer to Figure 5-26. Check to be certain that the information displayed is correct. If errors are found, close the window and go back to Patient Registration to make corrections as needed.

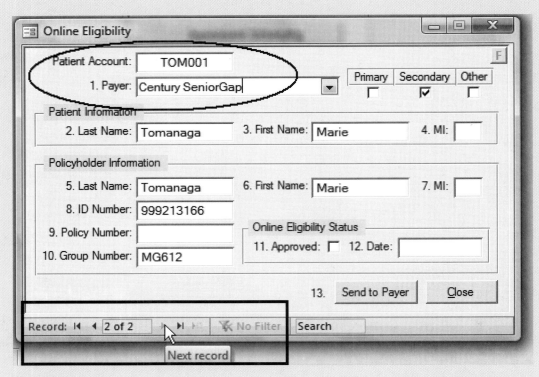

FIGURE 5-26

Delmar/Cengage Learning

STEP 3

Click on the *Send to Payer* button to begin the online verification process. A message displays indicating the session has disconnected and that the transfer is complete.

STEP 4

Click on the *View* button to see the results, as shown in Figure 5-27. Print the report for your records. Click the *Close* button when finished.

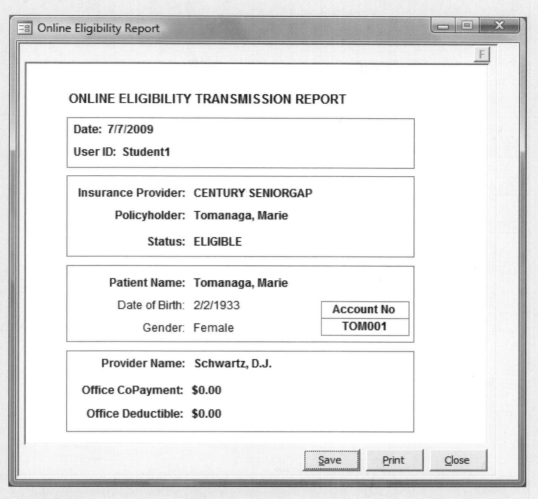

FIGURE 5-27
Delmar/Cengage Learning

CASE STUDY 5-F: VILLANOVA, RICKY

Today's Date: **October 27, 2009**

New patient: **Villanova, Ricky**

After being greeted by the office staff, patient Villanova is given a registration form to fill out and copies of his insurance card are made. The privacy notice is given to the patient and he is asked to sign, acknowledging receipt. He is complaining of being abnormally thirsty and frequent urination.

Refer to the Source Documents Appendix at the end of this book. Ricky Villanova's registration form (Source Document 5-10) and insurance card for Signal HMO (Source Document 5-11) will be needed for the following exercise.

Case Study 5-F Continues >>

Case Study 5-F Continued

STEP 1

Carefully review the information on the registration form and answer the following questions. *Cover the answers using the tear-off bookmark from the cover of your book. Check your work before entering data into MOSS.*

A.	What is the patient's date of birth?	**1/3/1979**
B.	Is the patient employed?	**Yes**
C.	What is the patient's marital status? If married, what is the spouse's name?	**Gina Villanova**
D.	Did another physician refer the patient? If yes, what is the physician's name?	**Joseph Reed**
E.	How many insurance policies is the patient covered by?	**1**
F.	What is the name of the primary health plan?	**Signal HMO**
G.	Who is the policyholder for the health plan?	**Gina Villanova**
H.	What is the policy ID number of the primary plan? Group number?	**ID: 999619923-02** **Group number: MA8991**

HINT: Click on *Start,* then *Programs,* then click on the *software title* to open it. If a desktop icon is available, you can also open the software by clicking on it.

STEP 2

If MOSS is running, continue to the next step. Otherwise, start MOSS and use your logon information to begin using the software.

STEP 3

Check the patient in for today's visit on 10/27/2009 using the appointment scheduler.

STEP 4

Open the Patient Registration screen and enter data from the registration form for Ricky Villanova. See Figure 5-28.

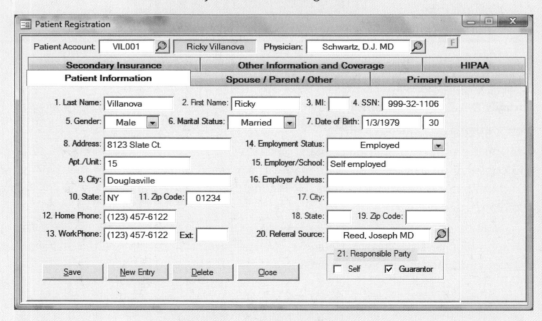

FIGURE 5-28

Delmar/Cengage Learning

STEP 5

Check your work to make sure it is complete and accurate. Did you remember the following items for Ricky's registration?

A. All demographic information?

B. Referring physician?

C. Spouse as guarantor? Input her home and work information. See Figure 5-29.

D. Primary insurance and policyholder information? See Figure 5-30.

E. HIPAA documentation?

STEP 6

Verify Ricky Villanova's insurance by using the online eligibility feature. Print the report for your records.

STEP 7

The patient is ready to have a superbill attached to his file and see the doctor. Close any open windows and return to the Main Menu of MOSS.

NT: For employment infor-tion, enter "Employed" in ld 14, and "Self-employed" Field 15 of the *Patient ormation* tab.

NT: Dr. Schwartz is an network physician for Signal MO and accepts assignment. ere is a $10.00 co-payment.

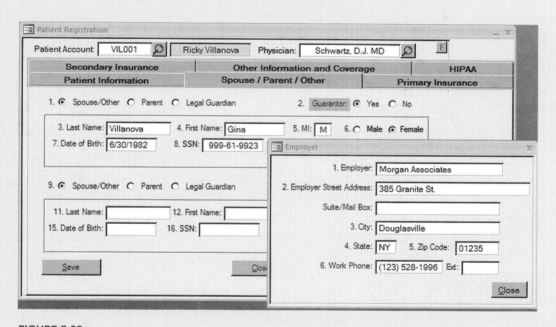

FIGURE 5-29

Delmar/Cengage Learning

Case Study 5-F Continues >>

Case Study 5-F Continued

Patient Registration

Patient Account: VIL001 | Ricky Villanova | Physician: Schwartz, D.J. MD | F

| Secondary Insurance | Other Information and Coverage | HIPAA |
| Patient Information | Spouse / Parent / Other | Primary Insurance |

1. Insurance Plan: Signal HMO

2. Patient's relationship to the policyholder
   ○ Self ● Spouse ○ Child ○ Other

Policyholder Information

3. Last Name: Villanova   4. First Name: Gina   5. MI: M   6. ○ Male ● Female

7. Date of Birth: 6 /30/1982   12. Office Co-pay: $10.00

8. ID Number: 999619923-02   13. Accept Assignment: ☑ YES ☐ NO

9. Policy Number: 14. Signature on File: ☑ YES ☐ NO

10. Group Number: MA8991   15. In-Network / PAR: ☑ YES ☐ NO

11. Employer Name: Morgan Associates   16. PCP:

Save   Close

FIGURE 5-30
Delmar/Cengage Learning

CASE STUDY 5–G: PRADHAN, KABIN

Today's Date: **November 3, 2009**

New patient: **Pradhan, Kabin**

After being greeted by the office staff, patient Pradhan is given a registration form to fill out and copies of his insurance card are made. The privacy notice is given to the patient and he is asked to sign, acknowledging receipt. He is complaining of heartburn and indigestion.

Refer to the Source Documents Section at the end of this book. Kabin Pradhan's registration form (Source Document 5-12) and insurance card for ConsumerONE (Source Document 5-13) will be needed for the following exercise.

STEP 1

Carefully review the information on the registration form and answer the following questions. *Cover the answers using the tear-off bookmark from the cover of your book. Check your work before entering data into MOSS.*

A.	What is the patient's date of birth?	**12/2/1951**
B.	Is the patient employed?	**Yes**
C.	What is the patient's marital status?	**Single**
D.	How many insurance policies is the patient covered by?	1
E.	What is the name of the primary health plan?	**ConsumerONE**
F.	Who is the policyholder for the health plan?	Kabin Pradhan
G.	What is the policy ID number of the primary plan? Group number?	ID: 999569844 Group number: ACM0211

NT: Click on *Start*, then *ograms*, then click on the *ftware title* to open it. If a *sktop icon is available, you* *n also open the software by* *cking on it.*

STEP 2

If MOSS is running, continue to the next step. Otherwise, start MOSS and use your logon information to begin using the software.

STEP 3

Check the patient in for today's visit on 11/03/2009, using the appointment scheduler.

STEP 4

Open the Patient Registration screen and enter data from the registration form for Kabin Pradhan.

STEP 5

Check your work to make sure it is complete and accurate. Did you remember the following items for Prahan's registration?

A. All demographic information?

B. Primary insurance and policyholder information?

C. HIPAA documentation?

NT: Dr. Schwartz is an *network physician for* *nsumerOne and accepts* *signment.*

STEP 6

Verify Kabin Pradhan's insurance by using the online eligibility feature. Print the report for your records.

STEP 7

The patient is ready to have a superbill attached to his file and see the doctor. Close any open windows and return to the Main Menu of MOSS.

CASE STUDY 5–H: BEALS, KIMBERLY

Today's Date: **November 3, 2009**

New patient: **Beals, Kimberly**

After being greeted by the office staff, patient Beals is given a registration form to fill out and copies of her insurance card are made. The privacy notice is given to the patient and she is asked to sign, acknowledging receipt. She is complaining of excessive weight loss.

Refer to the Source Documents Section at the end of this book. Kimberly Beals' registration form (Source Document 5-14) and insurance card for Signal HMO (Source Document 5-15) will be needed for the following exercise.

STEP 1

Carefully review the information on the registration form and answer the following questions. *Cover the answers using the tear-off bookmark from the cover of your book. Check your work before entering data into MOSS.*

Case Study 5-H Continues >>

A.	What is the patient's date of birth?	10/20/1969
B.	Is the patient employed?	Yes
C.	What is the patient's marital status?	Single
D.	How many insurance policies is the patient covered by?	1
E.	What is the name of the primary health plan?	Signal HMO
F.	Who is the policyholder for the health plan?	Kimberly Beals
G.	What is the policy ID number of the primary plan? Group number?	ID: 999229989-00 Group number: CLE5610

HINT: Click on *Start*, then *Programs*, then click on the *software title* to open it. If a desktop icon is available, you can also open the software by clicking on it.

STEP 2

If MOSS is running, continue to the next step. Otherwise, start MOSS and use your logon information to begin using the software.

STEP 3

Check the patient in for today's visit on 11/03/2009, using the appointment scheduler.

STEP 4

Open the Patient Registration screen and enter data from the registration form for Kimberly Beals.

STEP 5

Check your work to make sure it is complete and accurate. Did you remember the following items for patient Beal's registration?

HINT: Dr. Heath is an in-network physician for Signal HMO and accepts assignment. There is a $10.00 co-payment.

A. All demographic information?

B. Primary insurance and policyholder information?

C. HIPAA documentation?

STEP 6

Verify Kimberly Beals' insurance by using the online eligibility feature. Print the report for your records.

STEP 7

The patient is ready to have a superbill attached to her file and see the doctor. Close any open windows and return to the Main Menu of MOSS.

CASE STUDY 5–I: KINZLER, LINDA

Today's Date: **November 9, 2009**

New patient: **Kinzler, Linda**

After being greeted by the office staff, patient Kinzler is given a registration form to fill out and copies of her insurance card are made. The privacy notice is given to the patient and she is asked to sign, acknowledging receipt. She is in the office to receive a flu shot as a precaution, since she is asthmatic. A special note regarding this patient is that her insurance coverage is provided through her domestic partner, Jennifer Wade.

Refer to the Source Documents Section at the end of this book. Linda Kinzler's registration form (Source Document 5-16) and insurance card for FlexiHealth PPO (Source Document 5-17) will be needed for the following exercise.

STEP 1

Carefully review the information on the registration form and answer the following questions. *Cover the answers using the tear-off bookmark from the cover of your book. Check your work before entering data into MOSS.*

A.	What is the patient's date of birth?	2/27/1983
B.	Is the patient employed?	No
C.	What is the patient's marital status?	Single
D.	How many insurance policies is the patient covered by?	1
E.	What is the name of the primary health plan?	Flexihealth PPO
F.	Who is the policyholder for the health plan?	Jennifer Wade
G.	What is the policy ID number of the primary plan? Group number?	ID: 999125813-01 Group number: TCI015

STEP 2

If MOSS is running, continue to the next step. Otherwise, start MOSS and use your logon information to begin using the software.

STEP 3

Check the patient in for today's visit on 11/09/2009, using the appointment scheduler.

...NT: Click on *Start,* then ...grams, then click on the ...tware title to open it. If a ...sktop icon is available, you ...also open the software by ...king on it.

STEP 4

Open the Patient Registration screen and enter data from the registration form for Linda Kinzler.

STEP 5

Check your work to make sure it is complete and accurate. Did you remember the following items for Linda's registration?

A. All demographic information?

B. Referring physician?

...NT: Dr. Heath is an ...etwork physician for Flexi-...alth PPO and accepts ...ignment. There is a $20.00 ...payment.

C. Other (domestic partner) as guarantor? Input her home and work information.

D. Primary insurance and policyholder information?

E. HIPAA documentation?

STEP 6

Verify Linda Kinzler's insurance by using the online eligibility feature. Print the report for your records.

STEP 7

The patient is ready to have a superbill attached to her file and see the doctor. Close any open windows and return to the *Main Menu* of MOSS.

SERVICES RENDERED OUTSIDE THE OFFICE

Patients are usually scheduled to visit the physician in the medical office. However, the physician also renders services to patients outside the office in a variety of environments. Examples include hospitals, nursing homes, skilled nursing facilities, ambulatory surgical centers, and even house calls to the patient's home.

Hospitals provide 24-hour care to patients with the highest level of medical need. This includes those with serious illness, surgery and recovery, those who have suffered accidents, or require observation. Many hospitals offer outpatient services, especially with today's trend toward reducing time spent in the hospital. This, in turn, requires that the patient continue health services after discharge on an outpatient basis instead of in the hospital.

A **nursing home** is an entity that provides nursing care and rehabilitation services to people with illnesses, injuries, or functional disabilities. Most facilities serve the elderly; however, some facilities provide services to younger individuals with special needs. Such individuals may be developmentally disabled, mentally ill, or require drug and alcohol rehabilitation. Nursing homes are generally stand-alone facilities, but some are operated within a hospital or retirement community.

Skilled Nursing Facilities (SNFs) are for patients who need 24-hour nursing supervision in order to ensure their medical, psychological, or social needs are met. These facilities offer a full range of care including rehabilitation, specialized nutritional guidance, social services, and activity programs.

Ambulatory Surgical Centers provide a facility where surgery, medical procedures, or skilled rehabilitation services are performed and patients leave the center to return home the same day. With more effective and safer pain medications, and advances with anesthesia that produce fewer side effects for patients, same-day surgeries are more commonplace than ever before. Today, there are new surgery technologies that cause fewer traumas and provide for quicker recovery. This is allowing patients to return home and go back to work faster and more comfortably.

While there is a benefit in having the patient physically in the office to obtain necessary information for medical insurance billing, it becomes a challenging task if new patients receive services outside the office. The administrative medical staff still needs to secure demographic information as well as data needed for proper reimbursement, even if the patient has never been to the medical office itself. In this section, methods for securing new and established patient information for those receiving services at outside facilities are discussed.

THE PHYSICIAN AS AN INFORMATION SOURCE

The medical office staff is not always located near the facilities in which the physician provides services outside the office. In fact, the office depends on the physician to report to the staff which patients received services, including details of procedures and diagnoses for coding purposes. In addition, the physician must indicate at which facility and on what date the services were provided.

Medical practices have different policies regarding how this information is passed along to the staff. Some physicians maintain a pocket agenda or calendar book and make notes on each patient. The information is then transferred from the agenda book and logged into a record book or onto a computer document. The information is transferred on a daily or weekly basis by the billing staff. Other physicians prefer to call the office and give a verbal report on each patient to a staff member over the telephone. Again, information on each patient is documented in a record book or on the computer as it is received.

PDAs, such as the Palm, and Smartphones, such as the Blackberry, are proving to be tools for mobile physicians to easily record services provided to patients. With appropriate software, information can be transferred, either by media data card, cable, or wireless infrared, directly to the office computer files or to the medical software. Some practice management software programs come with features that produce documents and lists for physicians to track patients at outside facilities. Once the information is at the office, the medical biller can then begin preparing insurance claims for medical billing and reimbursement.

The medical specialty a physician practices usually dictates how much activity there is to report from outside facilities. For example, a general surgeon typically has a much higher workload at hospitals and ambulatory surgical centers than at the office. Most services involve performing surgery and following up patients after their procedures. This physician needs to stay in close contact with the office staff to report completed procedures for billing purposes, including hospital visits for the duration of a patient's inpatient stay. For surgeons, patients seen in the office are often limited to pre-operative consultations and routine follow-ups after discharge. A family medicine practitioner, however, sees the majority of her patients in the medical office. While there may be less activity at the hospital, there may be a heavy workload visiting nursing home patients.

In either case, the physician will be the primary information source for the medical office staff to post charges for services and properly bill medical insurance plans. Without accurate and timely input from the physician, proper reimbursement cannot be effectively accomplished.

NEW PATIENTS AT OUTSIDE FACILITIES

While the majority of the patients who receive services at outside facilities are established, there will be times when new patients are treated by the physician. These new patients usually do not have medical records at the physician's office and, therefore, little is known beyond the patient's name, diagnoses, and services rendered. Physicians generally do not know patient addresses, phone numbers, employer information, or insurance details, and will direct the staff to secure this information through the proper channels as needed.

As discussed in Unit 2, HIPAA requires a business associate agreement in order for PHI to be disclosed to another covered entity. Once the business associate obtains the information, use of it for business management and administration is permitted under the HIPAA guidelines, which include medical billing and reimbursement. Follow the office policy of your employer, and of associated medical facilities, in order to ensure that proper procedure is followed and patient privacy is maintained under HIPAA. The following list offers some tips for obtaining information on patients who receive services at outside facilities.

1. Many medical offices, hospitals, and associated facilities, such as diagnostic service providers, have access to dedicated networks where patient information can be obtained from a main database via the computer. If the patient has received services within the network, the information can be accessed by any of the providers in the network. However, if a provider is not part of the network, more traditional methods of obtaining a patient's registration information may be necessary, such as the ones that follow.

2. For inpatients at the hospital, or those admitted through the emergency room, the admissions department may provide a copy of the **face sheet,** also known as the *admission form, admitting sheet, data form,* or *patient information form.* The face sheet is a common document in medical facilities outside the private practice, such as hospitals. It is a variation of the registration form,

and derives its name from commonly being the first page of a medical record containing the demographic information for the patient. This information most likely was obtained during the check-in or registration process at the emergency room or admitting office.

Face sheets can be very complete or just have minimal information. The insurance information may reflect only details pertinent to coverage for hospital services and not physician services. At a minimum, the patient's address and phone number will be a good start if nothing else on the face sheet is useful. Figure 5-31 illustrates an example of a typical face sheet.

3. Once the patient's address is secured, a letter can be sent to the patient on practice letterhead requesting further information, such as copies of health insurance cards. A form letter, with a checklist of items, is useful and quick for this purpose. Include a self-addressed, stamped envelope for better results. If the patient is still in the hospital, it is likely a responsible party is taking care of correspondence and other important matters concerning the patient. Some medical offices have a staff member call the home to obtain patient information, if a phone number is available. A telephone request for information gives an opportunity for an introduction to the office and the physicians who provided services. Patients do not always remember every physician or specialist who visited them in the hospital. Many patients are not aware that physicians whom they never met bill separately for their services. A good example is the radiologist who reads an X-ray and provides the report showing the results. There is typically a charge from the facility for obtaining the X-ray and a charge from the radiologist for providing a diagnostic reading of the X-ray.

4. In most instances, you will have a directory in the medical office for every department and the hospital wards. A ward is a division of a hospital containing rooms, similar to a dormitory, used for the temporary accommodation of patients, either waiting for or recovering from operations or undergoing treatment. Each ward has a nurse's station and a health unit coordinator. **Health unit coordinators**, previously known as ward clerks, are individuals who manage the administrative tasks of the nurse's station, similar to the front-office staff of a medical practice. The health unit coordinator may be able to assist you with obtaining patient information, as well as the location of patients, especially when testing, surgeries, or room changes take place. The health unit coordinator is responsible for the patient medical record and can assist best with issues related to patient information.

5. Another resource for obtaining patient information is the medical offices of other physicians who provide care to the same patients. Patients who are new to your medical office probably have a family physician or other doctor they see on a regular basis. The office of the patient's regular physician should have a complete medical record. This is especially useful when medical billers for specialists need information on new patients in order to bill for consults and services requested by general practitioners. The doctor who has primary responsibility for the treatment and care of the patient is referred to as the **attending physician**. Often, this is the patient's regular physician; however, this could be another physician who has been assigned to the patient by the hospital. It is not uncommon for more than one physician to share responsibility for the care of a patient. If there is an attending or other physician listed on the patient's face sheet, their offices can be contacted for patient information, as needed.

6. In some unusual cases, the physician may not know the name of the patient who was treated. It may be a situation where the patient needed emergency care or surgery and details of patient information were not a priority at the time of service. In other circumstances, the patient may have been unconscious and did not have identification, often referred to as John Doe or Jane Doe cases.

RECORD OF ADMISSION

PATIENT NAME	ROOM NO.	HOSP. NO.	ADDRESS LINE - 1	ADDRESS LINE - 2

AGE	BIRTHDATE	SEX	BIRTHPLACE	CITY	STATE	ZIP CODE	COUNTRY CODE

SSAN	NATIONALITY	CIVIL ST.	MILITARY	RELIGION	CHURCH	PATIENT TELEPHONE

SPOUSE INFORMATION	NAME OF HUSBAND OR NAME OF WIFE	SPOUSE BIRTHPLACE	SPOUSE EMPLOYER NAME
	SPOUSE ADDRESS		SPOUSE EMPLOYER ADDRESS

NAME OF FATHER	BIRTHPLACE	NAME OF MOTHER	BIRTHPLACE

NOTIFY IN CASE OF EMERGENCY	NAME	RELATIONSHIP	ADDRESS	TELEPHONE

PATIENT EMPLOYER NAME	EMPLOYER ADDRESS	EMPLOYER TELEPHONE	GUARANTOR OCCUPATION

GUARANTOR NAME	GUARANTOR TELEPHONE	HOSPITALIZATION INSURANCE

GUARANTOR ADDRESS - 1	CITY	

GUARANTOR ADDRESS - 2	STATE	ZIP CODE	DATE	TIME	PLACE	EVENT	INJURY DUE TO ACCID.

ADMITTING PHYSICIAN	CONSULTING PHYSICIAN	ADMITTING SERVICE	SMOKER	ADMITTING DIAGNOSIS

ALLERGIES	DATE LAST ADM.	PREV. ADM. NO.	ADMISSION DATE	TIME OF ADMISSION	INITIALS	DISCHARGE DATE

FINANCIAL CLASS	MEDICAL RECORDS NUMBER	ADMISSION CODE	HOME 1	SHORT TERM HOSPITAL 2	SKILLED NURSING FACILITY 3	INTERMEDIATE CARE FACILITY 4	OTHER 5	LEFT AMA 7	EXPIRED 20	TIME

PRINCIPAL DIAGNOSIS: ADVANCE DIRECTIVE = CODE

SECONDARY DIAGNOSIS:

PRINCIPAL OPERATION/DATE:

SECONDARY OPERATIONS:

Consultation With _____

Results: ☐ Recovered ☐ Improved ☐ Not Improved ☐ Not Treated ☐ Diagnosis Only ☐ Died ☐ Released Against Advice

Cause of Death _____ Autopsy: ☐ Yes ☐ No

I have examined and approved this complete medical report on _____ 20 ____

Signed _____ Attending Physician

ADMISSION - SUMMARY SHEET

FIGURE 5-31

Sample of a patient information form, typically known as a face sheet. *Delmar/Cengage Learning*

Where surgery is concerned, the physician can provide the date of service, facility, and procedures performed along with the patient's diagnoses. With that information in hand, the operating room scheduling desk can be contacted, and the patient identified according to when the surgery was done and by which surgeon. After the patient's name is secured, follow the guidelines already discussed to obtain more information and a face sheet as needed.

Unidentified patients can be more challenging. Because there is no information, there may be a waiting period before medical claims can be submitted or a patient record can be formally created. Nonetheless, physicians continue to provide services for the patient as needed. If a long time passes before identification is made, contact the hospital's Department of Social Services. **Social Services** provides patient assistance in a number of areas, including assisting with information regarding financial resources to fit individual needs and eligibility. As such, unidentified patients may have been qualified for state or federal assistance medical programs through Social Services. If so, this helps offset some of the medical expenses.

Social Services also helps patients with discharge planning and arranging for available community resources. They provide assistance with identifying eligibility for special services and benefits, such as nursing home placement and alternate living arrangements.

LET'S TRY IT! 5-2 REGISTERING NEW PATIENTS WHO RECEIVE SERVICES OUT-OF-OFFICE

Objective: The case studies that follow are new patients who have received services from Dr. Heath or Dr. Schwartz outside the medical office. The office has received four admission forms (face sheets) and one emergency room outpatient record that contain demographic and insurance information for each patient. At a later time, the doctors will provide the office with information regarding actual services rendered. Until then, these patients will need to be registered and added to the software database so that the accounts are ready for medical billing.

NOTE: Until now, registration forms have been used to enter data into the software database for new patients. You will read the admission forms (face sheets) from the hospitals in order to input demographic and insurance information. Only the pertinent information from the admission form is required for data entry. Any data that is not normally used for registering patients in the office, such as religion or place of birth, can be disregarded.

MOSS NOTE: For these exercises, turn feedback mode off.

CASE STUDY 5–J: TATE, JASON

Refer to the Source Documents Section in the Appendix. Jason Tate's face sheet (Source Document 5-18) will be needed for the following exercise.

New patient: **Tate, Jason**

Facility: **Community General Hospital**

Status: **Inpatient**

Physician: **Heath**

STEP 1

Carefully review the information on the admission form from Community General Hospital and answer the following questions. *Cover the answers using the tear-off bookmark from the cover of your book. Check your work before entering data into MOSS.*

A.	What is the patient's date of birth?	3/5/1967
B.	Is the patient employed?	Yes
C.	What is the patient's marital status?	Single
D.	How many insurance policies is the patient covered by?	1
E.	What is the name of the primary health plan?	Flexihealth PPO In-Network
F.	Who is the policyholder for the health plan?	Jason Tate
G.	What is the policy ID number of the primary plan? Group number?	ID: 999561133 Group number: HRC321

NT: Click on *Start,* then *grams,* then click on the *tware title* to open. If a *ktop* icon is available, you *o* can open the software by *king* on it.

STEP 2

Start MOSS and use your logon information to begin using the software.

NT: Dr. Heath is the admit-*g* physician, participates with *xiHealth PPO,* and accepts *ignment.*

STEP 3

Open the Patient Registration screen. Check the database to make sure Jason Tate is not already in the system. If not, click *Add,* and then enter data from the admission form for patient Tate. Include demographic, employer, and insurance coverage information. Do not forget to enter the information that this in-network insurance plan has a $20.00 office co-payment. Check your work with Figure 5-32 and Figure 5-33.

Case Study 5-J Continues >>

Case Study 5-J Continued

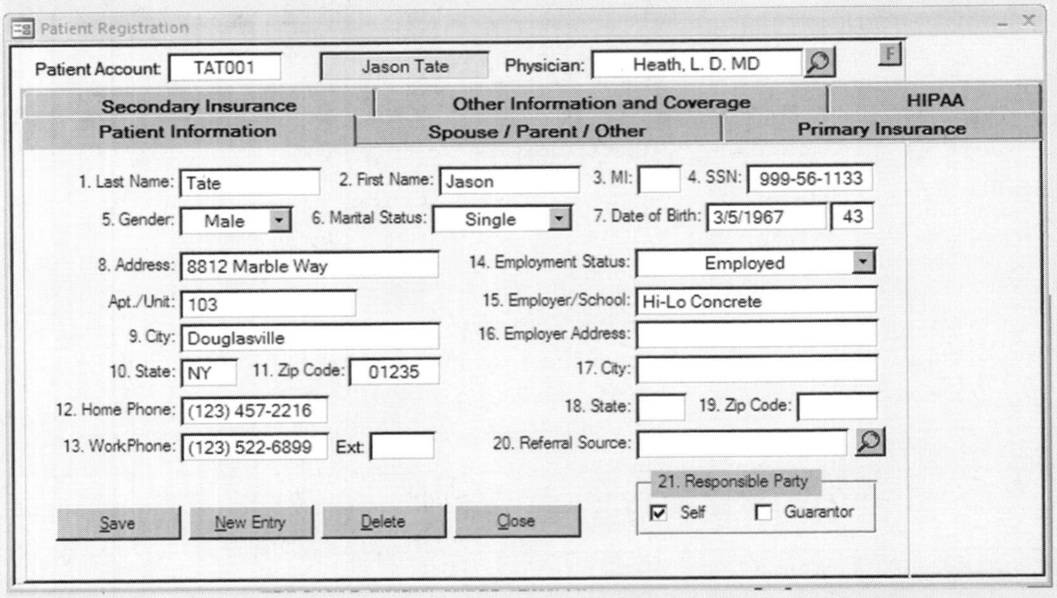

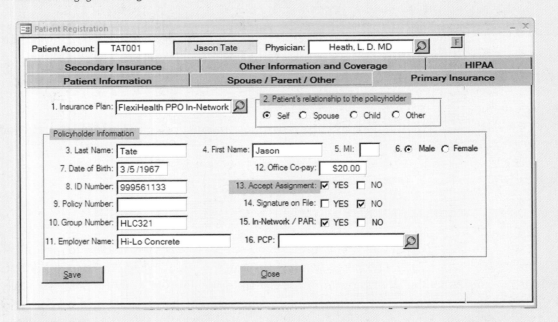

FIGURE 5-32

Delmar/Cengage Learning

FIGURE 5-33

Delmar/Cengage Learning

STEP 4

Since the patient was an inpatient at the hospital, we do not yet have a signature on file. The patient also has not received or signed for the privacy notice.

STEP 5

Check your work to make sure it is complete and accurate. Click the *Save* button when finished.

STEP 6

Verify Jason Tate's insurance by using the online eligibility feature. Print the report for your records, as shown in Figure 5–34.

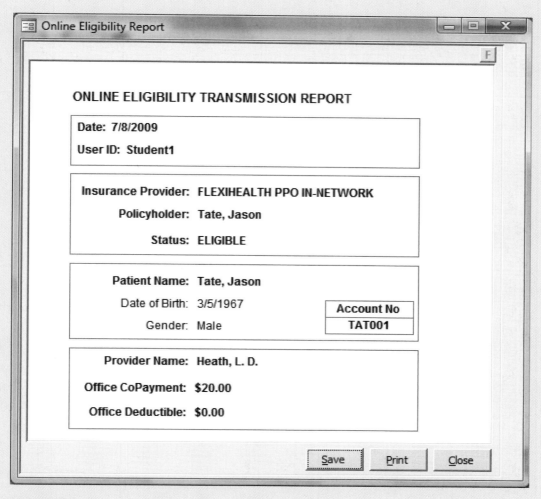

ONLINE ELIGIBILITY TRANSMISSION REPORT

Date: 7/8/2009

User ID: Student1

Insurance Provider: FLEXIHEALTH PPO IN-NETWORK

Policyholder: Tate, Jason

Status: ELIGIBLE

Patient Name: Tate, Jason

Date of Birth: 3/5/1967

Gender: Male

Account No

TAT001

Provider Name: Heath, L. D.

Office CoPayment: $20.00

Office Deductible: $0.00

Save   Print   Close

FIGURE 5-34

Delmar/Cengage Learning

CASE STUDY 5–K: MUÑOZ, GERALDO

Refer to the Source Documents Section at the end of this book. Geraldo Muñoz's face sheet (Source Document 5-19) will be needed for the following exercise.

New patient: **Muñoz, Geraldo**

Facility: **New York County Hospital**

Status: **Inpatient**

Physician: **Heath**

Case Study 5-K Continues >>

STEP 1

Carefully review the information on the admission form from New York County Hospital and answer the following questions. *Cover the answers using the tear-off bookmark from the cover of your book. Check your work before entering data into MOSS.*

A.	What is the patient's date of birth?	**3/28/1925**
B.	Is the patient employed?	**No, retired**
C.	What is the patient's marital status?	**Single**
D.	How many insurance policies is the patient covered by?	**2**
E.	What is the name of the primary health plan?	**Medicare**
F.	Is there a secondary health plan? If yes, what is the name of the plan?	**Century SeniorGap**
G.	Who is the policyholder for the health plan?	**Geraldo Muñoz**
H.	What is the policy ID number of the primary plan? Group number?	**ID: 999832166A** **Group number: None**
I.	What is the policy ID number of the secondary plan? Group number?	**ID: 999832166** **Group number: MG5121**

STEP 2

If MOSS is running, continue to the next step. Otherwise, start MOSS and use your logon information to begin using the software.

STEP 3

HINT: Dr. Heath is the admitting physician, participates with Medicare, and accepts assignment.

Open the Patient Registration screen. Check the database to make sure Geraldo Muñoz is not already in the system. If not, click *Add*, and then enter data from the admission form for patient Muñoz. Include demographic, employer, and insurance coverage information. Check your work with Figure 5-35, Figure 5-36, and Figure 5-37.

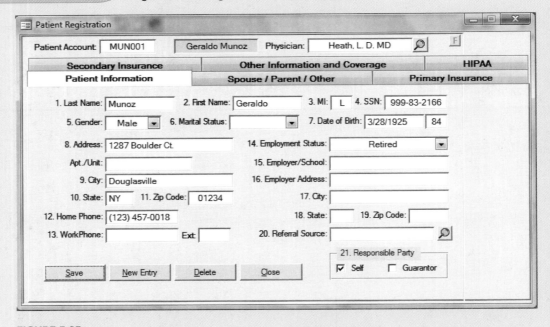

FIGURE 5-35

Delmar/Cengage Learning

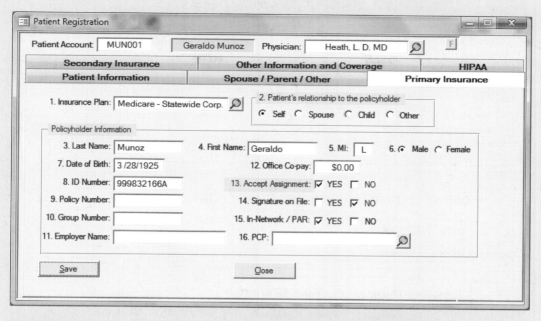

FIGURE 5-36

Delmar/Cengage Learning

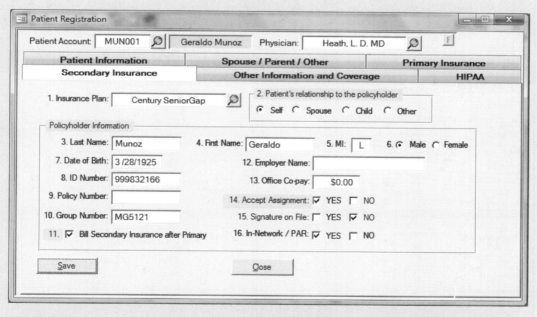

FIGURE 5-37

Delmar/Cengage Learning

STEP 4

Since the patient was an inpatient at the hospital, we do not have a signature on file yet. The patient also has not received or signed for the privacy notice.

STEP 5

Check your work to make sure it is complete and accurate. Click the *Save* button when finished.

Case Study 5-K Continues >>

STEP 6

Verify the secondary insurance (Century SeniorGap) for Geraldo Muñoz by using the online eligibility feature. Print the report for your records. Explain why Medicare is not verified, as shown in Figure 5-38.

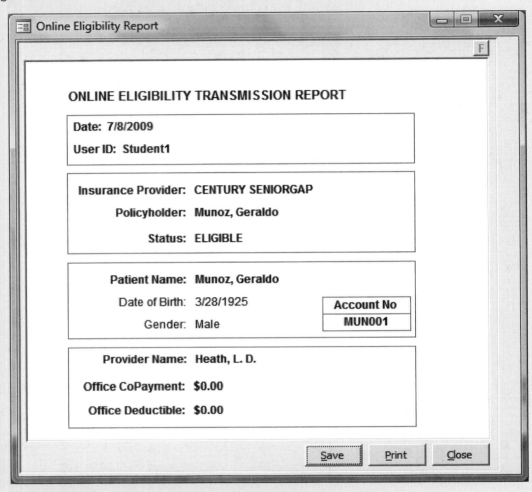

FIGURE 5-38
Delmar/Cengage Learning

CASE STUDY 5–L: RUHL, MARY

Refer to the Source Documents Section at the end of this book. Mary Ruhl's face sheet (Source Document 5-20) will be needed for the following exercise.

New patient: **Ruhl, Mary**

Facility: **New York County Hospital**

Status: **Inpatient**

Physician: **Heath**

STEP 1

Carefully review the information on the admission form from New York County Hospital and answer the following questions. *Cover the answers using the tear-off bookmark from the cover of your book. Check your work before entering data into MOSS.*

A.	What is the patient's date of birth?	**12/5/1935**
B.	Is the patient employed?	**No**
C.	What is the patient's marital status? If married, what is the spouse's name?	**Married; Robert M. Ruhl**
D.	How many insurance policies is the patient covered by?	**2**
E.	What is the name of the primary health plan?	**Flexihealth PPO**
F.	Is there a secondary health plan? If yes, what is the name of the plan?	**Medicare**
G.	Who is the policyholder for the health plan(s)?	**Robert M. Ruhl**
H.	What is the policy ID number of the primary plan? Group number?	**ID: 999321168-02 Group number: BH225**
I.	What is the identification number for the secondary plan? If Medicare, what do you know about this insurance based on the HIC number and suffix?	**ID: 999321168B**

NT: In this example, Robert guarantor and is the policy-der for the FlexiHealth plan.

STEP 2

If MOSS is running, continue to the next step. Otherwise, start MOSS and use your logon information to begin using the software.

STEP 3

NT: Dr. Heath is the admit-g physician, participates with th FlexiHealth and Medicare, d accepts assignment.

Open the Patient Registration screen. Check the database to make sure Mary Ruhl is not already in the system. If not, click *Add*, and then enter data from the admission form for patient Ruhl. Include demographic, spouse, and insurance coverage information. Do not forget to enter the information that this in-network insurance plan has a $20.00 office co-payment. The secondary insurance will be billed. Check your work with Figure 5-39, Figure 5-40, and Figure 5-41.

Case Study 5-L Continues >>

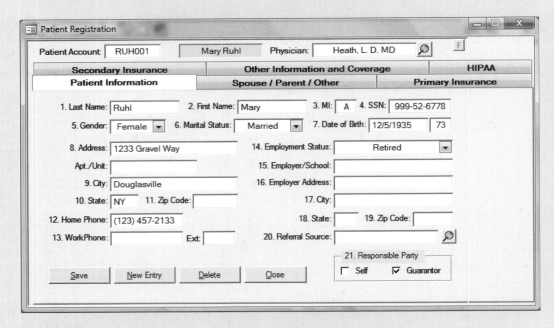

FIGURE 5-39

Delmar/Cengage Learning

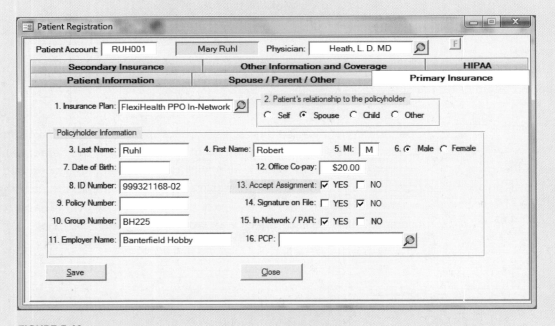

FIGURE 5-40

Delmar/Cengage Learning

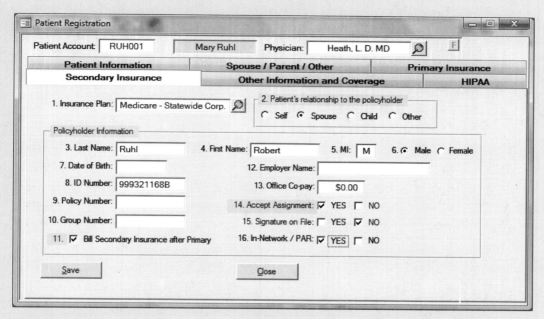

FIGURE 5-41

Delmar/Cengage Learning

STEP 4

Since the patient was an inpatient at the hospital, we do not yet have a signature on file. The patient also has not received or signed for the privacy notice.

STEP 5

Check your work to make sure it is complete and accurate. Click the *Save* button when finished.

STEP 6

Verify the primary insurance for Mary Ruhl by using the online eligibility feature. Print the report for your records.

CASE STUDY 5–M: MALLORY, CHRISTINA

Refer to the Source Documents Section at the end of this book. Christina Mallory's face sheet (Source Document 5-21) will be needed for the following exercise.

New patient:	**Mallory, Christina**
Facility:	**New York County Hospital**
Status:	**Inpatient**
Physician:	**Heath**

Case Study 5-M Continues >>

STEP 1

Carefully review the information on the admission form from New York County Hospital and answer the following questions. *Cover the answers using the tear-off bookmark from the cover of your book. Check your work before entering data into MOSS.*

A.	What is the patient's date of birth?	**2/20/1990**
B.	Is the patient employed?	**No**
C.	What is her student status?	**Full-time**
D.	What is the name of the school she attends?	**Central University**
E.	What is the patient's marital status?	**Single**
F.	How many insurance policies is the patient covered by?	**1**
G.	What is the name of the primary health plan?	**Flexihealth PPO**
H.	Who is the policyholder for the health plan?	**Michael Mallory**
I.	What is the policy ID number of the primary plan? Group number?	**ID: 999510226-B2** **Group number: PP2891**

STEP 2

If MOSS is running, continue to the next step. Otherwise, start MOSS and use your logon information to begin using the software.

STEP 3

Open the Patient Registration screen. Check the database to make sure Christina Mallory is not already in the system. If not, click *Add*, and then enter data from the admission form for patient Mallory. Include demographic, parent, and insurance coverage information. Do not forget to enter the information that this in-network insurance plan has a $20.00 office co-payment. Check you work with Figure 5-42, Figure 5-43, and Figure 5-44.

HINT: Dr. Heath is the admitting physician, participates with FlexiHealth, and accepts assignment.

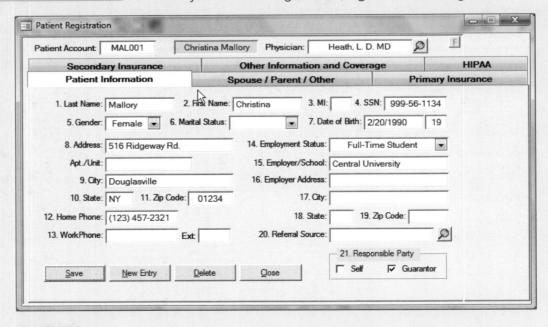

FIGURE 5-42

Delmar/Cengage Learning

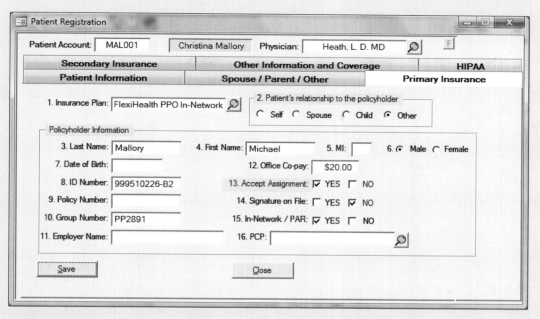

FIGURE 5-43

Delmar/Cengage Learning

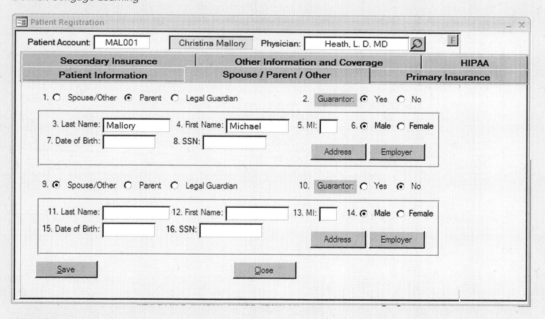

FIGURE 5-44

Delmar/Cengage Learning

STEP 4

Since the patient was an inpatient at the hospital, we do not have a signature on file yet. The patient also has not received or signed for the privacy notice.

STEP 5

Check your work to make sure it is complete and accurate. Click the *Save* button when finished.

STEP 6

Verify the primary insurance for Christina Mallory by using the online eligibility feature. Print the report for your records.

CASE STUDY 5–N: GOODNOW, LEONA

Refer to the Source Documents Section at the end of this book. Leona Goodnow's emergency outpatient record (Source Document 5-22) will be needed for the following exercise.

New patient: **Goodnow, Leona**

Facility: **Community General Hospital—Emergency Room**

Status: **Outpatient ER services; discharged same day.**

Physician: **Schwartz**

STEP 1

Carefully review the information on the emergency room outpatient record from Community General Hospital and answer the following questions. *Cover the answers using the tear-off bookmark from the cover of your book. Check your work before entering data into MOSS.*

HINT: If the patient's employment status is unknown, select "unemployed" until this information can be confirmed.

A.	What is the patient's date of birth?	7/31/1979
B.	Is the patient employed?	Unknown—select Unemployed
C.	What is the patient's marital status? If married, what is the spouse's name?	Married; Thomas L. Goodnow
D.	How many insurance policies is the patient covered by?	1
E.	What is the name of the primary health plan?	ConsumerONE HRA
F.	Who is the policyholder for the health plan?	Thomas L. Goodnow
G.	What is the policy ID number of the primary plan? Group number?	ID: 999151189-02 Group number: TRG01

STEP 2

If MOSS is running, continue to the next step. Otherwise, start MOSS and use your logon information to begin using the software.

STEP 3

HINT: Dr. Schwartz is the admitting physician, participates with ConsumerOne HRA, and does accept assignment.

Open the Patient Registration screen. Check the database to make sure Leona Goodnow is not already in the system. If not, click *Add*, and then enter as much data as is available from the admission form for patient Goodnow. Include demographic, spouse, and insurance coverage information. Check your work with Figure 5-45, Figure 5-46, and Figure 5-47.

STEP 4

Since the patient was an outpatient at the ER, we do not yet have a signature on file. The patient also has not received or signed for the privacy notice.

STEP 5

Check your work to make sure it is complete and accurate. Click the *Save* button when finished.

STEP 6

Verify the primary insurance for Leona Goodnow by using the online eligibility feature. Print the report for your records.

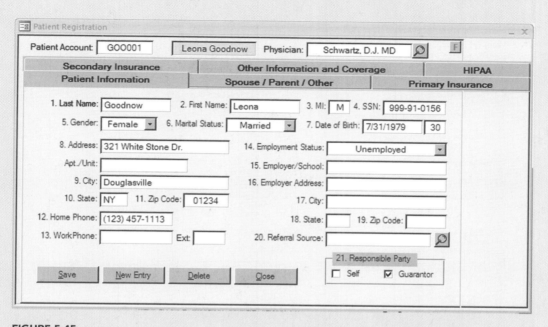

FIGURE 5-45

Delmar/Cengage Learning

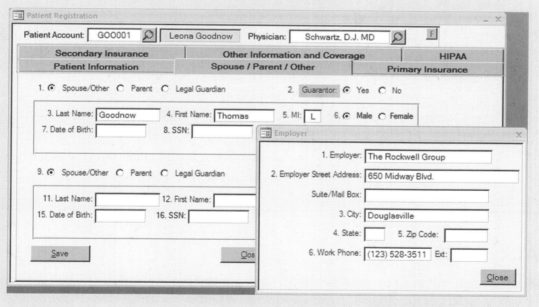

FIGURE 5-46

Delmar/Cengage Learning

Case Study 5-N Continues >>

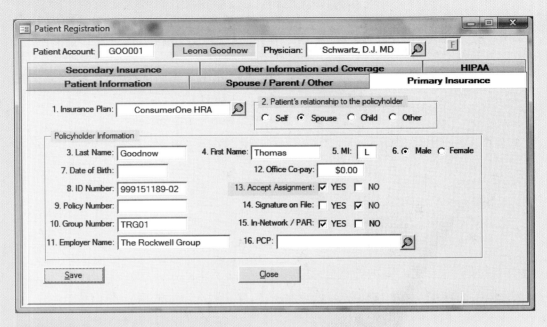

FIGURE 5-47

Delmar/Cengage Learning

STEP 7

Review the entire emergency room outpatient record (Source Document 5-22) for Leona Goodnow. Answer the following questions:

A. Why did the patient visit the emergency room?

HINT: Refer to the chief complaint.

B. What is the patient's description of her ailment?

C. What treatment was done at the emergency room?

D. What were the instructions to the patient from the physician?

E. Was the patient asked to see a doctor in follow-up? If yes, whom should she see, and when?

FINAL NOTES

The patient registration process is the single, most important process that lays out the foundation for excellent record keeping and reimbursement. Whether patients receive services in the office or at outside facilities, documentation is key, not only for proper follow-up and continuity of care for patients, but also to support every claim that is submitted to insurance companies.

Every member of the health care team has a responsibility to contribute to the overall accuracy and completeness of the patient record. Many individuals, in the course of their work in the office, reference patient records for many different tasks. Everything begins with patient registration, and continues as an ongoing process of maintenance, updating, and ensuring privacy.

CHECK YOUR KNOWLEDGE

Select the correct description for each of the following medical facilities.

a. Provides nursing care and rehabilitation services to people with illnesses, injuries, or functional disabilities

b. Provides 24-hour-care patients with the highest level of medical need

c. Provides a facility where surgical medical procedures or skilled rehabilitation services are performed and patients return home the same day

d. Provides service to patients who need 24-hour nursing supervision to ensure medical, psychological, or social needs are met

1. _____ Nursing Home

2. _____ Hospital

3. _____ Ambulatory Surgical Center

4. _____ Skilled Nursing Facility

5. Individuals who manage the administrative tasks of the nurse's station at hospitals are called

   a. office managers.

   b. health unit coordinators.

   c. medical receptionists.

   d. head nurses.

   e. none of the above.

6. The physician has rendered services to a new patient at the hospital. The only information available is the patient's name, location, and diagnosis.

   a. Describe examples where patient information can be obtained for registration and medical billing purposes.

   _____

   _____

   b. Explain the requirements of HIPAA for requesting and using information from medical providers and facilities.

   _____

   _____

7. The physician selected by or assigned to a patient who has primary responsibility for the treatment and care of the patient is called the

   a. referring physician.

   b. specialist.

   c. primary care physician.

   d. attending physician.

8. The equivalent of the registration form in a hospital setting is the face sheet, or admitting form.

   a. True

   b. False

Procedure Posting Routines

OBJECTIVES

Upon completion of this unit, the reader should be able to:

- Describe the parts of a superbill (encounter form) and the information it contains

- Using the superbill, demonstrate posting of procedure charges with *Medical Office Simulation Software* (MOSS)

- Demonstrate posting a payment made at the time of an office service, using MOSS

- Demonstrate opening and viewing the patient ledger to review charges and payments made on an account

- Demonstrate scheduling a follow-up appointment after a patient visit, following instructions from the physician

- Demonstrate posting of procedure charges for services performed outside the office for hospital and nursing home patients.

KEY TERMS

Block billing

Charges

Procedure posting

During patient hours on a typical day, several established and new patients will visit the medical office. Each patient, such as those registered in Unit 5, will receive services from the health care professionals in the clinical area. The superbill, also known as an encounter form, is used as a source document during office visits. Each procedure, and the diagnoses for which they are performed, is recorded on the superbill and returned to the front office. Next, the administrative staff reviews the superbill to be certain it is complete, and then applies the charges for services to the patient's account. The **charges** are the fees for each procedure performed. This process is referred to as entering procedure charges, or **procedure posting**.

The front-office administrative staff also collects payments from patients, as needed. Most offices require that applicable co-payments be paid at the time of the visit, either before or after. This is also the best time to collect past due balances, deductible portions, or any other balance due from the patient. The last task before the patient leaves the office is scheduling the follow-up appointment, as indicated by the physician.

In this unit, exercises that include procedure and payment posting will be completed using MOSS. Follow-up visits also will be scheduled as needed.

PARTS OF THE SUPERBILL

Recall that the superbill may also be known by other names. Among the most common are the encounter form, charge ticket, visit slip, and voucher. All are basically the same type of document with similar information. For simplicity, the term superbill is used in this book to refer collectively to this source document, regardless of other names used for it.

In order to properly review the superbill for completeness, it is important to understand the basic parts of this document. Douglasville Medicine Associates uses a standard superbill containing much of the information found in a typical family practice office. Each office must customize superbills according to type of practice and codes used; however, most of the information shown in Figure 6-1 is contained on all superbills. Refer to Figure 6-1 while reviewing each of the following components.

1. **Patient name.** The name of the patient receiving the service.

2. **Reference number.** Each superbill or encounter form has a sequential reference number, sometimes called a voucher number. This serves for identifying and matching the document to the services posted to the software. Medical offices may store superbills for record-keeping purposes, in case they need to be referenced in the future. A good example may be tracking a procedure that did not get posted because it was missed on the superbill at the time charges were entered.

3. **Place of service.** The location where services were rendered to the patient is indicated in this area. Procedures that took place outside the medical office can be recorded on the superbill and then posted to the software. Recall from Unit 5 that physicians need to report to the staff which patients received services outside the office, including where and when.

4. **Date of service.** Provides the date services were rendered to the patient.

5. **Procedure list.** This area lists the most common procedures for the practice, including CPT codes. Clinical staff will check off the services rendered to the patient.

6. **Miscellaneous.** Any procedures not on the list can be written in the "miscellaneous" section and, if needed, coded by the medical biller at a later time.

7. **Amount paid.** The total amount paid by the patient for services is entered here.

8. **Diagnoses not listed.** Any diagnosis not listed on the superbill is written in by the health care professional on this line. The medical biller codes the diagnosis, if needed.

9. **Diagnoses list.** Diagnoses most common to the medical practice are listed here. The physician indicates which diagnoses support the procedures performed by placing a "1," "2," or "3" on the line to the right. The numbers represent the primary diagnosis, secondary diagnosis, and even a tertiary diagnosis. The physician will write "4" if a fourth diagnosis also applies.

PLEASE RETURN THIS FORM TO RECEPTIONIST

NAME (1)

2330 (2)

(3)
PLACE OF
SERVICE:
( ) OFFICE
( ) NEW YORK COUNTY HOSPITAL
( ) COMMUNITY GENERAL HOSPITAL

( ) RETIREMENT INN NURSING HOME
( ) _____

DATE OF SERVICE _____ (4)

A. OFFICE VISITS - New Patient

Code	History	Exam	Dec.	Time
____ 99201	Prob. Foc.	Prob. Foc.	Straight	10 min. _____
____ 99202	Ex. Prob. Foc.	Ex. Prob. Foc.	Straight	20 min. _____
____ 99203	Detail	Detail	Low	30 min. _____
____ 99204	Comp.	Comp.	Mod.	45 min. _____
____ 99205	Comp.	Comp.	High	60 min. _____

B. OFFICE VISIT - Established Patient

Code	History	Exam	Dec.	Time
____ 99211	Minimal	Minimal	Minimal	5 min. _____
____ 99212	Prob. Foc.	Prob. Foc.	Straight	10min. _____
____ 99213	Ex. Prob. Foc.	Ex. Prob. Foc.	Low	15 min. _____
____ 99214	Detail	Detail	Mod.	25 min. _____
____ 99215	Comp.	Comp.	High	40 min. _____

C. HOSPITAL CARE   Dx Units

1. Initial Hospital Care (30 min) ____ ____ 99221 _____
2. Subsequent Care ____ ____ 99231 _____
3. Critical Care (30-74 min) ____ ____ 99291 _____
4. each additional 30 min. ____ ____ 99292 _____
5. Discharge Services ____ ____ 99238 _____
6. Emergency Room ____ ____ 99282 _____

D. NURSING HOME CARE

Dx Units

Initial Care - New Pt.
1. Expanded ____ ____ 99322 _____
2. Detailed ____ ____ 99323 _____

Subsequent Care - Estab. Pt.
3. Problem Focused ____ ____ 99307 _____
4. Expanded ____ ____ 99308 _____
5. Detailed ____ ____ 99309 _____
5. Comprehensive ____ ____ 99310 _____

E. PROCEDURES
1. Arthrocentesis, Small Jt. ____ 20600 _____
2. Colonoscopy ____ 45378 _____
3. EKG w/interpretation ____ 93000 _____
4. X-Ray Chest, PA/LAT ____ 71020 _____

F. LAB
1. Blood Sugar ____ 82947 _____
2. CBC w/differential ____ 85031 _____
3. Cholesterol ____ 82465 _____
4. Comprehensive Metabolic Panel ____ 80053 _____
5. ESR ____ 85651 _____
6. Hematocrit ____ 85014 _____
7. Mono Screen ____ 86308 _____
8. Pap Smear ____ 88150 _____
9. Potassium ____ 84132 _____
10. Preg. Test, Quantitative ____ 84702 _____
11. Routine Venipuncture ____ 36415 _____

F. Cont'd   Dx Units
12. Strep Screen ____ 87081 _____
13. UA, Routine w/Micro ____ 81000 _____
14. UA, Routine w/o Micro ____ 81002 _____
15. Uric Acid ____ 84550 _____
16. VDRL ____ 86592 _____
17. Wet Prep ____ 82710 _____
18. _____ ____ ____ _____

G. INJECTIONS
1. Influenza Virus Vaccine ____ 90658 _____
2. Pneumoccoccal Vaccine ____ 90772 _____
3. Tetanus Toxoids ____ 90703 _____
4. Therapeutic Subcut/IM ____ 90732 _____
5. Vaccine Administration ____ 90471 _____
6. Vaccine - each additional ____ 90472 _____

H. MISCELLANEOUS (6)
1. _____ ____
2. _____ ____

AMOUNT PAID $ ____ (7)

(5)

Mark diagnosis with
(1=Primary, 2=Secondary, 3=Tertiary)

DIAGNOSIS
NOT LISTED _____ (8)
BELOW _____

DIAGNOSIS	ICD-9-CM 1, 2, 3	DIAGNOSIS	ICD-9-CM 1, 2, 3	DIAGNOSIS	ICD-9-CM 1, 2, 3
Abdominal Pain	789.0_	Dehydration	276.51	Otitis Media, Acute NOS	382.9
Allergic Rhinitis, Unspec.	477.9	Depression, NOS	311	Peptic Ulcer Disease	536.9
Angina Pectoris, Unspec.	413.9	Diabetes Mellitus, Type II Controlled	250.00	Peripheral Vascular Disease NOS	443.9
Anemia, Iron Deficiency, Unspec.	280.9	Diabetes Mellitus, Type II Controlled	250.02	Pharyngitis, Acute	462
Anemia, NOS	285.9	Drug Reaction, NOS	995.29	Pneumonia, Organism Unspec.	486
Anemia, Pernicious	281.0	Dysuria	788.1	Prostatitis, NOS	601.9
Asthma w/ Exacerbation	493.92	Eczema, NOS	692.2	PVC	427.69
Asthmatic Bronchitis, Unspec.	493.90	Edema	782.3	Rash, Non Specific	782.1
Atrial Fibrillation	427.31	Fever, Unknown Origin	780.6	Seizure Disorder NOS	780.39
Atypical Chest Pain, Unspec.	786.59	Gastritis, Acute w/o Hemorrhage	535.00	Serous Otitis Media, Chronic, Unspec.	381.10
Bronchiolitis, due to RSV	466.11	Gastroenteritis, NOS	558.9	Sinusitis, Acute NOS	461.9
Bronchitis, Acute	466.0	Gastroesophageal Reflux	530.81	Tonsillitis, Acute	463.
Bronchitis, NOS	490	Hepatitis A, Infectious	070.1	Upper Respiratory Infection, Acute NOS	465.9
Cardiac Arrest	427.5	Hypercholesterolemia, Pure	272	Urinary Tract Infection, Unspec.	599.0
Cardiopulmonary Disease, Chronic, Unspec.	416.9	Hypertension, Unspec.	401.9	Urticaria, Unspec.	708.9
Cellulitis, NOS	682.9	Hypoglycemia NOS	251.2	Vertigo, NOS	780.4
Congestive Heart Failure, Unspec.	428.0	Hypokalemia	276.8	Viral Infection NOS	079.99
Contact Dermatitis NOS	692.9	Impetigo	684	Weakness, Generalized	780.79
COPD NOS	496	Lymphadenitis, Unspec.	289.3	Weight Loss, Abnormal	783.21
CVA, Acute, NOS	434.91	Mononucleosis	075		
CVA, Old or Healed	438.9	Myocardial Infarction, Acute, NOS	410.9		
Degenerative Arthritis		Organic Brain Syndrome	310.9		
(Specify Site)	715.9	Otitis Externa, Acute NOS	380.10		

(9)

(10) **ABN: I UNDERSTAND THAT MEDICARE PROBABLY WILL NOT COVER THE SERVICES LISTED BELOW**

A. _____ B. _____ C. _____
        Patient
Date _____ Signature _____

Doctor's
Signature (11) _____

(12) RETURN: _____ Days _____ Weeks _____ Months

REF# 122949 SB (05.07.09)   TO REORDER CALL INHEALTH RECORD SYSTEMS 800-477-7374

(13) **DOUGLASVILLE MEDICINE ASSOCIATES**
5076 BRAND BLVD., SUITE 401
DOUGLASVILLE, NY 01234
PHONE No. (123) 456-7890
☐ L.D. HEATH, M.D.   ☐ D.J. SCHWARTZ, M.D.
NPI# 9995010111   NPI# 9995020212
EIN# 00-1234560

FIGURE 6-1

Components of a superbill, or encounter form. *Used with permission. InHealth Record Systems, Inc., 5076 Winters Chapel Road, Atlanta, GA 30360, 800-477-7374. http://www.inhealthrecords.com*

10. **ABN notice.** An Advance Beneficiary Notice (ABN) advises Medicare beneficiaries, before items or services actually are provided, when Medicare is likely to deny payment for them. ABNs allow beneficiaries to make informed consumer decisions about receiving items or services for which they may have to pay out-of-pocket, and to be more active participants in their own health care treatment decisions. It is the responsibility of the provider to inform Medicare patients when a procedure is likely to be denied, and why. Signature on an ABN form confirms that this disclosure has taken place.

11. **Doctor's signature.** The physician signs the superbill, confirming the information it contains.

12. **Return.** The physician provides information indicating when the patient is to be seen again in follow-up. The front-desk staff uses this information to schedule the next appointment.

13. **Practice and physician information.** The practice information and relevant identification numbers are displayed in this area. There is also a check box in front of each physician's name used to indicate which one provided services to the patient.

In Unit 3, several new and established patients were scheduled for appointments. In Unit 5, new patients were registered when they arrived for appointments. Case studies in this unit will guide you through the procedure posting process as each patient checks out upon completion of his or her visit. If you have not completed the patient registration exercises from the case studies in Unit 5, *do not proceed.* These are required to continue.

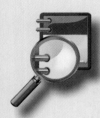

LET'S TRY IT! 6-1 **POSTING PROCEDURE CHARGES**

CASE STUDY 6–A: PRACTICE, PATTY

Objective: The reader will practice entering charges, posting a payment at the time of service, and scheduling a follow-up appointment, before proceeding with the simulation patients for Douglasville Medicine Associates.

Patient:	**Practice, Patty**
Service Date:	**October 28, 2009**
Superbill:	**Figure 6-2**
Physician:	**Heath**

Check-out Details

Today's date is 10/28/2009. The patient will pay her co-payment before leaving the office. The office will submit a claim to the insurance company. The patient will also schedule her follow-up appointment before leaving the office today.

STEP 1
Start MOSS.

STEP 2
Click on the *Procedure Posting button* on the Main Menu. Locate patient Practice from the Patient Selection window and then click on her *name*. Next, click the *Add button*, since you will be adding procedures to her account.

PLEASE RETURN THIS FORM TO RECEPTIONIST

NAME *Practice, Patty*

2331

PLACE OF SERVICE:	(X) OFFICE	( ) RETIREMENT INN NURSING HOME
	( ) NEW YORK COUNTY HOSPITAL	
	( ) COMMUNITY GENERAL HOSPITAL	( ) _____

DATE OF SERVICE *10/28/2009*

A. OFFICE VISITS - New Patient

Code	History	Exam	Dec.	Time	
___ 99201	Prob. Foc.	Prob. Foc.	Straight	10 min.	_____
___ 99202	Ex. Prob. Foc.	Ex. Prob. Foc.	Straight	20 min.	_____
___ 99203	Detail	Detail	Low	30 min.	_____
___ 99204	Comp.	Comp.	Mod.	45 min.	_____
___ 99205	Comp.	Comp.	High	60 min.	_____

B. OFFICE VISIT - Established Patient

Code	History	Exam	Dec.	Time	
___ 99211	Minimal	Minimal	Minimal	5 min.	_____
___ 99212	Prob. Foc.	Prob. Foc.	Straight	10min.	_____
___ 99213	Ex. Prob. Foc.	Ex. Prob. Foc.	Low	15 min.	_____
X 99214	Detail	Detail	Mod.	25 min.	1,2
___ 99215	Comp.	Comp.	High	40 min.	_____

C. HOSPITAL CARE   Dx   Units

1. Initial Hospital Care (30 min) ___ ___ 99221 _____
2. Subsequent Care ___ ___ 99231 _____
3. Critical Care (30-74 min) ___ ___ 99291 _____
4. each additional 30 min. ___ ___ 99292 _____
5. Discharge Services ___ ___ 99238 _____
6. Emergency Room ___ ___ 99282 _____

D. NURSING HOME CARE   Dx   Units

Initial Care - New Pt.

1. Expanded ___ ___ 99322 _____
2. Detailed ___ ___ 99323 _____

Subsequent Care - Estab. Pt.

3. Problem Focused ___ ___ 99307 _____
4. Expanded ___ ___ 99308 _____
5. Detailed ___ ___ 99309 _____
5. Comprehensive ___ ___ 99310 _____

E. PROCEDURES

1. Arthrocentesis, Small Jt. ___ 20600 _____
2. Colonoscopy ___ 45378 _____
3. EKG w/interpretation ___ 93000 _____
4. X-Ray Chest, PA/LAT ___ 71020 _____

F. LAB

1. Blood Sugar ___ 82947 _____
2. CBC w/differential 1 85031 X
3. Cholesterol ___ 82465 _____
4. Comprehensive Metabolic Panel ___ 80053 _____
5. ESR ___ 85651 _____
6. Hematocrit ___ 85014 _____
7. Mono Screen ___ 86308 _____
8. Pap Smear ___ 88150 _____
9. Potassium ___ 84132 _____
10. Preg. Test, Quantitative ___ 84702 _____
11. Routine Venipuncture ___ 36415 _____

F. Cont'd   Dx   Units

12. Strep Screen ___ 87081 _____
13. UA, Routine w/Micro ___ 81000 _____
14. UA, Routine w/o Micro ___ 81002 _____
15. Uric Acid ___ 84550 _____
16. VDRL ___ 86592 _____
17. Wet Prep ___ 82710 _____
18. ___ ___ _____

G. INJECTIONS

1. Influenza Virus Vaccine ___ 90658 _____
2. Pneumoccocal Vaccine ___ 90772 _____
3. Tetanus Toxoids ___ 90703 _____
4. Therapeutic Subcut/IM ___ 90732 _____
5. Vaccine Administration ___ 90471 _____
6. Vaccine - each additional ___ 90472 _____

H. MISCELLANEOUS

1. ___ ___ _____
2. ___ ___ _____

AMOUNT PAID $ *20.00*

Mark diagnosis with (1=Primary, 2=Secondary, 3=Tertiary)

DIAGNOSIS NOT LISTED BELOW _____

DIAGNOSIS	ICD-9-CM 1, 2, 3	DIAGNOSIS	ICD-9-CM 1, 2, 3	DIAGNOSIS	ICD-9-CM 1, 2, 3
Abdominal Pain	789.0	Dehydration	276.51 2	Otitis Media, Acute NOS	382.9
Allergic Rhinitis, Unspec.	477.9	Depression, NOS	311	Peptic Ulcer Disease	536.9
Angina Pectoris, Unspec.	413.9	Diabetes Mellitus, Type II Controlled	250.00	Peripheral Vascular Disease NOS	443.9
Anemia, Iron Deficiency, Unspec.	280.9	Diabetes Mellitus, Type II Controlled	250.02	Pharyngitis, Acute	462
Anemia, NOS	285.9	Drug Reaction, NOS	995.29	Pneumonia, Organism Unspec.	486
Anemia, Pernicious	281.0	Dysuria	788.1	Prostatitis, NOS	601.9
Asthma w/ Exacerbation	493.92	Eczema, NOS	692.2	PVC	427.69
Asthmatic Bronchitis, Unspec.	493.90	Edema	782.3	Rash, Non Specific	782.1
Atrial Fibrillation	427.31	Fever, Unknown Origin	780.6 1	Seizure Disorder NOS	780.39
Atypical Chest Pain, Unspec.	786.59	Gastritis, Acute w/o Hemorrhage	535.00	Serous Otitis Media, Chronic, Unspec.	381.10
Bronchiolitis, due to RSV	466.11	Gastroenteritis, NOS	558.9	Sinusitis, Acute NOS	461.9
Bronchitis, Acute	466.0	Gastroesophageal Reflux	530.81	Tonsillitis, Acute	463.
Bronchitis, NOS	490	Hepatitis A, Infectious	070.1	Upper Respiratory Infection, Acute NOS	465.9
Cardiac Arrest	427.5	Hypercholesterolemia, Pure	272.0	Urinary Tract Infection, Unspec.	599.0
Cardiopulmonary Disease, Chronic, Unspec.	416.9	Hypertension, Unspec.	401.9	Urticaria, Unspec.	708.9
Cellulitis, NOS	682.9	Hypoglycemia NOS	251.2	Vertigo, NOS	780.4
Congestive Heart Failure, Unspec.	428.0	Hypokalemia	276.8	Viral Infection NOS	079.99
Contact Dermatitis NOS	692.9	Impetigo	684	Weakness, Generalized	780.79
COPD NOS	496	Lymphadenitis, Unspec.	289.3	Weight Loss, Abnormal	783.21
CVA, Acute, NOS	434.91	Mononucleosis	075		
CVA, Old or Healed	438.9	Myocardial Infarction, Acute, NOS	410.9		
Degenerative Arthritis		Organic Brain Syndrome	310.9		
(Specify Site)	715.9	Otitis Externa, Acute NOS	380.10		

ABN: I UNDERSTAND THAT MEDICARE PROBABLY WILL NOT COVER THE SERVICES LISTED BELOW

A. _____ B. _____ C. _____

Patient

Date _____ Signature _____

Doctor's Signature *L.D. Heath* _____

RETURN: _2_ Days _____ Weeks _____ Months _____

REF# 122949 SB (05.07.09)   TO REORDER CALL INHEALTH RECORD SYSTEMS 800-477-7374

DOUGLASVILLE MEDICINE ASSOCIATES
5076 BRAND BLVD., SUITE 401
DOUGLASVILLE, NY 01234
PHONE No. (123) 456-7890

☒ L.D. HEATH, M.D.   ☐ D.J. SCHWARTZ, M.D.
NPI# 9995010111   NPI# 9995020212
EIN# 00-1234560

FIGURE 6-2

Superbill for Patty Practice. *Used with permission. InHealth Record Systems, Inc., 5076 Winters Chapel Road, Atlanta, GA 30360, 800-477-7374. http://www.inhealthrecords.com*

Case Study 6-A Continues >>

STEP 3

The Procedure Entry window opens. Next, refer to the superbill in Figure 6-2. Enter the superbill reference number in Field 1, as shown in Figure 6-3.

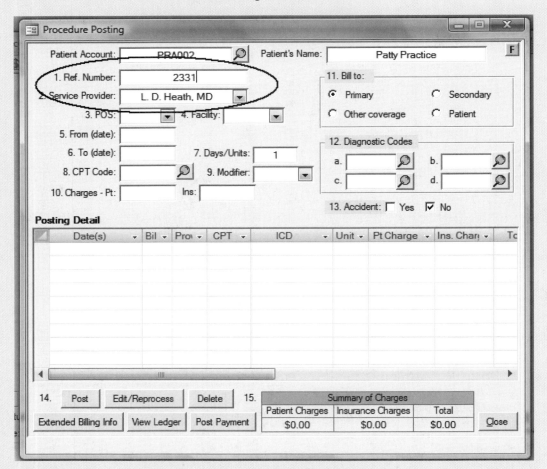

FIGURE 6-3

Delmar/Cengage Learning

STEP 4

Use the *Tab* key to move down to Field 3, POS, which stands for Place of Service. Drop down the box and select *Office.* Because the service was rendered in the office, it is not necessary to use Field 4 at this time.

STEP 5

Use the *Tab* key and move to Field 5. Notice there are two date fields; Field 5 reads "From" and Field 6 reads "To." For all procedures that take place on one date of service, use Field 5 only. Enter the service date for patient Practice in Field 5.

NOTE: It is not necessary to use Field 6 unless there is a range of dates to be charged, such as consecutive hospital visits. Use a range of dates only when the same CPT procedure code applies to each of the consecutive dates. This is referred to as **block billing**.

STEP 6

Refer to patient Practice's superbill and locate the procedures that have been checked off by the back office. Answer the following questions. *Cover the answers using the tear-off bookmark from the cover of your book. Check your work before entering data into MOSS to be sure you have correctly interpreted the source documents.*

A.	Which procedures were done for patient Practice?	**Office visit and CBC w/differential**
B.	What is the CPT code for each procedure?	**99214 and 85031**
C.	How many total procedures were performed?	**2**

Enter the CPT code for the first procedure in Field 8. Press the *Enter* key. The charges for this procedure should appear in Field 10. The patient's co-payment is in the left field, and the amount to be billed to the insurance company is in the right field. Check your work with Figure 6-4.

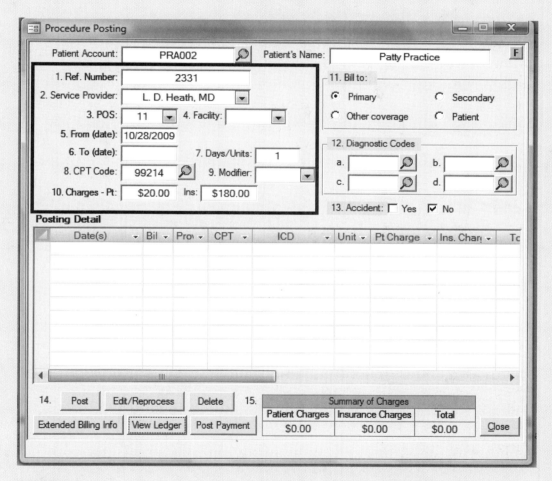

FIGURE 6-4

Delmar/Cengage Learning

Case Study 6-A Continues >>

Case Study 6-A Continued

STEP 7

Next, tab to Field 11. Bill Primary should be selected by default, indicating that the patient's primary insurance will be billed for these services.

STEP 8

Tab to Field 12a, Diagnostic Codes. Up to four diagnostic codes can be entered for a patient as indicated by the physician. Locate the diagnosis for patient Practice on the superbill. Answer the following questions.

| A. | How many diagnoses does this patient have? | 2 |
| B. | What is the description and code for each diagnosis for this patient? | 780.6 (fever, unknown origin) and 276.51 (dehydration) |

Enter the primary diagnostic code (marked "1") in Field 12a, and the secondary (marked "2") in Field 12b. Since the visit code (99214) is the first to be entered, all relevant diagnoses the patient came for will be entered. The Search icon next to the field can also be used to search and edit codes as needed.

STEP 9

The procedures for this case were not related to an accident, so be sure that Field 13 reads "No." Check your work with Figure 6-5.

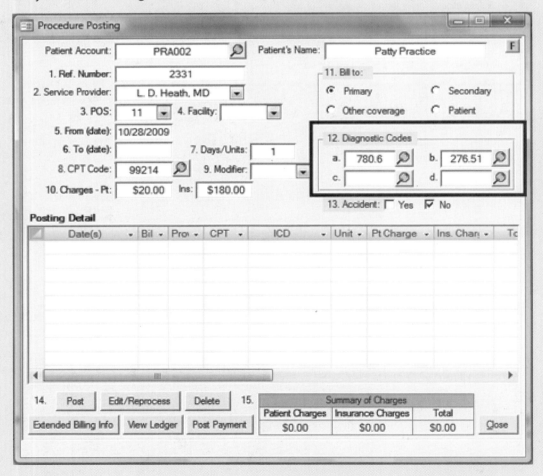

FIGURE 6-5

Delmar/Cengage Learning

STEP 10

When you are sure the entries are correct, click on the *Post button*. This will post the charges to the patient's account and display in the Posting Detail area in the middle of the window. See Figure 6-6.

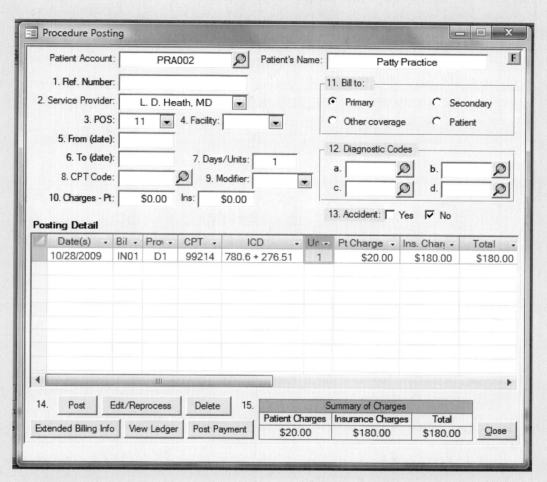

FIGURE 6-6

Delmar/Cengage Learning

Case Study 6-A Continues >>

MOSS NOTE: The Posting Detail displays only the current procedures that were posted. To view all charges, payments, and adjustments on a patient account, click on the *View Ledger button*. See Figure 6-7 for an example of the Patient Ledger screen. The Patient Ledger screen is meant to be viewed only; changes cannot be made to entries via the ledger. Click on the *Close button* to return to the Procedure Posting screen.

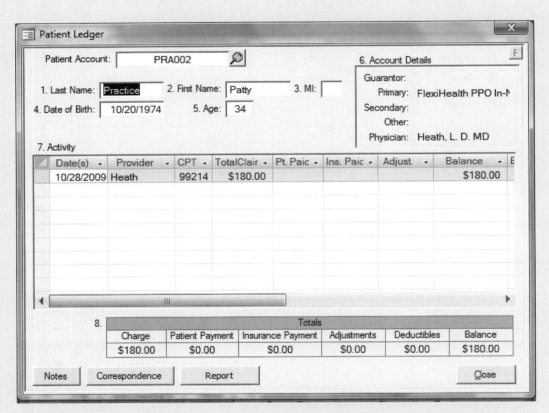

FIGURE 6-7
Delmar/Cengage Learning

STEP 11

Now that one set of charges has been entered and is displayed in the Posting Detail area, another charge can be entered. In Field 1, enter the reference number of the superbill (refer back to Figure 6-2). The physician indicated on the superbill that the "CBC w/differential" was provided for diagnosis "1," referring to the diagnoses in the lower area of the superbill. Enter the charge for this lab service using the methods you have just learned. Check your work with Figure 6-8.

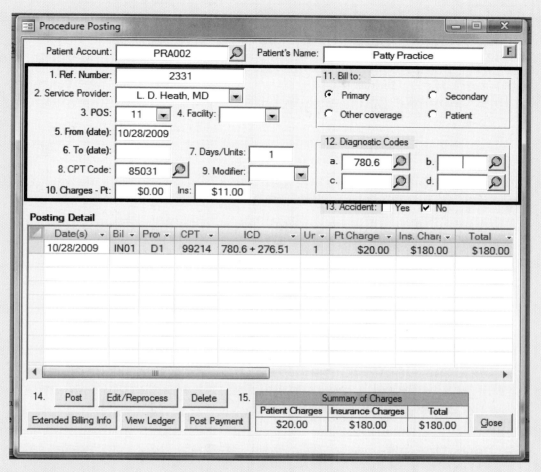

FIGURE 6-8

Delmar/Cengage Learning

STEP 12

When you are sure your entry is correct, click on the *Post button*. The Posting Detail area should display both of the charges for October 28, 2009 (see Figure 6-9). You can also view the entries by clicking on the *Patient Ledger button*.

STEP 13

Close all windows until you return to the Main Menu.

Case Study 6-A Continues >>

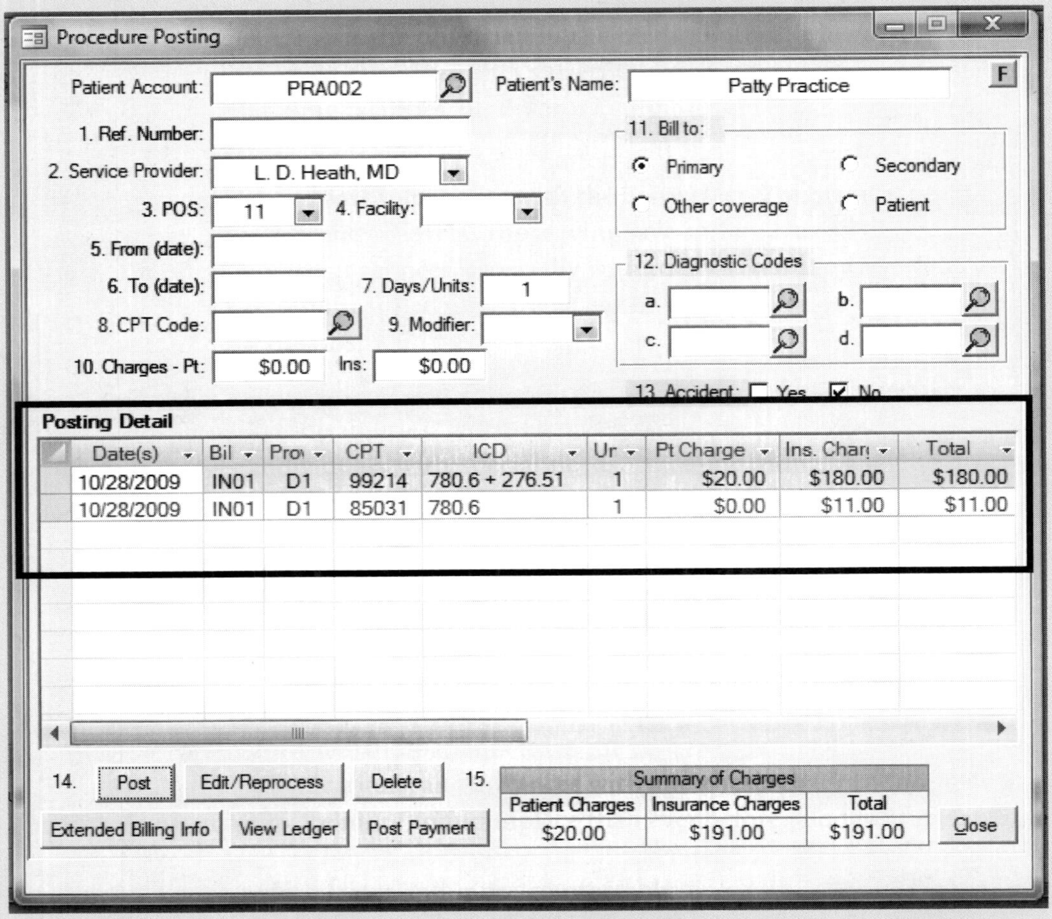

FIGURE 6-9
Delmar/Cengage Learning

CORRECTING ERRORS: CASE STUDY 6-A

Objective: While posting charges, you may discover that you have made an error. Editing is simple and can be done as long as the charges have not been sent to the insurance company using the Insurance Billing routine. Because MOSS is a training tool, it offers the ability to delete a procedure entry and start again. Follow the steps below for editing or deleting procedure entries prior to Insurance Billing.

STEP 1
Start MOSS.

STEP 2
Click on the *Procedure Posting button* on the Main Menu. Locate Patty Practice from the Patient Selection window, and then single click on her *name*. Next, click the *Select button*, since you want to view the procedures posted to her account in order to select the ones to be edited.

STEP 3

The Procedure Posting window opens with the "10/28/2009" procedures displayed in the Posting Detail area.

STEP 4

To select an entry to edit, single click the *line entry* desired and then click on the *Edit/Reprocess button*. For Patty Practice, select the posted procedure showing "CPT 99214." The data should move to the fields in the upper portion of the screen.

NT: If you do not see the cedures for this date, click the *Record bar* in the lower screen area until it displays.

STEP 5

Edit the procedure code for that visit by changing the CPT code to "99213." When finished, click on the *Post button*. The procedure entry should now show the "99213" edit in the Posting Detail area. Check your work with Figure 6-10.

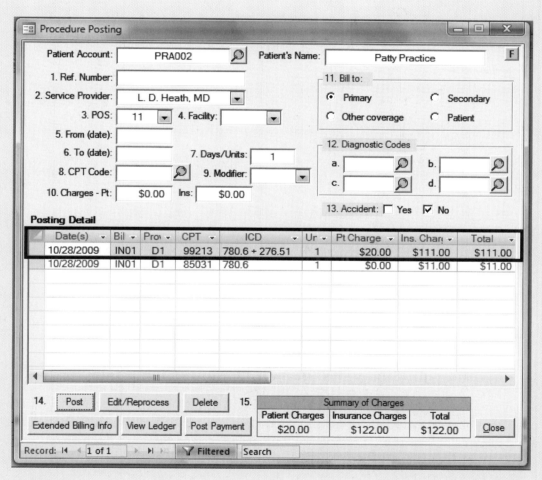

FIGURE 6-10
Delmar/Cengage Learning

Case Study 6-A Continues >>

STEP 6

Next, remove the lab charge from the account. Select the *line entry* with lab service "85031" by single clicking on it (do not double click). Click on the *Delete button*. Two prompts confirm that you are making a deletion. Click *Yes* to continue. Check your work with Figure 6-11.

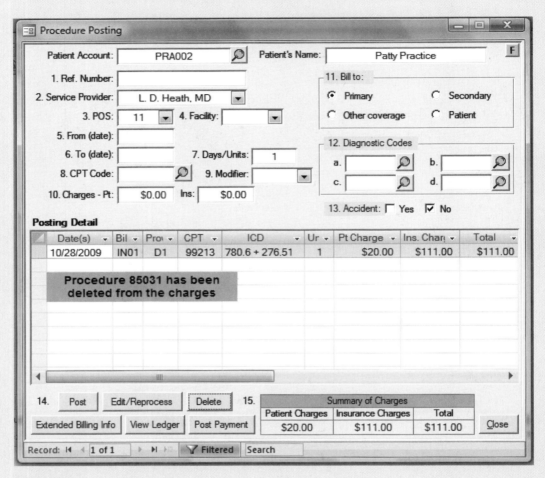

FIGURE 6-11

Delmar/Cengage Learning

POSTING PAYMENTS AT THE TIME OF SERVICE: CASE STUDY 6-A

You have learned how to post procedure charges to a patient's account. You also know how to edit and delete entries, as needed, for making corrections. As mentioned previously, patients will often make payments before or after their office visits, especially co-payments for managed-care health plans. The Procedure Entry window provides a convenient shortcut for posting payments by providing a Post Payment button at the bottom of the screen. See Figure 6-12.

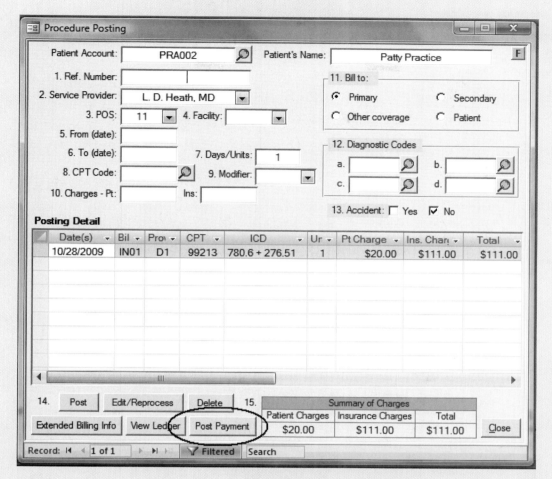

FIGURE 6-12

Delmar/Cengage Learning

NT: If you do not have the
ocedure Entry window on your
een, click on the *Procedure
sting button* from the Main
enu. Then, find Patty Practice
m the patient list and click
Select button.

Objective: The Procedure Entry window should still be open with the charge for CPT 99213 on 10/28/2009 for Patty Practice displayed. Using the Procedure Entry window, follow the steps below for posting a payment to this patient's account.

Case Study 6-A Continues >>

Case Study 6-A Continued

STEP 1

At the bottom of the Procedure Entry window, click on the *Post Payment button*. This opens the Posting Payments window. Check your screen with Figure 6-13.

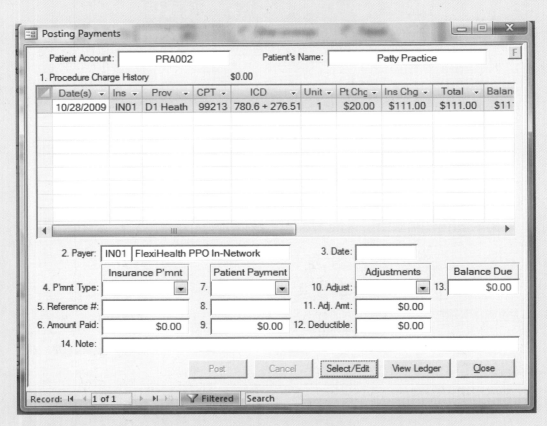

FIGURE 6-13

Delmar/Cengage Learning

STEP 2

> **HINT:** If the *line entry* is not selected, the Balance Due will remain at $0.

Before posting a payment, first select the *line entry* the payment will be applied to by single clicking on it. Next, click on the *Select/Edit button*. If done correctly, the Balance Due will display in the lower window next to Field 13. See Figure 6-14.

STEP 3

Field 2 shows the patient's insurance. Click in Field 3 and enter the date of posting. Since Patty will be paying her $20.00 co-payment at the time of visit, enter "10/28/2009."

STEP 4

There are no insurance payments at this time, so Fields 4, 5, and 6 will be skipped. Drop down the box in Field 7 under Patient Payment. Select *Payment Patient Check (PATCHECK)* from the list.

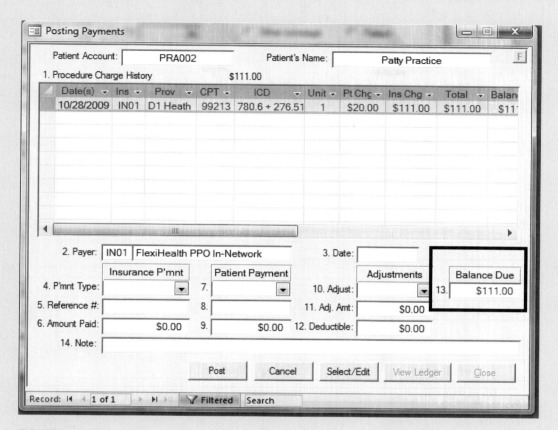

FIGURE 6-14

Delmar/Cengage Learning

STEP 5

Use the *Tab* key to move down to Field 8. Patty writes a check for $20.00 and gives it to you. The check is inspected to be sure it is correctly dated, shows the correct amount, and is signed. The check number is "601." Enter the check number in Field 8, Reference number.

HINT: Do not use the dollar sign.

STEP 6

Use the *Tab* key to move to Field 9. Type "20.00" in the Amount Paid field. Press the *Enter* key. There are no adjustments or deductibles that apply to this posting, so skip Fields 10, 11, and 12. Notice that the Balance Due now reads "$91.00." Check your screen with Figure 6-15. **Be sure all your entries are correct before proceeding.** If your entries are correct, apply the payment by clicking on the *Post button* at the bottom of the window.

STEP 7

After posting the payment, all figures in the lower part of the Payment Entry window display zeros. To view the payment on the patient's account, click on the *View Ledger button*. The $20.00 co-payment should be displayed, and a new balance of $91.00 is now due. The $91.00 balance will be billed to the insurance company. Check your work with the ledger for Patty Practice in Figure 6-16.

STEP 8

Close all windows until you return to the Main Menu.

Case Study 6-A Continues >>

Case Study 6-A Continued

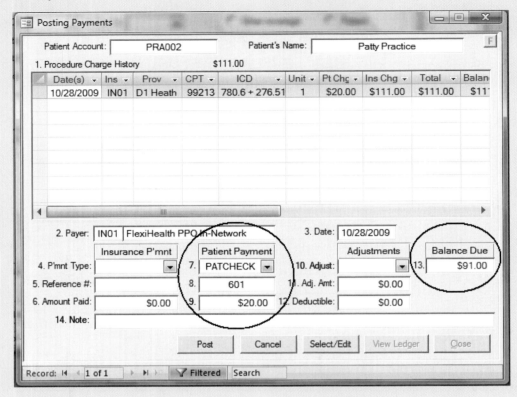

FIGURE 6-15

Delmar/Cengage Learning

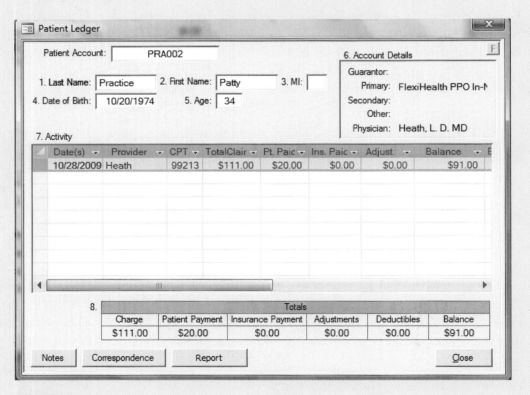

FIGURE 6-16

Delmar/Cengage Learning

SCHEDULING FOLLOW-UP APPOINTMENTS: CASE STUDY 6-A

Objective: The last task to complete for patients before they leave the office is scheduling the follow-up appointment. Scheduling an appointment is done exactly as learned in Unit 3. The physician indicates on the superbill when the patient is to return for a follow-up visit. Refer to the superbill for Patty Practice, Figure 6-2. Below the doctor's signature, Dr. Heath has indicated that the patient is to return in two days.

STEP 1

Click on the *Appointment Scheduling button* on the Main Menu. Using the small calendar on the scheduler, locate October 28, 2009 and click on the date two days later *(October 30, 2009)*. Does Dr. Heath have availability on that date?

STEP 2

NT: Double click on the *ppointment time*, search for *patient's name*, and then *k* on the *Add button* to *edule* a new appointment for *patient*.

After checking with the patient to be sure the date and time are convenient for her, schedule Patty Practice for a 15-minute visit on Friday, October 30, 2009 at 9:45 am. Enter the following reason in Field 6—"Office Visit." Enter "Follow-up fever and dehydration" in the note box for Field 9. Check your work with Figure 6-17 before saving the appointment. Figure 6-18 illustrates the completed appointment on the scheduler.

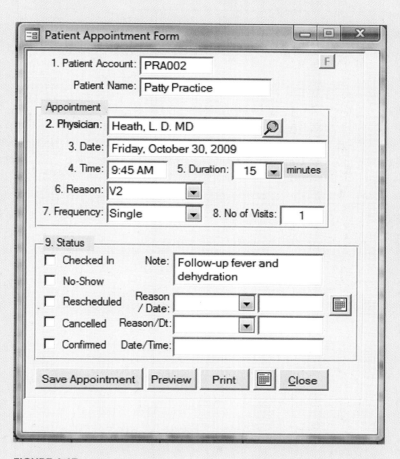

FIGURE 6-17

Delmar/Cengage Learning

Case Study 6-A Continues >>

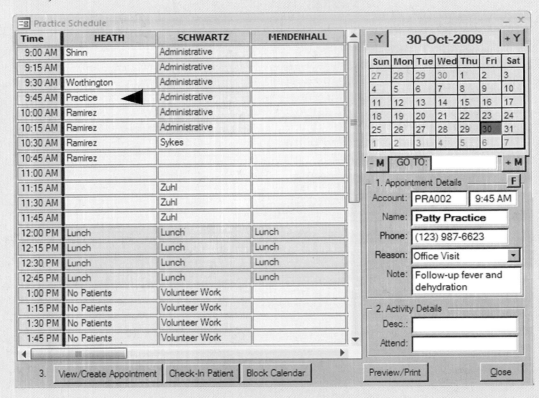

FIGURE 6-18

Delmar/Cengage Learning

STEP 3

If you want to give the patient a reminder slip, double click on Patty Practice's *name* on the appointment schedule. Click on the *Preview button* at the bottom of the patient appointment form to preview the appointment reminder slip before printing it. In the upper left corner, click on the *Printer icon*, as shown in Figure 6-19. When finished, click on the lower *Close button* in the upper right corner.

HINT: If the Main Menu is not visible, click on *File* in the drop-down menus and then click on *Main Menu*.

STEP 4

Close all windows and return to the Main Menu.

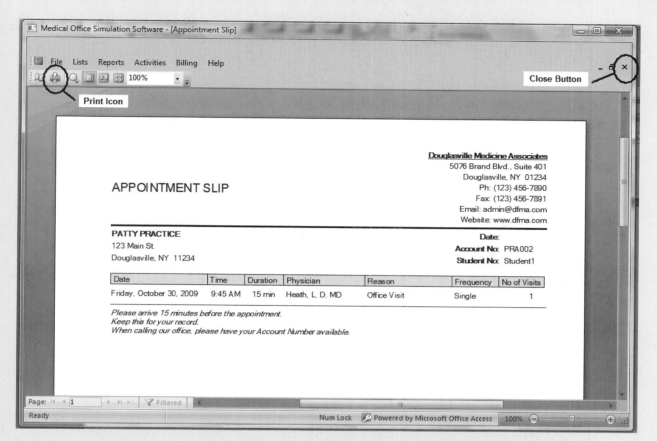

FIGURE 6-19
Delmar/Cengage Learning

CASE STUDY 6–B: MANALY, RICHARD

Patient:	**Manaly, Richard**
Service Date:	**October 21, 2009**
Check-in:	**Find this appointment on the scheduler and indicate the patient checked in.**
Superbill:	**Source Document 6-1**
Physician:	**Schwartz**

Check-out Details

No payment will be made by the patient. The office will submit a claim to patient Manaly's insurance and bill the balance to the patient later. The patient schedules his follow-up appointment before leaving the office.

Case Study 6-B Continues >>

STEP 1

Start MOSS.

STEP 2

Click on the *Procedure Posting button* on the Main Menu. Locate patient "Manaly" from the patient selection window and then click on his *name*. Next, click on the *Add button*, since you will be adding procedures to his account.

STEP 3

The Procedure Posting entry window opens. Next, refer to the superbill from the Source Document Appendix, Source Document 6-1. Enter the superbill number in Field 1.

STEP 4

Use the *Tab* key to move to Field 3, POS. Drop down the box and select *Office*. Because the services were rendered in the office, it is not necessary to use Field 4 at this time.

STEP 5

Use the *Tab* key to move to Field 5 and enter the Date of Service, "10/21/2009."

STEP 6

Use the *Tab* key and move to Field 8.

Refer to patient Manaly's superbill and locate the procedures that have been checked off by the back office. Answer the following questions.

A.	Which procedures apply to this patient?	**Office visit**
B.	What is the CPT code for each procedure?	**99213**
C.	How many procedures total were performed?	**Just the office visit**

Enter the CPT code for the procedure in Field 8. Press the *Enter* key. The charges for this procedure should appear in Field 10 in the Insurance (Ins) box, since this is the amount of the claim to be sent to the patient's health plan.

STEP 7

Next, tab to Field 11. Bill Primary should already be selected, indicating that the patient's primary insurance will be billed for these services.

STEP 8

Tab to Field 12a, Diagnostic Codes. Locate the diagnosis for patient Manaly on the superbill. Answer the following questions.

A.	How many diagnoses does this patient have?	**1**
B.	What is the description and code for each diagnosis for this patient?	**250.00 (Diabetes mellitus, non-insulin dependent)**

Enter the code for the diagnosis in Field 12a.

STEP 9

The procedures for this case were not related to an accident, so be sure that Field 13 reads "No." Check your work with Figure 6-20.

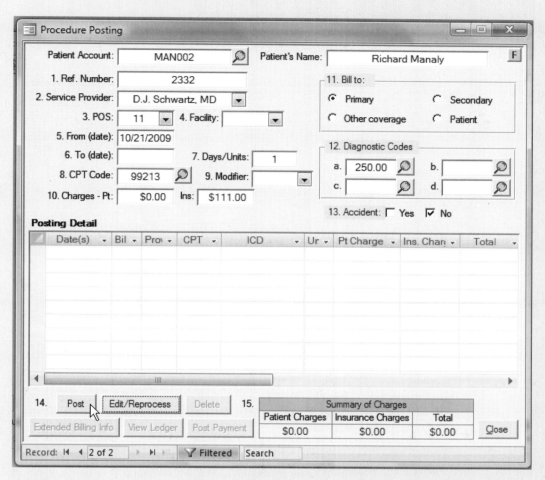

FIGURE 6-20
Delmar/Cengage Learning

STEP 10

When you are sure the entries are correct, click on the *Post button*. This will post the charges to the patient's account and display them in the Posting Detail area in the middle of the window.

MOSS NOTE: The posting detail displays only the current procedures that were posted. To view all charges, payments, and adjustments on a patient's account, click on the *Patient Ledger button*. When finished, close all windows and return to the Main Menu.

STEP 11

On the superbill for patient Manaly, locate the information where the doctor indicated when the patient is to return. How many days, weeks, or months from now does the patient need an appointment?

Case Study 6-B Continues >>

Case Study 6-B Continued

STEP 12

Click on the *Appointment Scheduling button* from the Main Menu. Click on the *dates* approximately three weeks from 10/21/2009 and check for availability with Dr. Schwartz.

Patient Manaly informs you that 10:00 a.m. on 11/11/09 is convenient for him. Using the methods you have learned, schedule a 15-minute appointment for an office visit. The note should read "Follow-up for diabetes." Check your work with Figure 6-21. Preview and print an appointment reminder slip for the patient to take.

HINT: After selecting the patient, click on *Add*.

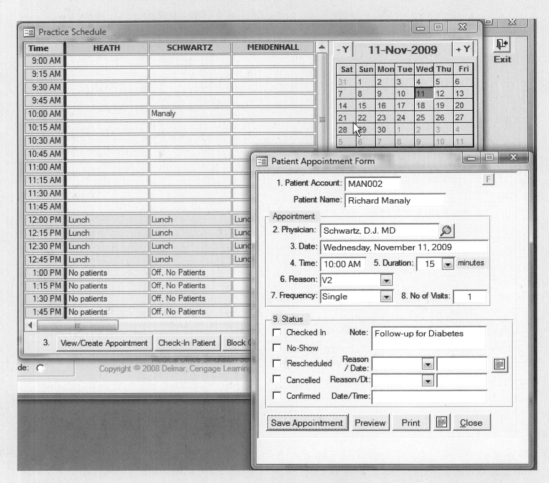

FIGURE 6-21

Delmar/Cengage Learning

STEP 13

Close all open windows and return to the Main Menu.

CASE STUDY 6–C: MONTNER, MARTIN

Patient: **Montner, Martin**
Service Date: **October 22, 2009**
Check-in: **Find this appointment on the scheduler and indicate the patient checked in.**
Superbill: **Source Document 6-2**
Physician: **Schwartz**

Check-out Details

The patient's mother will pay the $10.00 co-payment today. The patient also schedules his follow-up appointment before leaving the office.

STEP 1

Post procedure charges as shown on patient Montner's superbill (2333), Source Document 6-2. The office will submit a claim to the primary insurance. Before clicking on the *Post Payment button*, check your work with Figure 6-22.

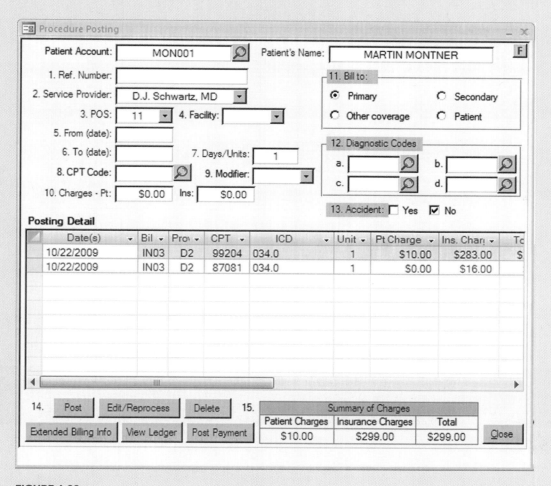

FIGURE 6-22

Delmar/Cengage Learning

Case Study 6-C Continues >>

Case Study 6-C Continued

STEP 2

A $10.00 co-payment is made for today's visit. The patient's mother pays on his behalf with a check. Inspect the check for the correct date, correct amount of payment, and signature. The check number is "1755." Enter the payment. Before posting the payment, check your work with Figure 6-23.

HINT: Use *PATCHECK*.

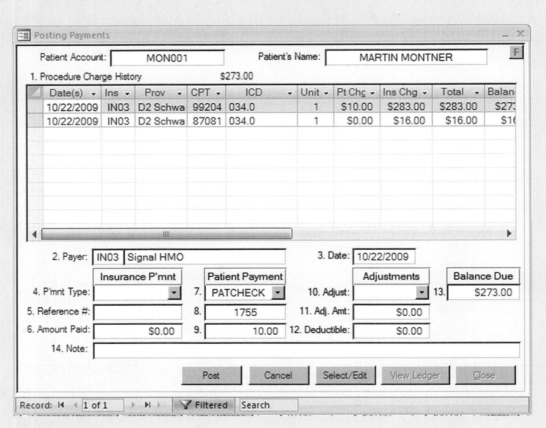

FIGURE 6-23

Delmar/Cengage Learning

MOSS NOTE: Recall that to post a payment, first select the *line entry* the payment will be applied to by single clicking on it. Next, click on the *Select/Edit button*. If done correctly, the Balance Due will display in the lower window next to Field 13.

STEP 3

View Patient Montner's Ledger and check your work with Figure 6-24. Close all windows and then open the appointment scheduler.

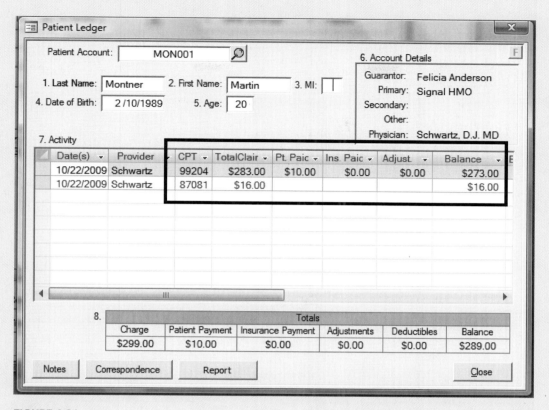

FIGURE 6-24

Delmar/Cengage Learning

NT: Refer to the superbill.

STEP 4

When does the doctor want to see the patient again? After checking with the patient, 10/29/2009 at 9:00 a.m. is convenient. Schedule the appointment for a 15-minute follow-up. The reason is "office visit." The note is "Recheck strep throat." Compare your scheduler to Figure 6-25 to check your work.

NT: Use the *Preview button* the bottom of patient ntner's appointment form.

STEP 5

Print an appointment slip to give to the patient. See Figure 6-26.

STEP 6

Close all windows and return to the Main Menu screen.

Case Study 6-C Continues >>

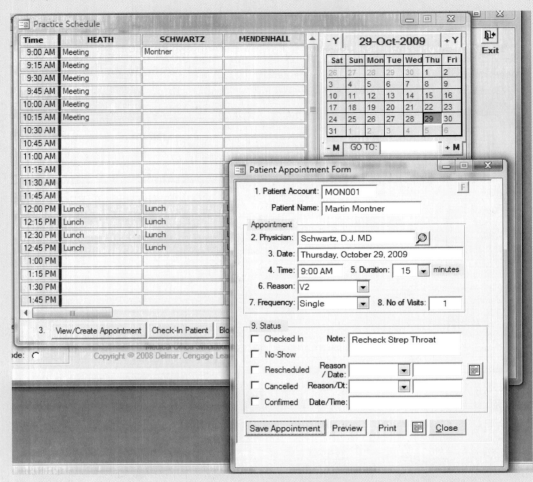

FIGURE 6-25

Delmar/Cengage Learning

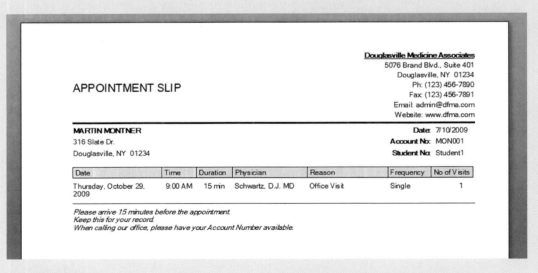

FIGURE 6-26

Delmar/Cengage Learning

CASE STUDY 6–D: CONWAY, JOHN

Patient:	**Conway, John**
Service Date:	**October 23, 2009**
Check-in:	**Find this appointment on the scheduler and indicate the patient checked in.**
Superbill:	**Source Document 6-3**
Physician:	**Heath**

Check-out Details

The patient will not make a payment today. The office will submit a claim to patient Conway's insurance company. The patient schedules his follow-up appointment before leaving the office.

STEP 1

Post procedure charges as shown on patient Conway's superbill (2334), Source Document 6-3. The office will submit a claim to the primary insurance. Check your work with Figure 6-27 after posting the charges.

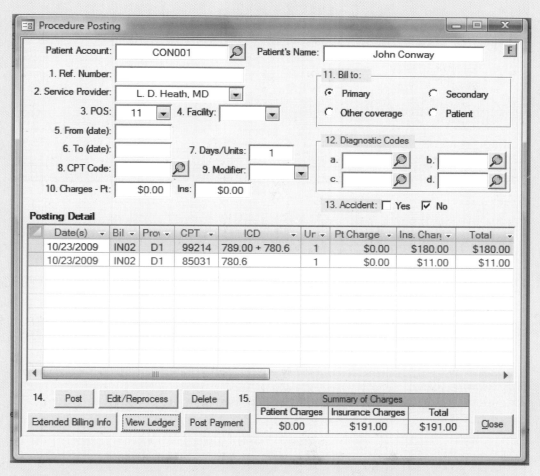

FIGURE 6-27

Delmar/Cengage Learning

Case Study 6-D Continues >>

Case Study 6-D Continued

STEP 2

Compare the Patient Ledger to Figure 6-28 to check your work. Close all windows, and then open the appointment scheduler.

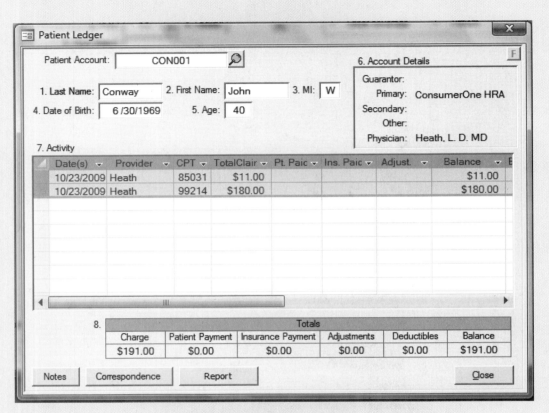

FIGURE 6-28
Delmar/Cengage Learning

HINT: Refer to the superbill.

STEP 3

When does the doctor want to see the patient again? After checking with the patient, 10/26/2009 at 11:00 a.m. is convenient. Schedule the appointment for a 15-minute office visit. The note is "Follow-up abdominal pain." Before posting the appointment, compare your scheduler to Figure 6-29 to check your work.

HINT: Use the *Preview button* at the bottom of patient Conway's appointment form.

STEP 4

Print an appointment slip to give to the patient. See Figure 6-30.

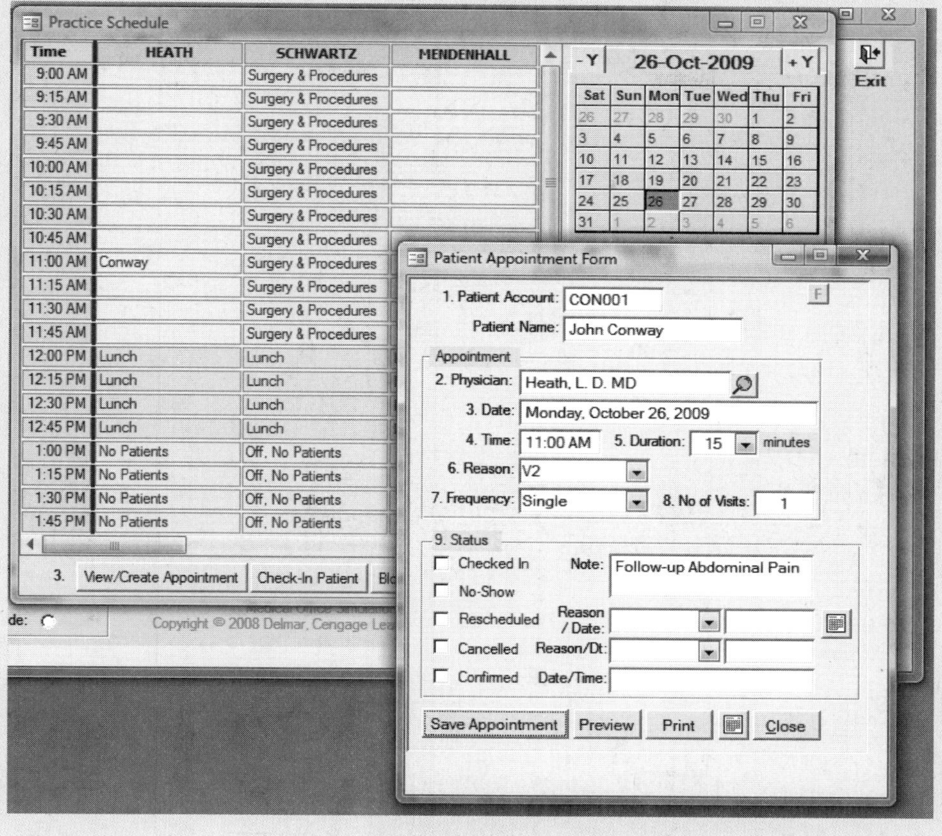

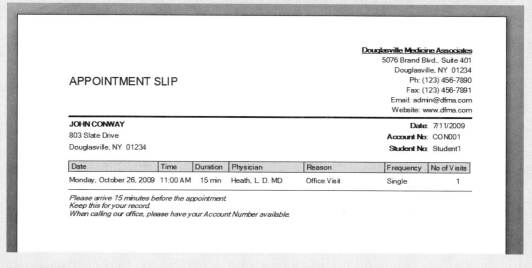

FIGURE 6-29
Delmar/Cengage Learning

FIGURE 6-30
Delmar/Cengage Learning

STEP 5

Close all windows and return to the Main Menu screen.

CASE STUDY 6–E: SHEKTAR, PAULA

Patient:	**Shektar, Paula**
Service Date:	**October 23, 2009**
Check-in:	**Find this appointment on the scheduler and indicate the patient checked in.**
Superbill:	**Source Document 6-4**
Physician:	**Schwartz**

Check-out Details

No payment is made by the patient. The office submits a claim to patient Shektar's insurance company and bills the balance to the secondary insurance. The patient schedules her follow-up appointment before leaving the office.

STEP 1

Post procedure charges as shown on patient Shektar's superbill (2335), Source Document 6-4. The office will submit a claim to the primary insurance. Check your work with Figure 6-31.

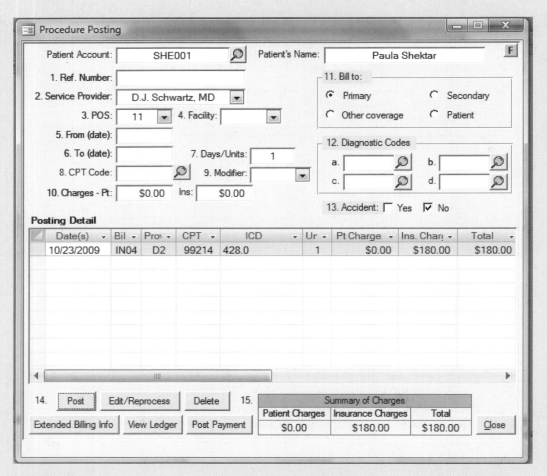

FIGURE 6-31

Delmar/Cengage Learning

STEP 2

This patient has Medicare, but her physician, Dr. Schwartz, is a non-PAR provider. He does not accept assignment on her health plans. The patient makes no payment today.

INT: Refer to the superbill.

STEP 3

When does the doctor want to see the patient again? Dr. Schwartz regularly sees Patient Shektar to monitor her condition and medications. Look at the dates approximately one month from 10/23/2009, and check availability for Dr. Schwartz. The patient informs you that 11/24/2009 at 3:00 p.m. is convenient. Schedule the appointment for a 30-minute office visit. The note is "CHF" (Congestive Heart Failure). Compare your scheduling screen to Figure 6-32 to check your work.

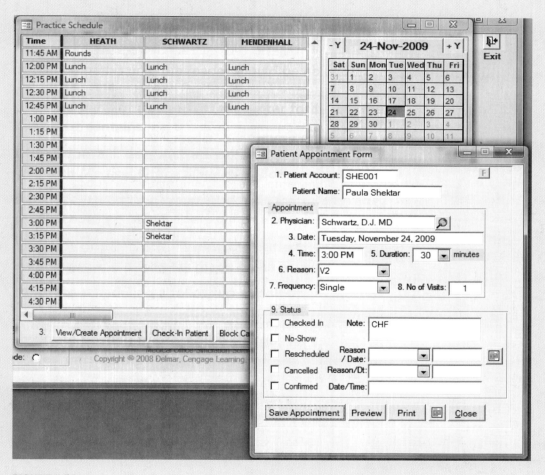

FIGURE 6-32

Delmar/Cengage Learning

Case Study 6-E Continues >>

STEP 4

Print an appointment slip to give to the patient. See Figure 6-33.

STEP 5

Close all windows and return to the Main Menu screen.

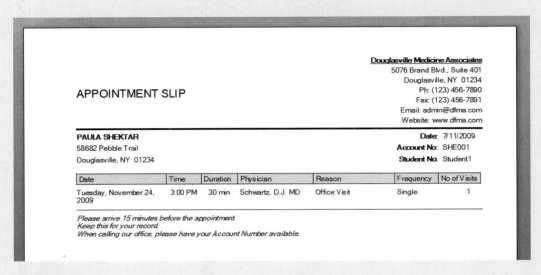

FIGURE 6-33
Delmar/Cengage Learning

CASE STUDY 6–F: VILLANOVA, RICKY

Patient:	**Villanova, Ricky**
Service Date:	**October 27, 2009**
Check-in:	**Find this appointment on the scheduler and indicate the patient checked in.**
Superbill:	**Source Document 6-5**
Physician:	**Schwartz**

Check-out Details

The patient will pay his $10.00 co-payment with cash. The office will submit a claim to patient Villanova's insurance company. The patient schedules his follow-up appointment before leaving the office.

STEP 1

Post procedure charges as shown on patient Villanova's superbill (2336), Source Document 6-5. The office will submit a claim to the primary insurance. Check your work with Figure 6-34 when finished.

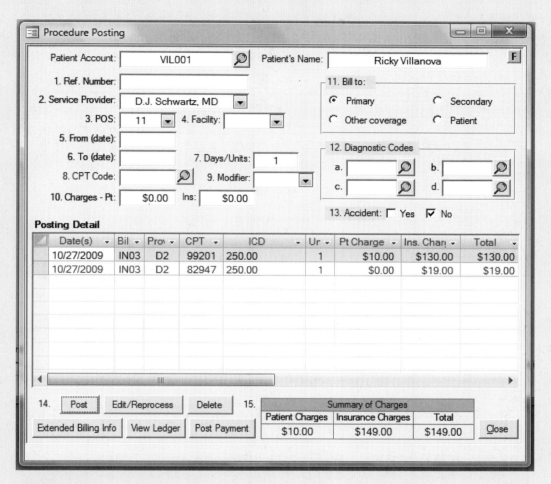

FIGURE 6-34

Delmar/Cengage Learning

Case Study 6-F Continues >>

Case Study 6-F Continued

STEP 2

The patient pays his $10.00 co-payment with cash. Enter the payment using the *Post Payment button*. Today's date is 10/27/2009. Single click on the first *line entry*, then click on the *Select/Edit button*. Post "$10.00" towards that charge, using *PATCASH* under Patient Payment. Compare your screen with Figure 6-35. Remember to click on the *Post button* to apply the payment.

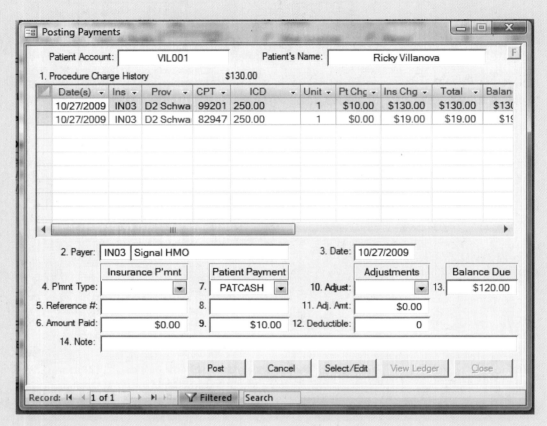

FIGURE 6-35

Delmar/Cengage Learning

STEP 3

Compare the Patient Ledger to Figure 6-36 to check your work. Close all windows, and then open the appointment scheduler.

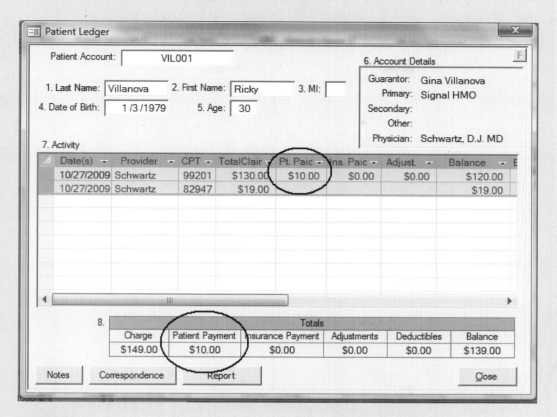

FIGURE 6-36
Delmar/Cengage Learning

STEP 4

When does the doctor want to see the patient again? Check the dates approximately one month from 10/27/2009. When is Dr. Schwartz available? The patient informs you that 11/24/2009 at 9:00 a.m. is convenient. Schedule the appointment for a 15-minute office visit. The note is "Repeat fasting blood glucose." Before posting the appointment, compare your scheduler to Figure 6-37 to check your work.

STEP 5

Print an appointment slip to give to the patient. See Figure 6-38.

STEP 6

Close all windows and return to the Main Menu screen.

Case Study 6-F Continues >>

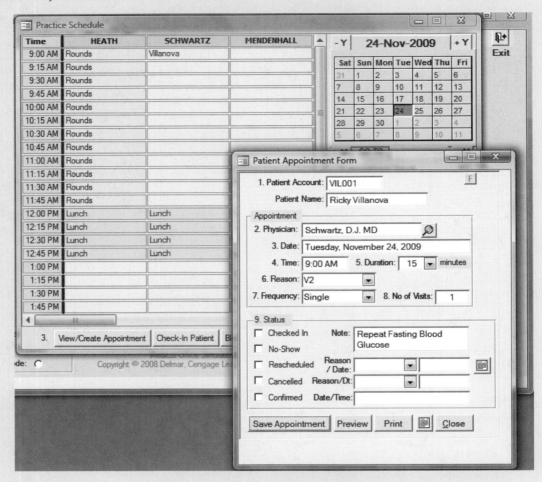

FIGURE 6-37
Delmar/Cengage Learning

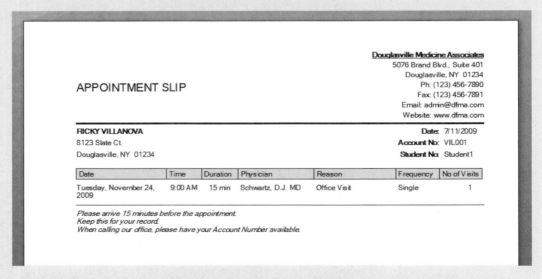

FIGURE 6-38
Delmar/Cengage Learning

CASE STUDY 6–G: ADAMS, MINNIE

Patient: **Adams, Minnie**
Service Date: **October 28, 2009**
Check-in: **Find this appointment on the scheduler and indicate the patient checked in.**
Superbill: **Source Document 6-6**
Physician: **Heath**

Dr. Heath will be patient Adams's new doctor since Douglasville Medicine Associates is closer to the patient's home. The doctor met the patient today, took a history, and performed a physical to become familiar with the patient's case.

Check-out Details

The patient will make no payment. The office will submit a claim to patient Adams's insurance plan.

STEP 1

Post procedure charges as shown on patient Adams's Superbill (2337), Source Document 6-6. The office will submit a claim to the primary insurance company. Check your work with Figure 6-39 for all three procedures posted. *Do not close the Procedure Posting window.*

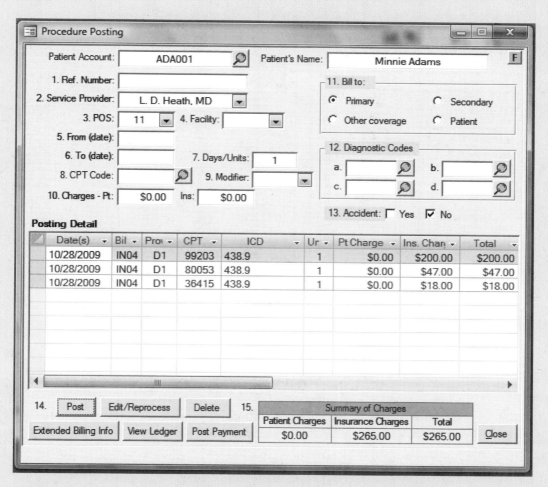

FIGURE 6-39

Delmar/Cengage Learning

Case Study 6-G Continues >>

STEP 2

This patient has Medicare. Her physician, Dr. Heath, is a PAR provider and accepts assignment on Medicare. The patient will be billed for the co-insurance after Medicare pays. If applicable, any deductible applied will be collected later, as well.

STEP 3

Patient Adams had laboratory work done today. These specimens will be sent out to BioPace Laboratory for analysis, but Douglasville Medicine Associates will be billing Medicare for the charges and collecting the payment. Medicare requires that the laboratory be identified on the claim for all services performed at an outside facility. The total charges for services must be included. This information will be entered using the *Extended Billing Info button.*

What were the total charges for the laboratory services (excluding venipuncture)? First, single click on the line that has *procedure CPT 80053* to select it. Next, click on the *Extended Billing Info button* and enter the information as shown on Figure 6-40. Click on *Save* when finished.

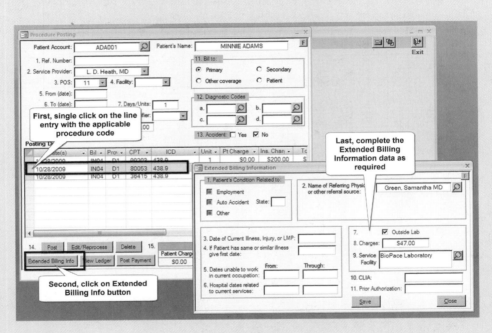

FIGURE 6-40

Delmar/Cengage Learning

By entering this information, it will now be included with the medical insurance claim when billed. When finished, close the window.

STEP 4

When does the doctor want to see the patient again? What does "prn" mean? Since Dr. Heath has indicated that the patient will return "prn," or as needed, no appointment is necessary at check-out today.

CASE STUDY 6–H: WORTHINGTON, CYNTHIA

Patient:	**Worthington, Cynthia**
Service Date:	**October 30, 2009**
Check-in:	**Find this appointment on the scheduler and indicate the patient checked in.**
Superbill:	**Source Document 6-7**
Physician:	**Heath**

Check-out Details

This patient was in the office a few days ago. Today's visit was for a reaction she had to the antibiotic given to her. The patient will pay the $20.00 co-payment by check. The office will submit a claim to patient Worthington's insurance company. The patient schedules a follow-up appointment before leaving the office.

STEP 1

Post procedure charges as shown on patient Worthington's superbill (2339), Source Document 6-7. The office will submit a claim to the primary insurance company. Check your work with Figure 6-41.

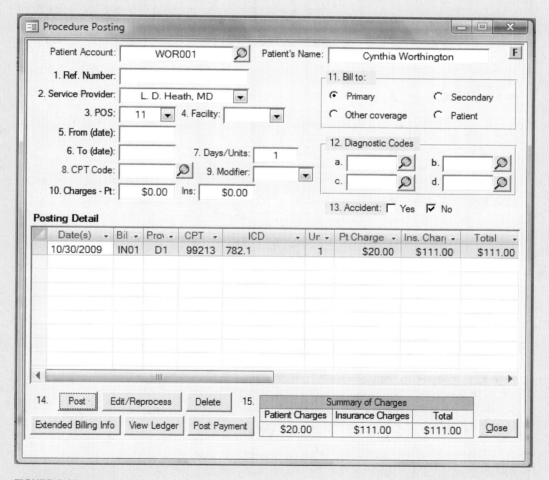

FIGURE 6-41

Delmar/Cengage Learning

Case Study 6-H Continues >>

Case Study 6-H Continued

STEP 2

Enter the payment using the *Post Payment button*. The patient pays her $20.00 co-payment with a check. Be sure to apply the payment to the 10/30/2009 service date. The check is inspected to be sure it is correctly dated, shows the correct amount, and is signed. The check number is "1563." Compare your screen with Figure 6-42 to check your work before clicking on the *Post button*.

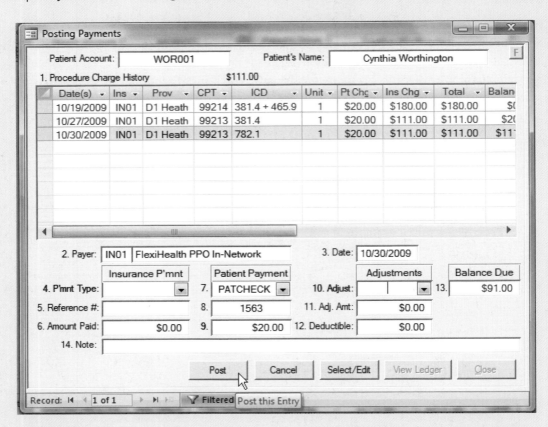

FIGURE 6-42

Delmar/Cengage Learning

STEP 3

Close all windows and then open the appointment scheduler. When does the doctor want to see the patient again? Check the dates approximately one week after 10/30/2009 for Dr. Heath's availability. The patient informs you that 11/05/2009 at 11:00 a.m. is convenient. Schedule the appointment for a 15-minute office visit. The note is "Follow-up rash post antibiotic treatment." Compare your work to Figure 6-43.

STEP 4

Print an appointment slip to give to the patient. See Figure 6-44.

STEP 5

Close all windows and return to the Main Menu screen.

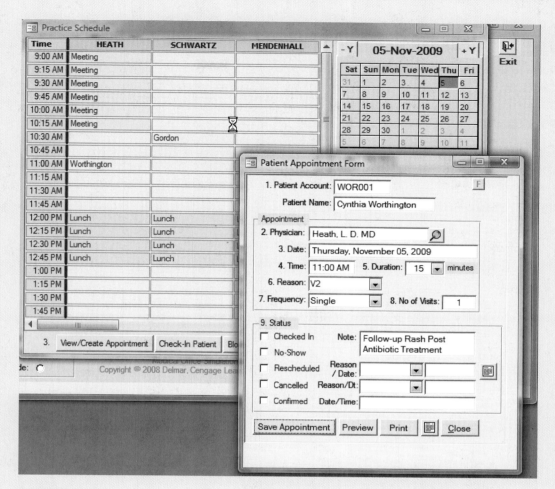

FIGURE 6-43

Delmar/Cengage Learning

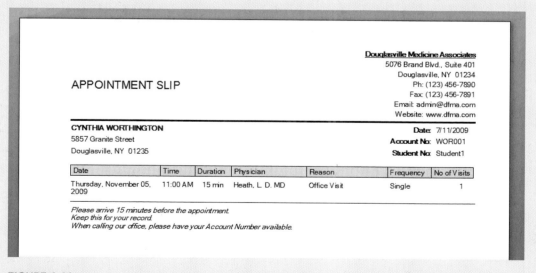

FIGURE 6-44

Delmar/Cengage Learning

CASE STUDY 6–I: ZUHL, RODNEY

Patient:	**Zuhl, Rodney**
Service Date:	**October 30, 2009**
Check-in:	**Find this appointment on the scheduler and indicate the patient checked in.**
Superbill:	**Source Document 6-8**
Physician:	**Schwartz**

Check-out Details

Patient Zuhl has no insurance coverage and is self-pay. The doctor will give him a 10% self-pay discount off the visit charge if services are paid for up front. The patient makes a follow-up appointment at the time of check out.

STEP 1

Post procedure charges as shown on patient Zuhl's superbill (2340), Source Document 6-8. What are the total charges for today's visit? What is the charge for only the office visit? Check your entries with Figure 6-45.

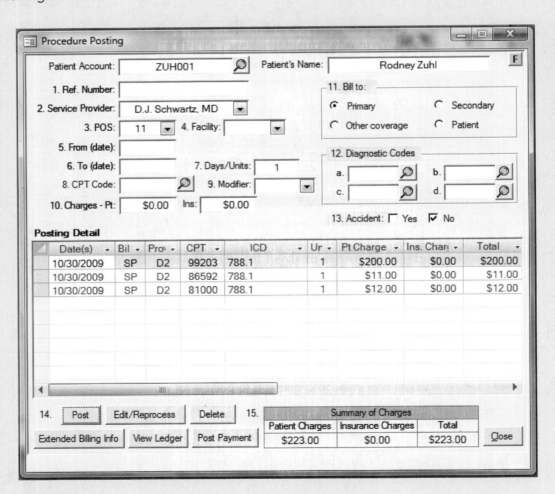

FIGURE 6-45

Delmar/Cengage Learning

STEP 2

Today, the patient will take advantage of the self-pay discount and pay for the office visit and laboratory work with a check.

What is the 10 percent discount off the office visit charge? Calculate as follows:

$200.00 × 10% (or .10) = $20.00

What is the 10 percent discount off the 86592 lab procedure? Calculate as follows:

$11.00 × 10% (or .10) = $1.10

What is the 10 percent discount off the 81000 lab procedure? Calculate as follows:

$12.00 × 10% (or .10) = $1.20

The patient will pay with one check (number 1200) in the amount of $200.70, as shown below:

$223.00	*(total charges)*
− $ 22.30	*(discount for cash payment)*
$200.70	**Total Payment**

STEP 3

Although the patient is paying with one check, the payment will need to be posted to each applicable procedure separately. Post the payment as follows.

Single click on the *line entry* for the office visit (99203) on 10/30/2009, and then click on the *Select/Edit button.* Select the drop down box for Patient Payment and select *PATCHECK.* Enter the check number ("1200") in Field 8, and then enter the payment amount "$180.00" in Field 9 ($200.00 charges minus $20.00 discount = $180.00).

STEP 4

Next, post the adjustment for the discount. In Field 10, drop down the box and select *Self-Pay discount.* Then, in Field 11, enter "$20.00." Check your work with Figure 6-46 before posting the payment. **Be sure all fields are correct prior to posting the payment.**

Case Study 6-I Continues >>

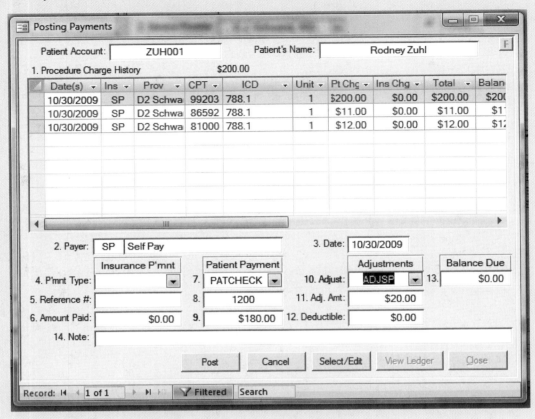

FIGURE 6-46

Delmar/Cengage Learning

STEP 5

Single click on the *line entry* for the lab procedure (86592) on 10/30/2009, and then click on the *Select/Edit button*. Select the drop down box for Patient Payment and select *PATCHECK*. Enter the check number ("1200") in Field 8, and then enter the payment amount "$9.90" in Field 9 ($11.00 charges minus $1.10 discount = $9.90).

Next, post the adjustment for the discount. In Field 10, drop down the box and select *Self-Pay discount*. Then, in Field 11, enter "$1.10." Check your work with Figure 6-47 before posting the payment.

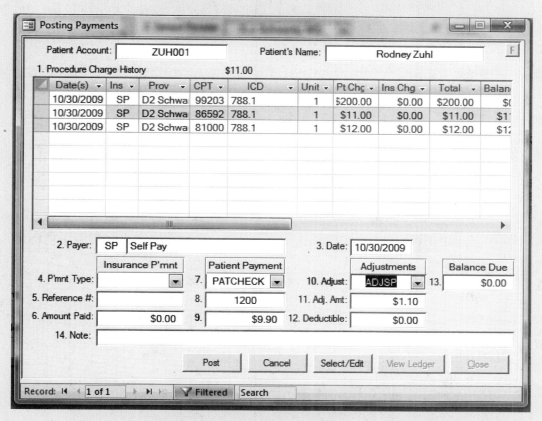

FIGURE 6-47

Delmar/Cengage Learning

Case Study 6-I Continues >>

Case Study 6-I Continued

STEP 6

Single click on the *line entry* for the lab procedure (81000) on 10/30/2009, and then click on the *Select/Edit button*. Select the drop down box for Patient Payment and select *PATCHECK*. Enter the check number ("1200") in Field 8, and then enter the payment amount "$10.80" in Field 9 ($12.00 charges minus $1.20 discount = $10.80).

Next, post the adjustment for the discount. In Field 10, drop down the box and select *Self-Pay discount*. Then, in Field 11, enter "$1.20." Check your work with Figure 6-48 before posting the payment.

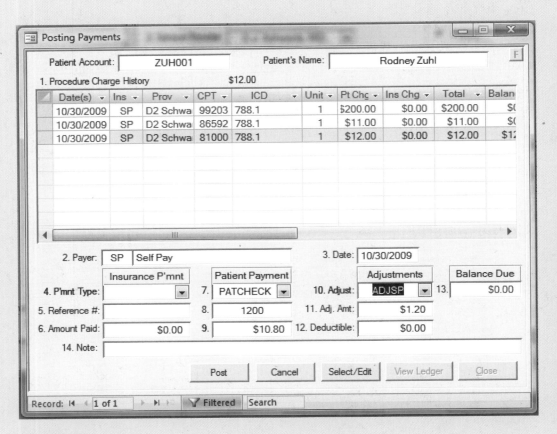

FIGURE 6-48
Delmar/Cengage Learning

STEP 7

Compare the Patient Ledger to Figure 6-49 to check your work. Close all windows and then open the appointment scheduler.

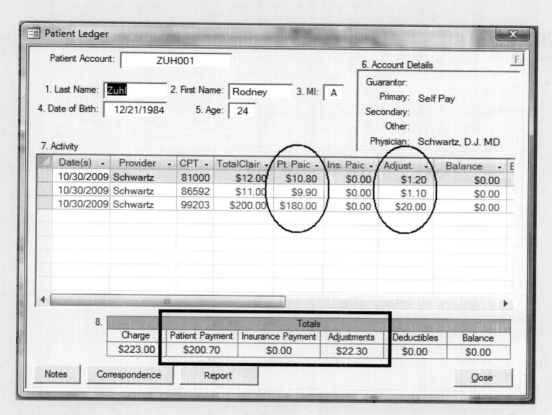

FIGURE 6-49

Delmar/Cengage Learning

STEP 8

When does the doctor want to see the patient again? Check the dates approximately five days after 10/30/2009 for Dr. Schwartz's availability. The patient informs you that 11/05/2009 at 9:30 a.m. is convenient. Schedule the appointment for a 30-minute office visit. The note is "Follow-up dysuria" (painful urination), "review lab results." Compare your scheduler to Figure 6-50 to check your work.

STEP 9

Print an appointment slip to give to the patient. See Figure 6-51.

STEP 10

Close all windows and return to the Main Menu screen.

Case Study 6-I Continues >>

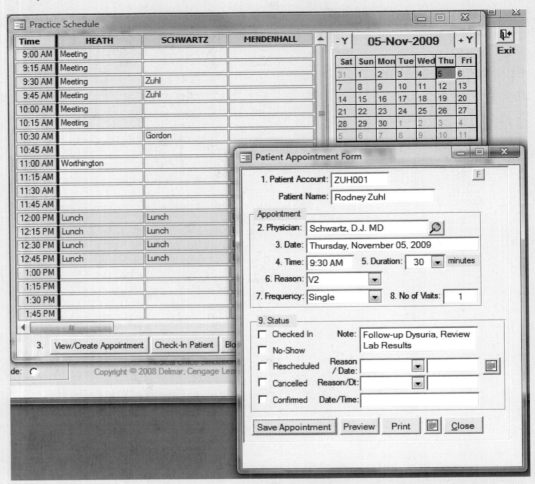

FIGURE 6-50

Delmar/Cengage Learning

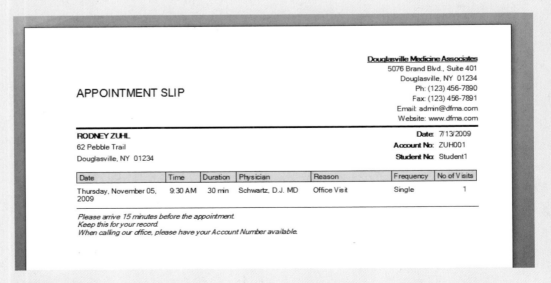

FIGURE 6-51

Delmar/Cengage Learning

CASE STUDY 6–J: SHINN, ROBERT

Patient: **Shinn, Robert**
Service Date: **October 30, 2009**
Check-in: **Find this appointment on the scheduler and indicate the patient checked in.**
Superbill: **Source Document 6-9**
Physician: **Heath**

Check-out Details

The patient's mother accompanied this minor to the office today for an earache. She will pay the co-payment and schedule a follow-up appointment for patient Shinn before leaving the office.

STEP 1

Post procedure charges as shown on patient Shinn's superbill (2341), Source Document 6-9. The office will submit a claim to the primary insurance company. Check your work with Figure 6-52.

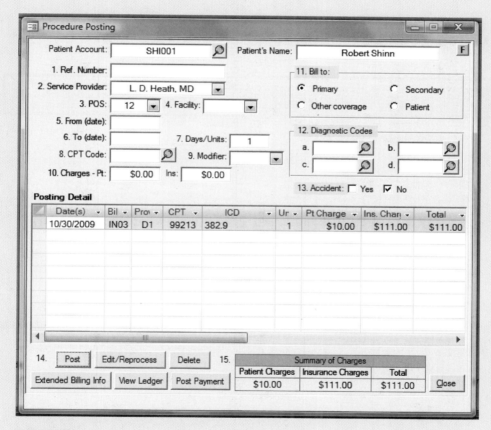

FIGURE 6-52

Delmar/Cengage Learning

Case Study 6-J Continues >>

Case Study 6-J Continued

HINT: Patient Shinn has other charges previously incurred. Be sure to select the 10/30/2009 line entry, to correctly post the payment. Remember to select *PATCHECK.*

STEP 2

Enter the payment using the *Post Payment button.* Single click on the *line entry* for 10/30/2009 and then click on the *Select/Edit button* and post $10.00 towards that charge. The patient's mother pays the $10.00 co-payment with a check. The check is inspected to be sure it is correctly dated, shows the correct amount, and is signed. The check number is "405."

STEP 3

Compare the Patient Ledger to Figure 6-53 to check your work. Close all windows and then open the appointment scheduler.

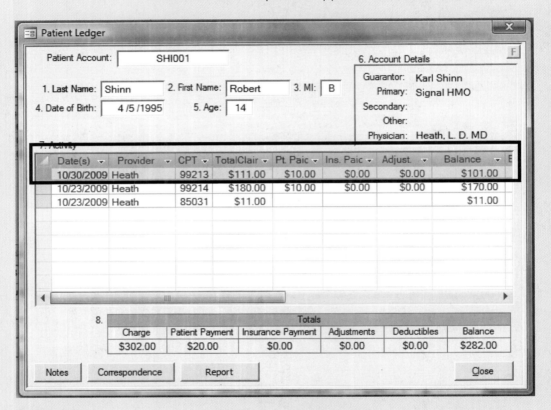

FIGURE 6-53

Delmar/Cengage Learning

STEP 4

When does the doctor want to see the patient again? Check the dates approximately one week after 10/30/2009 for Dr. Heath's availability. The patient's mother informs you that 11/06/2009 at 9:00 a.m. is convenient. Schedule the appointment for a 15-minute office visit. The note is "Follow-up earache." Before posting the appointment, compare your scheduler to Figure 6-54 to check your work.

STEP 5

Print an appointment slip to give to the patient. See Figure 6-55.

STEP 6

Close all windows and return to the Main Menu screen.

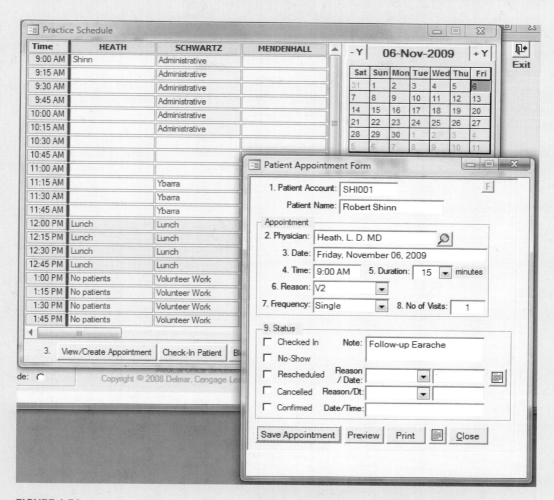

FIGURE 6-54

Delmar/Cengage Learning

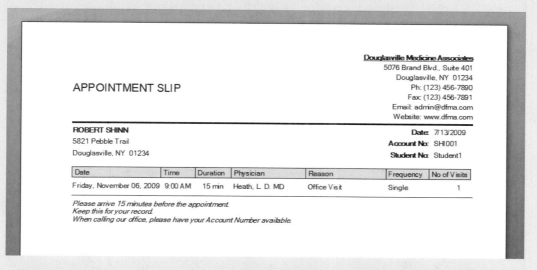

FIGURE 6-55

Delmar/Cengage Learning

CASE STUDY 6–K: PRADHAN, KABIN

Patient:	**Pradhan, Kabin**
Service Date:	**November 3, 2009**
Check-in:	**Find this appointment on the scheduler and indicate the patient checked in.**
Superbill:	**Source Document 6-10**
Physician:	**Schwartz**

Check-out Details

This patient will not make a payment today. The office will submit a claim to patient Pradhan's insurance company and bill any balances to the patient later. The patient schedules a follow-up appointment before leaving the office.

STEP 1

Post procedure charges as shown on patient Pradhan's superbill (2342), Source Document 6-10. The office will submit a claim to the primary insurance company. See Figure 6-56.

STEP 2

There are no payments to post. Close all windows and then open the appointment scheduler.

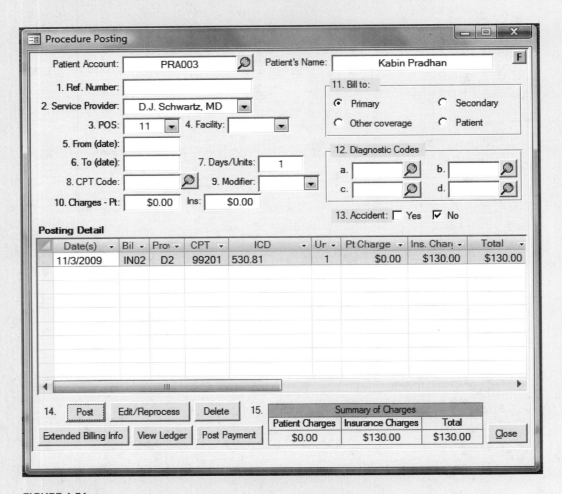

FIGURE 6-56

Delmar/Cengage Learning

STEP 3

When does the doctor want to see the patient again? Check the dates approximately one month after 11/03/2009 for Dr. Schwartz's availability. The patient informs you that 12/01/2009 at 4:00 p.m. is convenient. Schedule the appointment for a 15-minute office visit. The note is "Follow-up gastroesophageal reflux." See Figure 6-57.

INT: Use the *Preview button* the bottom of patient adhan's appointment entry reen.

STEP 4

Print an appointment slip to give to the patient. See Figure 6-58.

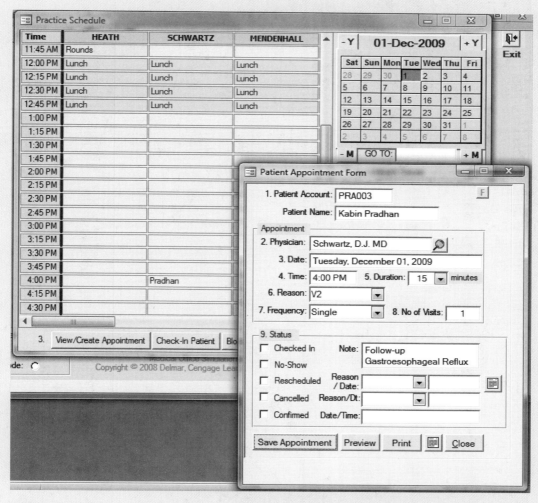

FIGURE 6-57

Delmar/Cengage Learning

STEP 5

Close all windows and return to the Main Menu screen.

Case Study 6-K Continues >>

```
                                                    Douglasville Medicine Associates
                                                      5076 Brand Blvd., Suite 401
                                                        Douglasville, NY  01234
     APPOINTMENT SLIP                                       Ph: (123) 456-7890
                                                           Fax: (123) 456-7891
                                                        Email: admin@dfma.com
                                                        Website: www.dfma.com

     KABIN PRADHAN                                    Date:  7/13/2009
     2213 Boulder Ct.                                 Account No:  PRA003
     Douglasville, NY  01235                          Student No:  Student1
```

Date	Time	Duration	Physician	Reason	Frequency	No of Visits
Tuesday, December 01, 2009	4:00 PM	15 min	Schwartz, D.J. MD	Office Visit	Single	1

Please arrive 15 minutes before the appointment.
Keep this for your record.
When calling our office, please have your Account Number available.

FIGURE 6-58

Delmar/Cengage Learning

CASE STUDY 6–L: TOMANAGA, MARIE

Patient:	**Tomanaga, Marie**
Service Date:	**November 3, 2009**
Check-in:	**Find this appointment on the scheduler and indicate the patient checked in.**
Superbill:	**Source Document 6-11**
Physician:	**Schwartz**

Check-out Details

Patient Tomanaga will not make a payment today since she has dual coverage with Medicare and a MediGap secondary insurance. The office will do the medical billing. The patient schedules a follow-up appointment before leaving the office.

STEP 1

Post procedure charges as shown on patient Tomanaga's superbill (2343), Source Document 6-11. Check your work with Figure 6-59.

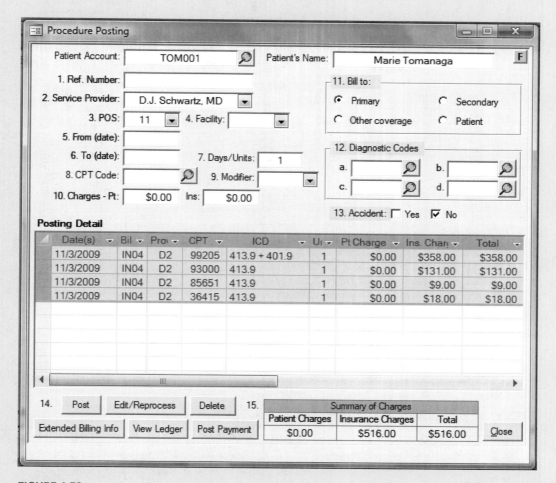

FIGURE 6-59

Delmar/Cengage Learning

STEP 2

Patient Tomanaga had laboratory work done today. These specimens will be sent out to BioPace Laboratory for analysis and Douglasville Medicine Associates will bill Medicare for the charges. As mentioned previously, Medicare requires that the laboratory be identified on the claim for all services performed at an outside facility, including total charges for services. What were the total charges for the laboratory services (excluding venipuncture)?

Click on the *line item* for CPT code 85651 in the Posting Detail. Next, click on the *Extended Billing Info button* and enter this information as shown on Figure 6-60. Click on *Save* when finished; then close the window.

STEP 3

No payments will be made today. Close all windows and then open the appointment scheduler.

Case Study 6-L Continues >>

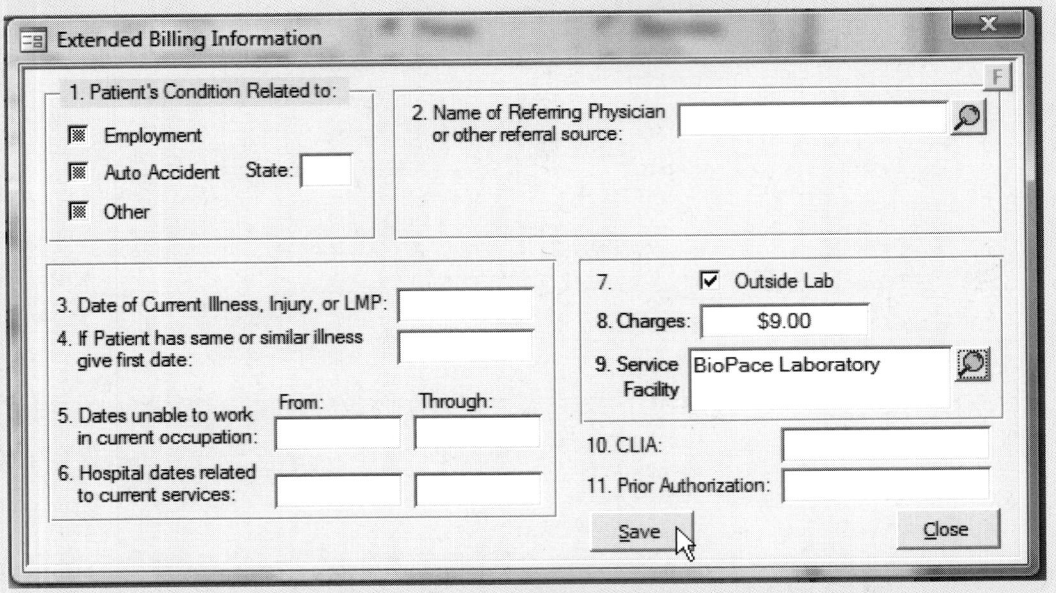

FIGURE 6-60

Delmar/Cengage Learning

STEP 4

When does the doctor want to see the patient again? Check the dates approximately three weeks after 11/03/2009 for Dr. Schwartz's availability. The patient informs you that 11/24/04 at 9:30 a.m. is convenient. Schedule the appointment for a 30-minute office visit. The note is "Follow-up angina and recheck blood pressure." Compare your scheduler to Figure 6-61 to check your work.

STEP 5

Print an appointment slip to give to the patient. See Figure 6-62.

STEP 6

Close all windows and return to the Main Menu screen.

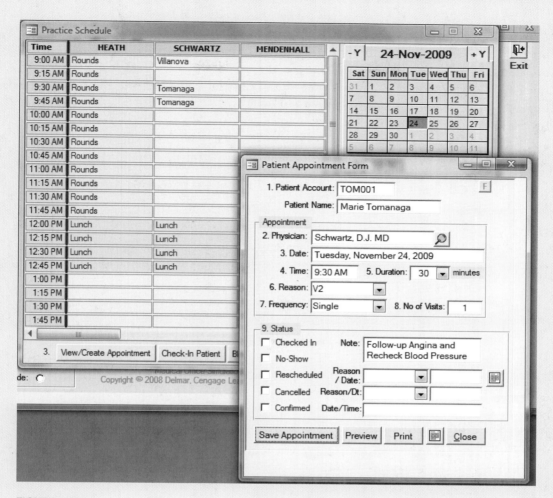

FIGURE 6-61

Delmar/Cengage Learning

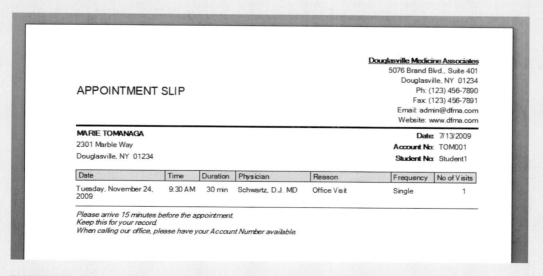

FIGURE 6-62

Delmar/Cengage Learning

CASE STUDY 6–M: BEALS, KIMBERLY

Patient:	**Beals, Kimberly**
Service Date:	**November 3, 2009**
Check-in:	**Find this appointment on the scheduler and indicate the patient checked in.**
Superbill:	**Source Document 6-12**
Physician:	**Heath**

Check-out Details

This patient will pay her co-payment after her visit when she leaves the office. The office will submit a claim to patient Beals's insurance company. The patient schedules a follow-up appointment before leaving the office.

STEP 1

Post procedure charges as shown on patient Beals's superbill (2344), Source Document 6-12. The office will submit a claim to the primary insurance company. Check your work with Figure 6-63.

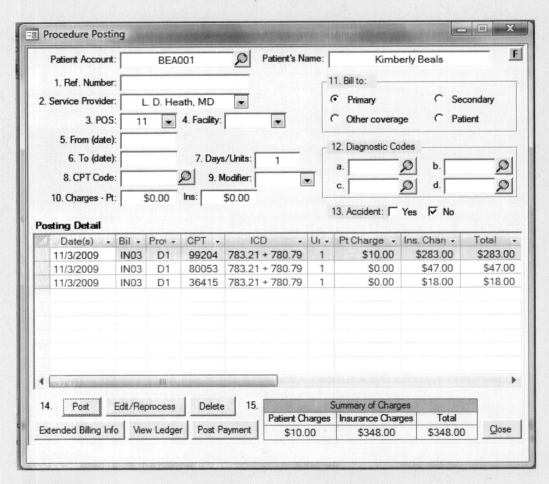

FIGURE 6-63

Delmar/Cengage Learning

STEP 2

Enter the payment using the *Post Payment button*. The patient pays her $10.00 co-payment with a check. The check is inspected to be sure it is correctly dated, shows the correct amount, and is signed. The check number is "557." Check your work with Figure 6-64.

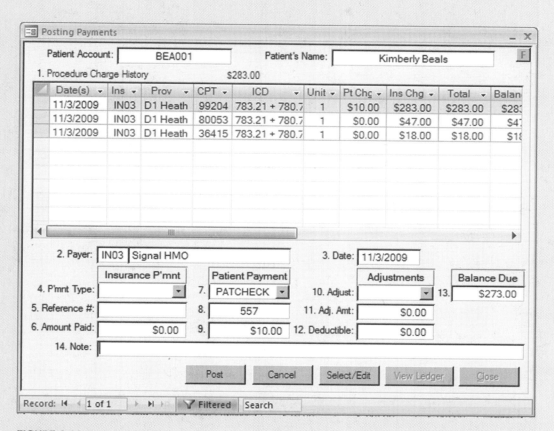

FIGURE 6-64

Delmar/Cengage Learning

Case Study 6-M Continues >>

STEP 3

Compare the Patient Ledger to Figure 6-65 to check your work. Close all windows and then open the appointment scheduler.

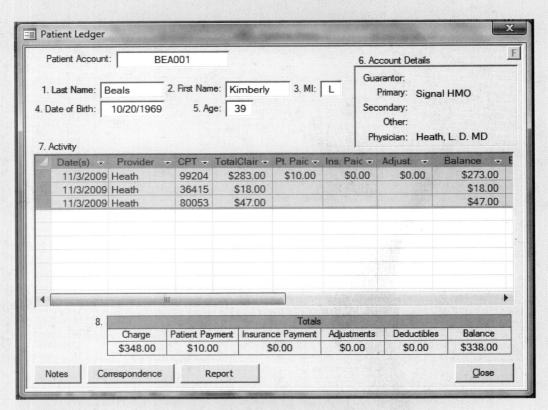

FIGURE 6-65
Delmar/Cengage Learning

STEP 4

When does the doctor want to see the patient again? Check dates approximately two weeks after 11/03/2009 for Dr. Heath's availability. The patient informs you that 11/19/2009 at 11:00 a.m. is convenient. Schedule the appointment for a 30-minute office visit. The note is "Weight loss, review lab results." See Figure 6-66.

STEP 5

Print an appointment slip to give to the patient. See Figure 6-67.

STEP 6

Close all windows and return to the Main Menu screen.

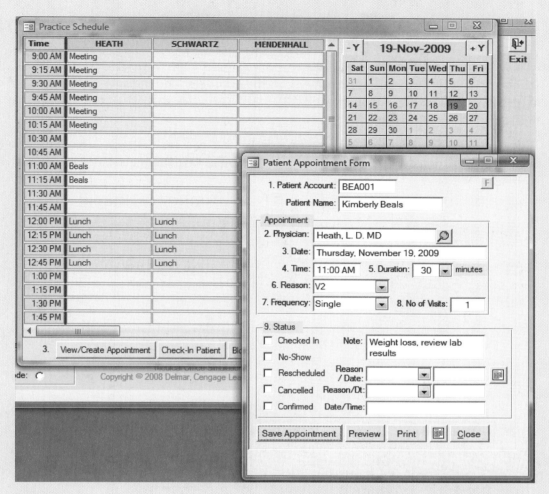

FIGURE 6-66
Delmar/Cengage Learning

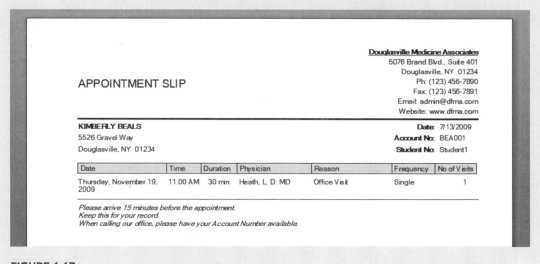

FIGURE 6-67
Delmar/Cengage Learning

CASE STUDY 6–N: GORDON, ERIC

Patient:	**Gordon, Eric**
Service Date:	**November 5, 2009**
Check-in:	**Find this appointment on the scheduler and indicate the patient checked in.**
Superbill:	**Source Document 6-13**
Physician:	**Schwartz**

Check-out Details

This patient will not make a payment today. The office will submit a claim to patient Gordon's insurance.

STEP 1

Post procedure charges as shown on patient Gordon's superbill (2345), Source Document 6-13. Check your work with Figure 6-68. Since there will be no payments, close all windows when finished.

STEP 2

When does the doctor want to see the patient again? Since the patient is to return only as needed, an appointment is not required at this time.

STEP 3

Close all windows and return to the Main Menu screen.

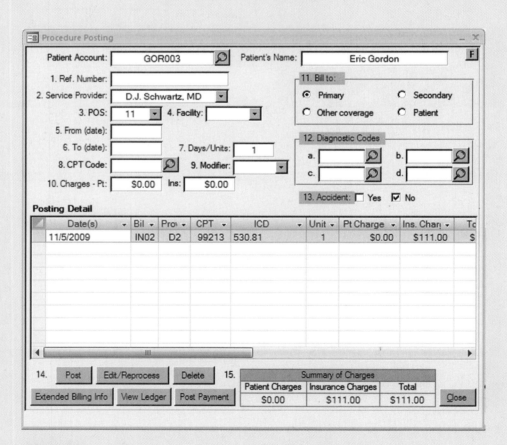

FIGURE 6-68

Delmar/Cengage Learning

CASE STUDY 6–O: YBARRA, ELANE

Patient: **Ybarra, Elane**
Service Date: **November 6, 2009**
Check-in: **Find this appointment on the scheduler and indicate the patient checked in.**
Superbill: **Source Document 6-14**
Physician: **Schwartz**

Check-out Details

This patient will not make a payment today. The office will submit a claim to patient Ybarra's insurance company. The patient schedules a follow-up appointment before leaving the office.

STEP 1

Post procedure charges as shown on patient Ybarra's superbill (2346), Source Document 6-14. Check your work with Figure 6-69.

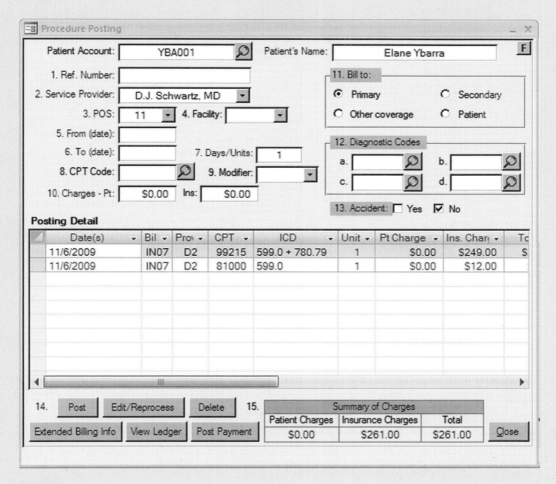

FIGURE 6-69
Delmar/Cengage Learning

Case Study 6-O Continues >>

Case Study 6-O Continued

STEP 2

When does the doctor want to see the patient again? The patient informs you that 11/13/2009 at 10:45 a.m. is convenient. Schedule the appointment for a 15-minute office visit. The note is "Follow-up UTI" (urinary tract infection). See Figure 6-70.

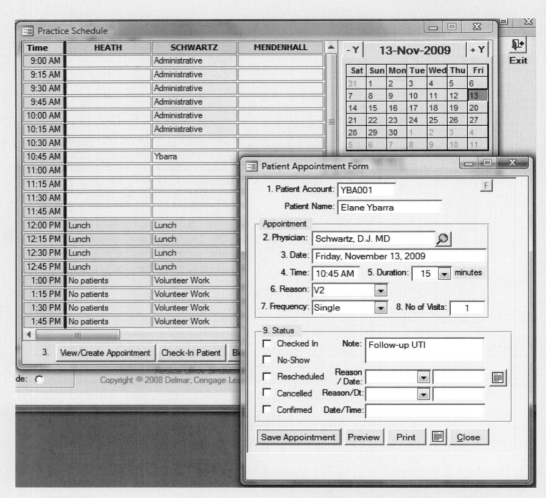

FIGURE 6-70

Delmar/Cengage Learning

STEP 3

Print an appointment slip to give to the patient. See Figure 6-71.

STEP 4

Close all windows and return to the Main Menu screen.

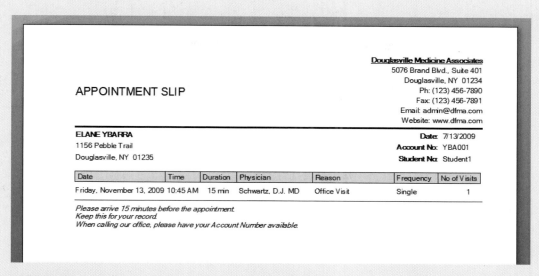

APPOINTMENT SLIP

Douglasville Medicine Associates
5076 Brand Blvd., Suite 401
Douglasville, NY 01234
Ph: (123) 456-7890
Fax: (123) 456-7891
Email: admin@dfma.com
Website: www.dfma.com

ELANE YBARRA
1156 Pebble Trail
Douglasville, NY 01235

Date: 7/13/2009
Account No: YBA001
Student No: Student1

Date	Time	Duration	Physician	Reason	Frequency	No of Visits
Friday, November 13, 2009	10:45 AM	15 min	Schwartz, D.J. MD	Office Visit	Single	1

Please arrive 15 minutes before the appointment.
Keep this for your record.
When calling our office, please have your Account Number available.

FIGURE 6-71

Delmar/Cengage Learning

CASE STUDY 6–P: KINZLER, LINDA

Patient:	**Kinzler, Linda**
Service Date:	**November 9, 2009**
Check-in:	**Find this appointment on the scheduler and indicate the patient checked in.**
Superbill:	**Source Document 6-15**
Physician:	**Heath**

Check-out Details

This patient will pay her co-payment and pay for her flu shot, which is an exclusion of her health plan. The office will submit a claim to patient Kinzler's insurance.

STEP 1

Post procedure charges as shown on patient Kinzler's superbill (2347), Source Document 6-15. Check your work with Figure 6-72.

STEP 2

Payment is made with one check, number "2266," in the amount of $42.00. The check is inspected to be sure it is correctly dated, shows the correct amount, and is signed. Single click on the *line entry* for 11/09/2009, office visit 99203, and then click on the *Select/Edit button*. Enter the check number in Field 8, Reference number. Post "$20.00" towards the co-payment amount.

Case Study 6-P Continues >>

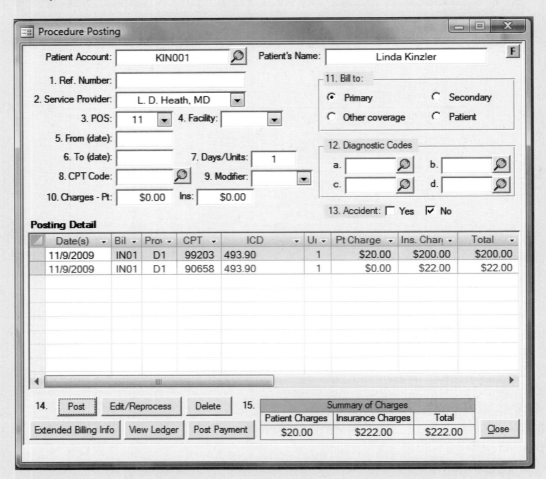

FIGURE 6-72

Delmar/Cengage Learning

STEP 3

Payment is made with the same check, number "2266," in the amount of $22.00 towards the flu shot charge. Post this payment, and then check your work with the Patient Ledger, as shown in Figure 6-73.

STEP 4

When does the doctor want to see the patient again? Since the patient is to come back only as needed, an appointment is not required at this time.

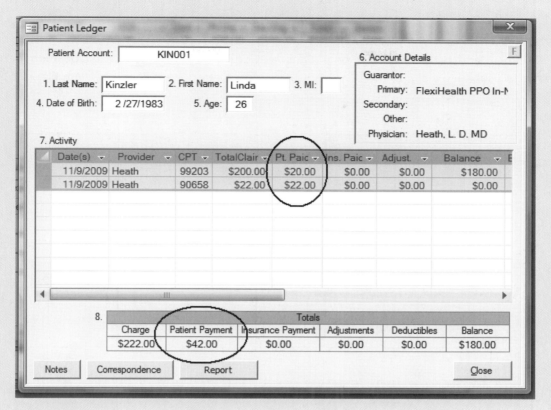

FIGURE 6-73
Delmar/Cengage Learning

CASE STUDY 6–Q: JAMES, DAVID

Patient:	**James, David**
Service Date:	**November 09, 2009**
Check-in:	**Find this appointment on the scheduler and indicate the patient checked in.**
Superbill:	**Source Document 6-16**
Physician:	**Heath**

Check-out Details

The patient's mother accompanied this minor to the office today for complaints of a tender abdomen and pain. She will pay the co-payment and schedule a follow-up appointment for patient James before leaving the office.

Case Study 6-Q Continues >>

STEP 1

Post procedure charges as shown on patient James's superbill (2348), Source Document 6-16. The office will submit a claim to the primary insurance company. Check your work with Figure 6-74.

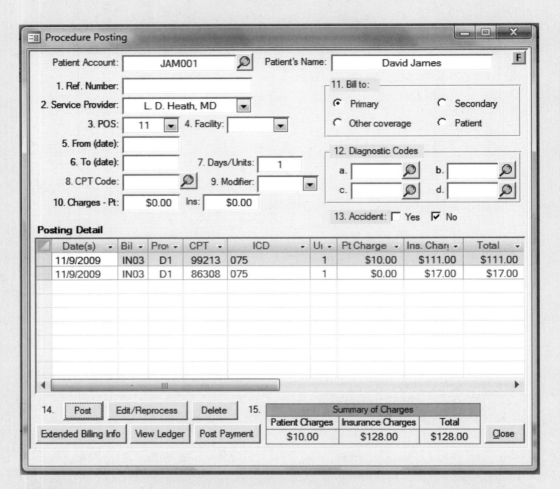

FIGURE 6-74

Delmar/Cengage Learning

STEP 2

Enter the payment using the *Post Payment button*. The patient's mother pays $10.00 with a check. The check is inspected to be sure it is correctly dated, shows the correct amount, and is signed. The check number is "786."

STEP 3

Compare the Patient Ledger to Figure 6-75 to check your work. Close all windows and then open the appointment scheduler.

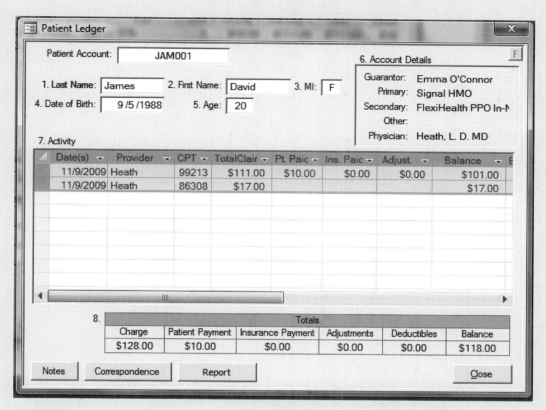

FIGURE 6-75

Delmar/Cengage Learning

STEP 4

When does the doctor want to see the patient again? Check the dates approximately two weeks after 11/09/2009 for Dr. Heath's availability. The patient's mother informs you that 11/24/2009 at 4:00 p.m. is convenient. Schedule the appointment for a 15-minute office visit. The note is "Follow-up mononucleosis." Check you work with Figure 6-76.

STEP 5

Print an appointment slip to give to the patient's mother. See Figure 6-77.

STEP 6

Close all windows and return to the Main Menu screen.

Case Study 6-Q Continues >>

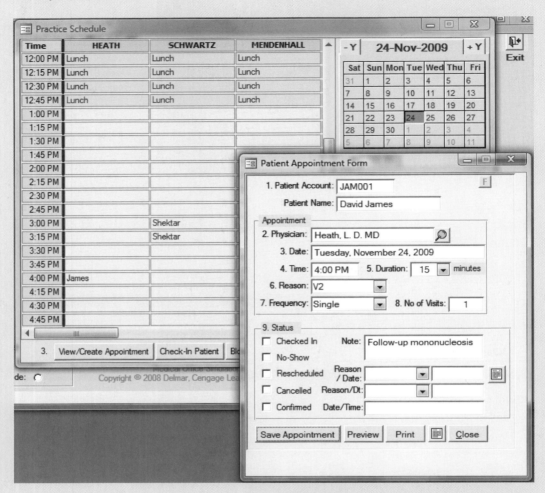

FIGURE 6-76
Delmar/Cengage Learning

APPOINTMENT SLIP

Douglasville Medicine Associates
5076 Brand Blvd., Suite 401
Douglasville, NY 01234
Ph: (123) 456-7890
Fax: (123) 456-7891
Email: admin@dfma.com
Website: www.dfma.com

DAVID JAMES
11690 Marble Way
Douglasville, NY 01234

Date: 7/13/2009
Account No: JAM001
Student No: Student1

Date	Time	Duration	Physician	Reason	Frequency	No of Visits
Tuesday, November 24, 2009	4:00 PM	15 min	Heath, L. D. MD	Office Visit	Single	1

Please arrive 15 minutes before the appointment.
Keep this for your record.
When calling our office, please have your Account Number available.

FIGURE 6-77
Delmar/Cengage Learning

POSTING CHARGES FOR SERVICES OUTSIDE THE OFFICE

Posting procedure charges for patients who receive services outside of the office is not that different from in-office patients. If you recall, the physician must inform the office which patients received services, provide the diagnoses, and advise where the procedures were performed. Each medical practice and physician has his or her own system for reporting outside services to the billing staff. Once the information is entered into the medical software, claims can be sent to insurance companies for payment. Because services are rendered in facilities other than the office, patients rarely make payments until after the insurance companies have been billed.

It is important to note that inpatients who are hospitalized for extended periods of time should have services billed to the insurance company consistently, such as on a per-week basis. For instance, if a patient is in the hospital for a serious medical condition for one month, claims can be submitted weekly. This will maintain cash flow and avoid backing up of claims.

OUTSIDE FACILITY CASE STUDIES

Doctors Heath and Schwartz have reported the procedures shown on the log illustrated in Source Document 6-17 from the Source Document Appendix. This log will now be used as a reference in order to post charges to each patient's account. Follow the steps as indicated in the following case studies.

LET'S TRY IT! 6-2 POSTING CHARGES FOR SERVICES OUTSIDE THE OFFICE

CASE STUDY 6–R: BLANC, FRANCOIS

Refer to Source Document 6-17 and locate patient Blanc. Using the information shown, answer the following questions. *Cover the answers using the tear-off bookmark from the cover of your book. Check your work before entering data into MOSS.*

A.	What is the date of service?	**11/24/2009**
B.	At which facility were the services rendered? What place of service (POS) code is this?	**Retirement Inn Nursing Home (POS 31)**
C.	Which doctor performed the services?	**Dr. Heath**

NT: Be sure to select CPT
des for the appropriate
-of-office encounter. These
vices were *not* rendered in
medical office.

Now refer to the blank superbill in Figure 6-1 and answer the following questions. When finished, you have gathered all of the information necessary to post charges for Francois Blanc.

D.	Which CPT code can be used for the service performed on 11/24/2009?	**99307 (Subsequent Care, Established Pt., Problem focused)**
E.	Which ICD codes can be used for the patient diagnoses?	**401.9 (Hypertension); 250.02 (Diabetes Mellitus, Type II, Uncontrolled)**

Case Study 6-R Continues >>

STEP 1

Start MOSS.

STEP 2

Click on the *Procedure Posting button* and locate patient Blanc on the list. Click on the *Add button* to open the Procedure Entry window.

STEP 3

Enter data regarding this procedure. Do not forget to include the reference number, as given on the log, and provide the place of service in Fields 3 and 4. Check your screen with Figure 6-78 before clicking on the *Post button*.

STEP 4

Post the procedure, and then close all windows when finished.

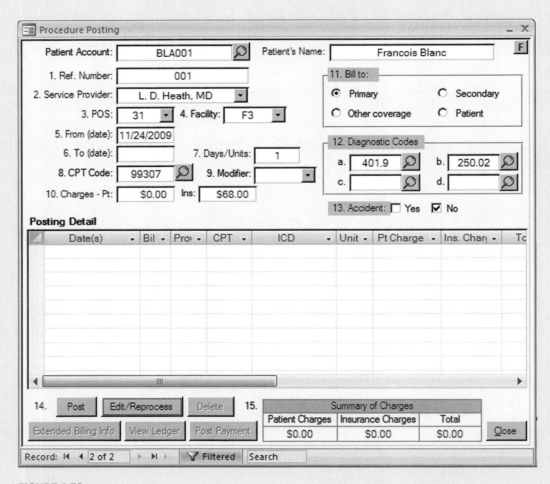

FIGURE 6-78

Delmar/Cengage Learning

CASE STUDY 6–S: CHANG, XAO

Refer to Source Document 6-17 and locate patient Chang. Using the information shown, answer the following questions.

A.	What is the date of service?	11/24/2009
B.	At which facility were the services rendered? What place of service (POS) code is this?	Retirement Inn Nursing Home (POS 31)
C.	Which doctor performed the services?	Dr. Heath

NT: Be sure to select CPT des for the appropriate t-of-office encounter. These vices were *not* rendered in e medical office.

Now refer to the blank superbill in Figure 6-1 and answer the following questions. When finished, you have gathered all of the information necessary to post charges for Xao Chang.

D.	Which CPT code can be used for the service performed on 11/24/2009?	99307 (Subsequent Care, Established Pt., Problem focused)
E.	Which ICD codes can be used for the patient diagnoses?	780.39 (Seizure Disorder)

STEP 1

Start MOSS.

STEP 2

Click on the *Procedure Posting button* and locate patient Chang on the list. Click on the *Add button* to open the Procedure Entry window.

STEP 3

Enter data regarding this procedure. Do not forget to include the reference number and place of service in Fields 3 and 4. Check your screen with Figure 6-79 before clicking on the *Post button*.

STEP 4

Post the procedure, and then close all windows when finished.

Case Study 6-S Continues >>

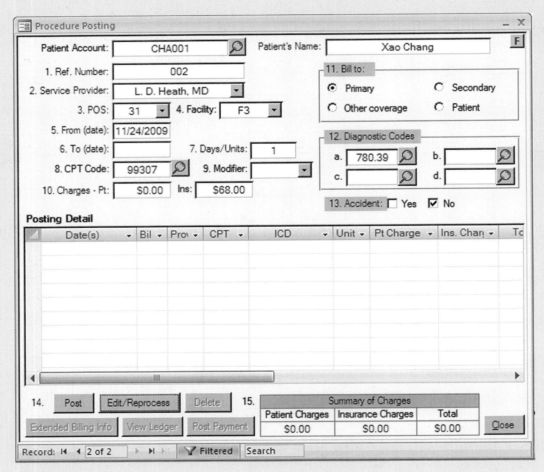

FIGURE 6-79
Delmar/Cengage Learning

CASE STUDY 6–T: PINKSTON, ANNA

Refer to Source Document 6-17 and locate patient Pinkston. Using the information shown, answer the following questions.

A.	What is the date of service?	**11/24/2009**
B.	At which facility were the services rendered? What place of service (POS) code is this?	**Retirement Inn Nursing Home (POS 31)**
C.	Which doctor performed the services?	**Dr. Heath**

NT: Be sure to select CPT
des for the appropriate
-of-office encounter. These
vices were *not* rendered in
medical office.

Now refer to the blank superbill in Figure 6-1 and answer the following questions. When finished, you have gathered all of the information necessary to post charges for Anna Pinkston.

D.	Which CPT code can be used for the service performed on 11/24/2009?	**99308 (Subsequent Care, Established Pt., Expanded)**
E.	Which ICD codes can be used for the patient diagnoses?	**443.9 (Peripheral vascular disease)**

STEP 1

Start MOSS.

STEP 2

Click on the *Procedure Posting button* and locate patient Pinkston on the list. Click on the *Add button* to open the Procedure Entry window.

STEP 3

Enter data regarding this procedure. Do not forget to include the reference number and place of service in Fields 3 and 4. Check your screen with Figure 6-80 before clicking on the *Post button*.

STEP 4

Post the procedure, and then close all windows when finished.

Case Study 6-T Continues >>

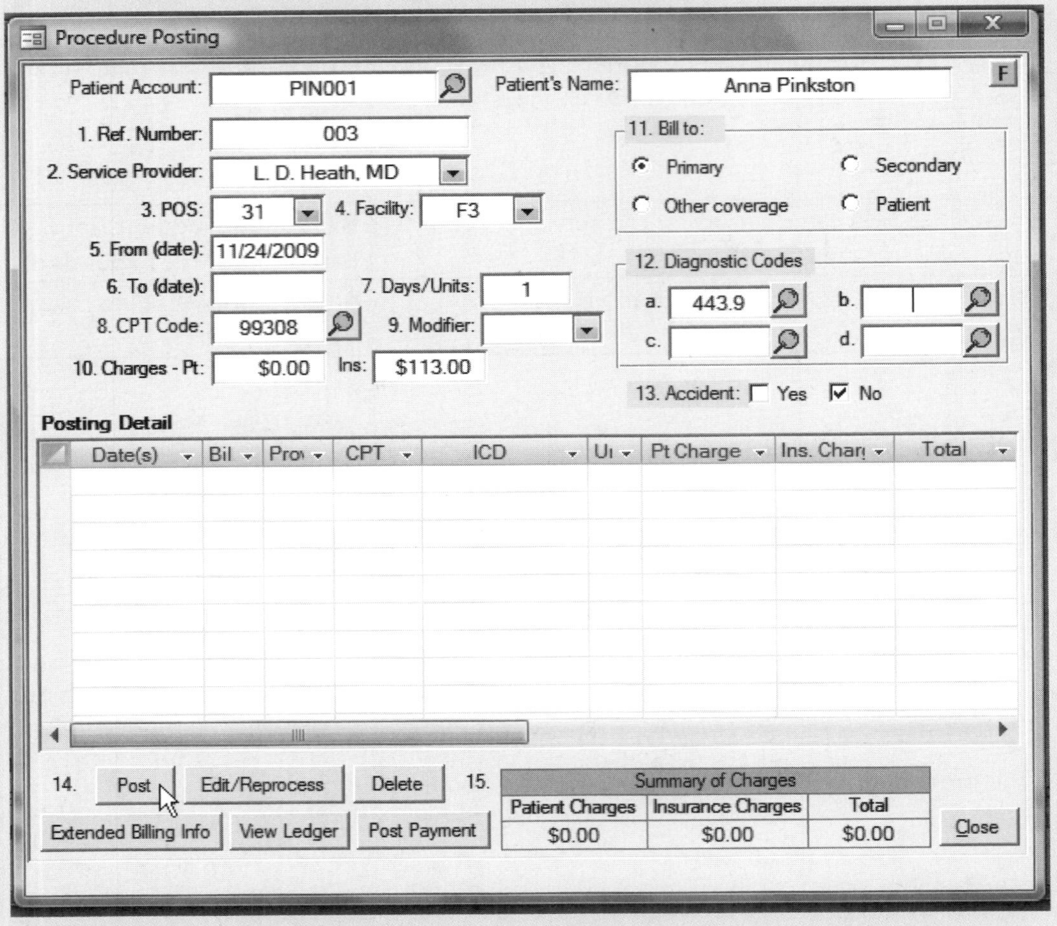

FIGURE 6-80

Delmar/Cengage Learning

USING EXTENDED BILLING INFORMATION

There are certain circumstances where additional information needs to be provided to insurance companies regarding claims. This additional data is critical for paying the claim; without it, the claim is likely to be denied.

Important information you have already been providing is the place of service. By indicating where services were rendered, such as the office, hospital, or nursing home, the information can be provided properly on a paper claim form, or transmitted electronically to insurance companies.

Hospitalization dates that apply to current services are another example of information that must be provided on a claim form. The Extended Billing Information button opens a dialog box for data entry of this information as required. The following case studies utilize extended billing information for hospitalized patients.

CASE STUDY 6–U: TATE, JASON

Refer to Source Document 6-17 and locate patient Tate. Using the information shown, answer the following questions.

A.	What are the dates of service?	11/3/2009 through 11/5/2009
B.	At which facility were the services rendered? What place of service (POS) code is this?	Community General Hospital (POS 21)
C.	Which doctor performed the services?	Dr. Heath

NT: Be sure to select CPT des for the appropriate t-of-office encounter. These vices were *not* rendered in e medical office.

Now refer to the blank superbill in Figure 6-1 and answer the following questions. When finished, you have gathered all of the information necessary to post charges for Jason Tate.

D.	Which CPT code can be used for the service performed on 11/3/2009?	99221 (Initial Hospital Care)
E.	Which CPT code can be used for the services performed on 11/04/2009?	99231 (Subsequent Care, Hospital)
F.	Which CPT code can be used for the services performed on 11/05/2009?	99238 (Discharge Services, Hospital)
G.	Which ICD codes can be used for the patient diagnoses?	536.9 (Peptic ulcer disease), 780.6 (Fever, unknown origin), 311 (Depression)

STEP 1

Start MOSS.

STEP 2

Click on the *Procedure Posting button* and locate patient Tate on the list. Click on the *Add button* to open the Procedure Entry window.

STEP 3

Enter data for the first procedure, rendered on 11/03/2009. Do not forget to include the reference number and the place of service in Fields 3 and 4. Check your screen with Figure 6-81 before clicking on the *Post button*.

NOTE: Although patient Tate has a PPO health plan and Dr. Heath is an in-network provider, the plan pays 80% after deductible for hospital services (see Unit 4, page 161). For this reason, there is no co-payment charge, as seen typically with procedures done in the medical office.

Case Study 6-U Continues >>

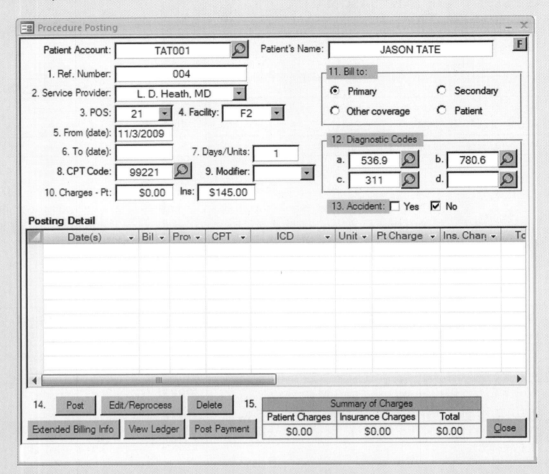

FIGURE 6-81

Delmar/Cengage Learning

STEP 4

Next, click on the *line for 11/03/2009* in the Posting Detail, as shown in Figure 6-82. Once the line has been selected by clicking on it, click on the *Extended Billing Information button*.

STEP 5

Notice on the log in Source Document 6-17 that we will be posting procedures done in the hospital for patient Tate on the dates from 11/03/2009 through 11/05/2009. In Field 6, enter these "From/To" dates, as shown in Figure 6-83.

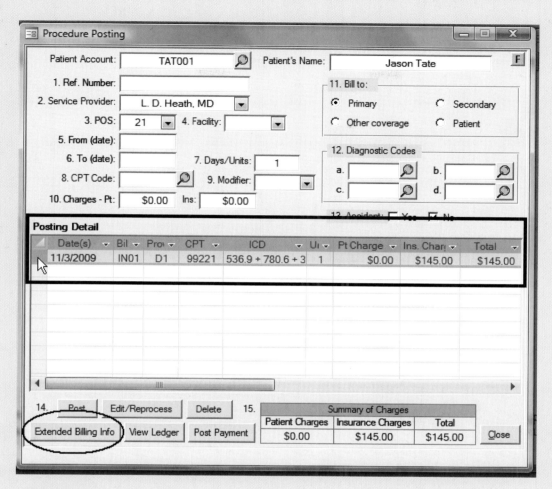

FIGURE 6-82

Delmar/Cengage Learning

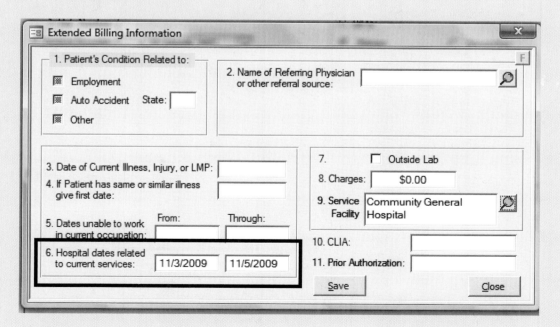

FIGURE 6-83

Delmar/Cengage Learning

Case Study 6-U Continues >>

STEP 6

Next, click on the *Search icon* at Field 9 to drop down the list of service facilities. See Figure 6-84. Select "Community General Hospital" from the list, so that it appears in Field 9.

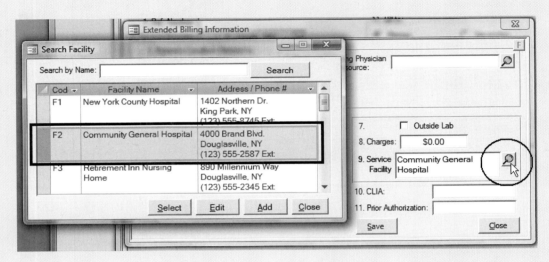

FIGURE 6-84

Delmar/Cengage Learning

STEP 7

Patient Tate has a PPO plan that requires preauthorization to approve admission to the hospital. At the time of admission, the health plan was contacted and authorization was obtained. The preauthorization number was recorded on the face sheet and appears on the log in Source Document 6-17. Enter the authorization number in Field 11. Check your work with Figure 6-85.

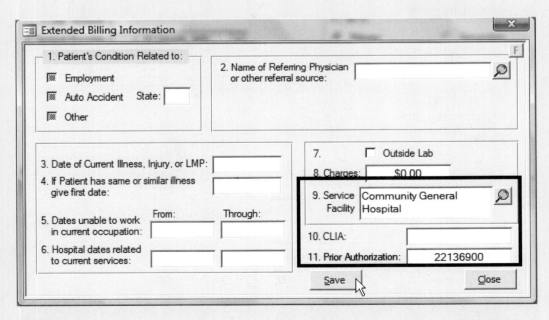

FIGURE 6-85

Delmar/Cengage Learning

STEP 8

Next, click on the *Save button* and close the window. This information will be retained in extended billing for the next procedures to be entered for patient Tate.

STEP 9

The Procedure Posting window should still be displayed on your screen, ready for input of the next services for patient Tate. Enter the procedures for 11/04/2009 and 11/05/2009, as shown on the log on Source Document 6-17. Check your screen with Figure 6-86 when finished.

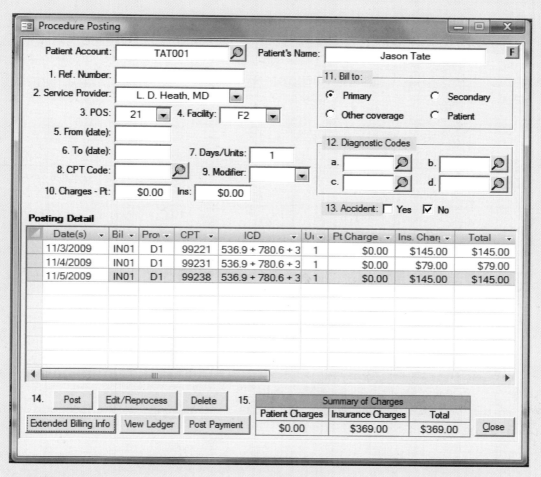

FIGURE 6-86

Delmar/Cengage Learning

STEP 10

Close all open windows until you return to the Procedure Posting patient list. You now are ready to select the next patient and post charges.

CASE STUDY 6–V: MUÑOZ, GERALDO

Refer to Source Document 6-17 and locate patient Muñoz. Using the information shown, answer the following questions.

A.	What are the dates of service?	**11/06/2009 through 11/09/2009**
B.	At which facility were the services rendered? What place of service (POS) code is this?	**New York County Hospital (POS 21)**
C.	Which doctor performed the services?	**Dr. Heath**

HINT: Be sure to select CPT codes for the appropriate out-of-office encounter. These services were *not* rendered in the medical office.

Now refer to the blank superbill in Figure 6-1 and answer the following questions. When finished, you have gathered all of the information necessary to post charges for Geraldo Muñoz.

D.	Which CPT code can be used for the service performed on 11/06/2009?	**99221 (Initial Hospital Care)**
E.	Which CPT code can be used for the services performed on 11/07 through 11/08/2009?	**99231 (Subsequent Care, Hospital)**
F.	Which CPT code can be used for the services performed on 11/09/2009?	**99238 (Discharge Services, Hospital)**
G.	Which ICD codes can be used for the patient diagnoses?	**427.31 (Atrial Fibrillation)**

STEP 1
Start MOSS.

STEP 2
Click on the *Procedure Posting button* and locate patient Muñoz on the list. Click on the *Add button* to open the Procedure Entry window.

STEP 3
Enter data for the first procedure, rendered on 11/06/2009. Do not forget to include the reference number and the place of service in Fields 3 and 4. Check your screen with Figure 6-87 before clicking on the *Post button.*

STEP 4
Next, click on the *line for 11/06/2009* in the Posting Detail. Once the line has been selected by clicking on it, click on the *Extended Billing Information button.*

STEP 5
Notice on the log in Source Document 6-17 that we will be posting procedures done in the hospital for patient Muñoz for dates from 11/06/2009 through 11/09/2009. In Field 6, enter these "From/To" dates.

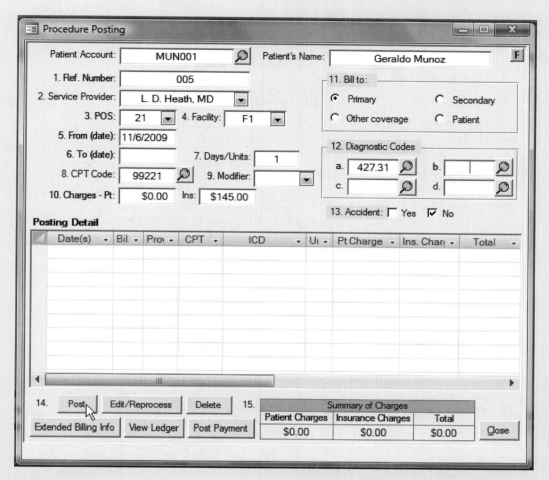

FIGURE 6-87

Delmar/Cengage Learning

STEP 6

Next, click on the *Search icon* at Field 9 to drop down the list of service facilities. Select "New York County Hospital" from the list, so that it appears in Field 9.

STEP 7

Patient Muñoz has Statewide Medicare, and no preauthorization number is needed. Check your work with Figure 6-88 before saving.

STEP 8

Next, click on the *Save button* and close the window. This information will be retained in extended billing for the next procedures to be entered for patient Muñoz.

STEP 9

The Procedure Posting window should still be displayed on your screen, ready for input of the next services for patient Muñoz. Enter the procedures for 11/07/2009 and 11/08/2009, as shown on the log on Source Document 6-17. Since these are two consecutive dates for the same CPT code, the services can be block billed using Fields 5 and 6. Check your screen with Figure 6-89 before saving your work.

Case Study 6-V Continues >>

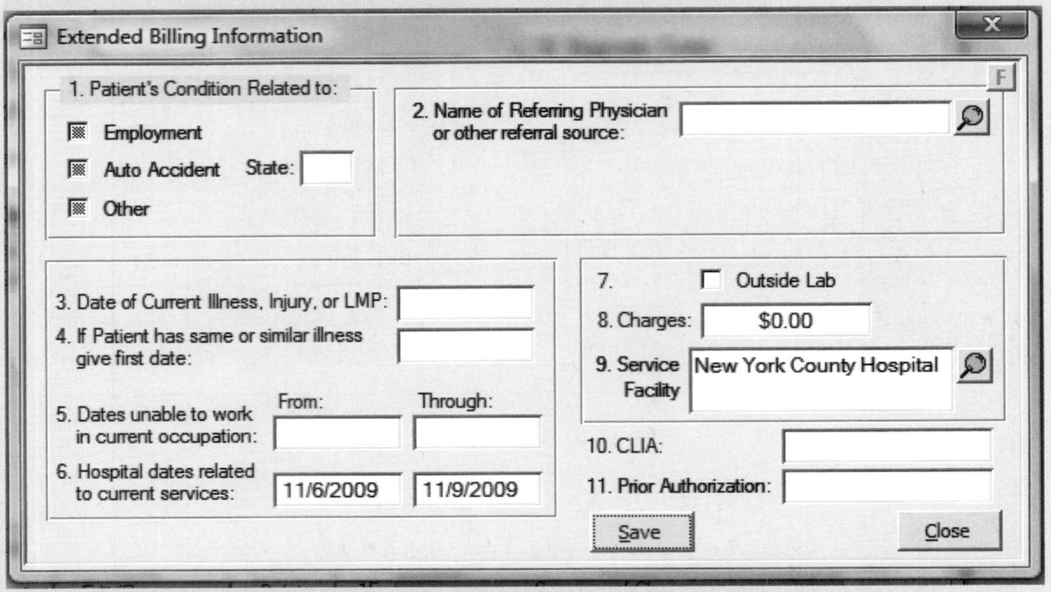

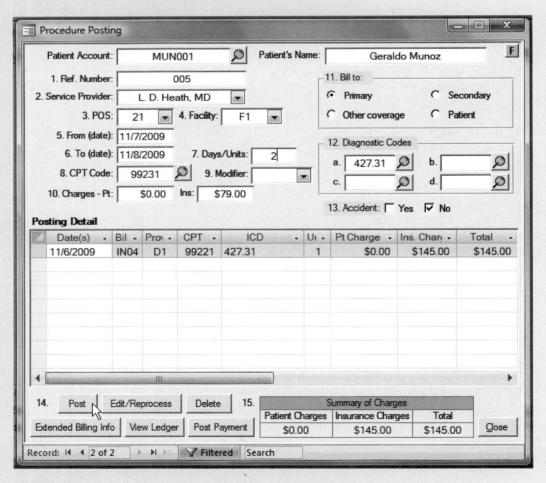

FIGURE 6-88

Delmar/Cengage Learning

FIGURE 6-89

Delmar/Cengage Learning

STEP 10

The Procedure Posting window should still be displayed on your screen, ready for input of the next service for patient Muñoz. Enter the procedure for 11/09/2009. Check your screen with Figure 6-90 when finished.

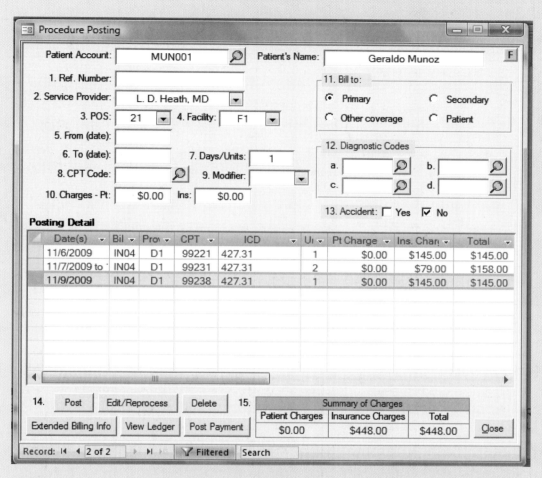

FIGURE 6-90

Delmar/Cengage Learning

STEP 11

Close all open windows until you return to the Procedure Posting patient list. You now are ready to select the next patient and post charges.

CASE STUDY 6–W: RUHL, MARY

Refer to Source Document 6-17 and locate patient Ruhl. Using the information shown, answer the following questions.

A.	What are the dates of service?	11/05/2009 through 11/10/2009
B.	At which facility were the services rendered? What place of service (POS) code is this?	New York County Hospital (POS 21)
C.	Which doctor performed the services?	Dr. Heath

HINT: Be sure to select CPT codes for the appropriate out-of-office encounter. These services were *not* rendered in the medical office.

Now refer to the blank superbill in Figure 6-1 and answer the following questions. When finished, you have gathered all of the information necessary to post charges for Mary Ruhl.

D.	Which CPT code can be used for the service performed on 11/05/2009?	99221 (Initial Hospital Care)
E.	Which CPT code can be used for the services performed on 11/06 through 11/09/2009?	99231 (Subsequent Care, Hospital)
F.	Which CPT code can be used for the services performed on 11/10/2009?	99238 (Discharge Services, Hospital)
G.	Which ICD codes can be used for the patient diagnoses?	558.9 (Gastroenteritis), 276.51 (Dehydration), 780.6 (Fever, unknown origin)

STEP 1
Start MOSS.

STEP 2
Click on the *Procedure Posting button* and locate patient Ruhl on the list. Click on the *Add button* to open the Procedure Entry window.

STEP 3
Enter data for the first procedure, rendered on 11/05/2009. Do not forget to include the reference number and the place of service in Fields 3 and 4. Check your screen with Figure 6-91 before clicking on the *Post button.*

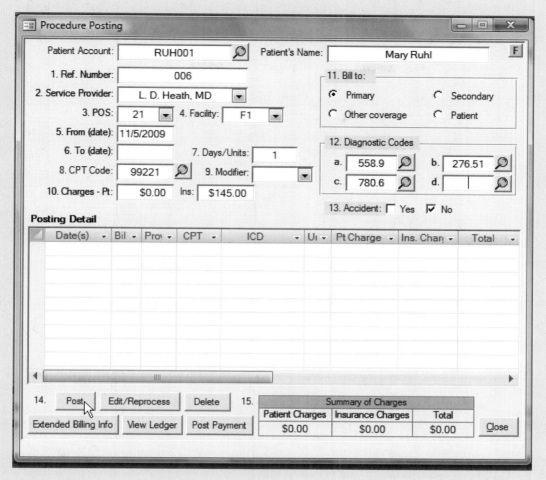

FIGURE 6-91

Delmar/Cengage Learning

STEP 4

Next, click on the *line for 11/05/2009* in the Posting Detail. Once the line has been selected by clicking on it, click on the *Extended Billing Information button*.

STEP 5

Notice on the log in Source Document 6-17 that we will be posting procedures done in the hospital for patient Ruhl for dates from 11/05/2009 through 11/10/2009. In Field 6, enter these "From/To" dates.

STEP 6

Next, click on the *Search icon* at Field 9 to drop down the list of service facilities. Select "New York County Hospital" from the list, so that it appears in Field 9.

Case Study 6-W Continues >>

STEP 7

Patient Ruhl has FlexiHealth PPO that requires preauthorization to approve admission to the hospital. At the time of admission, the health plan was contacted and authorization was obtained. The preauthorization number was recorded on the face sheet and appears on the log in Source Document 6-17. Enter the authorization number in Field 11. Check your work with Figure 6-92.

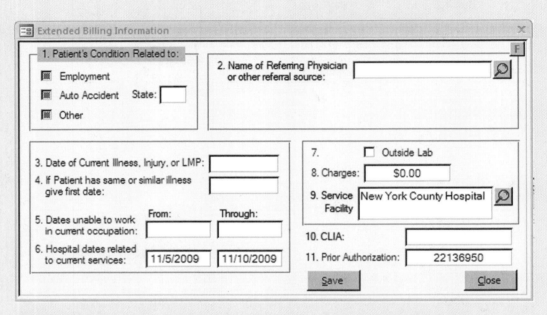

FIGURE 6-92

Delmar/Cengage Learning

STEP 8

Next, click on the *Save button* and close the window. This information will be retained in extended billing for the next procedures to be entered for patient Ruhl.

STEP 9

The Procedure Posting window should still be displayed on your screen, ready for input of the next services for patient Ruhl. Enter the procedures for 11/06/2009 and 11/09/2009, as shown on the log on Source Document 6-17. Since these are consecutive dates for the same CPT code, the services can be block billed using Fields 5 and 6. Check your screen with Figure 6-93 before saving your work.

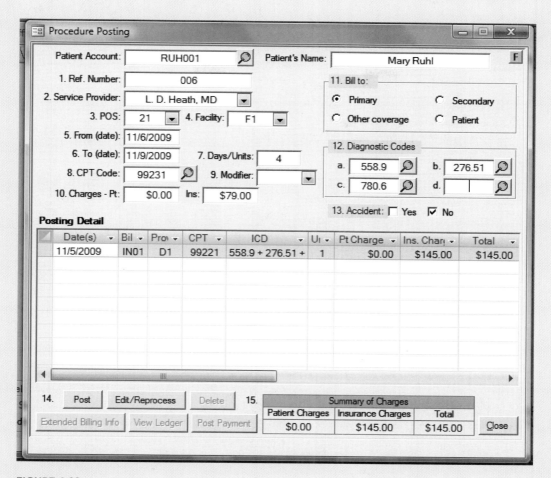

FIGURE 6-93

Delmar/Cengage Learning

STEP 10

The Procedure Posting window should still be displayed on your screen, ready for input of the next service for patient Ruhl. Enter the procedure for 11/10/2009. Check your screen with Figure 6-94 when finished.

STEP 11

Close all open windows until you return to the Procedure Posting patient list. You now are ready to select the next patient and post charges.

Case Study 6-W Continues >>

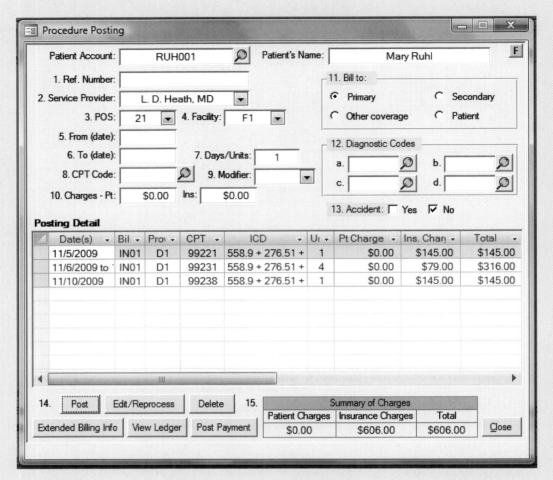

FIGURE 6-94

Delmar/Cengage Learning

CASE STUDY 6–X: MALLORY, CHRISTINA

Refer to Source Document 6-17 and locate patient Mallory. Using the information shown, answer the following questions.

A.	What are the dates of service?	**11/14/2009 through 11/15/2009**
B.	At which facility were the services rendered? What place of service (POS) code is this?	**New York County Hospital (POS 21)**
C.	Which doctor performed the services?	**Dr. Heath**

Now refer to the blank superbill in Figure 6-1 and answer the following questions. When finished, you have gathered all of the information necessary to post charges for Christina Mallory.

D.	Which CPT code can be used for the service performed on 11/14/2009?	99221 (Initial Hospital Care)
E.	Which CPT code can be used for the services performed on 11/15/2009?	99238 (Discharge Services, Hospital)
F.	Which ICD codes can be used for the patient diagnoses?	995.29 (Drug Reaction)

STEP 1

Start MOSS.

STEP 2

Click on the *Procedure Posting button* and locate patient Mallory on the list. Click on the *Add button* to open the Procedure Entry window.

STEP 3

Enter data for the first procedure, rendered on 11/14/2009. Do not forget to include the reference number and the place of service in Fields 3 and 4. Check your screen with Figure 6-95 before clicking on the *Post button.*

STEP 4

Next, click on the *line for 11/14/2009* in the Posting Detail. Once the line has been selected by clicking on it, click on the *Extended Billing Information button.*

STEP 5

Notice on the log in Source Document 6-17 that we will be posting procedures done in the hospital for patient Mallory for dates from 11/14/2009 through 11/15/2009. In Field 6, enter these "From/To" dates.

STEP 6

Next, click on the *Search icon* at Field 9 to drop down the list of service facilities. Select "New York County Hospital" from the list, so that it appears in Field 9.

STEP 7

Patient Mallory has FlexiHealth PPO that requires preauthorization to approve admission to the hospital. At the time of admission, the health plan was contacted and authorization was obtained. The preauthorization number was recorded on the face sheet and appears on the log in Source Document 6-17. Enter the authorization number in Field 11. Check your work with Figure 6-96.

STEP 8

Next, click on the *Save button* and close the window. This information will be retained in extended billing for the next procedures to be entered for patient Mallory.

Case Study 6-X Continues >>

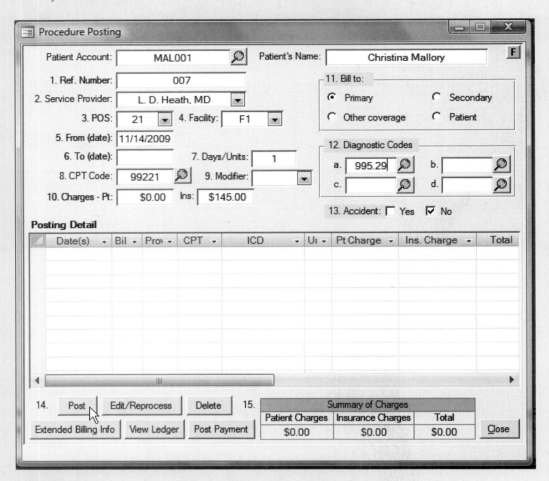

FIGURE 6-95

Delmar/Cengage Learning

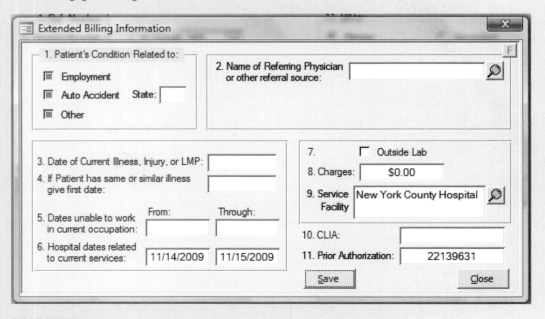

FIGURE 6-96

Delmar/Cengage Learning

STEP 9

The Procedure Posting window should still be displayed on your screen, ready for input of the next services for patient Mallory. Enter the procedure for 11/15/2009, as shown on the log on Source Document 6-17. Check your screen with Figure 6-97 before saving your work.

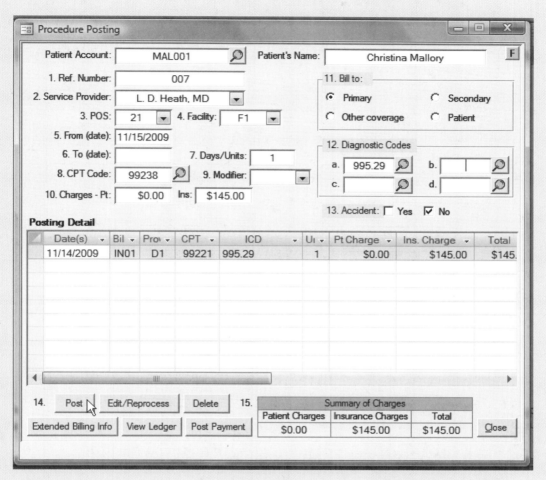

FIGURE 6-97

Delmar/Cengage Learning

STEP 10

Check your work with Figure 6-98 when finished.

STEP 11

Close all open windows until you return to the Procedure Posting patient list. You now are ready to select the next patient and post charges.

Case Study 6-X Continues >>

Case Study 6-X Continued

Procedure Posting

| Patient Account: | MAL001 | Patient's Name: | Christina Mallory | F |

1. Ref. Number:

2. Service Provider: L. D. Heath, MD

3. POS: 21   4. Facility: F1

5. From (date):

6. To (date):   7. Days/Units: 1

8. CPT Code: 9. Modifier:

10. Charges - Pt: $0.00   Ins: $0.00

11. Bill to:
- ⦿ Primary   ○ Secondary
- ○ Other coverage   ○ Patient

12. Diagnostic Codes
a.   b.
c.   d.

13. Accident: ☐ Yes ☑ No

Posting Detail

Date(s)	Bil	Prov	CPT	ICD	U	Pt Charge	Ins. Charge	Total
11/14/2009	IN01	D1	99221	995.29	1	$0.00	$145.00	$145.00
11/15/2009	IN01	D1	99238	995.29	1	$0.00	$145.00	$145.00

14. Post   Edit/Reprocess   Delete   15.

Extended Billing Info   View Ledger   Post Payment

Summary of Charges		
Patient Charges	Insurance Charges	Total
$0.00	$290.00	$290.00

Close

FIGURE 6-98

Delmar/Cengage Learning

CASE STUDY 6–Y: GOODNOW, LEONA

Refer to Source Document 6-17 and locate patient Goodnow. Using the information shown, answer the following questions.

A.	What are the dates of service?	**10/25/2009**
B.	At which facility were the services rendered? What place of service (POS) code is this?	**Community General Hospital Emergency Room (POS 23)**
C.	Was the patient hospitalized? If no, where did services take place?	**No**
D.	Which doctor performed the services?	**Dr. Schwartz**

INT: Be sure to select CPT des for the appropriate ut-of-office encounter. These rvices were *not* rendered in e medical office.

Now refer to the blank superbill in Figure 6-1 and answer the following questions. When finished, you have gathered all of the information necessary to post charges for Leona Goodnow.

E.	Which CPT code can be used for the service performed on 10/25/2009?	**99282**
F.	Which ICD codes can be used for the patient diagnoses?	**493.92**

STEP 1

Start MOSS.

STEP 2

Click on the *Procedure Posting button* and locate patient Goodnow on the list. Click on the *Add button* to open the Procedure Entry window.

STEP 3

Enter data for the procedure, rendered on 10/25/2009. Do not forget to include the reference number and the place of service in Fields 3 and 4. There is no extended billing information that needs to be entered. Check your screen with Figure 6-99 before clicking on the *Post button*.

Case Study 6-Y Continues >>

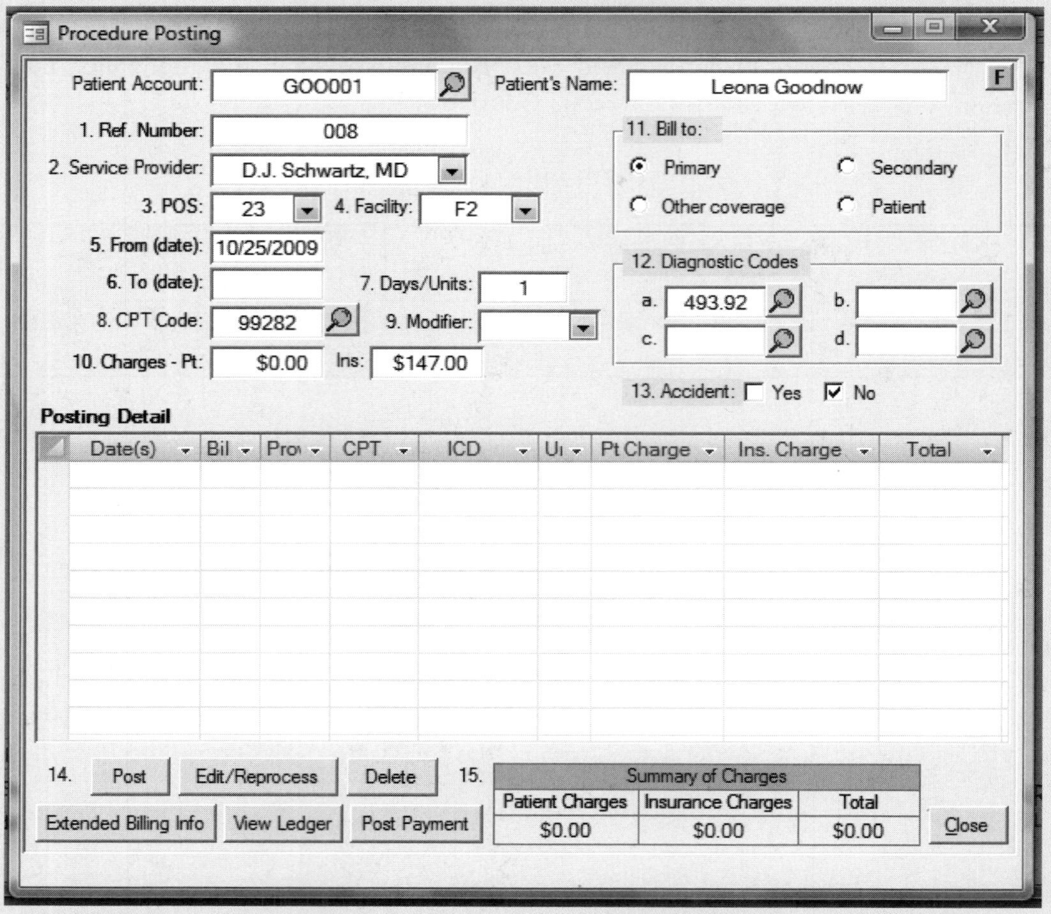

FIGURE 6-99

Delmar/Cengage Learning

STEP 4

Patient Goodnow has ConsumerOne HRA plan, and will not require preauthorization.

STEP 5

Open the Patient Ledger for patient Goodnow and compare your work with Figure 6-100 when finished.

STEP 6

Close all open windows until you return to the Main Menu of MOSS.

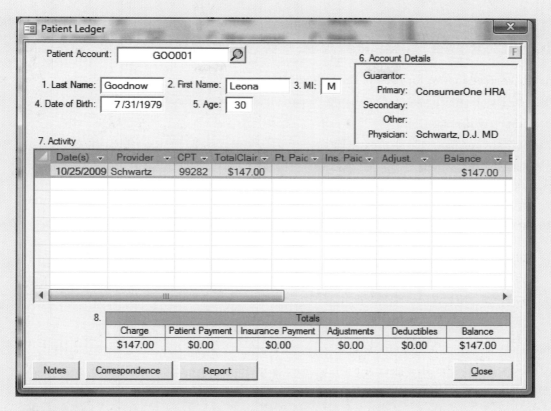

FIGURE 6-100

Delmar/Cengage Learning

FINAL NOTES

Posting procedures accurately is an important step prior to medical billing. Without proper application of charges to patients' accounts, including correct matching of CPT codes and ICD codes, claims will not reflect services rendered in a manner that promotes maximum reimbursement.

The administrative staff must handle each patient individually due to the various health plans, payment requirements, and even types of services rendered. These are factors that affect when and how much money is to be collected. It is preferable for patients to become accustomed to a routine, especially those who pay co-payments. Once a payment collection system is in place, and is enforced consistently, most patients will be prepared to settle their accounts in a timely fashion.

CHECK YOUR KNOWLEDGE

Provide the correct answer for each of the following.

1. The process of entering fees for services on a patient account is referred to as
   a. posting payments.
   b. procedure posting.
   c. registering the patient.
   d. none of the above.

2. How many diagnostic codes can be included on a procedure posting screen?
   a. 4
   b. 3
   c. 2
   d. 1

3. How will the medical staff know which diagnosis is primary, secondary, etc., for the patient?
   a. The back-office medical assistant will advise the administrative staff.
   b. The patient will inform the staff upon returning to the front desk.
   c. The physician will document details regarding the diagnosis on the superbill and in the patient file.
   d. The diagnosis is never provided to the administrative medical staff.

4. Under what circumstances does Medicare require the physician to report laboratory charges for work done at outside facilities?
   a. When the lab work charges total over $50.00
   b. When the lab work is done at an outside laboratory, but the physician is billing and collecting for the charges
   c. Medicare does not require reporting of laboratory charges under any circumstances.

5. When are co-payments due from patients with managed-care plans typically collected?
   a. At the time services are rendered
   b. Before the patient comes in for an office visit
   c. At the time a patient is sent a statement (bill)
   d. Co-payments are not typically collected from patients.

6. What is the purpose of the patient ledger?

   _____

   _____

   _____

7. Explain the purpose of having sequential reference numbers on a superbill (encounter form).

_____

_____

_____

8. Besides the physician's office, describe some locations where patients receive medical services from the doctor.

_____

_____

_____

9. A physician has treated a patient who has a diagnosis that is not listed on the superbill. How is this handled by the physician? The medical biller?

_____

_____

_____

10. Explain the purpose of the Advance Beneficiary Notice (ABN).

_____

_____

_____

11. When is it appropriate to use the "From/To" date fields when posting procedures?

_____

_____

_____

12. Explain the importance of having authorization from a health plan when providing and billing for services.

_____

_____

_____

Insurance Billing Routines

OBJECTIVES

Upon completion of this unit, the reader should be able to:

- Describe the procedure for preparing and processing paper and electronic claims

- Discuss the standard instructions for completing a CMS-1500 claim form, including special requirements for Medicare claims

- Demonstrate claims preparation using *Medical Office Simulation Software* (MOSS)

- Use the MOSS electronic claims submission simulator to process claims

- Print CMS-1500 claim forms for select insurance carriers

- Review reports generated by MOSS showing claims submitted to insurance companies for payment.

KEY TERMS

CMS-1500

National Provider Identifier (NPI)

Insurance claims management is a vital part of the reimbursement process for any medical facility. Claims management is the responsibility of the medical administrative staff, primarily the medical billers, although all staff participate in some part of the process. Some medical entities have a separate billing office that services many departments; this is common with very large group practices and hospitals. Other medical offices choose to outsource the billing and claims management to a medical billing service.

In preceding units, most of the tasks discussed ultimately contribute to providing all of the data required in order for each patient's health plan to be billed. Data needs to be accurate, and services rendered properly reflected, including the supporting diagnosis for each service. This will greatly decrease errors and reduce denied claims.

THE CLAIMS MANAGEMENT PROCESS

The claims management process involves three steps: claims preparation, claims editing, and claims submission. Each medical office determines how often claims are to be prepared for insurance billing. Some prepare claims daily, others weekly. Longer intervals are not recommended, especially for very busy offices. Not only will claims backlog, but also tracking and follow-up of slow paying and suspended claims will become more difficult. Patient billing, which is next in the reimbursement process after insurance billing, is also negatively affected. Overall, cash flow is unnecessarily slowed down if billing is not done on a frequent basis. Practice management software simplifies this task and makes the entire billing and follow-up process more efficient.

When using practice management software for claims preparation, the software user selects the settings the program refers to. This includes such data as which patient accounts are to be referenced from the database, and the insurance plans that are to be billed. The software, in turn, searches for records that meet the criteria and displays the claims that are ready for submission.

Because claims can be sent electronically or on paper, most practice management software accommodates both. The preferred method is electronic submission. Electronic submission offers editing features to make sure the claim is "clean," or free of errors, and meets the standard of each insurance carrier. Payment turnaround also is much faster, usually seven to 14 days, and may include electronic transfer of payments directly to bank accounts.

Paper claims need to be printed and sent by regular mail to the insurance carrier. Some clearinghouse transaction providers accept paper claims and submit them for a practice, providing proof of submission. This makes it easier, as all claims can be sent to just one place, the clearinghouse, and for a small fee plus postage, they will handle sending the claims to the various insurance plans. However, payment will take considerably longer, and tracking of the claims is more challenging. But there are circumstances under which paper claims are needed. These include secondary billing, where an EOB (Explanation of Benefits) must accompany the claim, requests from the insurance company for attachments, or insurance plans that require paper claims, usually on their own form(s). Using software to produce paper claims helps make them clean, reducing denials by insurance companies.

In addition to the edit checks the software makes, the user also has an opportunity to review the claims transactions that are in queue before they are sent. Obvious errors and omissions should be corrected immediately before claims submissions.

The last step is submitting the claims. Depending on the software, electronic claims can be sent either directly to the insurance carrier, or through a clearinghouse. A clearinghouse is a service agency that collects claims from many sources, "scrubs" the claims for errors, and then forwards them to the insurance carriers. Whether claims are sent directly to the carrier or through a clearinghouse, reports are generated that show which claims went through and which did not pass the scrub. Those that did not pass the scrub need to be corrected and resubmitted. For all claims that are accepted and transmitted, payment with an EOB or RA (remittance advice) will follow if the claim is deemed payable according to the guidelines of the health plan.

Once claims are billed electronically, or are printed for mailing, the transactions are identified as "sent," or processed, by the software. These transactions will not reappear on future claim preparation routines unless the user selects to rebill a claim.

It is worth adding a word of caution regarding rebilling of claims, especially paper claims that have already been sent to insurance companies. Some medical offices automatically rebill any claim that has not been paid in 30 to 45 days. However, for the few claims that do not get paid, it is more efficient to call the insurance company and investigate the reason for the delay. The payer holds some claims because more documentation is required, such as a copy of an operative report or specific diagnostic test results. In other cases, the claim is being reviewed. There could be several reasons why the claim has not been paid other than a denial or an assumption it was lost.

It is useful to look carefully at the reason codes provided with the EOB/RA for transactions showing a zero or reduced payment. These reason codes may offer explanations that save time, or pinpoint action required by the medical office. Simply rebilling every claim that has not been paid may result in duplicate denials and notices from insurance companies that the claim has been billed twice, or even already been paid by the time the rebill goes through the system. This practice causes confusion and double work for the medical billers and the administrative staff, and can be disruptive to the claims follow-up process.

REQUIREMENTS FOR INSURANCE CLAIMS SUBMISSION

Specific information is required for all claims submissions, regardless of which insurance carrier is being billed. The following list provides the items that should be available, at a minimum, prior to sending claims.

1. Patient's name, age, gender, identification number (Social Security number), and relation to the policyholder/insured

2. Policyholder's/insured's name and address (if different from patient) and identification number (Social Security number)

3. Information regarding health insurance plan(s) with policy numbers and group numbers, as applicable

4. Name of provider who rendered services with applicable provider identification number(s) as required

5. Name and identification number of the referring physician, if required by the insurance company

6. Date(s) that service(s) were provided

7. Proper CPT and ICD codes, as documented by the provider for each service rendered

8. Location where services were rendered, such as the office, hospital, nursing home, ambulatory surgical center, laboratory, etc. (The complete name and address of facilities outside the office is required.)

9. Authorization, pre-approval, or precertification numbers, if applicable.

Based on your experience working with MOSS, you recognize much, if not all, of the information in this list. These items comprise much of the information that you have been inputting and using as part of your work in this book. Practice-management software simplifies the task of creating insurance claims by using this information accordingly.

PROVIDER IDENTIFICATION NUMBERS

HIPAA has mandated the adoption of a **National Provider Identifier (NPI)**, which is a unique, government-issued identification number for individual health care providers and provider organizations, like clinics, hospitals, schools, and group practices that are defined as covered entities under

HIPAA. Any provider that uses standard electronic transactions, such as electronic claims, eligibility verification, and claims status inquiries were required to start including NPIs on electronic transactions no later than May 23, 2007.

The 10-digit NPI number is replacing identification numbers specific to insurance carriers (e.g., Medicare PIN and UPIN, private plan identification numbers, such as those issued by Blue Cross/Blue Shield, United Health Care, Cigna, etc.). Presently, the NPI does not replace the Social Security number, Employer Identification Number (EIN), or the Drug Enforcement Administration (DEA) number. Former identification numbers will be referred to as "Legacy" numbers, including Medicare's PIN and identifiers previously used by commercial health plans.

There are some advantages with using the NPI. Because the NPI will be accepted by all health plans, implementation of this identifier brings a new level of standardization to electronic transactions and should improve acceptance rates. It also eliminates the need to have several identifiers, as in years past, for the various health plans billed by providers.

INSURANCE CLAIM FORMS

At one time, paper claim forms were the only way for patients and medical providers to submit claims to insurance companies. Up through the mid-1980s, most Medicare patients were paying doctors at the time of office visits. They submitted their own claims, by attaching itemized bills to a simple Medicare form designed for patient use. Some medical offices even charged a nominal fee to bill the insurance provider on behalf of the patient.

With private health care plans, the most common type was indemnity plans, where patients made payments to providers when services were received. Insurance companies sent reimbursement directly to the patient. Obviously, reforms to Medicare, the popularity of managed-care plans, and other innovative plans, such as the consumer-driven health plans, have changed the reimbursement landscape. Today, medical offices are required to send claims to most of the insurance companies. Patients either pay co-payments or wait until claims are paid by their insurance before sending additional payments. It is clear that with coverage changes, coupled with the advent of computers and sophisticated software, the traditional ways of health insurance reimbursement in the United States are probably gone forever.

During the 1990s, the quest for implementing a standardized method for submitting claims, along with the shaping of HIPAA as we know it today, became more prevalent. While electronic billing is the preferred method for submitting claims, paper claim forms are still in use. It is important to understand the CMS-1500 claim form and its parts, even if electronic billing someday becomes the only way to submit claims. This form contains the critical components required by insurance companies in order for claims to be paid. Most of the fundamental data contained on the CMS-1500 paper claim form continues to be the required data for electronic billing.

THE CMS-1500 CLAIM FORM

The **CMS-1500** is the claim form approved by the Centers for Medicare & Medicaid Services (CMS). It is used by the Medicare program for submitting claims from physicians and suppliers. The CMS-1500 claim form is also accepted by the majority of insurance carriers whenever paper claims need to be submitted. Figure 7-1 illustrates the current CMS-1500 claim form.

1500

HEALTH INSURANCE CLAIM FORM

APPROVED BY NATIONAL UNIFORM CLAIM COMMITTEE 08/05

☐☐☐ PICA

PICA ☐☐☐

1. MEDICARE ☐ (Medicare #)   MEDICAID ☐ (Medicaid #)   TRICARE CHAMPUS ☐ (Sponsor's SSN)   CHAMPVA ☐ (Member ID#)   GROUP HEALTH PLAN ☐ (SSN or ID)   FECA BLK LUNG ☐ (SSN)   OTHER ☐ (ID)

1a. INSURED'S I.D. NUMBER   (For Program in Item 1)

2. PATIENT'S NAME (Last Name, First Name, Middle Initial)

3. PATIENT'S BIRTH DATE MM DD YY   SEX M ☐ F ☐

4. INSURED'S NAME (Last Name, First Name, Middle Initial)

5. PATIENT'S ADDRESS (No., Street)

6. PATIENT RELATIONSHIP TO INSURED   Self ☐ Spouse ☐ Child ☐ Other ☐

7. INSURED'S ADDRESS (No., Street)

CITY   STATE

8. PATIENT STATUS   Single ☐ Married ☐ Other ☐

CITY   STATE

ZIP CODE   TELEPHONE (Include Area Code) ( )

Employed ☐ Full-Time Student ☐ Part-Time Student ☐

ZIP CODE   TELEPHONE (Include Area Code) ( )

9. OTHER INSURED'S NAME (Last Name, First Name, Middle Initial)

10. IS PATIENT'S CONDITION RELATED TO:

11. INSURED'S POLICY GROUP OR FECA NUMBER

a. OTHER INSURED'S POLICY OR GROUP NUMBER

a. EMPLOYMENT? (Current or Previous) ☐ YES ☐ NO

a. INSURED'S DATE OF BIRTH MM DD YY   SEX M ☐ F ☐

b. OTHER INSURED'S DATE OF BIRTH MM DD YY   SEX M ☐ F ☐

b. AUTO ACCIDENT? ☐ YES ☐ NO   PLACE (State)

b. EMPLOYER'S NAME OR SCHOOL NAME

c. EMPLOYER'S NAME OR SCHOOL NAME

c. OTHER ACCIDENT? ☐ YES ☐ NO

c. INSURANCE PLAN NAME OR PROGRAM NAME

d. INSURANCE PLAN NAME OR PROGRAM NAME

10d. RESERVED FOR LOCAL USE

d. IS THERE ANOTHER HEALTH BENEFIT PLAN? ☐ YES ☐ NO *If yes*, return to and complete item 9 a-d.

READ BACK OF FORM BEFORE COMPLETING & SIGNING THIS FORM.

12. PATIENT'S OR AUTHORIZED PERSON'S SIGNATURE I authorize the release of any medical or other information necessary to process this claim. I also request payment of government benefits either to myself or to the party who accepts assignment below.

SIGNED_____ DATE_____

13. INSURED'S OR AUTHORIZED PERSON'S SIGNATURE I authorize payment of medical benefits to the undersigned physician or supplier for services described below.

SIGNED_____

14. DATE OF CURRENT: MM DD YY ☐ ILLNESS (First symptom) OR INJURY (Accident) OR PREGNANCY(LMP)

15. IF PATIENT HAS HAD SAME OR SIMILAR ILLNESS. GIVE FIRST DATE MM DD YY

16. DATES PATIENT UNABLE TO WORK IN CURRENT OCCUPATION FROM MM DD YY TO MM DD YY

17. NAME OF REFERRING PROVIDER OR OTHER SOURCE

17a.   17b. NPI

18. HOSPITALIZATION DATES RELATED TO CURRENT SERVICES FROM MM DD YY TO MM DD YY

19. RESERVED FOR LOCAL USE

20. OUTSIDE LAB? ☐ YES ☐ NO $ CHARGES

21. DIAGNOSIS OR NATURE OF ILLNESS OR INJURY (Relate Items 1, 2, 3 or 4 to Item 24E by Line)

1. |___.___   3. |___.___

2. |___.___   4. |___.___

22. MEDICAID RESUBMISSION CODE   ORIGINAL REF. NO.

23. PRIOR AUTHORIZATION NUMBER

24. A. DATE(S) OF SERVICE						B. PLACE OF SERVICE	C. EMG	D. PROCEDURES, SERVICES, OR SUPPLIES (Explain Unusual Circumstances)		E. DIAGNOSIS POINTER	F. $ CHARGES	G. DAYS OR UNITS	H. EPSDT Family Plan	I. ID. QUAL.	J. RENDERING PROVIDER ID. #
From MM	DD	YY	To MM	DD	YY			CPT/HCPCS	MODIFIER						
1														NPI	
2														NPI	
3														NPI	
4														NPI	
5														NPI	
6														NPI	

25. FEDERAL TAX I.D. NUMBER   SSN ☐ EIN ☐

26. PATIENT'S ACCOUNT NO.

27. ACCEPT ASSIGNMENT? (For govt. claims, see back) ☐ YES ☐ NO

28. TOTAL CHARGE $

29. AMOUNT PAID $

30. BALANCE DUE $

31. SIGNATURE OF PHYSICIAN OR SUPPLIER INCLUDING DEGREES OR CREDENTIALS (I certify that the statements on the reverse apply to this bill and are made a part thereof.)

SIGNED_____ DATE_____

32. SERVICE FACILITY LOCATION INFORMATION

a. NPI   b.

33. BILLING PROVIDER INFO & PH # ( )

a. NPI   b.

NUCC Instruction Manual available at: www.nucc.org

APPROVED OMB-0938-0999 FORM CMS-1500 (08/05)

CARRIER   *PATIENT AND INSURED INFORMATION*   *PHYSICIAN OR SUPPLIER INFORMATION*

FIGURE 7-1

The CMS-1500 Health Insurance Claim form. *Courtesy of the Centers for Medicare & Medicaid Services.*

Each insurance company may have slightly different requirements for data that is provided in some of the boxes of the form. Medicare claims are sent to fiscal intermediaries, or insurance carriers, that service Medicare claims in a particular region. A fiscal intermediary manages funds and makes payments on behalf of the beneficiary. The fiscal intermediary is also referred to as the Benefits Administrator and Part B Medicare carrier. The fiscal intermediary for Medicare in your region may have specific requirements for some of the boxes on the CMS-1500 form. In this book, the fiscal intermediary for Medicare in the locality of Douglasville Medicine Associates is Statewide Corporation. For the purposes of the exercises in this book, the fiscal intermediary name appears along with the Medicare title when selecting this insurance with MOSS.

It is important to note that more than one fiscal intermediary may be contracted to handle funds for Medicare beneficiaries in one region. For example, in the New York City area, Group Health Incorporated (GHI) handles funds for Medicare beneficiaries who receive services from providers in Queens County. Beneficiaries who receive services from providers in all other boroughs of New York City have funds handled by Empire Medicare Services Incorporated. Although technically, in this example, all Medicare patients receive services within New York City, two separate fiscal intermediaries exist. Claims are sent to one or the other depending on where, within the city, the service was provided.

Your instructor can guide you on special requirements, if any, that are pertinent to your area for the CMS-1500 claim form, including details about the fiscal intermediary for Medicare. Further information can be obtained on the Internet by using a search engine. Enter "Medicare (name of your state)," complete with quotation marks, in the search box. Then, click on relevant items in the results for more information.

CMS-1500 Claim Form Instructions

Refer to Figure 7-1 of the CMS-1500 form while reviewing the instructions for each box item presented in Figure 7-2. General and special instructions that apply to Medicare are provided where indicated.

Reminder for Date format on CSM 1500 form: For date fields other than date of birth, all fields shall be one or the other format, 6-digit: (MM | DD | YY) or 8-digit: (MM | DD | CCYY). Intermixing the two formats on the claim is not allowed.

Item 1	Show the type of health insurance coverage applicable to this claim by checking the appropriate box, e.g., if a Medicare claim is being filed, check the Medicare box.
Item 1a	Enter the patient's Medicare Health Insurance Claim (HIC) number whether Medicare is the primary or secondary payer. This is a required field.
Item 2	Enter the patient's last name, first name, and middle initial, if any, as shown on the patient's Medicare card. This is a required field.
Item 3	Enter the patient's 8-digit birth date (MM | DD | CCYY) and sex.
Item 4	If there is insurance primary to Medicare, either through the patient's or spouse's employment or any other source, list the name of the insured here. When the insured and the patient are the same, enter the word SAME. If Medicare is primary, leave blank.
Item 5	Enter the patient's mailing address and telephone number. On the first line enter the street address; the second line, the city and state; the third line, the ZIP code and phone number.
Item 6	Check the appropriate box for patient's relationship to insured when item 4 is completed.
Item 7	Enter the insured's address and telephone number. When the address is the same as the patient's, enter the word SAME. Complete this item only when items 4, 6, and 11 are completed.
Item 8	Check the appropriate box for the patient's marital status and whether employed or a student.

FIGURE 7-2

Instructions for the CMS-1500 claim form. *Delmar/Cengage Learning (continues)*

Item 9	Enter the last name, first name, and middle initial of the enrollee in a Medigap policy if it is different from that shown in item 2. Otherwise, enter the word SAME. If no Medigap benefits are assigned, leave blank. **This field may be used in the future for supplemental insurance plans**.
	Only participating physicians and suppliers are to complete item 9 and its subdivisions and only when the beneficiary wishes to assign his/her benefits under a MEDIGAP policy to the participating physician or supplier.
	Participating physicians and suppliers must enter information required in item 9 and its subdivisions if requested by the beneficiary. Participating physicians/suppliers sign an agreement with Medicare to accept assignment of Medicare benefits for **all** Medicare patients. A claim for which a beneficiary elects to assign his/her benefits under a Medigap policy to a participating physician/supplier is called a mandated Medigap transfer. (See chapter 28.)
	Do not list other supplemental coverage in item 9 and its subdivisions at the time a Medicare claim is filed. Other supplemental claims are forwarded automatically to the private insurer if the private insurer contracts with the carrier to send Medicare claim information electronically. If there is no such contract, the beneficiary must file his/her own supplemental claim.
Item 9a	Enter the policy and/or group number of the Medigap insured preceded by MEDIGAP, MG, or MGAP. (Item 9d must be completed, even when the provider enters a policy and/or group number in item 9a).
Item 9b	Enter the Medigap insured's 8-digit birth date (MM | DD | CCYY) and sex.
Item 9c	Leave blank if a Medigap PayerID is entered in item 9d. Otherwise, enter the claims processing address of the Medigap insurer. Use an abbreviated street address, two-letter postal code, and ZIP code copied from the Medigap insured's Medigap identification card.
	For example: 1257 Anywhere Street Baltimore, MD 21204 is shown as "1257 Anywhere St. MD 21204."
Item 9d	Enter the 9-digit PAYERID number of the Medigap insurer. If no PAYERID number exists, then enter the Medigap insurance program or plan name.
	If the beneficiary wants Medicare payment data forwarded to a Medigap insurer through the Medigap claim-based crossover process, the participating provider of service or supplier must accurately complete all of the information in items 9, 9a, 9b, and 9d.
	A Medicare participating provider or supplier shall **only** enter the COBA Medigap claim-based ID within item 9d when seeking to have the beneficiary's claim crossed over to a Medigap insurer. If a participating provider or supplier enters the PAYERID or the Medigap insurer program or its plan name within item 9d, the Medicare Part B contractor or Durable Medical Equipment Medicare Administrative Contractor (DMAC) will be unable to forward the claim information to the Medigap insurer prior to October 1, 2007, or to the Coordination of Benefits Contractor (COBC) for transfer to the Medicare insurer on or after October 1, 2007.
Items 10a through 10c	Check "YES" or "NO" to indicate whether employment, auto liability, or other accident involvement applies to one or more of the services described in item 24. Enter the State postal code. Any item checked "YES" indicates there may be other insurance primary to Medicare. Identify primary insurance information in item 11.
Item 10d	Use this item exclusively for Medicaid (MCD) information. If the patient is entitled to Medicaid, enter the patient's Medicaid number preceded by MCD.
Item 11	THIS ITEM MUST BE COMPLETED, IT IS A REQUIRED FIELD. By completing this item, the physician/supplier acknowledges having made a good faith effort to determine whether medicare is the primary or secondary payer.
	If there is insurance primary to Medicare, enter the insured's policy or group number and proceed to items 11a–11c. Items 4, 6, and 7 must also be completed.
	Enter the appropriate information in item 11c if insurance primary to Medicare is indicated in item 11. If there is no insurance primary to Medicare, enter the word "NONE" and proceed to item 12.
	If the insured reports a terminating event with regard to insurance which had been primary to Medicare (e.g., insured retired), enter the word "NONE" and proceed to item 11b.
Item 11a	Enter the insured's 8-digit birth date (MM | DD | CCYY) and sex if different from item 3.
Item 11b	Enter employer's name, if applicable. If there is a change in the insured's insurance status, e.g., retired, enter either a 6-digit (MM | DD | YY) or 8-digit (MM | DD | CCYY) retirement date preceded by the word "RETIRED."
Item 11c	Enter the 9-digit PAYERID number of the primary insurer. If no PAYERID number exists, then enter the **complete** primary payer's program or plan name. If the primary payer's EOB does not contain the claims processing address, record the primary payer's claims processing address directly on the EOB. This is required if there is insurance primary to Medicare that is indicated in item 11.
Item 11d	Leave blank. Not required by Medicare.

FIGURE 7-2

Instructions for the CMS-1500 claim form. *Delmar/Cengage Learning (continues)*

Item 12 The patient or authorized representative must sign and enter either a 6-digit date (MM | DD | YY), 8-digit date (MM | DD | CCYY), or an alpha-numeric date (e.g., January 1, 1998) unless the signature is on file. In lieu of signing the claim, the patient may sign a statement to be retained in the provider, physician, or supplier file. If the patient is physically or mentally unable to sign, a representative may sign on the patient's behalf and the statement's signature line must indicate the patient's name followed by "by" the representative's name, address, relationship to the patient, and the reason the patient cannot sign. The authorization is effective indefinitely unless the patient or the patient's representative revokes this arrangement.

Signature by Mark (X) - When an illiterate or physically handicapped enrollee signs by mark, a witness must enter his/her name and address next to the mark.

Item 13 The patient's signature or the statement "signature on file" in this item authorizes payment of medical benefits to the physician or supplier. The patient or his/her authorized representative signs this item or the signature must be on file separately with the provider as an authorization. However, note that when payment under the Act can only be made on an assignment-related basis or when payment is for services furnished by a participating physician or supplier, a patient's signature or a "signature on file" is not required in order for Medicare payment to be made directly to the physician or supplier.

The presence of or lack of a signature or "signature on file" in this field will be indicated as such to any downstream Coordination of Benefits trading partners (supplemental insurers) with whom CMS has a payer-to-payer coordination of benefits relationship. Medicare has no control over how supplemental claims are processed, so it is important that providers accurately address this field as it may affect supplemental payments to providers and/or their patients.

In addition, the signature in this item authorizes payment of mandated Medigap benefits to the participating physician or supplier if required Medigap information is included in item 9 and its subdivisions. The patient or his/her authorized representative signs this item or the signature must be on file as a separate Medigap authorization. The Medigap assignment on file in the participating provider of service/supplier's office must be insurer specific. It may state that the authorization applies to all occasions of service until it is revoked. It is permissible to write "Signature on File" and/or a computer generated signature.

Item 14 Enter either an 8-digit (MM | DD | CCYY) or 6-digit (MM | DD | YY) date of current illness, injury, or pregnancy. For chiropractic services, enter an 8-digit (MM | DD | CCYY) or 6-digit (MM | DD | YY) date of the initiation of the course of treatment and enter an 8-digit (MM | DD | CCYY) or 6-digit (MM | DD | YY) date in item 19.

Item 15 Leave blank. Not required by Medicare.

Item 16 If the patient is employed and is unable to work in his/her current occupation, enter an 8-digit (MM | DD | CCYY) or 6-digit (MM | DD | YY) date when patient is unable to work. An entry in this field may indicate employment related insurance coverage.

Item 17 Enter the name of the referring or ordering physician if the service or item was ordered or referred by a physician. All physicians who order services or refer Medicare beneficiaries must report this data. When a claim involves multiple referring and/or ordering physicians, a separate Form CMS-1500 shall be used for each ordering/referring physician.

Item 17a Effective May 23, 2008, 17a is not to be reported but 17b MUST be reported when a service was ordered or referred by a physician.

Item 17b Enter the NPI of the referring/ordering physician listed in item 17. All physicians who order services or refer Medicare beneficiaries must report this data.

Item 18 Enter either an 8-digit (MM | DD | CCYY) or a 6-digit (MM | DD | YY) date when a medical service is furnished as a result of, or subsequent to, a related hospitalization.

Item 19 Leave blank. Reserved for specialized use.

Item 20 Complete this item when billing for diagnostic tests subject to purchase price limitations. Enter the purchase price under charges if the "YES" block is checked. A "YES" check indicates that an entity other than the entity billing for the service performed the diagnostic test. A "NO" check indicates that "NO" purchased tests are included on the claim." When "YES" is annotated, item 32 must be completed. When billing for multiple purchased diagnostic tests, each test must be submitted on a separate claim form.

When billing for purchased services, the technical and professional components must be billed on separate lines of the claim (i.e., you may not bill globally for a purchased service).

Item 21 Enter the patient's diagnosis/condition. With the exception of claims submitted by ambulance suppliers (specialty type 59), all physician and nonphysician specialties (i.e., PA, NP, CNS, CRNA) use an ICD-9-CM code number and code to the highest level of specificity for the date of service. Enter up to four diagnoses in priority order. All narrative diagnoses for nonphysician specialties shall be submitted on an attachment.

Item 22 Leave blank. Not required by Medicare.

Item 23 Enter the Quality Improvement Organization (QIO) prior authorization number for those procedures requiring QIO prior approval.

Enter the Investigational Device Exemption (IDE) number when an investigational device is used in an FDA-approved clinical trial. Post Market Approval number should also be placed here when applicable.

FIGURE 7-2

Instructions for the CMS-1500 claim form. *Delmar/Cengage Learning* (*continues*)

For physicians performing care plan oversight services, enter the 6-digit Medicare provider number (or NPI) of the home health agency (HHA) or hospice when CPT code G0181 (HH) or G0182 (Hospice) is billed.

Enter the 10-digit Clinical Laboratory Improvement Act (CLIA) certification number for laboratory services billed by an entity performing CLIA covered procedures.

Item 23 can contain only one condition. Any additional conditions should be reported on a separate Form CMS-1500.

Item 24	The six service lines in section 24 have been divided horizontally to accommodate submission of both the NPI and legacy identifier during the NPI transition and to accommodate the submission of supplemental information to support the billed service. The top portion in each of the six service lines is shaded and is the location for reporting supplemental information. It is not intended to allow the billing of 12 service lines.
Item 24A	Enter a 6-digit or 8-digit (MMDDCCYY) date for each procedure, service, or supply. When "from" and "to" dates are shown for a series of identical services, enter the number of days or units in column G. This is a required field. Return as unprocessable if a date of service extends more than 1 day and a valid "to" date is not present.
Item 24B	Enter the appropriate place of service code(s) to identify the location for each item used or service performed. This is a required field. When a service is rendered to a hospital inpatient, use the "inpatient hospital" code.
Item 24C	Medicare providers are not required to complete this item.
Item 24D	Enter the procedures (CPT code), services, or supplies using the CMS Healthcare Common Procedure Coding System (HCPCS) code. When applicable, show HCPCS code modifiers with the HCPCS code. The CMS-1500 has the ability to capture up to four modifiers. Enter the specific procedure code without a narrative description. However, when reporting an "unlisted procedure code" or a "not otherwise classified" (NOC) code, include a narrative description in item 19 if a coherent description can be given within the confines of that box. Otherwise, an attachment shall be submitted with the claim. This is a required field. A claim shall be returned as unprocessable if an "unlisted procedure code" or an (NOC) code is indicated in item 24d, but an accompanying narrative is not present in item 19 or on an attachment.
Item 24E	Enter the diagnosis code reference number as shown in item 21 to relate the date of service and the procedures performed to the primary diagnosis. Enter only one reference number per line item. When multiple services are performed, enter the primary reference number for each service, either a 1, or a 2, or a 3, or a 4. This is a required field.
	If a situation arises where two or more diagnoses are required for a procedure code (e.g., pap smears), the provider shall reference only one of the diagnoses in item 21.
Item 24F	Enter the charge for each listed service.
Item 24G	Enter the number of days or units. This field is most commonly used for multiple visits, units of supplies, anesthesia minutes, or oxygen volume. If only one service is performed, the numeral 1 must be entered.
	Some services require that the actual number or quantity billed be clearly indicated on the claim form (e.g., multiple ostomy or urinary supplies, medication dosages, or allergy testing procedures). When multiple services are provided, enter the actual number provided.
	For anesthesia, show the elapsed time (minutes) in item 24g. Convert hours into minutes and enter the total minutes required for this procedure.
Item 24H	Leave blank. Not required by Medicare.
Item 24I	Effective May 23, 2008, the shaded portion of 24J is not to be reported.
Item 24J	Enter the rendering provider's NPI number in the lower unshaded portion. In the case of a service provided incident to the service of a physician or non-physician practitioner, when the person who ordered the service is not supervising, enter the NPI of the supervisor in the lower unshaded portion. This instruction does not apply to influenza virus and pneumococcal vaccine claims as they do not require a rendering provider NPI.
Item 25	Enter the provider of service or supplier Federal Tax ID (Employer Identification Number or Social Security Number) and check the appropriate check box. Medicare providers are not required to complete this item for crossover purposes since the Medicare contractor will retrieve the tax identification information from their internal provider file for inclusion on the COB outbound claim. However, tax identification information is used in the determination of accurate National Provider Identifier reimbursement. Reimbursement of claims submitted without tax identification information will/may be delayed.
Item 26	Enter the patient's account number assigned by the provider's of service or supplier's accounting system. This field is optional to assist the provider in patient identification. As a service, any account numbers entered here will be returned to the provider.
Item 27	Check the appropriate block to indicate whether the provider of service or supplier accepts assignment of Medicare benefits. If Medigap is indicated in item 9 and Medigap payment authorization is given in item 13, the provider of service or supplier shall also be a Medicare participating provider of service or supplier and accept assignment of Medicare benefits for all covered charges for all patients.

FIGURE 7-2

Instructions for the CMS-1500 claim form. *Delmar/Cengage Learning* (*continues*)

Item 28	Enter total charges for the services (i.e., total of all charges in item 24f).
Item 29	Enter the total amount the patient paid on the covered services only.
Item 30	Leave blank. Not required by Medicare.
Item 31	Enter the signature of provider of service or supplier, or his/her representative, and either the 6-digit date (MM | DD | YY), 8-digit date (MM | DD | CCYY), or alpha-numeric date (e.g., January 1, 1998) the form was signed.
	This is a required field, however the claim can be processed if a physician, supplier, or authorized person's signature is missing, but the signature is on file; or if any authorization is attached to the claim or if the signature field has "Signature on File" and/or a computer generated signature.
Item 32	Enter the name and address, and ZIP Code of the facility if the services were furnished in a hospital, clinic, laboratory, or facility other than the patient's home or physician's office. Only one name, address and ZIP Code may be entered in the block. If additional entries are needed, separate claim forms shall be submitted.
	Complete this item for all laboratory work performed outside a physician's office. If an independent laboratory is billing, enter the place where the test was performed.
Item 32a	If required by Medicare claims processing policy, enter the NPI of the service facility.
Item 32b	Effective May 23, 2008, Item 32b is not to be reported.
Item 33	Enter the provider of service/supplier's billing name, address, ZIP code, and telephone number. This is a required field.
Item 33a	Enter the NPI of the billing provider or group. This is a required field.
Item 33b	Effective May 23, 2008, Item 33b is not to be reported.

FIGURE 7-2

Instructions for the CMS-1500 claim form. *Delmar/Cengage Learning (continued)*

PREPARING CLAIMS FOR SUBMISSION

MOSS features a claim preparation window, as shown in Figure 7-3. This window allows the user to set criteria in order for the software to find and prepare claims ready to be submitted to insurance companies. Refer to the Claim Preparation window illustrated in Figure 7-3 as you review the function of each field for this window.

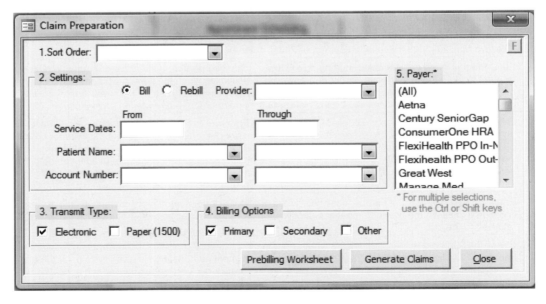

FIGURE 7-3

The Claim Preparation window in MOSS. *Delmar/Cengage Learning*

1. **Sort Order.** By using the drop-down box, claims can be sorted by patient's name, account number, or service dates.

2. **Settings.** The settings area consists of several components. By selecting "Bill," all claims being sent for the first time will be prepared. "Rebill" allows a specific claim for a patient to be re-sent to the carrier.

   In the "From" and "Through" fields, the user selects one service date, or a range of dates, pertaining to services that were rendered during that period. Individual or multiple patient names or account numbers are selected for billing.

3. **Transmit Type.** The method by which the claims will be billed and sent is selected here. By checking "Electronic," claims will be sent electronically to the insurance company or clearinghouse. By selecting "Paper (1500)," the claim will be produced on a CMS-1500 claim form and can be printed.

> **NOTE:** Whether "Electronic" or "Paper" is selected, the preview screen always displays the claims on a CMS-1500 first. This allows the user to review the information for errors or omissions. If errors are found, they should be corrected before proceeding with submission or printing the claims.

4. **Billing Options.** The user selects whether primary or secondary insurance plans are to be billed. "Other" is used to bill plans such as Workers Compensation or other third-party payers that are exclusive and separate from the patient's usual health plan. It is useful to note that patients who have coverage for specific services and diagnoses under Workers Compensation or No-Fault do not use their usual health plan to pay for these bills.

5. **Payer.** One or more of the insurance companies to be billed are selected in this area. If all insurance companies that meet the criteria in Fields 1 through 4 are to be billed, "All" is selected. Individual insurance companies can be selected by holding down the *Shift* or *Control* key while clicking on the plan names to be billed.

LET'S TRY IT! 7-1 PREPARING PAPER CLAIM FORMS FOR CONSUMERONE HRA

Objective: The reader selects ConsumerOne HRA patients of Drs. Heath and Schwartz and prints paper claim forms to be sent by mail to the insurance company.

STEP 1
Start MOSS by following your instructor's directions.

STEP 2
Click on the *Insurance Billing button* on the Main Menu.

STEP 3
Select the following settings:

NT: Drop down the box and ▸A. Sort by patient name (Field 1).
ect "Patient Name."

NT: Click in the radio but-
in front of "Bill," then drop ▸B. Bill for "All" providers (Field 2).
vn the box and select "All."

continues

PREPARING PAPER CLAIM FORMS FOR CONSUMERONE HRA *continued*

HINT: Drop down the box and make the selections.

C. Select service dates 10/01/2009 through 11/30/2009 by entering the dates in the "From" and "Through" fields.

D. Select "All" patient names and "All" patient accounts.

HINT: Click in the *box* in front of the selection "Paper."

E. Transmit type: Paper

HINT: Click in the *box* in front of "Primary."

F. Billing Options: Primary

G. Payer selection: Single click on *ConsumerOne HRA* so that only patients with that insurance plan are selected. Check your screen with Figure 7-4 before proceeding.

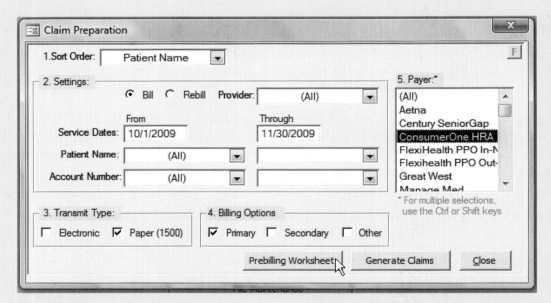

FIGURE 7-4

Delmar/Cengage Learning

STEP 4

Next, click the *Prebilling Worksheet button* to view a report of the claims that have been prepared for those dates and health plan. See Figure 7-5 to check your work. Be certain that if you see any errors, close the billing windows, and return to the patient account to make corrections where needed.

HINT: Top left corner.

STEP 5

Next, click on the *Print icon* so that you and your instructor may have a copy of the Insurance Prebilling Worksheet. See Figure 7-6. When done, close the window for the worksheet. This will return you to the Claim Preparation window.

HINT: Be careful not to close down MOSS.

INSURANCE PREBILLING WORKSHEET
Student1

Dates of Service	Diag Code	Proc Code	POS	Units	Dr	As	Bill Amt	Receipts	Net
ConsumerOne HRA									
Conway, John									
10/23/2009	789.00	85031	11	1.00	D1	Y	$11.00	$0.00	$11.00
10/23/2009	789.00	99214	12	1.00	D1	Y	$180.00	$0.00	$180.00
					Totals		$191.00	$0.00	$191.00
Goodnow, Leona									
10/25/2009	493.92	99282	23	1.00	D2	Y	$147.00	$0.00	$147.00
					Totals		$147.00	$0.00	$147.00
Gordon, Eric									
11/5/2009	530.81	99213	12	1.00	D2	Y	$111.00	$0.00	$111.00
					Totals		$111.00	$0.00	$111.00
Pradhan, Kabin									
11/3/2009	530.81	99201	11	1.00	D2	Y	$130.00	$0.00	$130.00
					Totals		$130.00	$0.00	$130.00
	TOTAL TO BE BILLED FOR ConsumerOne HRA							$579.00	
Grand Total			**Grand Total**					$579.00	

FIGURE 7-5

Delmar/Cengage Learning

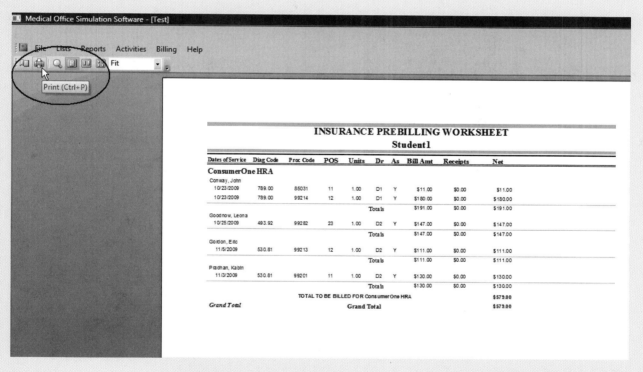

FIGURE 7-6

Delmar/Cengage Learning

STEP 6

The claim forms are now ready to be generated. Click on the *Claims Generation button.* You will have four CMS-1500 claim forms, one for each of the patients who appeared on the Insurance Billing Worksheet. View each patient's claim form by clicking on the *Record bar* at the lower left, as shown in Figure 7-7.

continues

PREPARING PAPER CLAIM FORMS FOR CONSUMERONE HRA *continued*

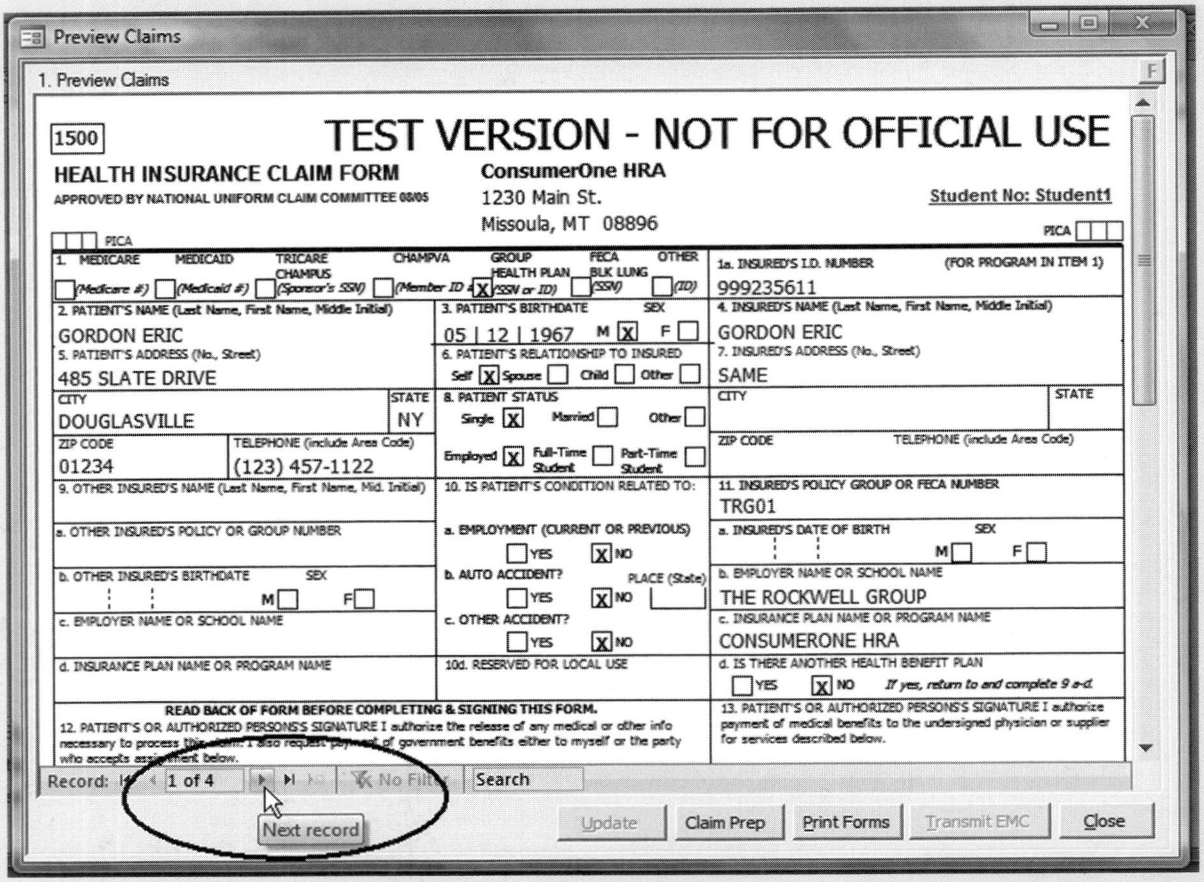

FIGURE 7-7

Delmar/Cengage Learning

STEP 7

Next, click on the *Print Forms button* to send the four forms to the printer, as shown in Figure 7-8. Check your claim forms with those in Figure 7-9 through Figure 7-12. In an actual office, these claim forms would be mailed to the insurance company to the address shown at the top of each form. Hand in the claim forms to your instructor.

STEP 8

Return to the Main Menu in MOSS.

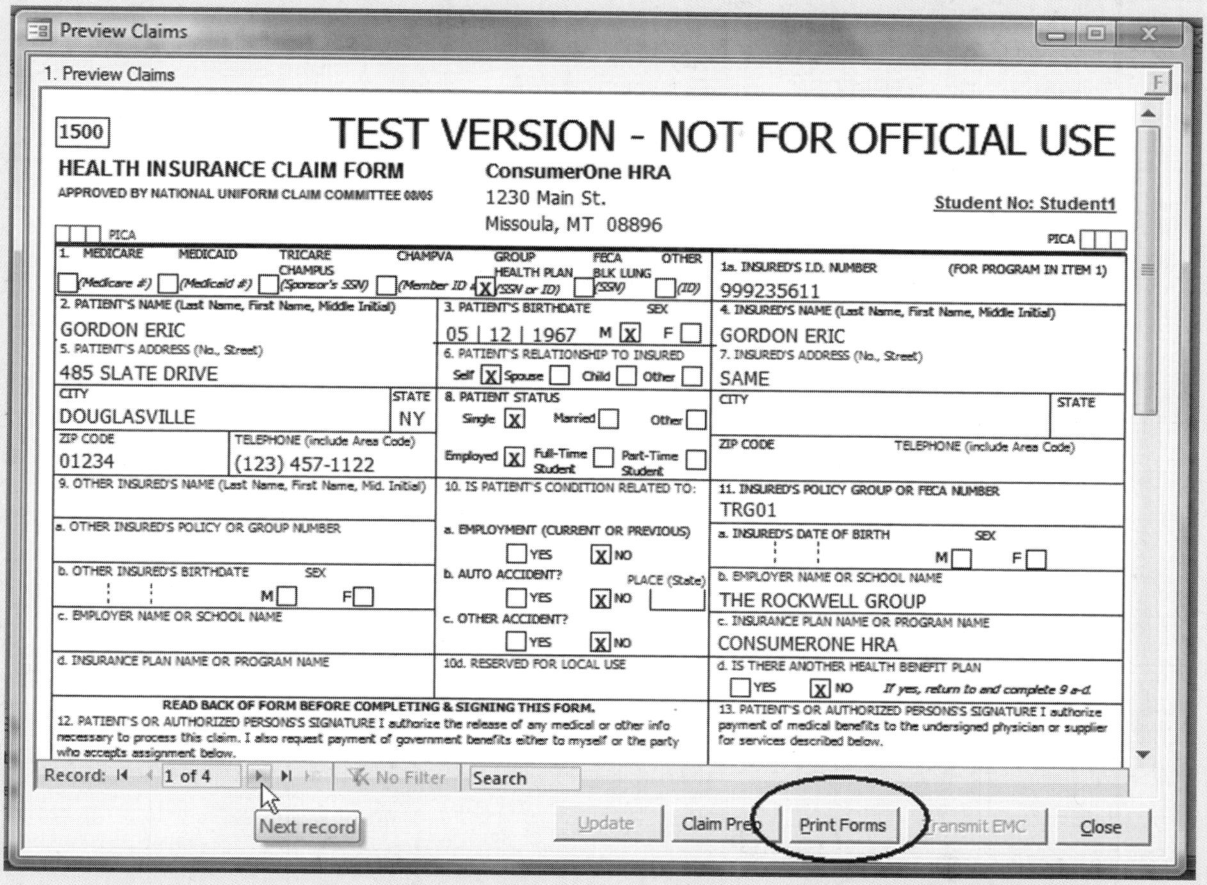

FIGURE 7-8

Delmar/Cengage Learning

continues

TEST VERSION - NOT FOR OFFICIAL USE

1500	**HEALTH INSURANCE CLAIM FORM**	**ConsumerOne HRA**

HEALTH INSURANCE CLAIM FORM
APPROVED BY NATIONAL UNIFORM CLAIM COMMITTEE 08/05

ConsumerOne HRA
1230 Main St.
Missoula, MT 08896

Student No: Student1

☐☐☐ PICA   PICA ☐☐☐

1. MEDICARE MEDICAID TRICARE CHAMPUS CHAMPVA GROUP HEALTH PLAN FECA BLK LUNG OTHER
☐(Medicare #) ☐(Medicaid #) ☐(Sponsor's SSN) ☐(Member ID) ☒(SSN or ID) ☐(SSN) ☐(ID)

1a. INSURED'S I.D. NUMBER (FOR PROGRAM IN ITEM 1)
999235611

2. PATIENT'S NAME (Last Name, First Name, Middle Initial)
GORDON ERIC

3. PATIENT'S BIRTHDATE SEX
05 | 12 | 1967 M ☒ F ☐

4. INSURED'S NAME (Last Name, First Name, Middle Initial)
GORDON ERIC

5. PATIENT'S ADDRESS (No., Street)
485 SLATE DRIVE

6. PATIENT'S RELATIONSHIP TO INSURED
Self ☒ Spouse ☐ Child ☐ Other ☐

7. INSURED'S ADDRESS (No., Street)
SAME

CITY **DOUGLASVILLE** STATE **NY**

8. PATIENT STATUS
Single ☒ Married ☐ Other ☐

CITY STATE

ZIP CODE **01234** TELEPHONE (include Area Code) **(123) 457-1122**

Employed ☒ Full-Time Student ☐ Part-Time Student ☐

ZIP CODE TELEPHONE (include Area Code)

9. OTHER INSURED'S NAME (Last Name, First Name, Mid. Initial)

10. IS PATIENT'S CONDITION RELATED TO:

11. INSURED'S POLICY GROUP OR FECA NUMBER
TRG01

a. OTHER INSURED'S POLICY OR GROUP NUMBER

a. EMPLOYMENT (CURRENT OR PREVIOUS)
☐YES ☒NO

a. INSURED'S DATE OF BIRTH SEX
M ☐ F ☐

b. OTHER INSURED'S BIRTHDATE SEX
M ☐ F ☐

b. AUTO ACCIDENT? PLACE (State)
☐YES ☒NO

b. EMPLOYER NAME OR SCHOOL NAME
THE ROCKWELL GROUP

c. EMPLOYER NAME OR SCHOOL NAME

c. OTHER ACCIDENT?
☐YES ☒NO

c. INSURANCE PLAN NAME OR PROGRAM NAME
CONSUMERONE HRA

d. INSURANCE PLAN NAME OR PROGRAM NAME

10d. RESERVED FOR LOCAL USE

d. IS THERE ANOTHER HEALTH BENEFIT PLAN
☐YES ☒NO *If yes, return to and complete 9 a-d.*

READ BACK OF FORM BEFORE COMPLETING & SIGNING THIS FORM.

12. PATIENT'S OR AUTHORIZED PERSONS'S SIGNATURE I authorize the release of any medical or other info necessary to process this claim. I also request payment of government benefits either to myself or the party who accepts assignment below.

SIGNED _____ SIGNATURE ON FILE _____ DATE _____ 11052009 _____

13. PATIENT'S OR AUTHORIZED PERSONS'S SIGNATURE I authorize payment of medical benefits to the undersigned physician or supplier for services described below.

SIGNED _____ SIGNATURE ON FILE _____

14. DATE OF CURRENT: ◀ ILLNESS (First symptom) OR INJURY (Accident) OR PREGRANCY (LMP)

15. IF PATIENT HAS HAD SAME ILLNESS, GIVE FIRST DATE

16. DATES PATIENT UNABLE TO WORK IN CURRENT OCCUPATION
FROM _____ TO _____

17. NAME OF REFERRING PROVIDER OR OTHER SOURCE
17a
17b NPI

18. HOSPITALIZATION DATES RELATED TO CURRENT SERVICES
FROM _____ TO _____

19. RESERVED FOR LOCAL USE

20. OUTSIDE LAB? ☐YES ☒NO $ CHARGES

21. DIAGNOSIS OR NATURE OF ILLNESS OR INJURY (RELATE ITEMS 1, 2, 3 OR 4 TO ITEM 24E BY LINE)
1. **530.81**
2. |
3. |
4. |

22. MEDICAID SUBMISSION CODE ORIGINAL REF. NO.

23. PRIOR AUTHORIZATION NUMBER

24. A DATE(S) OF SERVICE From MM DD YY	To MM DD YY	B. Place of Service	C. EMG	D. PROCEDURES, SERVICES OR SUPPLIES (Explain Unusual Circumstances) CPT/HCPCS	MODIFIER	E. DIAGNOSIS POINTER	F. $ CHARGES	G. DAYS OR UNITS	H. EPSDT Family Plan	I. ID. QUAL	J. RENDERING PROVIDER ID#
1	11 05 2009		11		99213		1	111 00	1		NPI	999502
2											NPI	
3											NPI	
4											NPI	
5											NPI	
6											NPI	

25. FEDERAL TAX I.D. NUMBER SSN EIN
00-1234560 ☐ ☒

26. PATIENT'S ACCOUNT NO
GOR003

27. ACCEPT ASSIGNMENT?
☒YES ☐NO

28. TOTAL CHARGE $ **111 00**

29. AMOUNT PAID $

30. BALANCE DUE $

31. SIGNATURE OF PHYSICIAN OR SUPPLIER INCLUDING DEGREES OR CREDENTIALS (I certify that the statements on the reverse apply to this bill and are made a part thereof.)
11052009
SIGNED **D.J. SCHWARTZ, MD** DAT

32. SERVICE FACILITY LOCATION INFORMATION
DOUGLASVILLE MEDICINE ASSOCIATES
5076 BRAND BLVD., SUITE 401
DOUGLASVILLE, NY 01234
a. **9995020212** b.

33. BILLING PROVIDER INFO PH # **(123) 456-7892**
DOUGLASVILLE MEDICINE ASSOCIATES
5076 BRAND BLVD., SUITE 401
DOUGLASVILLE, NY 01234
a. **9995020212** b.

NUCC Instruction Manual available at: www.nucc.org

OMB APPROVAL PENDING

FIGURE 7-9

Courtesy of the Centers for Medicare & Medicaid Services

TEST VERSION - NOT FOR OFFICIAL USE

HEALTH INSURANCE CLAIM FORM

ConsumerOne HRA

APPROVED BY NATIONAL UNIFORM CLAIM COMMITTEE 08/05

1230 Main St.
Missoula, MT 08896

Student No: Student1

| | PICA | | | PICA | | |

1. MEDICARE MEDICAID TRICARE CHAMPUS CHAMPVA GROUP HEALTH PLAN FECA BLK LUNG OTHER	1a. INSURED'S I.D. NUMBER (FOR PROGRAM IN ITEM 1)
☐(Medicare #) ☐(Medicaid #) ☐(Sponsor's SSN) ☐(Member ID) ☒(SSN or ID) ☐(SSN) ☐(ID)	999385562

2. PATIENT'S NAME (Last Name, First Name, Middle Initial)	3. PATIENT'S BIRTHDATE SEX	4. INSURED'S NAME (Last Name, First Name, Middle Initial)
CONWAY JOHN W	06 | 30 | 1969 M ☒ F ☐	CONWAY JOHN W

5. PATIENT'S ADDRESS (No., Street)	6. PATIENT'S RELATIONSHIP TO INSURED	7. INSURED'S ADDRESS (No., Street)
803 SLATE DRIVE	Self ☒ Spouse ☐ Child ☐ Other ☐	SAME

CITY DOUGLASVILLE	STATE NY	8. PATIENT STATUS Single ☐ Married ☒ Other ☐	CITY	STATE

ZIP CODE 01234	TELEPHONE (include Area Code) (123) 457-8123	Employed ☒ Full-Time Student ☐ Part-Time Student ☐	ZIP CODE	TELEPHONE (include Area Code)

9. OTHER INSURED'S NAME (Last Name, First Name, Mid. Initial)	10. IS PATIENT'S CONDITION RELATED TO:	11. INSURED'S POLICY GROUP OR FECA NUMBER MIS015

a. OTHER INSURED'S POLICY OR GROUP NUMBER	a. EMPLOYMENT (CURRENT OR PREVIOUS) ☐YES ☒NO	a. INSURED'S DATE OF BIRTH SEX M ☐ F ☐

b. OTHER INSURED'S BIRTHDATE SEX M ☐ F ☐	b. AUTO ACCIDENT? ☐YES ☒NO PLACE (State)	b. EMPLOYER NAME OR SCHOOL NAME MIDWAY INVESTMENTS

c. EMPLOYER NAME OR SCHOOL NAME	c. OTHER ACCIDENT? ☐YES ☒NO	c. INSURANCE PLAN NAME OR PROGRAM NAME CONSUMERONE HRA

d. INSURANCE PLAN NAME OR PROGRAM NAME	10d. RESERVED FOR LOCAL USE	d. IS THERE ANOTHER HEALTH BENEFIT PLAN ☐ YES ☒ NO If yes, return to and complete 9 a-d.

READ BACK OF FORM BEFORE COMPLETING & SIGNING THIS FORM.

12. PATIENT'S OR AUTHORIZED PERSONS'S SIGNATURE I authorize the release of any medical or other info necessary to process this claim. I also request payment of government benefits either to myself or the party who accepts assignment below.

SIGNED _____ SIGNATURE ON FILE _____ DATE _____ 10232009 _____

13. PATIENT'S OR AUTHORIZED PERSONS'S SIGNATURE I authorize payment of medical benefits to the undersigned physician or supplier for services described below.

SIGNED _____ SIGNATURE ON FILE _____

14. DATE OF CURRENT: ◄ ILLNESS (First symptom) OR INJURY (Accident) OR PREGNANCY (LMP)	15. IF PATIENT HAS HAD SAME ILLNESS, GIVE FIRST DATE	16. DATES PATIENT UNABLE TO WORK IN CURRENT OCCUPATION FROM _____ TO _____

17. NAME OF REFERRING PROVIDER OR OTHER SOURCE	17a 17b NPI	18. HOSPITALIZATION DATES RELATED TO CURRENT SERVICES FROM _____ TO _____

19. RESERVED FOR LOCAL USE	20. OUTSIDE LAB? ☐ YES ☒ NO $ CHARGES

21. DIAGNOSIS OR NATURE OF ILLNESS OR INJURY (RELATE ITEMS 1, 2, 3 OR 4 TO ITEM 24E BY LINE)	22. MEDICAID SUBMISSION CODE ORIGINAL REF. NO.
1. | 789.00 3. | 2. | 780.6 4. |	23. PRIOR AUTHORIZATION NUMBER

24. A DATE(S) OF SERVICE From / To MM DD YY / MM DD YY	B. Place of Service	C. EMG	D. PROCEDURES, SERVICES OR SUPPLIES (Explain Unusual Circumstances) CPT/HCPCS MODIFIER	E. DIAGNOSIS POINTER	F. $ CHARGES	G. DAYS OR UNITS	H. EPSDT Family Plan	I. ID. QUAL	J. RENDERING PROVIDER ID#
1	10 23 2009	11		99214		1 2	180 00	1		NPI	999501
2	10 23 2009	11		85031		2	11 00	1		NPI	999501
3										NPI	
4										NPI	
5										NPI	
6										NPI	

25. FEDERAL TAX I.D. NUMBER 00-1234560	SSN EIN ☐ ☒	26. PATIENT'S ACCOUNT NO CON001	27. ACCEPT ASSIGNMENT? ☒ YES ☐ NO	28. TOTAL CHARGE $ 191 00	29. AMOUNT PAID $	30. BALANCE DUE $

31. SIGNATURE OF PHYSICIAN OR SUPPLIER INCLUDING DEGREES OR CREDENTIALS (I certify that the statements on the reverse apply to this bill and are made a part thereof.) 10232009 SIGNED L. D. HEATH, MD DAT	32. SERVICE FACILITY LOCATION INFORMATION DOUGLASVILLE MEDICINE ASSOCIATES 5076 BRAND BLVD., SUITE 401 DOUGLASVILLE, NY 01234 a. 9995010111 b.	33. BILLING PROVIDER INFO PH # (123) 456-7890 DOUGLASVILLE MEDICINE ASSOCIATES 5076 BRAND BLVD., SUITE 401 DOUGLASVILLE, NY 01234 a. 9995010111 b.

NUCC Instruction Manual available at: www.nucc.org

OMB APPROVAL PENDING

FIGURE 7-10

Courtesy of the Centers for Medicare & Medicaid Services

continues

PREPARING PAPER CLAIM FORMS FOR CONSUMERONE HRA *continued*

TEST VERSION - NOT FOR OFFICIAL USE

1500	

HEALTH INSURANCE CLAIM FORM
APPROVED BY NATIONAL UNIFORM CLAIM COMMITTEE 08/05

ConsumerOne HRA
1230 Main St.
Missoula, MT 08896

Student No: Student1

□□□ PICA   PICA □□□

1. MEDICARE	MEDICAID	TRICARE CHAMPUS	CHAMPVA	GROUP HEALTH PLAN	FECA BLK LUNG	OTHER	1a. INSURED'S I.D. NUMBER (FOR PROGRAM IN ITEM 1)
☐ (Medicare #)	☐ (Medicaid #)	☐ (Sponsor's SSN)	☐ (Member ID)	☒ (SSN or ID)	☐ (SSN)	☐ (ID)	999569844

2. PATIENT'S NAME (Last Name, First Name, Middle Initial)	3. PATIENT'S BIRTHDATE SEX	4. INSURED'S NAME (Last Name, First Name, Middle Initial)
PRADHAN KABIN	12	02	1951 M ☒ F ☐	PRADHAN KABIN

5. PATIENT'S ADDRESS (No., Street)	6. PATIENT'S RELATIONSHIP TO INSURED	7. INSURED'S ADDRESS (No., Street)
2213 BOULDER COURT	Self ☒ Spouse ☐ Child ☐ Other ☐	SAME

CITY	STATE	8. PATIENT STATUS	CITY	STATE
DOUGLASVILLE	NY	Single ☒ Married ☐ Other ☐		

ZIP CODE	TELEPHONE (include Area Code)		ZIP CODE	TELEPHONE (include Area Code)
01234	(123) 528-9772	Employed ☒ Full-Time Student ☐ Part-Time Student ☐		

9. OTHER INSURED'S NAME (Last Name, First Name, Mid. Initial)	10. IS PATIENT'S CONDITION RELATED TO:	11. INSURED'S POLICY GROUP OR FECA NUMBER
		ACM0211

a. OTHER INSURED'S POLICY OR GROUP NUMBER	a. EMPLOYMENT (CURRENT OR PREVIOUS) ☐ YES ☒ NO	a. INSURED'S DATE OF BIRTH SEX M ☐ F ☐

b. OTHER INSURED'S BIRTHDATE SEX M ☐ F ☐	b. AUTO ACCIDENT? PLACE (State) ☐ YES ☒ NO	b. EMPLOYER NAME OR SCHOOL NAME ALLCITY MORTGAGE CO

c. EMPLOYER NAME OR SCHOOL NAME	c. OTHER ACCIDENT? ☐ YES ☒ NO	c. INSURANCE PLAN NAME OR PROGRAM NAME CONSUMERONE HRA

d. INSURANCE PLAN NAME OR PROGRAM NAME	10d. RESERVED FOR LOCAL USE	d. IS THERE ANOTHER HEALTH BENEFIT PLAN ☐ YES ☒ NO If yes, return to and complete 9 a-d.

READ BACK OF FORM BEFORE COMPLETING & SIGNING THIS FORM.

12. PATIENT'S OR AUTHORIZED PERSONS'S SIGNATURE I authorize the release of any medical or other info necessary to process this claim. I also request payment of government benefits either to myself or the party who accepts assignment below.

SIGNED _____SIGNATURE ON FILE_____ DATE _11032009_

13. PATIENT'S OR AUTHORIZED PERSONS'S SIGNATURE I authorize payment of medical benefits to the undersigned physician or supplier for services described below.

SIGNED _____SIGNATURE ON FILE_____

14. DATE OF CURRENT: ◄ ILLNESS (First symptom) OR INJURY (Accident) OR PREGNANCY (LMP)	15. IF PATIENT HAS HAD SAME ILLNESS, GIVE FIRST DATE	16. DATES PATIENT UNABLE TO WORK IN CURRENT OCCUPATION FROM TO

17. NAME OF REFERRING PROVIDER OR OTHER SOURCE	17a	18. HOSPITALIZATION DATES RELATED TO CURRENT SERVICES
	17b NPI	FROM TO

19. RESERVED FOR LOCAL USE	20. OUTSIDE LAB? $ CHARGES ☐ YES ☒ NO

21. DIAGNOSIS OR NATURE OF ILLNESS OR INJURY (RELATE ITEMS 1, 2, 3 OR 4 TO ITEM 24E BY LINE)

1. | 530.81   3. |_____
2. |_____   4. |_____

22. MEDICAID SUBMISSION CODE   ORIGINAL REF. NO.
23. PRIOR AUTHORIZATION NUMBER

24. A DATE(S) OF SERVICE From / To MM DD YY MM DD YY	B. Place of Service	C. EMG	D. PROCEDURES, SERVICES OR SUPPLIES (Explain Unusual Circumstances) CPT/HCPCS MODIFIER	E. DIAGNOSIS POINTER	F. $ CHARGES	G. DAYS OR UNITS	H. EPSDT Family Plan	I. ID. QUAL	J. RENDERING PROVIDER ID#
1	11 03 2009	11		99201		1	130 00	1		NPI	999502
2									NPI	
3									NPI	
4									NPI	
5									NPI	
6									NPI	

25. FEDERAL TAX I.D. NUMBER SSN EIN	26. PATIENT'S ACCOUNT NO	27. ACCEPT ASSIGNMENT?	28. TOTAL CHARGE	29. AMOUNT PAID	30. BALANCE DUE
00-1234560 ☐ ☒	PRA003	☒ YES ☐ NO	$ 130 00	$	$

31. SIGNATURE OF PHYSICIAN OR SUPPLIER INCLUDING DEGREES OR CREDENTIALS (I certify that the statements on the reverse apply to this bill and are made a part thereof.) 11032009 SIGNED D.J. SCHWARTZ, MD DAT	32. SERVICE FACILITY LOCATION INFORMATION DOUGLASVILLE MEDICINE ASSOCIATES 5076 BRAND BLVD., SUITE 401 DOUGLASVILLE, NY 01234 a. 9995020212 b.	33. BILLING PROVIDER INFO PH # (123) 456-7892 DOUGLASVILLE MEDICINE ASSOCIATES 5076 BRAND BLVD., SUITE 401 DOUGLASVILLE, NY 01234 a. 9995020212 b.

NUCC Instruction Manual available at: www.nucc.org   OMB APPROVAL PENDING

FIGURE 7-11

Courtesy of the Centers for Medicare & Medicaid Services

| 1500 | | TEST VERSION - NOT FOR OFFICIAL USE |

HEALTH INSURANCE CLAIM FORM
APPROVED BY NATIONAL UNIFORM CLAIM COMMITTEE 08/05

ConsumerOne HRA
1230 Main St.
Missoula, MT 08896

Student No: Student1

PICA

1. MEDICARE MEDICAID TRICARE CHAMPUS CHAMPVA GROUP HEALTH PLAN FECA BLK LUNG OTHER
(Medicare #) (Medicaid #) (Sponsor's SSN) (Member ID) [X](SSN or ID) (SSN) (ID)

1a. INSURED'S I.D. NUMBER (FOR PROGRAM IN ITEM 1)
99915118902

2. PATIENT'S NAME (Last Name, First Name, Middle Initial)
GOODNOW LEONA M

3. PATIENT'S BIRTHDATE 07 | 31 | 1979 SEX M [ ] F [X]

4. INSURED'S NAME (Last Name, First Name, Middle Initial)
GOODNOW THOMAS L

5. PATIENT'S ADDRESS (No., Street)
321 WHITE STONE DRIVE

6. PATIENT'S RELATIONSHIP TO INSURED
Self [ ] Spouse [X] Child [ ] Other [ ]

7. INSURED'S ADDRESS (No., Street)
321 WHITE STONE DRIVE

CITY DOUGLASVILLE STATE NY

8. PATIENT STATUS
Single [ ] Married [X] Other [ ]
Employed [ ] Full-Time Student [ ] Part-Time Student [ ]

CITY DOUGLASVILLE STATE NY

ZIP CODE 01234 TELEPHONE (123) 457-1113

ZIP CODE 01234 TELEPHONE (123) 457-1113

9. OTHER INSURED'S NAME (Last Name, First Name, Mid. Initial)

10. IS PATIENT'S CONDITION RELATED TO:

11. INSURED'S POLICY GROUP OR FECA NUMBER
TRG01

a. OTHER INSURED'S POLICY OR GROUP NUMBER

a. EMPLOYMENT (CURRENT OR PREVIOUS) [ ]YES [X]NO

a. INSURED'S DATE OF BIRTH SEX M [X] F [ ]

b. OTHER INSURED'S BIRTHDATE SEX M[ ] F[ ]

b. AUTO ACCIDENT? [ ]YES [X]NO PLACE (State)

b. EMPLOYER NAME OR SCHOOL NAME
THE ROCKWELL GROUP

c. EMPLOYER NAME OR SCHOOL NAME

c. OTHER ACCIDENT? [ ]YES [X]NO

c. INSURANCE PLAN NAME OR PROGRAM NAME
CONSUMERONE HRA

d. INSURANCE PLAN NAME OR PROGRAM NAME

10d. RESERVED FOR LOCAL USE

d. IS THERE ANOTHER HEALTH BENEFIT PLAN
[ ]YES [X]NO If yes, return to and complete 9 a-d.

READ BACK OF FORM BEFORE COMPLETING & SIGNING THIS FORM.
12. PATIENT'S OR AUTHORIZED PERSON'S SIGNATURE ...
SIGNED _____ DATE 10252009

13. PATIENT'S OR AUTHORIZED PERSON'S SIGNATURE ...
SIGNED SIGNATURE ON FILE

14. DATE OF CURRENT: ILLNESS/INJURY/PREGNANCY (LMP)

15. IF PATIENT HAS HAD SAME ILLNESS, GIVE FIRST DATE

16. DATES PATIENT UNABLE TO WORK FROM TO

17. NAME OF REFERRING PROVIDER OR OTHER SOURCE
17a / 17b NPI

18. HOSPITALIZATION DATES FROM TO

19. RESERVED FOR LOCAL USE

20. OUTSIDE LAB? [ ]YES [X]NO $ CHARGES

21. DIAGNOSIS OR NATURE OF ILLNESS OR INJURY
1. 493.92   3.
2.   4.

22. MEDICAID SUBMISSION CODE ORIGINAL REF. NO.

23. PRIOR AUTHORIZATION NUMBER

24. A DATE(S) OF SERVICE From MM DD YY / To MM DD YY	B. Place	C. EMG	D. CPT/HCPCS MODIFIER	E. DIAG PTR	F. $ CHARGES	G. UNITS	H.	I. QUAL	J. RENDERING PROVIDER ID#
1	10 25 2009	23		99282	1	147 00	1		NPI	999502
2									NPI	
3									NPI	
4									NPI	
5									NPI	
6									NPI	

25. FEDERAL TAX I.D. NUMBER 00-1234560 SSN[ ] EIN[X]

26. PATIENT'S ACCOUNT NO. GOO001

27. ACCEPT ASSIGNMENT? [X]YES [ ]NO

28. TOTAL CHARGE $ 147 00

29. AMOUNT PAID $

30. BALANCE DUE $

31. SIGNATURE OF PHYSICIAN OR SUPPLIER
SIGNED D.J. SCHWARTZ, MD DATE 10252009

32. SERVICE FACILITY LOCATION INFORMATION
COMMUNITY GENERAL HOSPITAL
4000 BRAND BLVD.
DOUGLASVILLE, NY 01234
a. 9997794511 b.

33. BILLING PROVIDER INFO PH # (123) 456-7892
DOUGLASVILLE MEDICINE ASSOCIATES
5076 BRAND BLVD., SUITE 401
DOUGLASVILLE, NY 01234
a. 9995020212 b.

NUCC Instruction Manual available at: www.nucc.org OMB APPROVAL PENDING

FIGURE 7-12
Courtesy of the Centers for Medicare & Medicaid Services

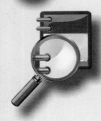

LET'S TRY IT! 7-2 SENDING MEDICARE CLAIMS ELECTRONICALLY

Objective: The reader selects Medicare patients of Drs. Heath and Schwartz and submits claims electronically.

STEP 1
Start MOSS by following your instructor's directions.

STEP 2
Click on the *Insurance Billing button* on the Main Menu.

STEP 3
Select the following settings:

    A.   Sort by patient name (Field 1).

    B.   Bill for "All" providers (Field 2).

    C.   Select service dates 10/01/2009 through 11/30/2009 by entering the dates in the "From" and "Through" fields.

    D.   Select "All" patient names and "All" patient accounts.

    E.   Transmit type: Electronic

    F.   Billing Options: Primary

HINT: Remember, the fiscal intermediary for Medicare is Statewide Corporation.

    G.   Payer selection: Single click on *Medicare Statewide* so that only patients with that insurance plan are selected.

Check your screen with Figure 7-13 before proceeding.

STEP 4
Next, click the *Prebilling Worksheet button* to view the two-page report of the claims that have been prepared for those dates and health plan. See Figure 7-14 and Figure 7-15 to check your work. Be certain that if you see any errors, close the billing windows, and return to the patient account to make corrections where needed.

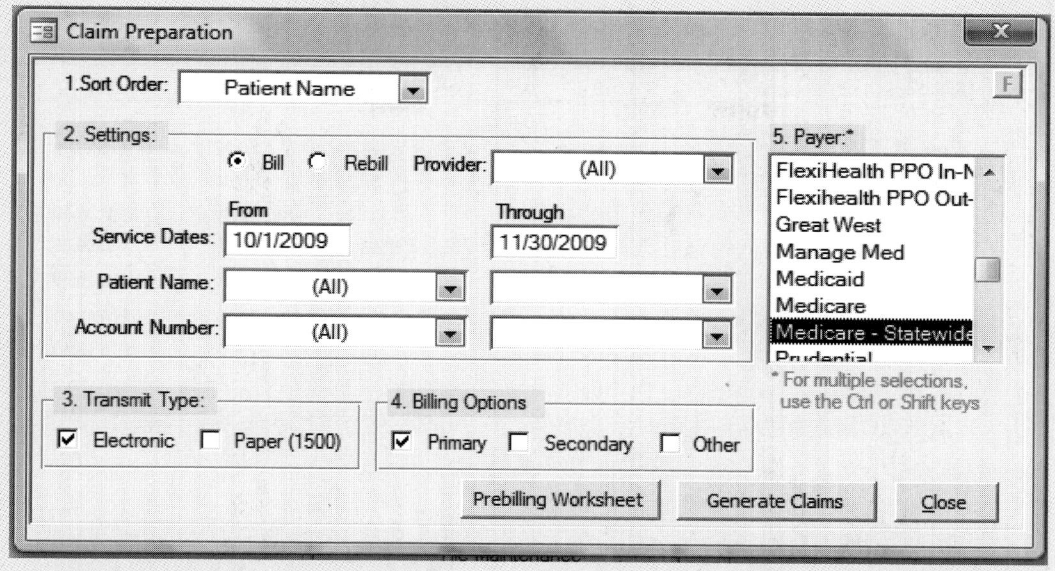

FIGURE 7-13

Delmar/Cengage Learning

INSURANCE PREBILLING WORKSHEET
Student1

Dates of Service	Diag Code	Proc Code	POS	Units	Dr	As	Bill Amt	Receipts	Net
Medicare - Statewide Corp.									
Adams, Minnie									
10/28/2009	438.9	36415	11	1.00	D1	Y	$18.00	$0.00	$18.00
10/28/2009	438.9	80053	11	1.00	D1	Y	$47.00	$0.00	$47.00
10/28/2009	438.9	99203	11	1.00	D1	Y	$200.00	$0.00	$200.00
					Totals		$265.00	$0.00	$265.00
Blanc, Francois									
11/24/2009	401.9	99307	32	1.00	D1	Y	$68.00	$0.00	$68.00
					Totals		$68.00	$0.00	$68.00
Chang, Xao									
10/16/2009	250.00	99307	31	1.00	D1	Y	$60.00	$0.00	$60.00
11/24/2009	780.39	99307	31	1.00	D1	Y	$68.00	$0.00	$68.00
					Totals		$128.00	$0.00	$128.00
Munoz, Geraldo									
11/6/2009	427.31	99221	21	1.00	D1	Y	$145.00	$0.00	$145.00
11/7/2009	427.31	99231	21	2.00	D1	Y	$158.00	$0.00	$158.00
11/9/2009	427.31	99238	21	1.00	D1	Y	$145.00	$0.00	$145.00
					Totals		$448.00	$0.00	$448.00
Pinkston, Anna									
11/24/2009	443.9	99308	31	1.00	D1	Y	$113.00	$0.00	$113.00
					Totals		$113.00	$0.00	$113.00
Shektar, Paula									
10/23/2009	428.0	99214	11	1.00	D2	N	$180.00	$0.00	$180.00
					Totals		$180.00	$0.00	$180.00

FIGURE 7-14

Delmar/Cengage Learning

continues

SENDING MEDICARE CLAIMS ELECTRONICALLY *continued*

Dates of Service	Diag Code	Proc Code	POS	Units	Dr	As	Bill Amt	Receipts	Net
Tomanaga, Marie									
11/3/2009	413.9	36415	11	1.00	D2	Y	$18.00	$0.00	$18.00
11/3/2009	413.9	85651	11	1.00	D2	Y	$9.00	$0.00	$9.00
11/3/2009	413.9	93000	11	1.00	D2	Y	$131.00	$0.00	$131.00
11/3/2009	413.9	99205	11	1.00	D2	Y	$358.00	$0.00	$358.00
						Totals	$516.00	$0.00	$516.00
			TOTAL TO BE BILLED FOR Medicare - Statewide Corp.						$1,718.00
Grand Total			*Grand Total*						$1,718.00

FIGURE 7-15

Delmar/Cengage Learning

STEP 5

Next, click on the *Print icon* so that you and your instructor may have a copy of the Insurance Prebilling Worksheet. When done, close the window for the worksheet. This will return you to the Claim Preparation window.

> **HINT:** Be careful not to close down MOSS.

STEP 6

The claim forms are now ready to be generated. Click on the *Generate Claims button*. Once the CMS-1500 claim forms are displayed, scroll to the bottom half of each patient's claim and check the dates, procedures, and fees being charged with the information on the Insurance Prebilling Worksheet you printed in Step 5. (Patient Chang will have two forms, one for DOS 10/16/2009 and the other for DOS 11/24/2009.) View each patient's claim form by clicking on the *Record bar* at the lower left. Check your claim forms with those in Figure 7-16 through Figure 7-23. If any errors are found, click on the *Claim Prep button* and then close any open windows and return to the areas of MOSS where corrections are required.

TEST VERSION - NOT FOR OFFICIAL USE

1500

HEALTH INSURANCE CLAIM FORM
APPROVED BY NATIONAL UNIFORM CLAIM COMMITTEE 08/05

Medicare - Statewide Corp.

200 Tech Center
Queens City, NY 01135

Student No: Student1

☐☐☐ PICA	PICA ☐☐☐

1. MEDICARE [X] (Medicare #) **MEDICAID** ☐ (Medicaid #) **TRICARE CHAMPUS** ☐ (Sponsor's SSN) **CHAMPVA** ☐ (Member ID) **GROUP HEALTH PLAN** ☐ (SSN or ID) **FECA BLK LUNG** ☐ (SSN) **OTHER** ☐ (ID)

1a. INSURED'S I.D. NUMBER (FOR PROGRAM IN ITEM 1)
999135611A

2. PATIENT'S NAME (Last Name, First Name, Middle Initial)
BLANC FRANCOIS

3. PATIENT'S BIRTHDATE 12 | 25 | 1917   **SEX** M [X] F ☐

4. INSURED'S NAME (Last Name, First Name, Middle Initial)

5. PATIENT'S ADDRESS (No., Street)
890 MILLENNIUM WAY

6. PATIENT'S RELATIONSHIP TO INSURED Self [X] Spouse ☐ Child ☐ Other ☐

7. INSURED'S ADDRESS (No., Street)

CITY DOUGLASVILLE   **STATE** NY

8. PATIENT STATUS Single [X] Married ☐ Other ☐

CITY   **STATE**

ZIP CODE 01234   **TELEPHONE** (include Area Code) (123) 528-0012

Employed ☐ Full-Time Student ☐ Part-Time Student ☐

ZIP CODE   **TELEPHONE** (include Area Code)

9. OTHER INSURED'S NAME (Last Name, First Name, Mid. Initial)

10. IS PATIENT'S CONDITION RELATED TO:

11. INSURED'S POLICY GROUP OR FECA NUMBER
NONE

a. OTHER INSURED'S POLICY OR GROUP NUMBER

a. EMPLOYMENT (CURRENT OR PREVIOUS) ☐ YES [X] NO

a. INSURED'S DATE OF BIRTH   **SEX** M ☐ F ☐

b. OTHER INSURED'S BIRTHDATE   **SEX** M ☐ F ☐

b. AUTO ACCIDENT? ☐ YES [X] NO   **PLACE (State)**

b. EMPLOYER NAME OR SCHOOL NAME

c. EMPLOYER NAME OR SCHOOL NAME

c. OTHER ACCIDENT? ☐ YES [X] NO

c. INSURANCE PLAN NAME OR PROGRAM NAME

d. INSURANCE PLAN NAME OR PROGRAM NAME

10d. RESERVED FOR LOCAL USE

d. IS THERE ANOTHER HEALTH BENEFIT PLAN ☐ YES ☐ NO   If yes, return to and complete 9 a-d.

READ BACK OF FORM BEFORE COMPLETING & SIGNING THIS FORM.
12. PATIENT'S OR AUTHORIZED PERSONS'S SIGNATURE I authorize the release of any medical or other info necessary to process this claim. I also request payment of government benefits either to myself or the party who accepts assignment below.

SIGNED ___SIGNATURE ON FILE___   DATE ___11242009___

13. PATIENT'S OR AUTHORIZED PERSONS'S SIGNATURE I authorize payment of medical benefits to the undersigned physician or supplier for services described below.

SIGNED _____

14. DATE OF CURRENT: ILLNESS (First symptom) OR INJURY (Accident) OR PREGRACY (LMP)

15. IF PATIENT HAS HAD SAME ILLNESS, GIVE FIRST DATE

16. DATES PATIENT UNABLE TO WORK IN CURRENT OCCUPATION FROM   TO

17. NAME OF REFERRING PROVIDER OR OTHER SOURCE   17a   17b NPI

18. HOSPITALIZATION DATES RELATED TO CURRENT SERVICES FROM   TO

19. RESERVED FOR LOCAL USE

20. OUTSIDE LAB? ☐ YES [X] NO   **$ CHARGES**

21. DIAGNOSIS OR NATURE OF ILLNESS OR INJURY (RELATE ITEMS 1, 2, 3 OR 4 TO ITEM 24E BY LINE)
1. | 401.9
2. | 250.02
3. |
4. |

22. MEDICAID SUBMISSION CODE   ORIGINAL REF. NO.

23. PRIOR AUTHORIZATION NUMBER

24. A. DATE(S) OF SERVICE From MM DD YY	To MM DD YY	B. Place of Service	C. EMG	D. PROCEDURES, SERVICES OR SUPPLIES (Explain Unusual Circumstances) CPT/HCPCS MODIFIER	E. DIAGNOSIS POINTER	F. $ CHARGES	G. DAYS OR UNITS	H. EPSDT Family Plan	I. ID. QUAL	J. RENDERING PROVIDER ID#
1	11 24 2009		31		99307	1 2	68 00	1		NPI	999501
2										NPI	
3										NPI	
4										NPI	
5										NPI	
6										NPI	

25. FEDERAL TAX I.D. NUMBER 00-1234560 SSN ☐ EIN [X]

26. PATIENT'S ACCOUNT NO. BLA001

27. ACCEPT ASSIGNMENT? ☐ YES [X] NO

28. TOTAL CHARGE $ 68 00

29. AMOUNT PAID $

30. BALANCE DUE $

31. SIGNATURE OF PHYSICIAN OR SUPPLIER INCLUDING DEGREES OR CREDENTIALS (I certify that the statements on the reverse apply to this bill and are made a part thereof.)
SIGNED L. D. HEATH, MD   11242009 DAT

32. SERVICE FACILITY LOCATION INFORMATION
RETIREMENT INN NURSING HOME
890 MILLENNIUM WAY
DOUGLASVILLE, NY 01234
a. 9990928531   b.

33. BILLING PROVIDER INFO PH # (123) 456-7890
DOUGLASVILLE MEDICINE ASSOCIATES
5076 BRAND BLVD., SUITE 401
DOUGLASVILLE, NY 01234
a. 9995010111   b.

NUCC Instruction Manual available at: www.nucc.org

OMB APPROVAL PENDING

FIGURE 7-16

Courtesy of the Centers for Medicare & Medicaid Services

continues

SENDING MEDICARE CLAIMS ELECTRONICALLY *continued*

1500	**TEST VERSION - NOT FOR OFFICIAL USE**	

HEALTH INSURANCE CLAIM FORM
APPROVED BY NATIONAL UNIFORM CLAIM COMMITTEE 08/05

Medicare - Statewide Corp.
200 Tech Center
Queens City, NY 01135

<u>Student No: Student1</u>

☐☐☐ PICA   PICA ☐☐☐

1. MEDICARE ☒ *(Medicare #)* MEDICAID ☐ *(Medicaid #)* TRICARE CHAMPUS ☐ *(Sponsor's SSN)* CHAMPVA ☐ *(Member ID)* GROUP HEALTH PLAN ☐ *(SSN or ID)* FECA BLK LUNG ☐ *(SSN)* OTHER ☐ *(ID)*	1a. INSURED'S I.D. NUMBER (FOR PROGRAM IN ITEM 1) 999412131A

2. PATIENT'S NAME (Last Name, First Name, Middle Initial) SHEKTAR PAULA M	3. PATIENT'S BIRTHDATE SEX 03	18	1939 M ☐ F ☒	4. INSURED'S NAME (Last Name, First Name, Middle Initial)

5. PATIENT'S ADDRESS (No., Street) 58682 PEBBLE TRAIL	6. PATIENT'S RELATIONSHIP TO INSURED Self ☐ Spouse ☐ Child ☐ Other ☐	7. INSURED'S ADDRESS (No., Street)

CITY DOUGLASVILLE	STATE NY	8. PATIENT STATUS Single ☐ Married ☒ Other ☐	CITY	STATE

ZIP CODE 01234	TELEPHONE (include Area Code) (123) 456-1118	Employed ☐ Full-Time Student ☐ Part-Time Student ☐	ZIP CODE	TELEPHONE (include Area Code)

9. OTHER INSURED'S NAME (Last Name, First Name, Mid. Initial)	10. IS PATIENT'S CONDITION RELATED TO:	11. INSURED'S POLICY GROUP OR FECA NUMBER NONE

a. OTHER INSURED'S POLICY OR GROUP NUMBER	a. EMPLOYMENT (CURRENT OR PREVIOUS) ☐ YES ☒ NO	a. INSURED'S DATE OF BIRTH SEX M ☐ F ☐

b. OTHER INSURED'S BIRTHDATE SEX M ☐ F ☐	b. AUTO ACCIDENT? PLACE (State) ☐ YES ☒ NO	b. EMPLOYER NAME OR SCHOOL NAME

c. EMPLOYER NAME OR SCHOOL NAME	c. OTHER ACCIDENT? ☐ YES ☒ NO	c. INSURANCE PLAN NAME OR PROGRAM NAME

d. INSURANCE PLAN NAME OR PROGRAM NAME	10d. RESERVED FOR LOCAL USE	d. IS THERE ANOTHER HEALTH BENEFIT PLAN ☐ YES ☐ NO *If yes, return to and complete 9 a-d.*

READ BACK OF FORM BEFORE COMPLETING & SIGNING THIS FORM.

12. PATIENT'S OR AUTHORIZED PERSONS'S SIGNATURE I authorize the release of any medical or other info necessary to process this claim. I also request payment of government benefits either to myself or the party who accepts assignment below. SIGNED _SIGNATURE ON FILE_ DATE _10232009_	13. PATIENT'S OR AUTHORIZED PERSONS'S SIGNATURE I authorize payment of medical benefits to the undersigned physician or supplier for services described below. SIGNED _____

14. DATE OF CURRENT: ◀ ILLNESS (First symptom) OR INJURY (Accident) OR PREGRANCY (LMP)	15. IF PATIENT HAS HAD SAME ILLNESS, GIVE FIRST DATE	16. DATES PATIENT UNABLE TO WORK IN CURRENT OCCUPATION FROM TO

17. NAME OF REFERRING PROVIDER OR OTHER SOURCE	17a. 17b. NPI	18. HOSPITALIZATION DATES RELATED TO CURRENT SERVICES FROM TO

19. RESERVED FOR LOCAL USE	20. OUTSIDE LAB? $ CHARGES ☐ YES ☒ NO

21. DIAGNOSIS OR NATURE OF ILLNESS OR INJURY (RELATE ITEMS 1, 2, 3 OR 4 TO ITEM 24E BY LINE ┐ 1. 428.0 3. |_____ 2. |_____ 4. |_____	22. MEDICAID SUBMISSION CODE ORIGINAL REF. NO.
	23. PRIOR AUTHORIZATION NUMBER

24. A. DATE(S) OF SERVICE From MM DD YY To MM DD YY	B. Place of Service	C. EMG	D. PROCEDURES, SERVICES OR SUPPLIES (Explain Unusual Circumstances) CPT/HCPCS MODIFIER	E. DIAGNOSIS POINTER	F. $ CHARGES	G. DAYS OR UNITS	H. EPSDT Family Plan	I. ID. QUAL	J. RENDERING PROVIDER ID#
1	10 23 2009	11		99214	1	180 00	1		NPI	999502
2									NPI	
3									NPI	
4									NPI	
5									NPI	
6									NPI	

25. FEDERAL TAX I.D. NUMBER SSN EIN 00-1234560 ☐ ☒	26. PATIENT'S ACCOUNT NO. SHE001	27. ACCEPT ASSIGNMENT? ☐ YES ☒ NO	28. TOTAL CHARGE $ 180 00	29. AMOUNT PAID $	30. BALANCE DUE $

31. SIGNATURE OF PHYSICIAN OR SUPPLIER INCLUDING DEGREES OR CREDENTIALS (I certify that the statements on the reverse apply to this bill and are made a part thereof.) 10232009 SIGNED D.J. SCHWARTZ, MD DAT	32. SERVICE FACILITY LOCATION INFORMATION DOUGLASVILLE MEDICINE ASSOCIATES 5076 BRAND BLVD., SUITE 401 DOUGLASVILLE, NY 01234 a. 9995020212 b.	33. BILLING PROVIDER INFO PH # (123) 456-7892 DOUGLASVILLE MEDICINE ASSOCIATES 5076 BRAND BLVD., SUITE 401 DOUGLASVILLE, NY 01234 a. 9995020212 b.

NUCC Instruction Manual available at: www.nucc.org   OMB APPROVAL PENDING

FIGURE 7-17

Courtesy of the Centers for Medicare & Medicaid Services

| 1500 | TEST VERSION - NOT FOR OFFICIAL USE |

HEALTH INSURANCE CLAIM FORM
APPROVED BY NATIONAL UNIFORM CLAIM COMMITTEE 08/05

Medicare - Statewide Corp.
200 Tech Center
Queens City, NY 01135

Student No: Student1

☐☐☐ PICA

PICA ☐☐☐

| 1. MEDICARE   MEDICAID   TRICARE   CHAMPVA   GROUP   FECA   OTHER | 1a. INSURED'S I.D. NUMBER   (FOR PROGRAM IN ITEM 1) |
| | |

CHAMPUS   HEALTH PLAN   BLK LUNG
[X](Medicare #) ☐(Medicaid #) ☐(Sponsor's SSN) ☐(Member ID) ☐(SSN or ID) ☐(SSN) ☐(ID)

1a. INSURED'S I.D. NUMBER   (FOR PROGRAM IN ITEM 1)
999210132D

2. PATIENT'S NAME (Last Name, First Name, Middle Initial)
PINKSTON ANNA

3. PATIENT'S BIRTHDATE   SEX
07 | 28 | 1922   M ☐ F [X]

4. INSURED'S NAME (Last Name, First Name, Middle Initial)

5. PATIENT'S ADDRESS (No., Street)
690 PARK ROSE AVE

6. PATIENT'S RELATIONSHIP TO INSURED
Self ☐ Spouse ☐ Child ☐ Other ☐

7. INSURED'S ADDRESS (No., Street)

CITY
DOUGLASVILLE   STATE NY

8. PATIENT STATUS
Single [X] Married ☐ Other ☐

CITY   STATE

ZIP CODE   TELEPHONE (include Area Code)
01235   (123) 528-0112

Employed ☐ Full-Time ☐ Part-Time ☐
                Student   Student

ZIP CODE   TELEPHONE (include Area Code)

9. OTHER INSURED'S NAME (Last Name, First Name, Mid. Initial)

10. IS PATIENT'S CONDITION RELATED TO:

11. INSURED'S POLICY GROUP OR FECA NUMBER
NONE

a. OTHER INSURED'S POLICY OR GROUP NUMBER

a. EMPLOYMENT (CURRENT OR PREVIOUS)
☐YES [X]NO

a. INSURED'S DATE OF BIRTH   SEX
M ☐ F ☐

b. OTHER INSURED'S BIRTHDATE   SEX
M ☐ F ☐

b. AUTO ACCIDENT?   PLACE (State)
☐YES [X]NO

b. EMPLOYER NAME OR SCHOOL NAME

c. EMPLOYER NAME OR SCHOOL NAME

c. OTHER ACCIDENT?
☐YES [X]NO

c. INSURANCE PLAN NAME OR PROGRAM NAME

d. INSURANCE PLAN NAME OR PROGRAM NAME

10d. RESERVED FOR LOCAL USE

d. IS THERE ANOTHER HEALTH BENEFIT PLAN
☐YES ☐NO   If yes, return to and complete 9 a-d.

READ BACK OF FORM BEFORE COMPLETING & SIGNING THIS FORM.
12. PATIENT'S OR AUTHORIZED PERSONS'S SIGNATURE I authorize the release of any medical or other info necessary to process this claim. I also request payment of government benefits either to myself or the party who accepts assignment below.

SIGNED _____ SIGNATURE ON FILE _____   DATE _____ 11242009 _____

13. PATIENT'S OR AUTHORIZED PERSONS'S SIGNATURE I authorize payment of medical benefits to the undersigned physician or supplier for services described below.

SIGNED _____

14. DATE OF CURRENT: ◄ ILLNESS (First symptom) OR
                          INJURY (Accident) OR
                          PREGRANCY (LMP)

15. IF PATIENT HAS HAD SAME ILLNESS,
    GIVE FIRST DATE

16. DATES PATIENT UNABLE TO WORK IN CURRENT OCCUPATION
FROM _____ TO _____

17. NAME OF REFERRING PROVIDER OR OTHER SOURCE

17a
17b NPI

18. HOSPITALIZATION DATES RELATED TO CURRENT SERVICES
FROM _____ TO _____

19. RESERVED FOR LOCAL USE

20. OUTSIDE LAB? $ CHARGES
☐YES [X]NO

21. DIAGNOSIS OR NATURE OF ILLNESS OR INJURY (RELATE ITEMS 1, 2, 3 OR 4 TO ITEM 24E BY LINE

1. | 443.9   3. |
2. | 4. |

22. MEDICAID SUBMISSION
    CODE   ORIGINAL REF. NO.

23. PRIOR AUTHORIZATION NUMBER

24. A DATE(S) OF SERVICE						B. Place of Service	C. EMG	D. PROCEDURES, SERVICES OR SUPPLIES (Explain Unusual Circumstances)		E. DIAGNOSIS POINTER	F. $ CHARGES	G. DAYS OR UNITS	H. EPSDT Family Plan	I. ID. QUAL	J. RENDERING PROVIDER ID#
From			To					CPT/HCPCS	MODIFIER						
MM	DD	YY	MM	DD	YY										
11	24	2009				31		99308		1	113	00	1		NPI	999501
															NPI	
															NPI	
															NPI	
															NPI	
															NPI	

| 25. FEDERAL TAX I.D. NUMBER   SSN EIN | 26. PATIENT'S ACCOUNT NO | 27. ACCEPT ASSIGNMENT? | 28. TOTAL CHARGE | 29. AMOUNT PAID | 30. BALANCE DUE |
| 00-1234560   ☐ [X] | PIN001 | [X]YES ☐NO | $ 113 00 | $ | $ |

31. SIGNATURE OF PHYSICIAN OR SUPPLIER INCLUDING DEGREES OR CREDENTIALS
(I certify that the statements on the reverse apply to this bill and are made a part thereof.)

SIGNED L. D. HEATH, MD   DAT 11242009

32. SERVICE FACILITY LOCATION INFORMATION
RETIREMENT INN NURSING HOME
890 MILLENNIUM WAY
DOUGLASVILLE, NY 01234
a. 9990928531   b.

33. BILLING PROVIDER INFO PH #   (123) 456-7890
DOUGLASVILLE MEDICINE ASSOCIATES
5076 BRAND BLVD., SUITE 401
DOUGLASVILLE, NY 01234
a. 9995010111   b.

NUCC Instruction Manual available at: www.nucc.org

OMB APPROVAL PENDING

FIGURE 7-18
Courtesy of the Centers for Medicare & Medicaid Services

continues

SENDING MEDICARE CLAIMS ELECTRONICALLY *continued*

1500	TEST VERSION - NOT FOR OFFICIAL USE

HEALTH INSURANCE CLAIM FORM
APPROVED BY NATIONAL UNIFORM CLAIM COMMITTEE 08/05

Medicare - Statewide Corp.
200 Tech Center
Queens City, NY 01135

Student No: **Student1**

☐☐☐ PICA   PICA ☐☐☐

1. MEDICARE	MEDICAID	TRICARE CHAMPUS	CHAMPVA	GROUP HEALTH PLAN	FECA BLK LUNG	OTHER	1a. INSURED'S I.D. NUMBER (FOR PROGRAM IN ITEM 1)
☒ (Medicare #)	☐ (Medicaid #)	☐ (Sponsor's SSN)	☐ (Member ID)	☐ (SSN or ID)	☐ (SSN)	☐ (ID)	999321156A

2. PATIENT'S NAME (Last Name, First Name, Middle Initial)
CHANG XAO

3. PATIENT'S BIRTHDATE   11 | 13 | 1926   SEX M ☒ F ☐

4. INSURED'S NAME (Last Name, First Name, Middle Initial)

5. PATIENT'S ADDRESS (No., Street)
890 MILLENNIUM WAY

6. PATIENT'S RELATIONSHIP TO INSURED
Self ☐ Spouse ☐ Child ☐ Other ☐

7. INSURED'S ADDRESS (No., Street)

CITY
DOUGLASVILLE   STATE NY

8. PATIENT STATUS
Single ☒   Married ☐   Other ☐

CITY   STATE

ZIP CODE   01234   TELEPHONE (include Area Code)   (123) 528-0112

Employed ☐   Full-Time Student ☐   Part-Time Student ☐

ZIP CODE   TELEPHONE (include Area Code)

9. OTHER INSURED'S NAME (Last Name, First Name, Mid. Initial)

10. IS PATIENT'S CONDITION RELATED TO:

11. INSURED'S POLICY GROUP OR FECA NUMBER
NONE

a. OTHER INSURED'S POLICY OR GROUP NUMBER

a. EMPLOYMENT (CURRENT OR PREVIOUS)
☐ YES   ☒ NO

a. INSURED'S DATE OF BIRTH   SEX M ☐ F ☐

b. OTHER INSURED'S BIRTHDATE   SEX M ☐ F ☐

b. AUTO ACCIDENT?   PLACE (State)
☐ YES   ☒ NO

b. EMPLOYER NAME OR SCHOOL NAME

c. EMPLOYER NAME OR SCHOOL NAME

c. OTHER ACCIDENT?
☐ YES   ☒ NO

c. INSURANCE PLAN NAME OR PROGRAM NAME

d. INSURANCE PLAN NAME OR PROGRAM NAME

10d. RESERVED FOR LOCAL USE

d. IS THERE ANOTHER HEALTH BENEFIT PLAN
☐ YES   ☐ NO   *If yes, return to and complete 9 a-d.*

READ BACK OF FORM BEFORE COMPLETING & SIGNING THIS FORM.

12. PATIENT'S OR AUTHORIZED PERSONS'S SIGNATURE I authorize the release of any medical or other info necessary to process this claim. I also request payment of government benefits either to myself or the party who accepts assignment below.

SIGNED ___ SIGNATURE ON FILE ___   DATE ___ 10162009 ___

13. PATIENT'S OR AUTHORIZED PERSONS'S SIGNATURE I authorize payment of medical benefits to the undersigned physician or supplier for services described below.

SIGNED _____

14. DATE OF CURRENT: ◄ ILLNESS (First symptom) OR INJURY (Accident) OR PREGRACY (LMP)

15. IF PATIENT HAS HAD SAME ILLNESS, GIVE FIRST DATE

16. DATES PATIENT UNABLE TO WORK IN CURRENT OCCUPATION
FROM   TO

17. NAME OF REFERRING PROVIDER OR OTHER SOURCE
17a
17b NPI

18. HOSPITALIZATION DATES RELATED TO CURRENT SERVICES
FROM   TO

19. RESERVED FOR LOCAL USE

20. OUTSIDE LAB?   ☐ YES   ☒ NO $ CHARGES

21. DIAGNOSIS OR NATURE OF ILLNESS OR INJURY (RELATE ITEMS 1, 2, 3 OR 4 TO ITEM 24E BY LINE)
1. 250.00
2. |
3. |
4. |

22. MEDICAID SUBMISSION CODE   ORIGINAL REF. NO.

23. PRIOR AUTHORIZATION NUMBER

24. A DATE(S) OF SERVICE From MM DD YY	To MM DD YY	B. Place of Service	C. EMG	D. PROCEDURES, SERVICES OR SUPPLIES (Explain Unusual Circumstances) CPT/HCPCS	MODIFIER	E. DIAGNOSIS POINTER	F. $ CHARGES	G. DAYS OR UNITS	H. EPSDT Family Plan	I. ID. QUAL	J. RENDERING PROVIDER ID#
1 10 16 2009		31		99307		1	60 00	1		NPI	999501
2										NPI	
3										NPI	
4										NPI	
5										NPI	
6										NPI	

25. FEDERAL TAX I.D. NUMBER   SSN ☐ EIN ☒
00-1234560

26. PATIENT'S ACCOUNT NO
CHA001

27. ACCEPT ASSIGNMENT?
☒ YES   ☐ NO

28. TOTAL CHARGE
$ 60 00

29. AMOUNT PAID
$

30. BALANCE DUE
$

31. SIGNATURE OF PHYSICIAN OR SUPPLIER INCLUDING DEGREES OR CREDENTIALS (I certify that the statements on the reverse apply to this bill and are made a part thereof.)
10162009
SIGNED   L. D. HEATH, MD   DAT

32. SERVICE FACILITY LOCATION INFORMATION
RETIREMENT INN NURSING HOME
890 MILLENNIUM WAY
DOUGLASVILLE, NY 01234
a. 9990928531   b.

33. BILLING PROVIDER INFO PH #   (123) 456-7890
DOUGLASVILLE MEDICINE ASSOCIATES
5076 BRAND BLVD., SUITE 401
DOUGLASVILLE, NY 01234
a. 9995010111   b.

NUCC Instruction Manual available at: www.nucc.org

OMB APPROVAL PENDING

FIGURE 7-19

Courtesy of the Centers for Medicare & Medicaid Services

1500	TEST VERSION - NOT FOR OFFICIAL USE

HEALTH INSURANCE CLAIM FORM

Medicare - Statewide Corp.

APPROVED BY NATIONAL UNIFORM CLAIM COMMITTEE 08/05

200 Tech Center

Queens City, NY 01135

Student No: Student1

| | | | | | | | PICA | | | | PICA | | |

1. MEDICARE	MEDICAID	TRICARE CHAMPUS	CHAMPVA	GROUP HEALTH PLAN	FECA BLK LUNG	OTHER	1a. INSURED'S I.D. NUMBER (FOR PROGRAM IN ITEM 1)
[X] (Medicare #)	☐ (Medicaid #)	☐ (Sponsor's SSN)	☐ (Member ID)	☐ (SSN or ID)	☐ (SSN)	☐ (ID)	999321156A

2. PATIENT'S NAME (Last Name, First Name, Middle Initial)	3. PATIENT'S BIRTHDATE SEX	4. INSURED'S NAME (Last Name, First Name, Middle Initial)
CHANG XAO	11 | 13 | 1926 M [X] F ☐	

5. PATIENT'S ADDRESS (No., Street)	6. PATIENT'S RELATIONSHIP TO INSURED	7. INSURED'S ADDRESS (No., Street)
890 MILLENNIUM WAY	Self ☐ Spouse ☐ Child ☐ Other ☐	

CITY	STATE	8. PATIENT STATUS	CITY	STATE
DOUGLASVILLE	NY	Single [X] Married ☐ Other ☐		

ZIP CODE	TELEPHONE (include Area Code)		ZIP CODE	TELEPHONE (include Area Code)
01234	(123) 528-0112	Employed ☐ Full-Time Student ☐ Part-Time Student ☐		

9. OTHER INSURED'S NAME (Last Name, First Name, Mid. Initial)	10. IS PATIENT'S CONDITION RELATED TO:	11. INSURED'S POLICY GROUP OR FECA NUMBER
		NONE

a. OTHER INSURED'S POLICY OR GROUP NUMBER	a. EMPLOYMENT (CURRENT OR PREVIOUS)	a. INSURED'S DATE OF BIRTH SEX
	☐ YES [X] NO	M ☐ F ☐

b. OTHER INSURED'S BIRTHDATE SEX	b. AUTO ACCIDENT? PLACE (State)	b. EMPLOYER NAME OR SCHOOL NAME
M ☐ F ☐	☐ YES [X] NO	

c. EMPLOYER NAME OR SCHOOL NAME	c. OTHER ACCIDENT?	c. INSURANCE PLAN NAME OR PROGRAM NAME
	☐ YES [X] NO	

d. INSURANCE PLAN NAME OR PROGRAM NAME	10d. RESERVED FOR LOCAL USE	d. IS THERE ANOTHER HEALTH BENEFIT PLAN
		☐ YES ☐ NO If yes, return to and complete 9 a-d.

READ BACK OF FORM BEFORE COMPLETING & SIGNING THIS FORM.

12. PATIENT'S OR AUTHORIZED PERSONS'S SIGNATURE I authorize the release of any medical or other info necessary to process this claim. I also request payment of government benefits either to myself or the party who accepts assignment below.

SIGNED _SIGNATURE ON FILE_   DATE _11242009_

13. PATIENT'S OR AUTHORIZED PERSONS'S SIGNATURE I authorize payment of medical benefits to the undersigned physician or supplier for services described below.

SIGNED _____

14. DATE OF CURRENT: ◄ ILLNESS (First symptom) OR INJURY (Accident) OR PREGRACY (LMP)	15. IF PATIENT HAS HAD SAME ILLNESS, GIVE FIRST DATE	16. DATES PATIENT UNABLE TO WORK IN CURRENT OCCUPATION
		FROM TO

17. NAME OF REFERRING PROVIDER OR OTHER SOURCE	17a		18. HOSPITALIZATION DATES RELATED TO CURRENT SERVICES
	17b NPI		FROM TO

19. RESERVED FOR LOCAL USE	20. OUTSIDE LAB? $ CHARGES
	☐ YES [X] NO

21. DIAGNOSIS OR NATURE OF ILLNESS OR INJURY (RELATE ITEMS 1, 2, 3 OR 4 TO ITEM 24E BY LINE)

1. | 780.39   3. |_____

2. |_____   4. |_____

22. MEDICAID SUBMISSION CODE	ORIGINAL REF. NO.

23. PRIOR AUTHORIZATION NUMBER

24. A DATE(S) OF SERVICE From / To						B. Place of Service	C. EMG	D. PROCEDURES, SERVICES OR SUPPLIES (Explain Unusual Circumstances) CPT/HCPCS MODIFIER		E. DIAGNOSIS POINTER	F. $ CHARGES		G. DAYS OR UNITS	H. EPSDT Famly Plan	I. ID. QUAL	J. RENDERING PROVIDER ID#
MM	DD	YY	MM	DD	YY											
1 11	24	2009				31		99307		1	68	00	1		NPI	999501
2															NPI	
3															NPI	
4															NPI	
5															NPI	
6															NPI	

25. FEDERAL TAX I.D. NUMBER SSN EIN	26. PATIENT'S ACCOUNT NO.	27. ACCEPT ASSIGNMENT?	28. TOTAL CHARGE	29. AMOUNT PAID	30. BALANCE DUE
00-1234560 ☐ [X]	CHA001	[X] YES ☐ NO	$ 68 00	$	$

31. SIGNATURE OF PHYSICIAN OR SUPPLIER INCLUDING DEGREES OR CREDENTIALS (I certify that the statements on the reverse apply to this bill and are made a part thereof.)	32. SERVICE FACILITY LOCATION INFORMATION	33. BILLING PROVIDER INFO PH # (123) 456-7890
11242009	RETIREMENT INN NURSING HOME	DOUGLASVILLE MEDICINE ASSOCIATES
SIGNED L. D. HEATH, MD DAT	890 MILLENNIUM WAY DOUGLASVILLE, NY 01234	5076 BRAND BLVD., SUITE 401 DOUGLASVILLE, NY 01234
	a. 9990928531 b.	a. 9995010111 b.

NUCC Instruction Manual available at: www.nucc.org

OMB APPROVAL PENDING

FIGURE 7-20

Courtesy of the Centers for Medicare & Medicaid Services

continues

SENDING MEDICARE CLAIMS ELECTRONICALLY *continued*

1500

TEST VERSION - NOT FOR OFFICIAL USE

HEALTH INSURANCE CLAIM FORM
APPROVED BY NATIONAL UNIFORM CLAIM COMMITTEE 08/05

Medicare - Statewide Corp.
200 Tech Center
Queens City, NY 01135

Student No: Student1

PICA | PICA

1. MEDICARE [X] (Medicare #) MEDICAID (Medicaid #) TRICARE CHAMPUS (Sponsor's SSN) CHAMPVA (Member ID) GROUP HEALTH PLAN (SSN or ID) FECA BLK LUNG (SSN) OTHER (ID)
1a. INSURED'S I.D. NUMBER (FOR PROGRAM IN ITEM 1): 999571266A

2. PATIENT'S NAME (Last Name, First Name, Middle Initial): ADAMS MINNIE
3. PATIENT'S BIRTHDATE: 09 | 04 | 1928 SEX M [ ] F [X]
4. INSURED'S NAME (Last Name, First Name, Middle Initial)

5. PATIENT'S ADDRESS (No., Street): 1287 SLATE DRIVE
6. PATIENT'S RELATIONSHIP TO INSURED: Self [ ] Spouse [ ] Child [ ] Other [ ]
7. INSURED'S ADDRESS (No., Street)

CITY: DOUGLASVILLE STATE: NY
8. PATIENT STATUS: Single [X] Married [ ] Other [ ]
CITY | STATE

ZIP CODE: 01234 TELEPHONE (include Area Code): (123) 457-3688
Employed [ ] Full-Time Student [ ] Part-Time Student [ ]
ZIP CODE | TELEPHONE (include Area Code)

9. OTHER INSURED'S NAME (Last Name, First Name, Mid. Initial)
10. IS PATIENT'S CONDITION RELATED TO:
11. INSURED'S POLICY GROUP OR FECA NUMBER: NONE

a. OTHER INSURED'S POLICY OR GROUP NUMBER
a. EMPLOYMENT (CURRENT OR PREVIOUS)? [ ] YES [X] NO
a. INSURED'S DATE OF BIRTH SEX M [ ] F [ ]

b. OTHER INSURED'S BIRTHDATE SEX M [ ] F [ ]
b. AUTO ACCIDENT? [ ] YES [X] NO PLACE (State)
b. EMPLOYER NAME OR SCHOOL NAME

c. EMPLOYER NAME OR SCHOOL NAME
c. OTHER ACCIDENT? [ ] YES [X] NO
c. INSURANCE PLAN NAME OR PROGRAM NAME

d. INSURANCE PLAN NAME OR PROGRAM NAME
10d. RESERVED FOR LOCAL USE
d. IS THERE ANOTHER HEALTH BENEFIT PLAN? [ ] YES [ ] NO *If yes, return to and complete 9 a-d.*

READ BACK OF FORM BEFORE COMPLETING & SIGNING THIS FORM.
12. PATIENT'S OR AUTHORIZED PERSONS'S SIGNATURE I authorize the release of any medical or other info necessary to process this claim. I also request payment of government benefits either to myself or the party who accepts assignment below.
SIGNED: SIGNATURE ON FILE DATE: 10282009

13. PATIENT'S OR AUTHORIZED PERSONS'S SIGNATURE I authorize payment of medical benefits to the undersigned physician or supplier for services described below.
SIGNED:

14. DATE OF CURRENT: ILLNESS (First symptom) OR INJURY (Accident) OR PREGRANCY (LMP)
15. IF PATIENT HAS HAD SAME ILLNESS, GIVE FIRST DATE
16. DATES PATIENT UNABLE TO WORK IN CURRENT OCCUPATION FROM | TO

17. NAME OF REFERRING PROVIDER OR OTHER SOURCE: SAMANTHA GREEN
17a
17b NPI 9995598741
18. HOSPITALIZATION DATES RELATED TO CURRENT SERVICES FROM | TO

19. RESERVED FOR LOCAL USE
20. OUTSIDE LAB? [X] YES [ ] NO $ CHARGES 47.00

21. DIAGNOSIS OR NATURE OF ILLNESS OR INJURY (RELATE ITEMS 1, 2, 3 OR 4 TO ITEM 24E BY LINE)
1. 438.9
2.
3.
4.
22. MEDICAID SUBMISSION CODE | ORIGINAL REF. NO.
23. PRIOR AUTHORIZATION NUMBER

24. A. DATE(S) OF SERVICE From MM DD YY	To MM DD YY	B. Place of Service	C. EMG	D. PROCEDURES, SERVICES OR SUPPLIES (Explain Unusual Circumstances) CPT/HCPCS	MODIFIER	E. DIAGNOSIS POINTER	F. $ CHARGES	G. DAYS OR UNITS	H. EPSDT Family Plan	I. ID. QUAL	J. RENDERING PROVIDER ID#
1	10 28 2009		11		99203		1	200 00	1		NPI	999501
2	10 28 2009		11		80053		1	47 00	1		NPI	999501
3	10 28 2009		11		36415		1	18 00	1		NPI	999501
4											NPI	
5											NPI	
6											NPI	

25. FEDERAL TAX I.D. NUMBER: 00-1234560 SSN [ ] EIN [X]
26. PATIENT'S ACCOUNT NO: ADA001
27. ACCEPT ASSIGNMENT? [X] YES [ ] NO
28. TOTAL CHARGE $ 265 00
29. AMOUNT PAID $
30. BALANCE DUE $

31. SIGNATURE OF PHYSICIAN OR SUPPLIER INCLUDING DEGREES OR CREDENTIALS (I certify that the statements on the reverse apply to this bill and are made a part thereof.)
SIGNED: L. D. HEATH, MD DAT 10282009

32. SERVICE FACILITY LOCATION INFORMATION
BIOPACE LABORATORY
1600 MIDWAY AVE.
DOUGLASVILLE, NY 01234
a. 9992849492 b.

33. BILLING PROVIDER INFO PH # (123) 456-7890
DOUGLASVILLE MEDICINE ASSOCIATES
5076 BRAND BLVD., SUITE 401
DOUGLASVILLE, NY 01234
a. 9995010111 b.

NUCC Instruction Manual available at: www.nucc.org
OMB APPROVAL PENDING

FIGURE 7-21

Courtesy of the Centers for Medicare & Medicaid Services

TEST VERSION - NOT FOR OFFICIAL USE

1500

HEALTH INSURANCE CLAIM FORM
APPROVED BY NATIONAL UNIFORM CLAIM COMMITTEE 08/05

Medicare - Statewide Corp.
200 Tech Center
Queens City, NY 01135

Student No: Student1

[ ][ ][ ] PICA

PICA [ ][ ]

1. MEDICARE / MEDICAID / TRICARE CHAMPUS / CHAMPVA / GROUP HEALTH PLAN / FECA BLK LUNG / OTHER	1a. INSURED'S I.D. NUMBER (FOR PROGRAM IN ITEM 1)
[X] (Medicare #) [ ] (Medicaid #) [ ] (Sponsor's SSN) [ ] (Member ID) [ ] (SSN or ID) [ ] (SSN) [ ] (ID)	999213166A

2. PATIENT'S NAME (Last Name, First Name, Middle Initial)
TOMANAGA MARIE

3. PATIENT'S BIRTHDATE   SEX
02 | 02 | 1933   M [ ] F [X]

4. INSURED'S NAME (Last Name, First Name, Middle Initial)

5. PATIENT'S ADDRESS (No., Street)
2301 MARBLE WAY

6. PATIENT'S RELATIONSHIP TO INSURED
Self [ ] Spouse [ ] Child [ ] Other [ ]

7. INSURED'S ADDRESS (No., Street)

CITY   DOUGLASVILLE   STATE NY

8. PATIENT STATUS
Single [ ] Married [X] Other [ ]

CITY   STATE

ZIP CODE 01234   TELEPHONE (include Area Code) (123) 457-2110

Employed [ ] Full-Time Student [ ] Part-Time Student [ ]

ZIP CODE   TELEPHONE (include Area Code)

9. OTHER INSURED'S NAME (Last Name, First Name, Mid. Initial)

10. IS PATIENT'S CONDITION RELATED TO:

11. INSURED'S POLICY GROUP OR FECA NUMBER
NONE

a. OTHER INSURED'S POLICY OR GROUP NUMBER

a. EMPLOYMENT (CURRENT OR PREVIOUS)
[ ] YES [X] NO

a. INSURED'S DATE OF BIRTH   SEX
M [ ] F [ ]

b. OTHER INSURED'S BIRTHDATE   SEX
M [ ] F [ ]

b. AUTO ACCIDENT?   PLACE (State)
[ ] YES [X] NO

b. EMPLOYER NAME OR SCHOOL NAME

c. EMPLOYER NAME OR SCHOOL NAME

c. OTHER ACCIDENT?
[ ] YES [X] NO

c. INSURANCE PLAN NAME OR PROGRAM NAME

d. INSURANCE PLAN NAME OR PROGRAM NAME

10d. RESERVED FOR LOCAL USE

d. IS THERE ANOTHER HEALTH BENEFIT PLAN
[ ] YES [ ] NO   If yes, return to and complete 9 a-d.

READ BACK OF FORM BEFORE COMPLETING & SIGNING THIS FORM.

12. PATIENT'S OR AUTHORIZED PERSONS'S SIGNATURE I authorize the release of any medical or other info necessary to process this claim. I also request payment of government benefits either to myself or the party who accepts assignment below.

SIGNED   SIGNATURE ON FILE   DATE   11032009

13. PATIENT'S OR AUTHORIZED PERSONS'S SIGNATURE I authorize payment of medical benefits to the undersigned physician or supplier for services described below.

SIGNED

14. DATE OF CURRENT: ILLNESS (First symptom) OR INJURY (Accident) OR PREGRANCY (LMP)

15. IF PATIENT HAS HAD SAME ILLNESS, GIVE FIRST DATE

16. DATES PATIENT UNABLE TO WORK IN CURRENT OCCUPATION
FROM   TO

17. NAME OF REFERRING PROVIDER OR OTHER SOURCE
17a
17b NPI

18. HOSPITALIZATION DATES RELATED TO CURRENT SERVICES
FROM   TO

19. RESERVED FOR LOCAL USE

20. OUTSIDE LAB? $ CHARGES
[X] YES [ ] NO   9.00

21. DIAGNOSIS OR NATURE OF ILLNESS OR INJURY (RELATE ITEMS 1, 2, 3 OR 4 TO ITEM 24E BY LINE
1. | 413.9
2. | 401.9
3. |
4. |

22. MEDICAID SUBMISSION CODE   ORIGINAL REF. NO.

23. PRIOR AUTHORIZATION NUMBER

24. A DATE(S) OF SERVICE From			To			B. Place of Service	C. EMG	D. PROCEDURES, SERVICES OR SUPPLIES (Explain Unusual Circumstances) CPT/HCPCS MODIFIER	E. DIAGNOSIS POINTER	F. $ CHARGES		G. DAYS OR UNITS	H. EPSDT Family Plan	I. ID. QUAL	J. RENDERING PROVIDER ID#
MM	DD	YY	MM	DD	YY										
11	03	2009				11		99205	1 2	358	00	1		NPI	999502
11	03	2009				11		93000	1	131	00	1		NPI	999502
11	03	2009				11		85651	1	9	00	1		NPI	999502
11	03	2009				11		36415	1	18	00	1		NPI	999502
														NPI	
														NPI	

25. FEDERAL TAX I.D. NUMBER   SSN EIN
00-1234560   [ ] [X]

26. PATIENT'S ACCOUNT NO
TOM001

27. ACCEPT ASSIGNMENT?
[X] YES [ ] NO

28. TOTAL CHARGE
$ 516 00

29. AMOUNT PAID
$

30. BALANCE DUE
$

31. SIGNATURE OF PHYSICIAN OR SUPPLIER INCLUDING DEGREES OR CREDENTIALS (I certify that the statements on the reverse apply to this bill and are made a part thereof.)
11032009
SIGNED   D.J. SCHWARTZ, MD   DAT

32. SERVICE FACILITY LOCATION INFORMATION
BIOPACE LABORATORY
1600 MIDWAY AVE.
DOUGLASVILLE, NY 01234
a. 9992849492   b.

33. BILLING PROVIDER INFO PH #   (123) 456-7892
DOUGLASVILLE MEDICINE ASSOCIATES
5076 BRAND BLVD., SUITE 401
DOUGLASVILLE, NY 01234
a. 9995020212   b.

NUCC Instruction Manual available at: www.nucc.org

OMB APPROVAL PENDING

FIGURE 7-22

Courtesy of the Centers for Medicare & Medicaid Services

continues

1500	TEST VERSION - NOT FOR OFFICIAL USE

HEALTH INSURANCE CLAIM FORM
APPROVED BY NATIONAL UNIFORM CLAIM COMMITTEE 08/05

Medicare - Statewide Corp.
200 Tech Center
Queens City, NY 01135

Student No: Student1

☐☐☐ PICA   PICA ☐☐☐

1. MEDICARE ☒ *(Medicare #)*	MEDICAID ☐ *(Medicaid #)*	TRICARE CHAMPUS ☐ *(Sponsor's SSN)*	CHAMPVA ☐ *(Member ID)*	GROUP HEALTH PLAN ☐ *(SSN or ID)*	FECA BLK LUNG ☐ *(SSN)*	OTHER ☐ *(ID)*	1a. INSURED'S I.D. NUMBER (FOR PROGRAM IN ITEM 1) 999832166A

2. PATIENT'S NAME (Last Name, First Name, Middle Initial) MUNOZ GERALDO L	3. PATIENT'S BIRTHDATE 03 | 28 | 1925 SEX M ☒ F ☐	4. INSURED'S NAME (Last Name, First Name, Middle Initial)

5. PATIENT'S ADDRESS (No., Street) 1287 BOULDER COURT	6. PATIENT'S RELATIONSHIP TO INSURED Self ☐ Spouse ☐ Child ☐ Other ☐	7. INSURED'S ADDRESS (No., Street)

CITY DOUGLASVILLE	STATE NY	8. PATIENT STATUS Single ☒ Married ☐ Other ☐	CITY	STATE

ZIP CODE 01234	TELEPHONE (include Area Code) (123) 457-0018	Employed ☐ Full-Time Student ☐ Part-Time Student ☐	ZIP CODE	TELEPHONE (include Area Code)

9. OTHER INSURED'S NAME (Last Name, First Name, Mid. Initial)	10. IS PATIENT'S CONDITION RELATED TO:	11. INSURED'S POLICY GROUP OR FECA NUMBER NONE

a. OTHER INSURED'S POLICY OR GROUP NUMBER	a. EMPLOYMENT (CURRENT OR PREVIOUS) ☐ YES ☒ NO	a. INSURED'S DATE OF BIRTH SEX M ☐ F ☐

b. OTHER INSURED'S BIRTHDATE SEX M ☐ F ☐	b. AUTO ACCIDENT? ☐ YES ☒ NO PLACE (State)	b. EMPLOYER NAME OR SCHOOL NAME

c. EMPLOYER NAME OR SCHOOL NAME	c. OTHER ACCIDENT? ☐ YES ☒ NO	c. INSURANCE PLAN NAME OR PROGRAM NAME

d. INSURANCE PLAN NAME OR PROGRAM NAME	10d. RESERVED FOR LOCAL USE	d. IS THERE ANOTHER HEALTH BENEFIT PLAN? ☐ YES ☐ NO If yes, return to and complete 9 a-d.

READ BACK OF FORM BEFORE COMPLETING & SIGNING THIS FORM.

12. PATIENT'S OR AUTHORIZED PERSONS'S SIGNATURE I authorize the release of any medical or other info necessary to process this claim. I also request payment of government benefits either to myself or the party who accepts assignment below. SIGNED SIGNATURE ON FILE DATE 11092009	13. PATIENT'S OR AUTHORIZED PERSONS'S SIGNATURE I authorize payment of medical benefits to the undersigned physician or supplier for services described below. SIGNED

14. DATE OF CURRENT: ◄ ILLNESS (First symptom) OR INJURY (Accident) OR PREGNANCY (LMP)	15. IF PATIENT HAS HAD SAME ILLNESS, GIVE FIRST DATE	16. DATES PATIENT UNABLE TO WORK IN CURRENT OCCUPATION FROM TO

17. NAME OF REFERRING PROVIDER OR OTHER SOURCE	17a. 17b. NPI	18. HOSPITALIZATION DATES RELATED TO CURRENT SERVICES FROM 11 06 2009 TO 11 09 2009

19. RESERVED FOR LOCAL USE	20. OUTSIDE LAB? ☐ YES ☒ NO $ CHARGES

21. DIAGNOSIS OR NATURE OF ILLNESS OR INJURY (RELATE ITEMS 1, 2, 3 OR 4 TO ITEM 24E BY LINE) 1. 427.31 3. 2. 4.	22. MEDICAID SUBMISSION CODE ORIGINAL REF. NO. 23. PRIOR AUTHORIZATION NUMBER

24. A. DATE(S) OF SERVICE From MM DD YY	To MM DD YY	B. Place of Service	C. EMG	D. PROCEDURES, SERVICES OR SUPPLIES (Explain Unusual Circumstances) CPT/HCPCS	MODIFIER	E. DIAGNOSIS POINTER	F. $ CHARGES	G. DAYS OR UNITS	H. EPSDT Family Plan	I. ID. QUAL	J. RENDERING PROVIDER ID#
1	11 06 2009		21		99221		1	145 00	1		NPI	999501
2	11 07 2009	11 08 2009	21		99231		1	158 00	2		NPI	999501
3	11 09 2009		21		99238		1	145 00	1		NPI	999501
4											NPI	
5											NPI	
6											NPI	

25. FEDERAL TAX I.D. NUMBER 00-1234560 SSN ☐ EIN ☒	26. PATIENT'S ACCOUNT NO. MUN001	27. ACCEPT ASSIGNMENT? ☒ YES ☐ NO	28. TOTAL CHARGE $ 448 00	29. AMOUNT PAID $	30. BALANCE DUE $

31. SIGNATURE OF PHYSICIAN OR SUPPLIER INCLUDING DEGREES OR CREDENTIALS (I certify that the statements on the reverse apply to this bill and are made a part thereof.) 11092009 SIGNED L. D. HEATH, MD DAT	32. SERVICE FACILITY LOCATION INFORMATION NEW YORK COUNTY HOSPITAL 1402 NORTHERN DR. KING PARK, NY 01238 a. 9997894320 b.	33. BILLING PROVIDER INFO PH # (123) 456-7890 DOUGLASVILLE MEDICINE ASSOCIATES 5076 BRAND BLVD., SUITE 401 DOUGLASVILLE, NY 01234 a. 9995010111 b.

NUCC Instruction Manual available at: www.nucc.org

OMB APPROVAL PENDING

FIGURE 7-23

Courtesy of the Centers for Medicare & Medicaid Services

STEP 7

Next, click on the *Transmit EMC button* to send the claims electronically to the clearinghouse/insurance carrier. An automated (simulated) upload will start and display a Transmission Status window, similar to the one shown in Figure 7-24.

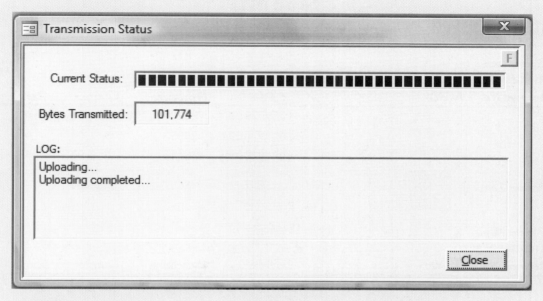

FIGURE 7-24

Delmar/Cengage Learning

STEP 8

When the transmission is complete, and the window reads that it has disconnected as shown in Figure 7-25, click on the *View button* to display the two-page report. Check your work with Figure 7-26 and Figure 7-27.

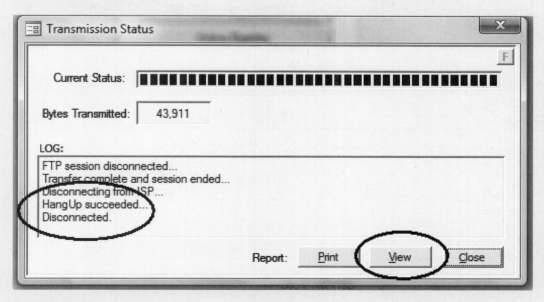

FIGURE 7-25

Delmar/Cengage Learning

continues

SENDING MEDICARE CLAIMS ELECTRONICALLY *continued*

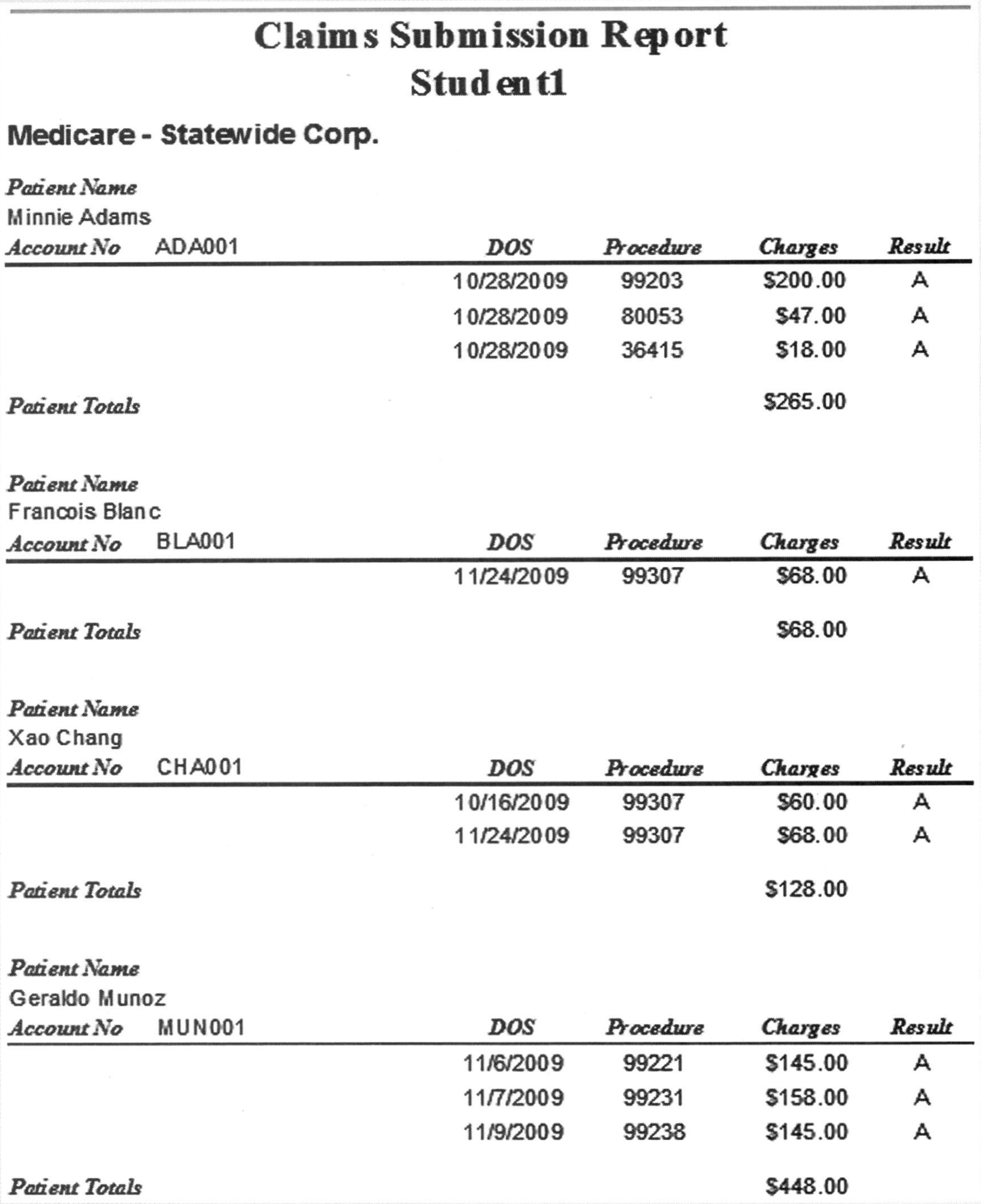

Claims Submission Report
Student1

Medicare - Statewide Corp.

Patient Name
Minnie Adams

Account No	ADA001	DOS	Procedure	Charges	Result
		10/28/2009	99203	$200.00	A
		10/28/2009	80053	$47.00	A
		10/28/2009	36415	$18.00	A
Patient Totals				$265.00	

Patient Name
Francois Blanc

Account No	BLA001	DOS	Procedure	Charges	Result
		11/24/2009	99307	$68.00	A
Patient Totals				$68.00	

Patient Name
Xao Chang

Account No	CHA001	DOS	Procedure	Charges	Result
		10/16/2009	99307	$60.00	A
		11/24/2009	99307	$68.00	A
Patient Totals				$128.00	

Patient Name
Geraldo Munoz

Account No	MUN001	DOS	Procedure	Charges	Result
		11/6/2009	99221	$145.00	A
		11/7/2009	99231	$158.00	A
		11/9/2009	99238	$145.00	A
Patient Totals				$448.00	

FIGURE 7-26

Delmar/Cengage Learning

Patient Name
Anna Pinkston

Account No	PIN001	DOS	Procedure	Charges	Result
		11/24/2009	99308	$113.00	A
Patient Totals				$113.00	

Patient Name
Paula Shektar

Account No	SHE001	DOS	Procedure	Charges	Result
		10/23/2009	99214	$180.00	A
Patient Totals				$180.00	

Patient Name
Marie Tomanaga

Account No	TOM001	DOS	Procedure	Charges	Result
		11/3/2009	99205	$358.00	A
		11/3/2009	93000	$131.00	A
		11/3/2009	85651	$9.00	A
		11/3/2009	36415	$18.00	A
Patient Totals				$516.00	

FIGURE 7-27
Delmar/Cengage Learning

STEP 9

Next, print pages one and two of the report to turn in to your instructor. When finished, close the open windows and return to the Main Menu.

LET'S TRY IT! 7-3 SENDING SIGNAL HMO CLAIMS ELECTRONICALLY

Objective: The reader selects Signal HMO patients of Drs. Heath and Schwartz and submits claims electronically.

STEP 1

Start MOSS by following your instructor's directions.

STEP 2

Click on the *Insurance Billing button* on the Main Menu.

STEP 3

Select the following settings:

continues

SENDING SIGNAL HMO CLAIMS ELECTRONICALLY *continued*

A. Sort by patient name (Field 1).

B. Bill for "All" providers (Field 2).

C. Select service dates 10/01/2009 through 11/30/2009 by entering the dates in the "From" and "Through" fields.

D. Select "All" patient names and "All" patient accounts.

E. Transmit type: Electronic

F. Billing Options: Primary

G. Payer selection: Single click on *Signal HMO* so that only patients with that insurance plan are selected. Check your screen with Figure 7-28 before proceeding.

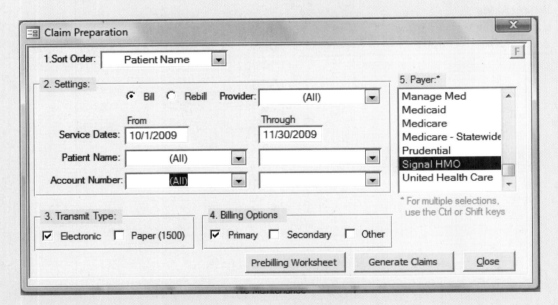

FIGURE 7-28

Delmar/Cengage Learning

STEP 4

Next, click the *Prebilling Worksheet button* to view the report of the claims that have been prepared for those dates and health plan. See Figure 7-29 to check your work. Be certain that if you see any errors, close the billing windows, and return to the patient account to make corrections where needed.

INSURANCE PREBILLING WORKSHEET
Student1

Dates of Service	Diag Code	Proc Code	POS	Units	Dr	As	Bill Amt	Receipts	Net
Signal HMO									
Beals, Kimberly									
11/3/2009	783.21	36415	11	1.00	D1	Y	$18.00	$0.00	$18.00
11/3/2009	783.21	80053	11	1.00	D1	Y	$47.00	$0.00	$47.00
11/3/2009	783.21	99204	11	1.00	D1	Y	$283.00	$10.00	$273.00
				Totals			$348.00	$10.00	$338.00
James, David									
11/9/2009	075	86308	11	1.00	D1	Y	$17.00	$0.00	$17.00
11/9/2009	075	99213	11	1.00	D1	Y	$111.00	$10.00	$101.00
				Totals			$128.00	$10.00	$118.00
Montner, Martin									
10/22/2009	034.0	87081	12	1.00	D2	Y	$16.00	$0.00	$16.00
10/22/2009	034.0	99204	11	1.00	D2	Y	$283.00	$10.00	$273.00
				Totals			$299.00	$10.00	$289.00
Shinn, Robert									
10/30/2009	382.9	99213	12	1.00	D1	Y	$111.00	$10.00	$101.00
				Totals			$111.00	$10.00	$101.00
Villanova, Ricky									
10/27/2009	250.00	82947	11	1.00	D2	Y	$19.00	$0.00	$19.00
10/27/2009	250.00	99201	11	1.00	D2	Y	$130.00	$10.00	$120.00
				Totals			$149.00	$10.00	$139.00
	TOTAL TO BE BILLED FOR Signal HMO								$985.00
Grand Total			Grand Total						$985.00

FIGURE 7-29

Delmar/Cengage Learning

STEP 5

Next, click on the *Print icon* (top left corner) so that you and your instructor may have a copy of the Insurance Prebilling Worksheet. When done, close the window for the worksheet. This will return you to the Claim Preparation window.

STEP 6

The claim forms are now ready to be generated. Click on the *Generate Claims button*. Once the CMS-1500 claim forms are displayed, scroll to the bottom half of each patient's form and check the dates, procedures, and fees being charged with the information on the Insurance Prebilling Worksheet you printed in Step 5. Again, if any errors are found, click on the *Claim Prep button* and then close any open windows and return to the areas of MOSS where corrections are required. If all data is correct, continue to Step 7.

continues

SENDING SIGNAL HMO CLAIMS ELECTRONICALLY *continued*

STEP 7

Next, click on the *Transmit EMC button* to send the claims electronically to the clearinghouse/insurance carrier. An automated (simulated) upload will start and display a Transmission Status window.

STEP 8

When the transmission is complete, and the window reads that it has disconnected, click on the *View button* to display the two-page report. Check your work with Figure 7-30 and Figure 7-31.

Claims Submission Report
Student1

Signal HMO

Patient Name
Kimberly Beals

Account No	BEA001	DOS	Procedure	Charges	Result
		11/3/2009	99204	$283.00	A
		11/3/2009	80053	$47.00	A
		11/3/2009	36415	$18.00	A
Patient Totals				$348.00	

Patient Name
David James

Account No	JAM001	DOS	Procedure	Charges	Result
		11/9/2009	99213	$111.00	A
		11/9/2009	86308	$17.00	A
Patient Totals				$128.00	

Patient Name
Martin Montner

Account No	MON001	DOS	Procedure	Charges	Result
		10/22/2009	99204	$283.00	A
		10/22/2009	87081	$16.00	A
Patient Totals				$299.00	

Patient Name
Robert Shinn

Account No	SHI001	DOS	Procedure	Charges	Result
		10/30/2009	99213	$111.00	A
Patient Totals				$111.00	

FIGURE 7-30

Delmar/Cengage Learning

Patient Name					
Ricky Villanova					
Account No VIL001		DOS	Procedure	Charges	Result
		10/27/2009	99201	$130.00	A
		10/27/2009	82947	$19.00	A
Patient Totals				$149.00	

FIGURE 7-31

Delmar/Cengage Learning

STEP 9

Next, print pages one and two of the report to turn in to your instructor. When finished, close the open windows and return to the Main Menu.

LET'S TRY IT! 7-4 SENDING FLEXIHEALTH PPO IN-NETWORK CLAIMS ELECTRONICALLY

Objective: The reader selects FlexiHealth PPO In-Network patients of Dr. Heath and submits claims electronically.

STEP 1
Start MOSS by following your instructor's directions.

STEP 2
Click on the *Insurance Billing button* on the Main Menu.

STEP 3
Select the following settings:

A.   Sort by patient name (Field 1).

> **NT:** Recall that Dr. Heath cepts FlexiHealth PPO insur- ce as a participating provider, t not Dr. Schwartz.

B.   Bill for "Dr. Heath" as provider (Field 2).

C.   Select service dates 10/01/2009 through 11/30/2009 by entering the dates in the "From" and "Through" fields.

D.   Select "All" patient names and "All" patient accounts.

E.   Transmit type: Electronic

F.   Billing Options: Primary

G.   Payer selection: Single click on *FlexiHealth PPO In-Network* so that only patients with that insurance plan are selected. Check your screen with Figure 7-32 before proceeding.

continues

SENDING FLEXIHEALTH PPO IN-NETWORK CLAIMS ELECTRONICALLY *continued*

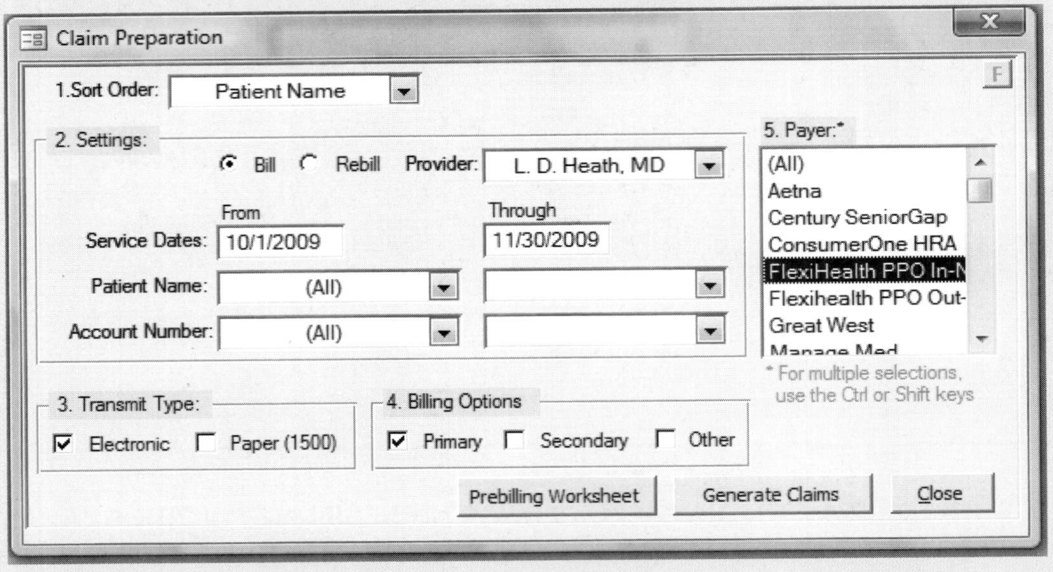

FIGURE 7-32

Delmar/Cengage Learning

STEP 4

Next, click the *Prebilling Worksheet button* to view the report of the claims that have been prepared for those dates and health plan. See Figure 7-33 and Figure 7-34 to check your work. Be certain that if you see any errors, to close any open windows and return to the areas of MOSS where corrections are needed.

STEP 5

Next, click on the *Print icon* so that you and your instructor may have a copy of the Insurance Prebilling Worksheet. When done, close the window for the worksheet. This will return you to the Claim Preparation window.

STEP 6

The claim forms are now ready to be generated. Click on the *Generate Claims button*. Once the CMS-1500 claim forms are displayed, scroll to the bottom half of each patient's form and check the dates, procedures, and fees being charged with the information on the Insurance Prebilling Worksheet you printed in Step 5. Again, if any errors are found, click on the *Claim Prep button* and then close any open windows and return to the areas of MOSS where corrections are required. If all data is correct, continue to Step 7.

STEP 7

Next, click on the *Transmit EMC button* to send the claims electronically to the clearinghouse/insurance carrier. An automated (simulated) upload will start and display a Transmission Status window.

INSURANCE PREBILLING WORKSHEET
Student1

Dates of Service	Diag Code	Proc Code	POS	Units	Dr	As	Bill Amt	Receipts	Net
FlexiHealth PPO In-Network									
Kinzler, Linda									
11/9/2009	493.90	90658	11	1.00	D1	Y	$22.00	$22.00	$0.00
11/9/2009	493.90	99203	11	1.00	D1	Y	$200.00	$20.00	$180.00
					Totals		$222.00	$42.00	$180.00
Mallory, Christina									
11/14/2009	995.29	99221	21	1.00	D1	Y	$145.00	$0.00	$145.00
11/15/2009	995.29	99238	21	1.00	D1	Y	$145.00	$0.00	$145.00
					Totals		$290.00	$0.00	$290.00
Practice, Patty									
10/28/2009	780.6	99213	11	1.00	D1	Y	$111.00	$20.00	$91.00
					Totals		$111.00	$20.00	$91.00
Ruhl, Mary									
11/5/2009	558.9	99221	21	1.00	D1	Y	$145.00	$0.00	$145.00
11/6/2009	558.9	99231	21	4.00	D1	Y	$316.00	$0.00	$316.00
11/10/2009	558.9	99238	21	1.00	D1	Y	$145.00	$0.00	$145.00
					Totals		$606.00	$0.00	$606.00
Tate, Jason									
11/3/2009	536.9	99221	21	1.00	D1	Y	$145.00	$0.00	$145.00
11/4/2009	536.9	99231	21	1.00	D1	Y	$79.00	$0.00	$79.00
11/5/2009	536.9	99238	21	1.00	D1	Y	$145.00	$0.00	$145.00
					Totals		$369.00	$0.00	$369.00
Worthington, Cynthia									
10/30/2009	782.1	99213	11	1.00	D1	Y	$111.00	$20.00	$91.00
					Totals		$111.00	$20.00	$91.00

FIGURE 7-33

Delmar/Cengage Learning

Dates of Service	Diag Code	Proc Code	POS	Units	Dr	As	Bill Amt	Receipts	Net
		TOTAL TO BE BILLED FOR FlexiHealth PPO In-Network							$1,627.00
Grand Total		**Grand Total**							$1,627.00

FIGURE 7-34

Delmar/Cengage Learning

continues

SENDING FLEXIHEALTH PPO IN-NETWORK CLAIMS
ELECTRONICALLY *continued*

STEP 8

When the transmission is complete, and the window reads that it has disconnected, click on the View button to display the two-page report. Check your work with Figure 7-35 and Figure 7-36.

STEP 9

Next, print pages one and two of the report to turn in to your instructor. When finished, close the open windows and return to the Main Menu.

Claims Submission Report
Student1

FlexiHealth PPO In-Network

Patient Name
Linda Kinzler

Account No KIN001	*DOS*	*Procedure*	*Charges*	*Result*
	11/9/2009	99203	$200.00	A
	11/9/2009	90658	$22.00	A
Patient Totals			$222.00	

Patient Name
Christina Mallory

Account No MAL001	*DOS*	*Procedure*	*Charges*	*Result*
	11/14/2009	99221	$145.00	A
	11/15/2009	99238	$145.00	A
Patient Totals			$290.00	

Patient Name
Patty Practice

Account No PRA002	*DOS*	*Procedure*	*Charges*	*Result*
	10/28/2009	99213	$111.00	A
Patient Totals			$111.00	

Patient Name
Mary Ruhl

Account No RUH001	*DOS*	*Procedure*	*Charges*	*Result*
	11/5/2009	99221	$145.00	A
	11/6/2009	99231	$316.00	A
	11/10/2009	99238	$145.00	A
Patient Totals			$606.00	

FIGURE 7-35

Delmar/Cengage Learning

Patient Name
Jason Tate

Account No TAT001	DOS	Procedure	Charges	Result
	11/3/2009	99221	$145.00	A
	11/4/2009	99231	$79.00	A
	11/5/2009	99238	$145.00	A
Patient Totals			$369.00	

Patient Name
Cynthia Worthington

Account No WOR001	DOS	Procedure	Charges	Result
	10/30/2009	99213	$111.00	A
Patient Totals			$111.00	

FIGURE 7-36

Delmar/Cengage Learning

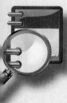

LET'S TRY IT! 7-5 SENDING FLEXIHEALTH PPO OUT-OF-NETWORK CLAIMS ELECTRONICALLY

Objective: The reader selects FlexiHealth PPO out-of-network patients of Dr. Schwarz and submits claims electronically.

STEP 1
Start MOSS by following your instructor's directions.

STEP 2
Click on the *Insurance Billing button* on the Main Menu.

STEP 3
Select the following settings:

A. Sort by patient name (Field 1).

> **HINT:** Recall that Dr. Schwartz does not accept FlexiHealth PPO insurance and is a non-participating provider.

B. Bill for "Dr. Schwartz" as provider (Field 2).

C. Select service dates 10/01/2009 through 11/30/2009 by entering the dates in the "From" and "Through" fields.

D. Select "All" patient names and "All" patient accounts.

E. Transmit type: Electronic

F. Billing Options: Primary

continues

SENDING FLEXIHEALTH PPO OUT-OF-NETWORK CLAIMS
ELECTRONICALLY *continued*

G. Payer selection: Single click on *FlexiHealth PPO Out-of-Network* so that only patients with that insurance plan are selected. Check your screen with Figure 7-37 before proceeding.

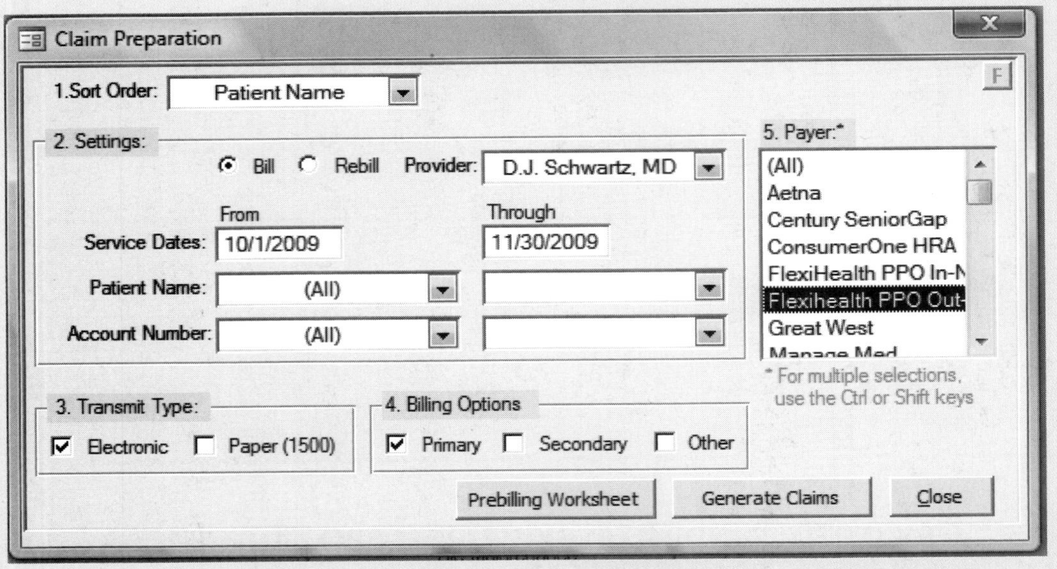

FIGURE 7-37

Delmar/Cengage Learning

STEP 4

Next, click the *Prebilling Worksheet button* to view the report of the claims that have been prepared for those dates and health plan. See Figure 7-38 to check your work. Be certain that if you see any errors, close any open windows and return to the areas of MOSS where corrections are needed.

INSURANCE PREBILLING WORKSHEET
Student1

Dates of Service	Diag Code	Proc Code	POS	Units	Dr	As	Bill Amt	Receipts	Net
Flexihealth PPO Out-of-Netwo									
Kramer, Stanley									
10/29/2009	486	99231	11	2.00	D2	N	$158.00	$0.00	$158.00
10/30/2009	486	99212	11	1.00	D2	N	$80.00	$0.00	$80.00
						Totals	$238.00	$0.00	$238.00
Manaly, Richard									
10/21/2009	250.00	99213	11	1.00	D2	N	$111.00	$0.00	$111.00
						Totals	$111.00	$0.00	$111.00
Ybarra, Elane									
10/16/2009	034.0	87081	11	1.00	D2	N	$16.00	$0.00	$16.00
10/16/2009	034.0	99214	11	1.00	D2	N	$180.00	$0.00	$180.00
11/6/2009	599.0	81000	11	1.00	D2	N	$12.00	$0.00	$12.00
11/6/2009	599.0	99215	11	1.00	D2	N	$249.00	$0.00	$249.00
						Totals	$457.00	$0.00	$457.00
		TOTAL TO BE BILLED FOR Flexihealth PPO Out-of-Network							$806.00
Grand Total		Grand Total							$806.00

FIGURE 7-38

Delmar/Cengage Learning

STEP 5

Next, click on the Print icon so that you and your instructor may have a copy of the Insurance Prebilling Worksheet. When done, close the window for the worksheet. This will return you to the Claim Preparation window.

STEP 6

The claim forms are now ready to be generated. Click on the *Generate Claims button*. Once the CMS-1500 claim forms are displayed, scroll to the bottom half of each patient's form and check the dates, procedures, and fees being charged with the information on the Insurance Prebilling Worksheet you printed in Step 5. Again, if any errors are found, click on the *Claim Prep button* and then close any open windows and return to the areas of MOSS where corrections are required. If all data is correct, continue to Step 7.

STEP 7

Next, click on the *Transmit EMC button* to send the claims electronically to the clearinghouse/insurance carrier. An automated (simulated) upload will start and display a Transmission Status window.

STEP 8

When the transmission is complete, and the window reads that it has disconnected, click on the View button to display the two-page report. Check your work with Figure 7-39.

Claims Submission Report
Student1

Flexihealth PPO Out-of-Network

Patient Name
Stanley Kramer

Account No	KRA001	DOS	Procedure	Charges	Result
		10/29/2009	99231	$158.00	A
		10/30/2009	99212	$80.00	A
Patient Totals				$238.00	

Patient Name
Richard Manaly

Account No	MAN002	DOS	Procedure	Charges	Result
		10/21/2009	99213	$111.00	A
Patient Totals				$111.00	

Patient Name
Elane Ybarra

Account No	YBA001	DOS	Procedure	Charges	Result
		10/16/2009	99214	$180.00	A
		10/16/2009	87081	$16.00	A
		11/6/2009	99215	$249.00	A
		11/6/2009	81000	$12.00	A
Patient Totals				$457.00	

FIGURE 7-39

Delmar/Cengage Learning

continues

SENDING FLEXIHEALTH PPO OUT-OF-NETWORK CLAIMS ELECTRONICALLY *continued*

STEP 9
Next, print page one to turn in to your instructor. When finished, close the open windows and return to the Main Menu.

FINAL NOTES

Whether billing medical claims using paper or electronic transmission, the importance of all tasks that came before becomes clear when reviewing claims for submission. Any error or omission along the way, be it an error in the patient's or insured's name, identification numbers, health plan entries, or even procedure posting, will have a significant effect on medical billing. Diligent and accurate collection of information, and the proper use of that information within the practice management software, is essential for good reimbursement.

Additionally, good management of office procedures and software use greatly reduces denied or problem claims. This, in turn, limits the amount of insurance follow-up and tracing to be done. It is far better to use time and energy to pursue insurance claims that require legitimate attention, rather than those that result from poor administrative practices.

As mentioned previously, the medical staff, including you as a new employee, will become familiar with the health plans and billing nuances of a particular specialty or area. Be sure to read the insurance provider manuals located in your office. Furthermore, seek guidance from a supervisor when needed, and always follow the office policies of your employer. Each medical specialty is sure to have its own specific requirements.

CHECK YOUR KNOWLEDGE

1. Name the three steps involved in the claims management process.

_____
_____
_____

2. Explain, and give examples, why timely submission of claims to insurance companies is recommended for a medical office.

_____
_____
_____

3. Explain the differences, advantages, or disadvantages of electronic claims submission versus billing with paper claims.

_____

_____

_____

4. Provide examples where paper claims might be necessary over electronic claims submissions.

_____

_____

_____

5. Explain why it is not recommended to automatically rebill outstanding claims every 30 to 45 days.

_____

_____

_____

6. There are a number of items insurance companies require in order to process medical billing claims. List at least eight of these items.

_____

_____

_____

7. Describe the NPI number.

_____

_____

_____

8. Describe the advantages of the implementation of the NPI.

_____

_____

_____

9. What type of provider must use the NPI?

_____

_____

_____

10. Describe two specific factors that greatly reduce denied claims and limit the amount of insurance follow-up and tracing to be done.

_____

_____

_____

Refer to the CMS-1500 claim form in Figure 7-1. Use the form to answer questions 11 through 19.

11. In which box is the insured's identification number provided?

_____

_____

_____

12. Which box provides the name of the patient for whom services are being billed?

_____

_____

_____

13. If a patient receives benefits as a dependent on a health plan, in which box will the policyholder's name appear?

_____

_____

_____

14. Which boxes are used to provide the dates a patient was hospitalized related to the services being billed?

_____

_____

_____

15. The diagnoses for the patient are provided in which box?

_____

_____

_____

16. Which box is used to enter the dates of service for each procedure being billed?

_____

_____

_____

17. Medicare providers must always answer YES or NO in Box 27. Is this a true statement? Explain your answer.

_____

_____

_____

18. The CPT code for each procedure being billed is provided in which box?

_____

_____

_____

19. Which box identifies the provider/practice information?

_____

_____

_____

Posting Payments and Secondary Insurance Billing

OBJECTIVES

Upon completion of this unit, the reader should be able to:

- **Describe the components of a Medicare Remittance Advice (RA) and a general Explanation of Benefits (EOB)**

- **Read and decipher a sample Medicare RA and general EOBs in preparation for payment posting**

- **Demonstrate posting payments as indicated on the Medicare RA and PPO/HRA EOBs, using *Medical Office Simulation Software* (MOSS)**

- **Prepare and process claims for secondary billing using MOSS.**

Throughout the month, various payments are received by the medical office. These include reimbursement from insurance companies for claims that were submitted either electronically, or on paper claim forms. Patients also send payments for portions that are due from them. Each of these payments needs to be properly applied to the respective patient account. For patients with dual insurance coverage, payment from the primary health plan initiates the process for the secondary health plan to be billed. For patients with one health plan, there may be remaining balances due that need to be billed directly to the patient. Of course, any adjustments, discounts, or other write-offs should be accounted for according to contractual (or other) agreement.

While learning to enter procedure charges in Unit 7, you had an opportunity to begin using the posting payment window to record payments made at the time of service. In this unit, you will use the methods you learned to post these payments and take it a step further, using

KEY TERMS

Birthday Rule

Coordination of Benefits (COB)

Electronic payment and statement (EPS) system

Explanation of Benefits (EOB)

Large group health plan (LGHP)

Liability insurance

No-fault

Remittance Advice (RA)

Usual, customary, and reasonable (UCR) expenses

Workers' compensation

MOSS. Here, you receive payments from insurance companies, read the explanation of benefits, and then post the payments, including adjustments, accordingly.

PAYMENTS FROM INSURANCE COMPANIES

Information regarding claims that were sent either electronically or on paper claim forms is documented and returned to the medical office by the insurance carrier. These documents are referred to as the **Explanation of Benefits (EOB)**, or a **Remittance Advice (RA)**. The EOB, or RA, is accompanied by a check for the payment, unless the medical office has arranged to participate in an **Electronic Payment and Statement (EPS) system**. This type of service will transfer payments made on claims directly to the medical provider's financial institution by way of a clearinghouse. In addition, an electronic version of the RA can be downloaded, and is often easily integrated with most practice management software programs, including automated payment posting capabilities. Even if the office prefers manual posting of payments to patient accounts, it is possible to view, download, and print hard copies of the RA for this purpose.

Often, the payment made by an insurance company will be a lump sum, a portion of which applies to several patients. The EOB or RA lists the individual patients and details about the payment. Typically, only certain staff members, perhaps even the office manager, are responsible for posting payments. The person who posts payments ensures that the correct portion that applies to each patient is posted. Accuracy is very important so that secondary billing and patient billing for any balance due can be completed.

COMPONENTS OF THE EXPLANATION OF BENEFITS

While EOBs from various insurance carriers may look different from each other, they have several basic components in common. These include the following:

1. Patient's name who received service(s), including identification number

2. Provider or practice name that rendered services

3. Dates the service(s) was/were rendered, as provided on the claim

4. CPT codes, or a description, for each service for which a claim was submitted

5. Amount approved, and payment made, toward each service, including applicable adjustments

6. Reason codes or notes which provide additional details explaining the payment, or why a claim was denied, or its status

7. Additional information may be provided, according to the requirements of the health plan or contracts.

The sample Medicare RA illustrated in Figure 8-1 is a good place to begin orientation for reading insurance EOBs. This sample illustrates only the most pertinent sections of a Medicare RA and contains essential information for posting payments. Your instructor may have examples of actual Medicare RAs that best illustrate local carriers, reason codes, and procedures from various specialty practices.

The list that follows guides you through each section of the Medicare RA. Refer to Figure 8-1 while reviewing each item and its purpose.

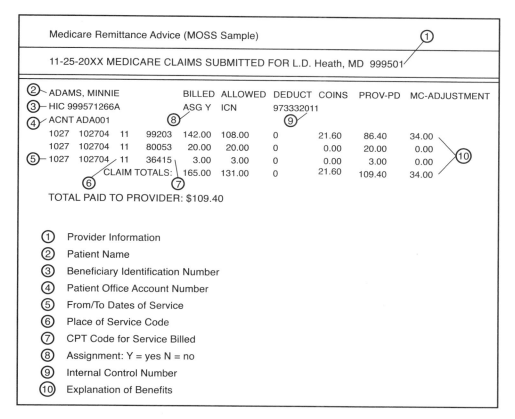

FIGURE 8-1

Basic components of the Medicare Remittance Advice (RA). *Delmar/Cengage Learning*

1. **Provider information.** This line identifies the Medicare provider for which payment details have been sent.

2. **Patient name.** Identifies the Medicare beneficiary this claim pertains to.

3. **Health Insurance Claim (HIC) number.** As discussed in a previous unit, this is the identification number of the Medicare beneficiary.

4. **ACNT number.** This is the Medicare beneficiary's account number at the medical office. The medical office provided this number on the claim form. It can be used to easily retrieve the patient account from the software database.

5. **Date of Service (DOS).** The first date is the "From" date, representing the month and day. As shown in this example, 1027 is October 27. The date directly to the right is the "To" date and includes the year: 102704, or October 27, 2004. Since the "From" and "To" dates are exactly the same, it means the service was provided on that date only.

6. **Place of Service (POS) code.** The POS code indicates where the service was provided. These codes are the same as those submitted on the claim form by the medical office and follow the Center for Medicare & Medicaid Services guidelines.

7. **CPT code.** Each procedure billed is listed with the corresponding CPT code.

8. **Assignment (ASG).** A "Y" for yes or "N" for no indicates whether the provider accepts assignment on the claim.

9. **Internal Control Number (ICN).** A number used internally by Medicare to identify the claim.

10. **Explanation of benefits.** There are five columns that explain details of the claim for each service, as follows:

   A. **BILLED.** This column shows the amount billed as submitted on the claim for each CPT code.

   B. **ALLOWED.** This column shows the amount allowed by Medicare for each service. Most insurance plans, including Medicare, pay a percentage of this amount, based on the health plan's usual, customary, and reasonable (UCR) expenses, approved fee schedule, or other negotiated payment agreements.

   C. **DEDUCT.** If any amount was applied towards the deductible, it appears in this column.

   D. **COINS.** Shows the co-insurance portion due from the patient. This amount may also be billed to the secondary insurance plan if the patient has dual coverage.

   E. **PROV-PD.** The amount the provider was paid for each individual procedure listed in the column. Notice the "Claim Totals" line along the bottom.

   F. **MC-ADJUSTMENT.** Shows the amount that must be written off the account as required by Medicare. This usually includes amounts over the Medicare allowable that cannot be collected by participating Medicare providers (or providers located in states that do not permit collecting any amount over the allowable).

As mentioned previously, EOBs from different carriers are formatted differently. However, the Medicare sample contains most of the basic components found on EOBs in general. Included in this unit are EOBs from Medicare, the FlexiHealth PPO Plan, and ConsumerONE HRA, containing benefits and payment information for services billed in Unit 7. If you have not completed the *Let's Try It!* exercises from Unit 7, *do not proceed.* These are required to continue.

POSTING MEDICARE PAYMENTS

The exercises that follow begin with posting Medicare payments. It is still common to post payments using the RA that accompanies the reimbursement check from Medicare. However, there are an increasing number of automated posting systems available that interface with practice management software. Nevertheless, learning to interpret and post payments directly from the RA will help in identifying errors and problems that may arise with automated posting systems. In addition, knowledge of posting will help you understand customized settings for these systems.

LET'S TRY IT! 8-1 POSTING MEDICARE PAYMENTS—ADAMS, MINNIE

Objective: The user reads the Medicare RA notice for patient Minnie Adams (Source Document 8-1) and posts payments, as indicated, to the patient's account.

STEP 1
Start MOSS.

STEP 2
Refer to the Medicare RA notice shown in Source Document 8-1 in the Source Document Appendix. There are three beneficiaries listed. Locate Minnie Adams and review the following. *Cover the answers using the tear-off bookmark from the cover of your book. Check your work before entering data into MOSS to be sure you have correctly interpreted the source documents.*

A.	What is patient Adams's Medicare number? What is her account number at the medical office?	**Medicare Number: 999571266A. ADA001 is the account number.**
B.	Which provider is listed for these services and was assignment accepted?	**L.D. Heath, MD. Assignment was accepted.**
C.	What is the Internal Control Number for these services? This number is used as a reference for posting payments.	**ICN 973332011**
D.	Find the date(s) of service. On which date(s) was service provided?	**10/28/2009**
E.	What code for POS is indicated for patient Adams? What type of place does this code represent?	**11. Office**
F.	To the right of each POS code is the CPT code that was billed for services rendered. Which three CPT service codes are listed?	**99203, 80053, 36415**

Finally, to the right of the CPT codes are columns which contain the amount billed, how much Medicare allowed, the amount that was applied to the deductible (DEDUCT), the patient's co-insurance responsibility (COINS), how much the provider was paid (PROV-PD), and the required Medicare adjustment (MC-ADJUSTMENT). **Identify these amounts in the spaces below to be used in the following steps to post the payment.** *Cover the answers below using the tear-off bookmark from the cover of your book.*

Code:	Billed:	Allowed:	Deductible:	Co-ins:	Provider paid:	Adjustment:

Code:	Billed:	Allowed:	Deductible:	Co-ins:	Provider paid:	Adjustment:
99203	$200.00	$106.99	$0.00	$21.40	$85.59	$93.01
80053	$47.00	$14.77	$0.00	$0.00	$14.77	$32.23
36415	$18.00	$3.00	$0.00	$0.00	$3.00	$15.00

continues

POSTING MEDICARE PAYMENTS—ADAMS, MINNIE *continued*

STEP 3

Click on the **Posting Payments button** on the Main Menu. The Patient Selection window opens.

STEP 4

Select Minnie Adams from the patient list by single clicking on her *name*, then clicking on the *Apply Payment button*. You may also retrieve her account by using the account number provided on the Medicare RA. Compare your screen to Figure 8-2.

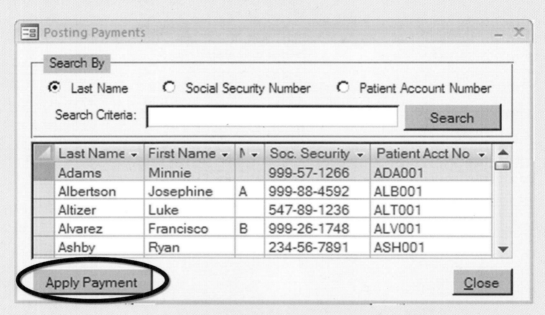

FIGURE 8-2

Delmar/Cengage Learning

STEP 5

Start by reading across the first line for CPT 99203 on the RA for patient Adams. The amount billed was $200.00 (which is shown for this procedure code on Source Document 8-1). Of that amount, $106.99 was allowed. Medicare pays 80% of the allowed amount, so the provider was paid $85.59. The patient's co-insurance is $21.40, which will be billed to a secondary insurance, if there is one, or directly to the patient. Since Dr. Heath is PAR and has agreed to accept the Medicare allowable as the full charge for services, the $93.01 in the adjustment column is the write-off. These components will now be posted to the patient account.

STEP 6

Single click the *line entry* in the Procedure Charge History area that contains CPT 99203 on 10/28/2009. Then, click on the *Select/Edit button*. The Balance Due Field 13 should show $200.00. Check your screen with Figure 8-3.

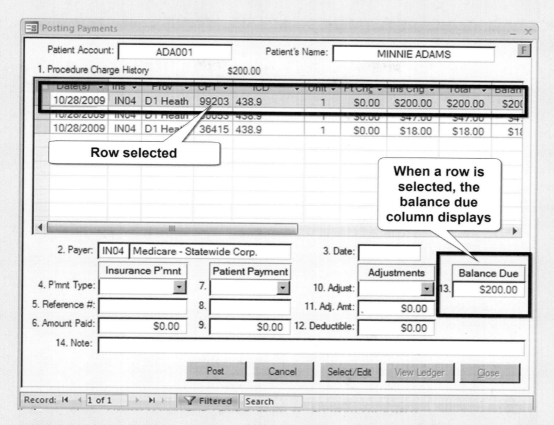

FIGURE 8-3

Delmar/Cengage Learning

STEP 7

Next, enter the date of posting in Field 3, which is 11/30/2009. Drop down the box for Field 4 on the Payment Entry window. Select *PAYINS*, since this is a Medicare payment. In Field 5, Reference #, enter the ICN provided on the RA for patient Adams. See Figure 8-4.

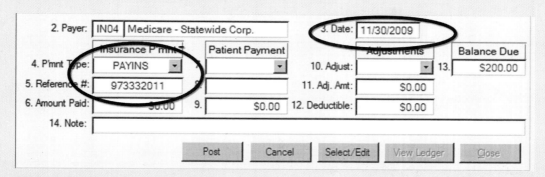

FIGURE 8-4

Delmar/Cengage Learning

continues

POSTING MEDICARE PAYMENTS—ADAMS, MINNIE *continued*

STEP 8

In Field 6, Amount Paid, enter the Medicare payment of $85.59. Press *Enter*. The Balance Due should now show a balance of $114.41.

STEP 9

The patient is not going to pay anything at this time, so Fields 7, 8, and 9 are not used. The adjustment is entered next. Drop down the box at Field 10 and select *ADJINS*, meaning this is an insurance adjustment. Click *Enter* or *Tab* to move to Field 11 and enter the $93.01 adjustment, as indicated on the RA. Press *Enter*. The balance due should now reflect $21.40, which is the patient's co-insurance amount. Check your work with Figure 8-5 before proceeding and make corrections if needed.

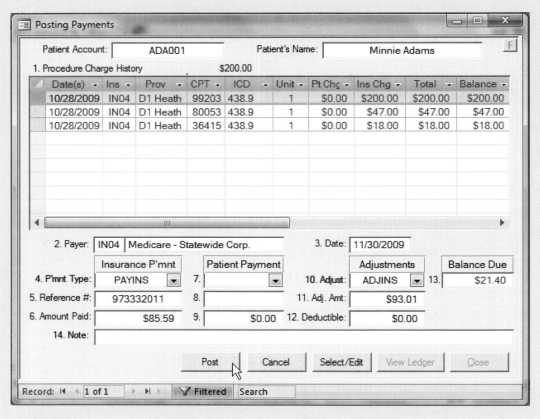

FIGURE 8-5

Delmar/Cengage Learning

MOSS NOTE: MOSS 2.0 does not allow corrections to posted payments. Be sure all information is correct prior to posting.

STEP 10

Next, click on the *Post button* to apply the payment and adjustment. Click on the *View Ledger button* to review the posting. Check your screen with Figure 8-6. Close the ledger when finished.

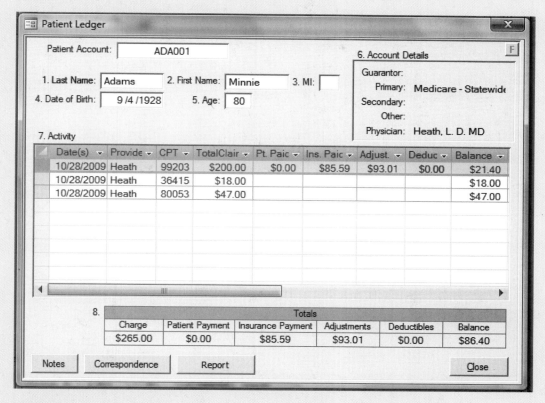

FIGURE 8-6

Delmar/Cengage Learning

STEP 11

There are still two more services with payments to be posted for patient Adams. Using the same methods just learned, post the payment for each line entry. Continue to use the posting date of 11/30/2009. Take care that the correct line has been selected for payment application. Compare your Completed Payment entry screen for procedure code 80053 with Figure 8-7. Make corrections before posting the payment.

continues

POSTING MEDICARE PAYMENTS—ADAMS, MINNIE *continued*

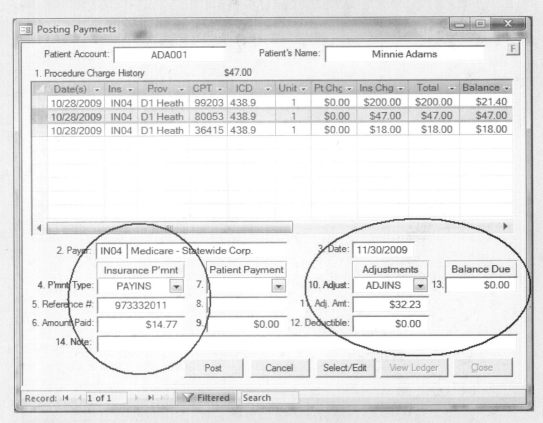

FIGURE 8-7

Delmar/Cengage Learning

STEP 12

View the Patient Ledger, and compare your work to Figure 8-8.

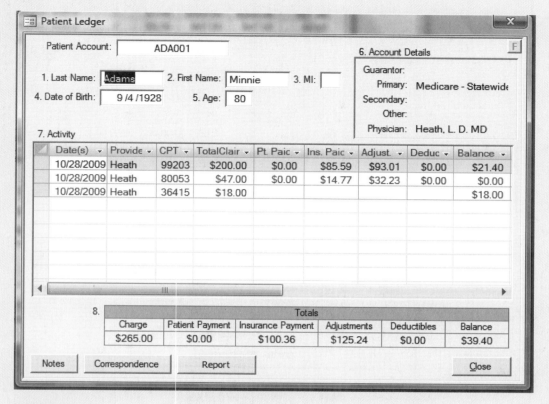

FIGURE 8-8

Delmar/Cengage Learning

STEP 13

Post the last procedure 36415 for patient Adams. Continue to use the posting date of 11/30/2009. Take care that the correct line has been selected for payment application.

STEP 14

Compare your Completed Payment entry screen for procedure code 36415 with Figure 8-9. Make corrections before posting the payment.

continues

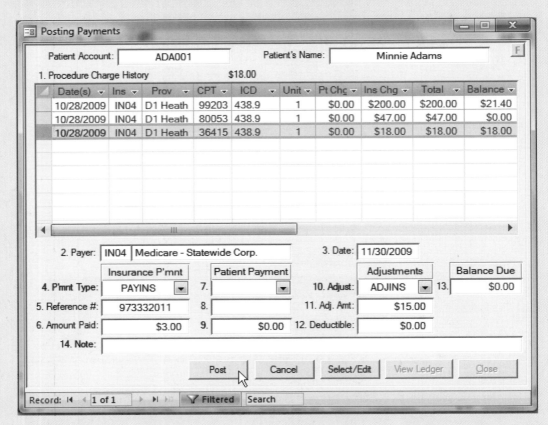

FIGURE 8-9

Delmar/Cengage Learning

STEP 15

View the Patient Ledger, and compare your work to Figure 8-10.

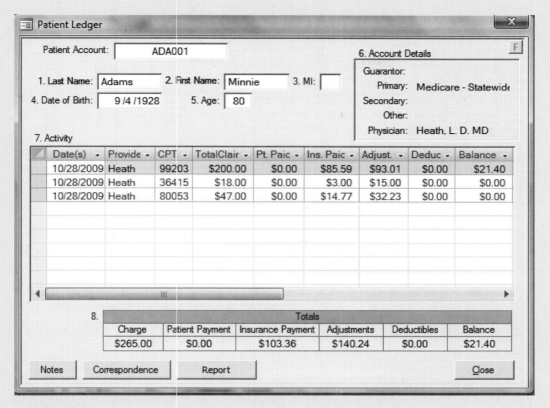

FIGURE 8-10

Delmar/Cengage Learning

STEP 16

All payments for Medicare have been completed for patient Adams. Click on the *Close button* on all open windows and return to the Main Menu.

LET'S TRY IT! 8-2 **POSTING MEDICARE PAYMENTS—BLANC, FRANCOIS**

Objective: The user reads the Medicare RA notice for Francois Blanc (Source Document 8-1) and posts payments as indicated to the patient's account.

STEP 1

Start MOSS.

continues

POSTING MEDICARE PAYMENTS—BLANC, FRANCOIS *continued*

STEP 2
Refer to the Medicare RA notice in Source Document 8-1. Locate Francois Blanc and review the following.

A.	What is patient Blanc's Medicare number? What is his account number at the medical office?	The Medicare number is: 999135611A. BLA001 is the account number.
B.	Which provider is listed for these services and was assignment accepted?	L.D. Heath, MD. Assignment was accepted.
C.	What is the Internal Control Number for these services? This number is used as a reference for posting payments.	ICN 973332012
D.	Find the date(s) of service. On which date(s) was service provided?	10/27/2009 and 11/24/2009
E.	What code for POS is indicated for patient Blanc? What type of place does this code represent?	31. Skilled Nursing Facility
F.	To the right of each POS code is the CPT code that was billed for services rendered. Which two CPT service codes are listed?	99307

Finally, to the right of the CPT codes are columns which contain the amount billed, how much Medicare allowed, the amount that was applied to the deductible (DEDUCT), the patient's co-insurance responsibility (COINS), how much the provider was paid (PROV-PD), and the required Medicare adjustment (MC-ADJUSTMENT). **Identify these amounts in the spaces below to be used in the following steps to post the payment.** *Cover the answers below using the tear-off bookmark from the cover of your book.*

Code:	Billed:	Allowed:	Deductible:	Co-ins:	Provider paid:	Adjustment:

Code:	Billed:	Allowed:	Deductible:	Co-ins:	Provider paid:	Adjustment:
99307	$60.00	$35.62	$0.00	$7.12	$28.50	$24.38
99307	$68.00	$35.62	$0.00	$7.12	$28.50	$32.38

STEP 3
Click on the *Posting Payments button* on the Main Menu. The Patient Selection window opens.

STEP 4
Select Francois Blanc from the patient list by single clicking on his name, then clicking on the Apply Payment button. You may also retrieve his account by using the account number provided on the Medicare RA. Compare your screen to Figure 8-11.

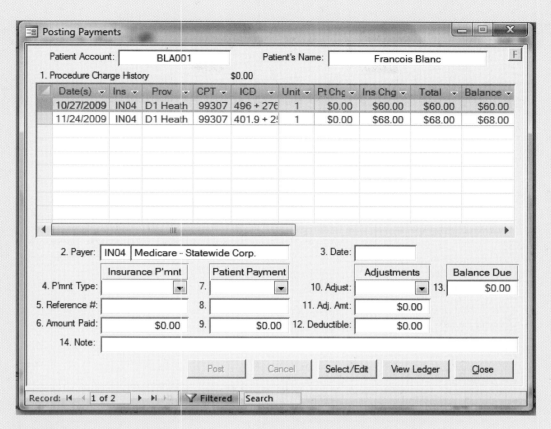

FIGURE 8-11

Delmar/Cengage Learning

STEP 5

Start by reading across the first line on the RA for CPT 99307 on DOS 10/27/09 for patient Blanc. The amount billed was $60.00 (which is shown for this procedure code on Source Document 8-1). Of that amount, $35.62 was allowed. Medicare pays 80% of the allowed amount, so the provider was paid $28.50. The patient's co-insurance is $7.12, which in this case, the Medicare RA shows a message that the claim information has been forwarded to Medicaid. This indicates *crossover* of the claim by the primary insurance to the secondary for the remainder balance due, and no further secondary billing is needed. Since Dr. Heath is PAR and has agreed to accept the Medicare allowable as the full charge for services, the $24.38 in the adjustment column is the write-off. These components will now be posted to the patient account.

STEP 6

Single click the *line entry* in the Procedure Charge History area that contains CPT 99307 on 10/27/2009. Then, click on the *Select/Edit button*. The Balance Due Field 13 should show $60.00. Next, enter the date of posting in Field 3, which is 11/30/2009. Check your screen with Figure 8-12.

continues

POSTING MEDICARE PAYMENTS—BLANC, FRANCOIS *continued*

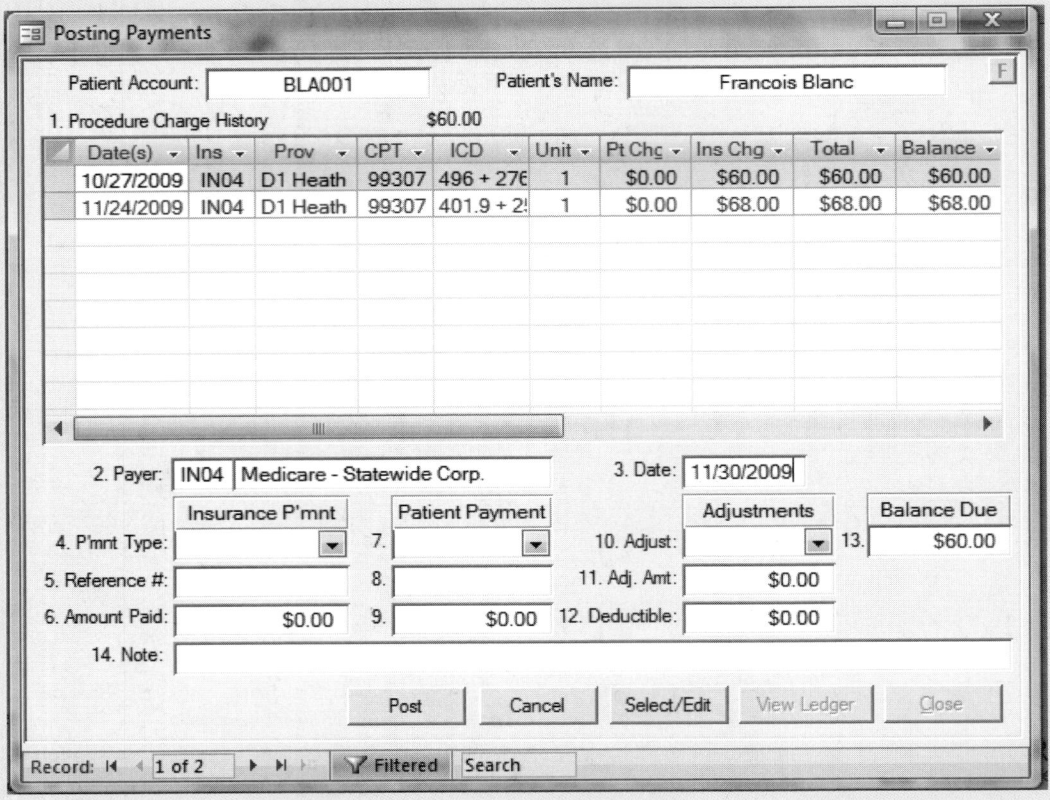

FIGURE 8-12

Delmar/Cengage Learning

STEP 7

Drop down the box for Field 4 on the Payment Entry window. Select *PAYINS*, since this is a Medicare payment. In Field 5, Reference #, enter the ICN provided on the RA for patient Blanc.

STEP 8

In Field 6, Amount Paid, enter the Medicare payment of $28.50. Press *Enter*. The balance due should now show a balance of $31.50.

STEP 9

The patient is not going to pay anything at this time, so Fields 7, 8, and 9 are not used. The adjustment is entered next. Drop down the box at Field 10 and select *ADJINS*, meaning this is an insurance adjustment. Click *Enter* or *Tab* to move to Field 11 and enter the $24.38 adjustment, as indicated on the RA. Press *Enter*. The Balance Due should now reflect $7.12, which is the patient's co-insurance amount.

STEP 10

Check your work with Figure 8-13 before proceeding and make corrections if needed. Next, click on the *Post button* to apply the payment and adjustment. Click on the *View Ledger button* to review the posting. Check your screen with Figure 8-14. Close the ledger when finished.

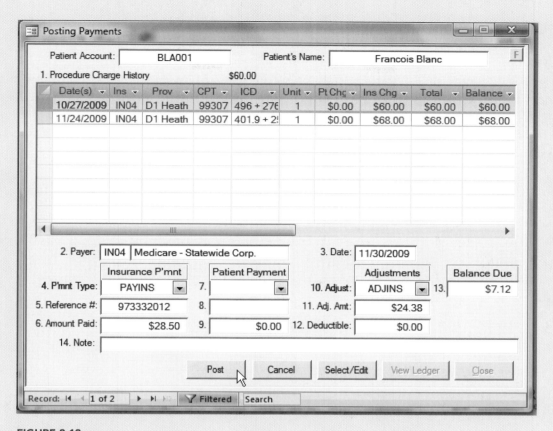

FIGURE 8-13

Delmar/Cengage Learning

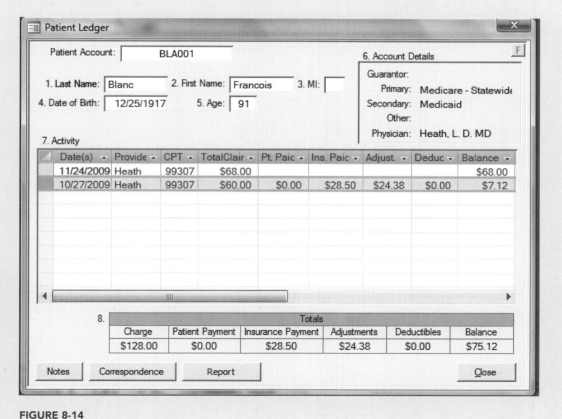

FIGURE 8-14

Delmar/Cengage Learning

continues

POSTING MEDICARE PAYMENTS—BLANC, FRANCOIS *continued*

STEP 11

There is one more service to be posted for patient Blanc. Using the same methods, post the payment for the service on 11/24/2009. Continue to use the posting date of 11/30/2009. Take care that the correct line has been selected for payment application. Compare your completed Payment Entry screen for procedure code 99307 on 11/24/2009 with Figure 8-15. Make corrections before posting the payment.

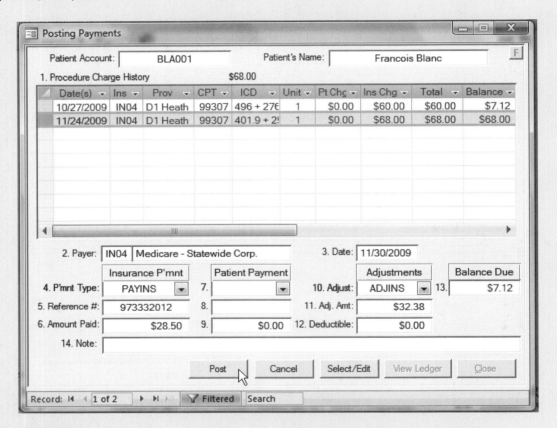

FIGURE 8-15

Delmar/Cengage Learning

STEP 12

View the Patient Ledger, and compare your work to Figure 8-16.

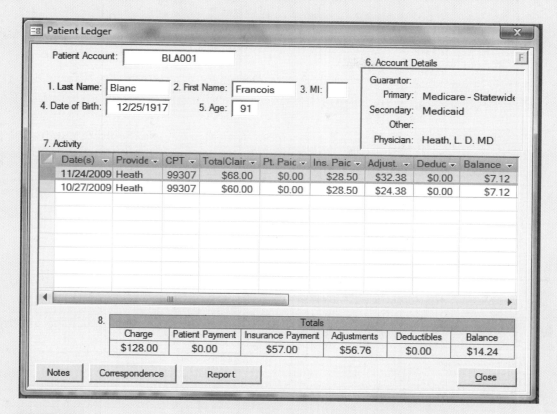

FIGURE 8-16

Delmar/Cengage Learning

STEP 13

All payments for Medicare have been completed for patient Blanc. Click on the *Close button* on all open windows and return to the Main Menu.

LET'S TRY IT! 8-3 POSTING MEDICARE PAYMENTS—CHANG, XAO

Objective: The user reads the Medicare RA notice for Xao Chang (Source Document 8-1) and posts payments as indicated to the patient's account.

STEP 1

Start MOSS.

continues

STEP 2

Refer to the Medicare RA notice in Source Document 8-1. Locate Xao Chang and review the following.

A.	What is patient Chang's Medicare number? What is his account number at the medical office?	The Medicare number is: 999321156A. CHA001 is the account number.
B.	Which provider is listed for these services and was assignment accepted?	L.D. Heath, MD. Assignment was accepted.
C.	What is the Internal Control Number for these services? This number is used as a reference for posting payments.	ICN 973332013
D.	Find the date(s) of service. On which date(s) was service provided?	10/16/2009 and 11/24/2009
E.	What code for POS is indicated for patient Chang? What type of place does this code represent?	31. Skilled Nursing Facility
F.	To the right of each POS code is the CPT code that was billed for services rendered. Which two CPT service codes are listed?	99307

Finally, to the right of the CPT codes are columns which contain the amount billed, how much Medicare allowed, the amount that was applied to the deductible (DEDUCT), the patient's co-insurance responsibility (COINS), how much the provider was paid (PROV-PD), and the required Medicare adjustment (MC-ADJUSTMENT). **Identify these amounts in the spaces below to be used in the following steps to post the payment.** *Cover the answers below using the tear-off bookmark from the cover of your book.*

Code:	Billed:	Allowed:	Deductible:	Co-ins:	Provider paid:	Adjustment:

Code:	Billed:	Allowed:	Deductible:	Co-ins:	Provider paid:	Adjustment:
99307	$60.00	$35.62	$0.00	$7.12	$28.50	$24.38
99307	$68.00	$35.62	$0.00	$7.12	$28.50	$32.38

STEP 3

Click on the *Posting Payments button* on the Main Menu. The Patient Selection window opens.

STEP 4

Select Xao Chang from the patient list by single clicking on his *name*, then clicking on the *Apply Payment button*. You may also retrieve his account by using the account number provided on the Medicare RA.

STEP 5

Start by reading across the first line on the RA for CPT 99307 on DOS 10/16/09 for patient Chang. The amount billed was $60.00 (which is shown for this procedure code on Source Document 8-1). Of that amount, $35.62 was allowed. Medicare pays 80% of the allowed amount, so the provider was paid $28.50. The patient's co-insurance is $7.12, which again, is showing on this Medicare RA that the claim information has been forwarded to Medicaid. This indicates *crossover* of the claim by the primary insurance to the secondary for the remainder balance due, and no further secondary billing is needed. Since Dr. Heath is PAR and has agreed to accept the Medicare allowable as the full charge for services, the $24.38 in the adjustment column is the write-off. These components will now be posted to the patient account.

STEP 6

Single click the *line entry* in the Procedure Charge History area that contains CPT 99307 on 10/16/2009. Then, click on the *Select/Edit button*. The Balance Due Field 13 should show $60.00. Next, enter the date of posting in Field 3, which is 11/30/2009.

STEP 7

Drop down the box for Field 4 on the Payment Entry window. Select *PAYINS*, since this is a Medicare payment. In Field 5, Reference #, enter the ICN provided on the RA for patient Blanc.

STEP 8

In Field 6, Amount Paid, enter the Medicare payment of $28.50. Press *Enter*. The Balance Due should now show a balance of $31.50.

STEP 9

The patient is not going to pay anything at this time, so Fields 7, 8, and 9 are not used. The adjustment is entered next. Drop down the box at Field 10 and select *ADJINS*, meaning this is an insurance adjustment. Click *Enter* or *Tab* to move to Field 11 and enter the $24.38 adjustment, as indicated on the RA. Press *Enter*. The Balance Due should now reflect $7.12, which is the patient's co-insurance amount.

STEP 10

Check your work with Figure 8-17 before proceeding and make corrections if needed. Next, click on the *Post button* to apply the payment and adjustment. Click on the *View Ledger button* to review the posting. Check your screen with Figure 8-18. Close the ledger when finished.

continues

POSTING MEDICARE PAYMENTS—CHANG, XAO *continued*

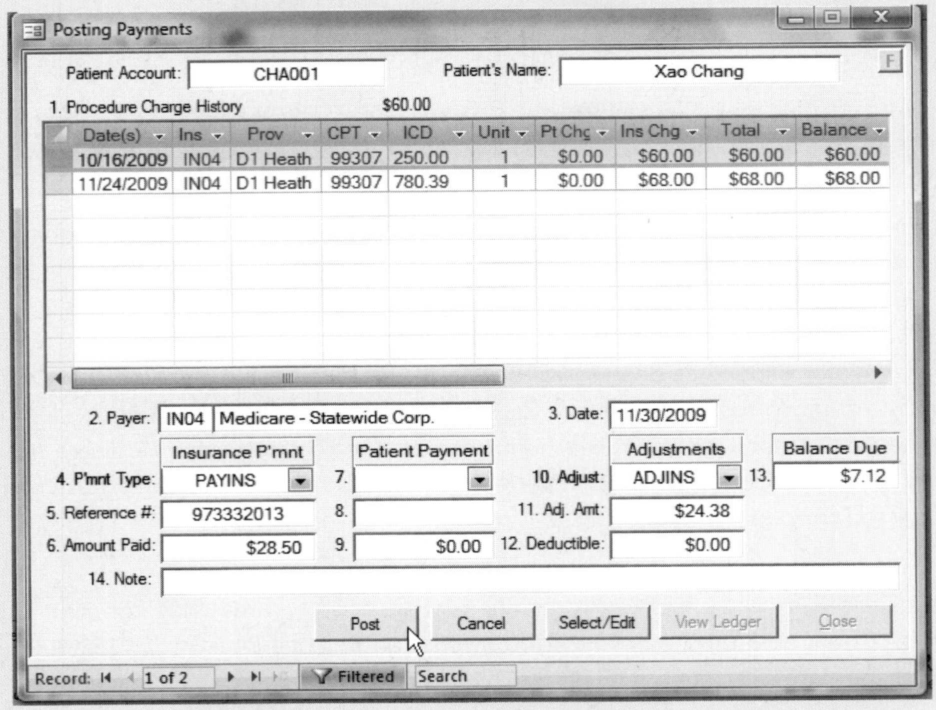

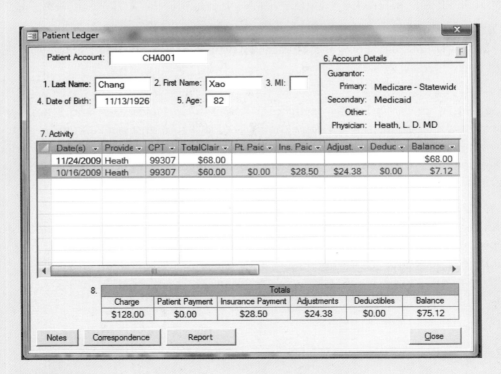

FIGURE 8-17

Delmar/Cengage Learning

FIGURE 8-18

Delmar/Cengage Learning

STEP 11

There is one more service to be posted for patient Chang. Using the same methods, post the payment for the service on 11/24/2009. Continue to use the posting date of 11/30/2009. Take care that the correct line has been selected for payment application. Compare your completed Payment Entry screen for procedure code 99307 on 11/24/2009 with Figure 8-19. Make corrections before posting the payment.

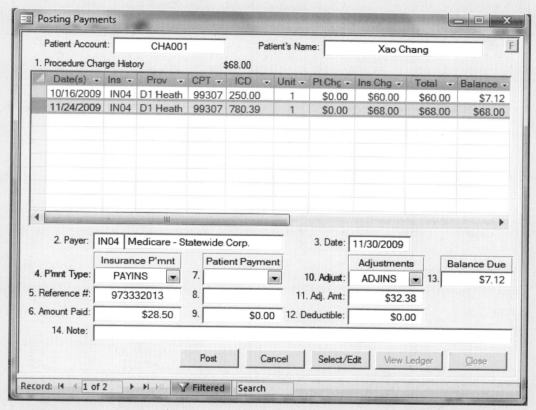

FIGURE 8-19

Delmar/Cengage Learning

STEP 12

View the Patient Ledger, and compare your work to Figure 8-20.

continues

POSTING MEDICARE PAYMENTS—CHANG, XAO *continued*

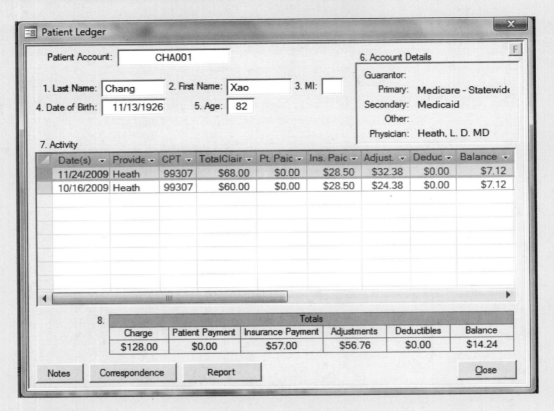

FIGURE 8-20

Delmar/Cengage Learning

STEP 13

All payments for Medicare have been completed for patient Blanc. Click on the *Close button* on all open windows and return to the Main Menu.

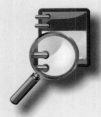

LET'S TRY IT! 8-4 POSTING MEDICARE PAYMENTS—ALL PATIENTS

Objective: The user reads the Medicare RA notices for select patients (Source Document 8-2) and posts payments as indicated to the respective patient accounts.

STEP 1

Start MOSS.

STEP 2

Refer to the Medicare RA notice in Source Document 8-2. There are three patients on this RA: Manuel Ramirez, Geraldo Muñoz and Anna Pinkston. Review each patient's payment details for each of the following.

A.	What is each patient's Medicare number?	**Ramirez: 999512136A** **Muñoz: 999832166A** **Pinkston: 999210132D**
B.	Which provider is listed for these services and was assignment accepted?	**L.D. Heath, MD. Assignment was accepted.**
C.	What is the Internal Control Number for these services?	**Ramirez: 973332020** **Muñoz: 973332021** **Pinkston: 973332022**
D.	Find the date(s) of service. On which date(s) was service provided?	**Ramirez: 10/30/2009** **Muñoz: 11/6/2009 through 11/9/2009 (consecutive days)** **DOS for Pinkston: 10/20/2009 and 11/24/2009**
E.	What POS code was billed for each procedure?	**Ramirez: 11** **Muñoz: 21** **Pinkston: 31**
F.	What CPT code that was billed for each service rendered for each patient?	**Ramirez: 99215, 45378** **Muñoz: 99221, 99231, 99238** **Pinkston: 99308**
G.	Have any claims been crossover? Explain your answer.	**Yes, the co-insurance claim information was crossed over to Medicaid for payment for Patient Anna Pinkston.**

Finally, to the right of the CPT codes are columns which contain the amount billed, how much Medicare allowed, the amount that was applied to the deductible (DEDUCT), the patient's co-insurance responsibility (COINS), how much the provider was paid (PROV-PD), and the required Medicare adjustment (MC-ADJUSTMENT). **Identify these amounts in the spaces below to be used in the following steps to post the payment.** *Cover the answers below using the tear-off bookmark from the cover of your book.*

Ramirez

Code:	Billed:	Allowed:	Deductible:	Co-ins:	Provider paid:	Adjustment:

continues

POSTING MEDICARE PAYMENTS—ALL PATIENTS *continued*

Muñoz

Code:	Billed:	Allowed:	Deductible:	Co-ins:	Provider paid:	Adjustment:

Pinkston

Code:	Billed:	Allowed:	Deductible:	Co-ins:	Provider paid:	Adjustment:

Ramirez

Code:	Billed:	Allowed:	Deductible:	Co-ins:	Provider paid:	Adjustment:
99215	$249.00	$140.31	$0.00	$28.06	$112.25	$108.69
45378	$1518.00	$451.54	$0.00	$90.30	$361.24	$1066.46

Muñoz

Code:	Billed:	Allowed:	Deductible:	Co-ins:	Provider paid:	Adjustment:
99221	$145.00	$92.33	$0.00	$18.47	$73.86	$52.67
99231	$158.00	$78.14	$0.00	$15.63	$62.51	$79.86
99238	$145.00	$73.16	$0.00	$14.63	$58.53	$71.84

Pinkston

Code:	Billed:	Allowed:	Deductible:	Co-ins:	Provider paid:	Adjustment:
99308	$78.00	$74.00	$0.00	$14.80	$59.20	$4.00
99308	$113.00	$59.06	$0.00	$11.81	$47.25	$53.94

STEP 3
Click on the *Posting Payments button* on the Main Menu. The Patient Selection window opens.

STEP 4
With the information that you gathered in Step 2, post the payment for each procedure for patients Ramirez, Muñoz, and Pinkston. The date of posting is 11/30/2009. Be sure to check your work before posting each payment with Figure 8-21 through Figure 8-30.

STEP 5
When all payments for Medicare have been completed for each patient, click on the *Close button* on all open windows and return to the Main Menu.

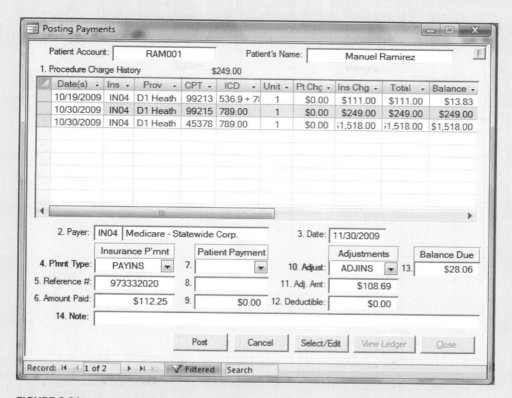

FIGURE 8-21

Delmar/Cengage Learning

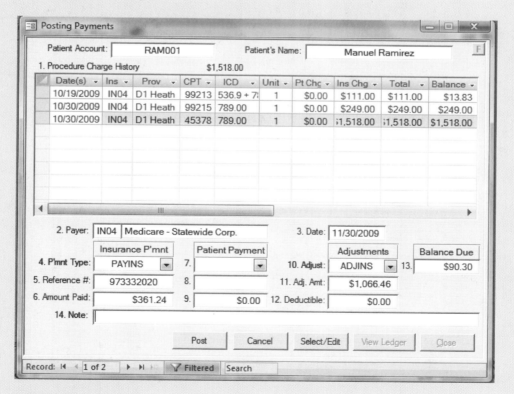

FIGURE 8-22

Delmar/Cengage Learning

continues

POSTING MEDICARE PAYMENTS—ALL PATIENTS *continued*

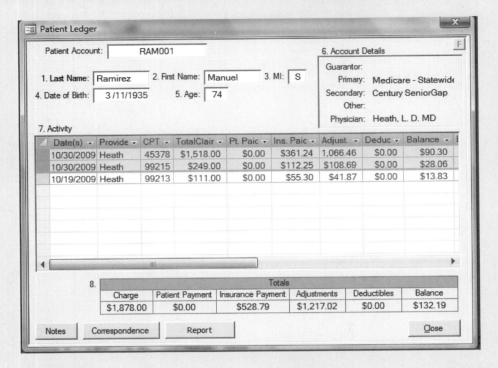

FIGURE 8-23

Delmar/Cengage Learning

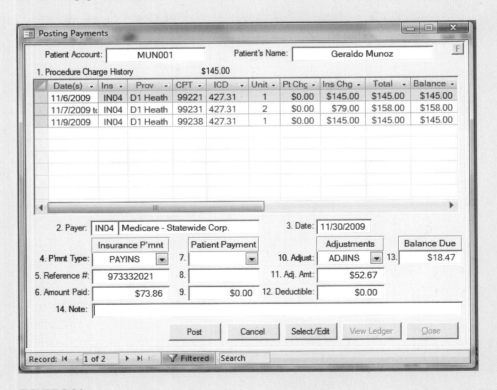

FIGURE 8-24

Delmar/Cengage Learning

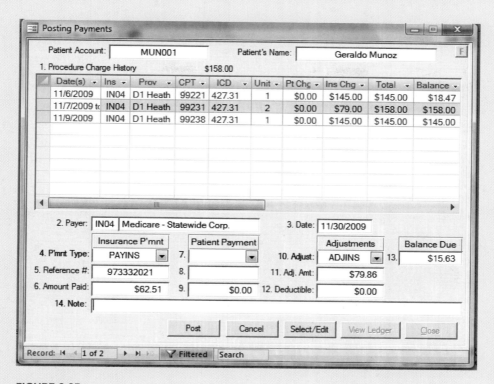

FIGURE 8-25

Delmar/Cengage Learning

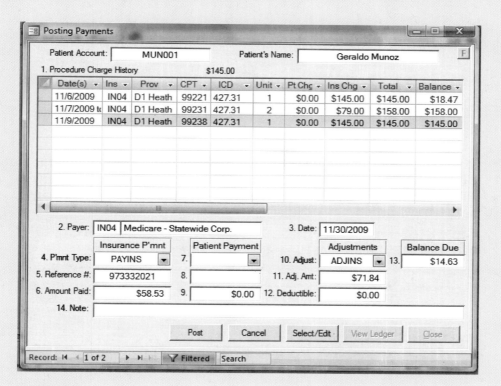

FIGURE 8-26

Delmar/Cengage Learning

continues

POSTING MEDICARE PAYMENTS—ALL PATIENTS *continued*

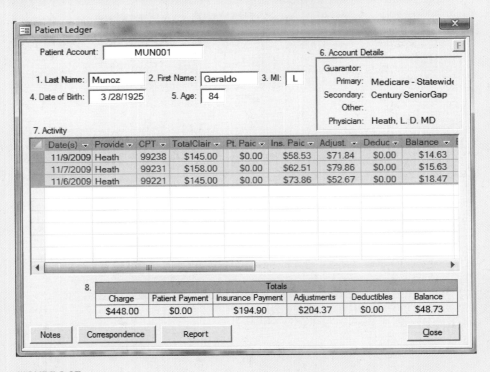

FIGURE 8-27

Delmar/Cengage Learning

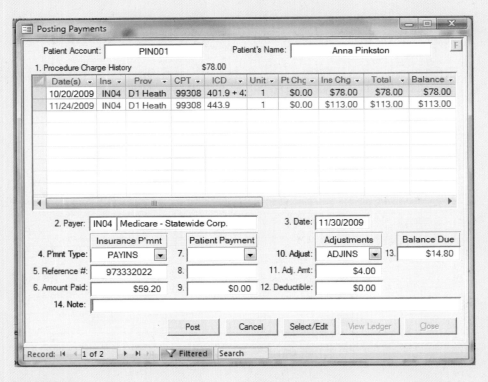

FIGURE 8-28

Delmar/Cengage Learning

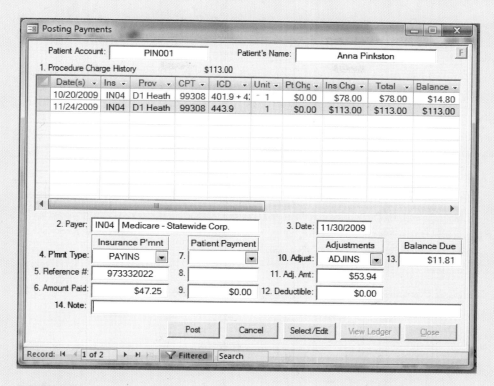

FIGURE 8-29

Delmar/Cengage Learning

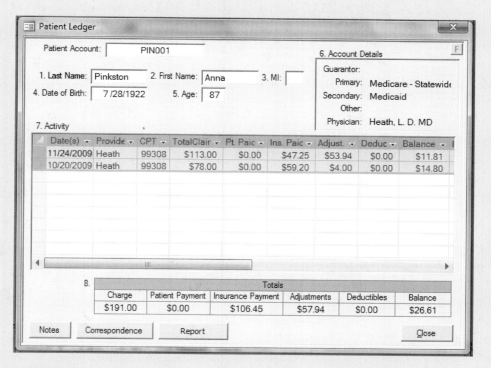

FIGURE 8-30

Delmar/Cengage Learning

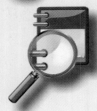

LET'S TRY IT! 8-5 APPLYING DEDUCTIBLES FOR MEDICARE

Objective: The user reads the Medicare RA notices for payments received for patients Mangano and Tomanaga (Source Document 8-3). Deductibles and payments are posted as indicated to the respective patient accounts.

STEP 1

Open the Payment Entry window by clicking on the *Posting Payments button* on the Main Menu. Select Vito Mangano from the patient list.

STEP 2

Review the first entry for patient Mangano on the Medicare RA, Source Document 8-3 from the Source Document Appendix. As you read the RA for date 10/27/2009, you will notice that $75.00 was applied to the Medicare deductible. Since Medicare currently has a $135.00 deductible, this means the deductible is now met for the year.

NOTE: Because the billed charges totaled $180.00, if there was more deductible to be met, it would have been applied. This is how we know the deductible has been met.

STEP 3

On the Posting Payments window, select the line entry for 10/27/2009 and CPT 99214. Use 11/30/2009 as the date of posting. Enter the payment and adjustment in the same manner as before. The amount applied to the deductible is entered in Field 12. Before clicking on the *Post button*, check your work with Figure 8-31.

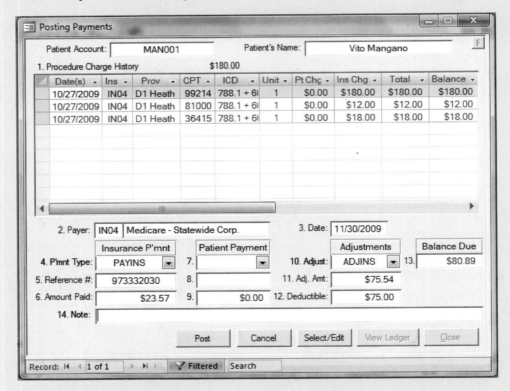

FIGURE 8-31

Delmar/Cengage Learning

Notice the Balance Due shows $80.89. This represents the patient's co-insurance of $5.89 plus the $75.00 which was applied to the deductible. Since the patient does not have secondary insurance, both of these amounts are billed to the patient at a later time. Click on the *Post button*. Open the Patient's Ledger and check your work with Figure 8-32.

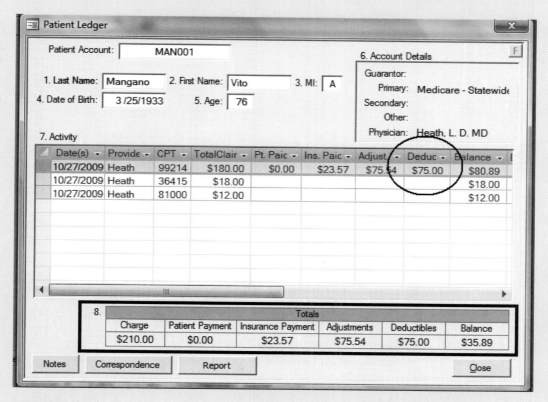

FIGURE 8-32
Delmar/Cengage Learning

STEP 4

It is sometimes useful to document special situations regarding patient accounts. For instance, it might be handy for other staff members to be able to view notes when patient statements are prepared. With a quick check of the notes, the fact patient Mangano owes the deductible saves time. These types of notes remind the staff of special circumstances that might otherwise be easily forgotten, or are time-consuming to go back and research.

The Patient's Ledger should still be open; if not, click on the View Ledger button for patient Mangano, and then click on the **Notes button** at the bottom of the window. On the Patient Notes window, click on the **Add button** and click inside the note box next to the asterisk. Type the following: "Patient owes a $75.00 deductible applied to CPT 99214, 10/27/2009." See Figure 8-33. Click the **Close button**. The software automatically saves the notes upon closing the window.

continues

APPLYING DEDUCTIBLES FOR MEDICARE *continued*

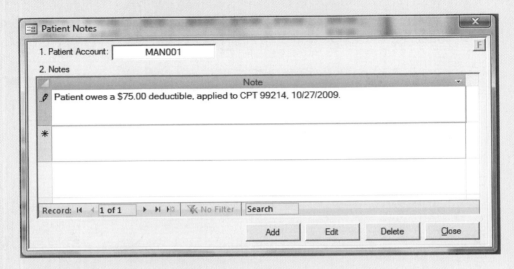

FIGURE 8-33

Delmar/Cengage Learning

HINT: Do not forget to use the Medicare ICN as your reference number and 11/30/2009 as the date of posting.

STEP 5

Post the other two payments for patient Mangano, procedures CPT 81000 and 36415, using the same method you have already learned. Check your payment posting work with Figure 8-34 through Figure 8-36 before posting each payment.

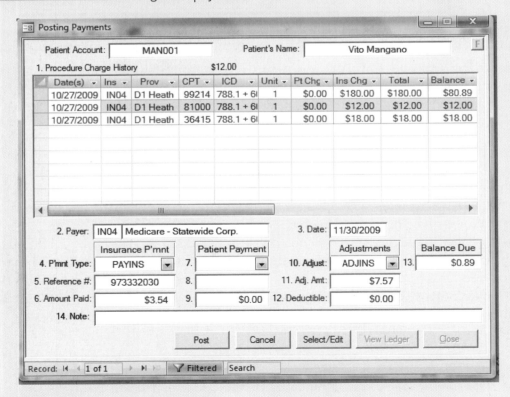

FIGURE 8-34

Delmar/Cengage Learning

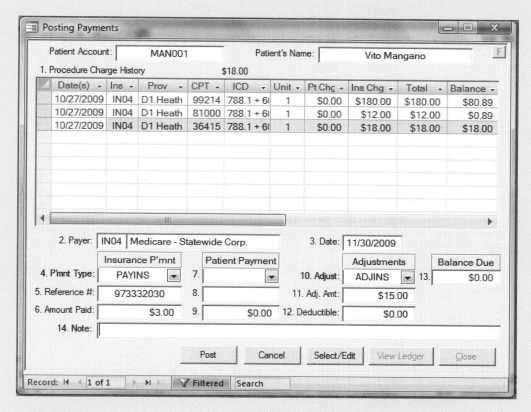

FIGURE 8-35

Delmar/Cengage Learning

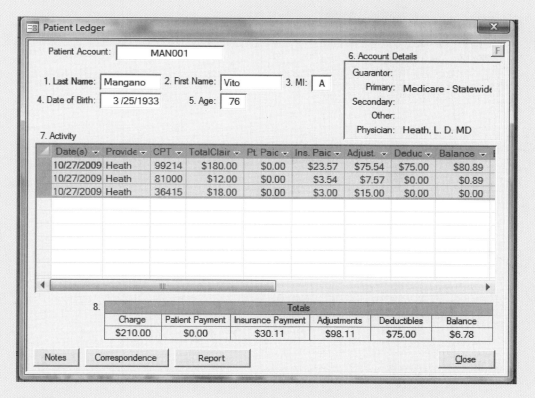

FIGURE 8-36

Delmar/Cengage Learning

continues

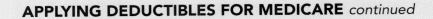

APPLYING DEDUCTIBLES FOR MEDICARE *continued*

STEP 6

Close all open windows and return to the Posting Payments Patient Selection window. Refer to Source Document 8-3 and answer the following questions regarding patient Tomanaga. *Cover the answers using the tear-off bookmark from the cover of your book. Check your work before entering data into MOSS.*

A.	Was any portion of her charges applied to the deductible? If yes, how much?	**$135.00**
B.	What is the date of service and CPT code for the service the deductible was applied to?	**11/03/2009 to CPT 99205**
C.	Is patient Tomanaga's Medicare deductible now met as of 11/3/2009?	**Yes**

NOTE: What is the current Medicare deductible, at the time of this book's writing?

STEP 8

Refer to CPT code 99205 on 11/03/2009 on the RA. Fill in the following blanks, then do the math indicated by the parentheses ( ).

A.	Fee billed to Medicare for 99205:		$_____	**$358.00**
B.	Payment to provider:	(-)	$_____	**$51.82**
C.	Adjustment amount:	(-)	$_____	**$158.22**
D.	Co-insurance amount:	(-)	$_____	**$12.96**
E.	ANSWER =		$_____	**$135.00** **(The deductible amount)**

STEP 9

Open the Posting Payments window for patient Tomanaga. Post the deductible, payments, and applicable adjustments for all services on 11/03/2009 as previously learned. Before clicking on the *Post button* for each payment posting, check your work with Figure 8-37 through Figure 8-41.

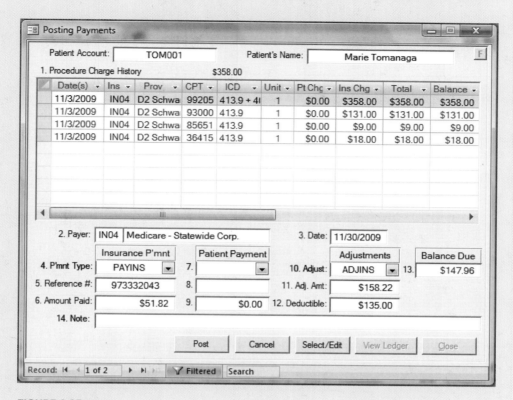

FIGURE 8-37

Delmar/Cengage Learning

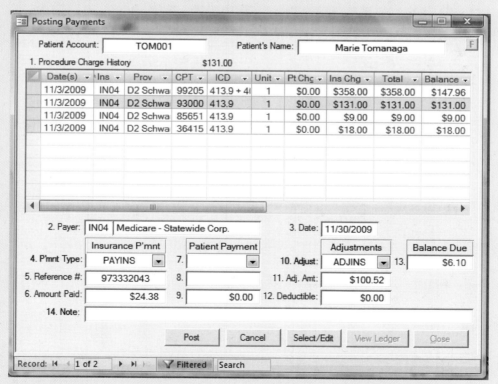

FIGURE 8-38

Delmar/Cengage Learning

continues

APPLYING DEDUCTIBLES FOR MEDICARE *continued*

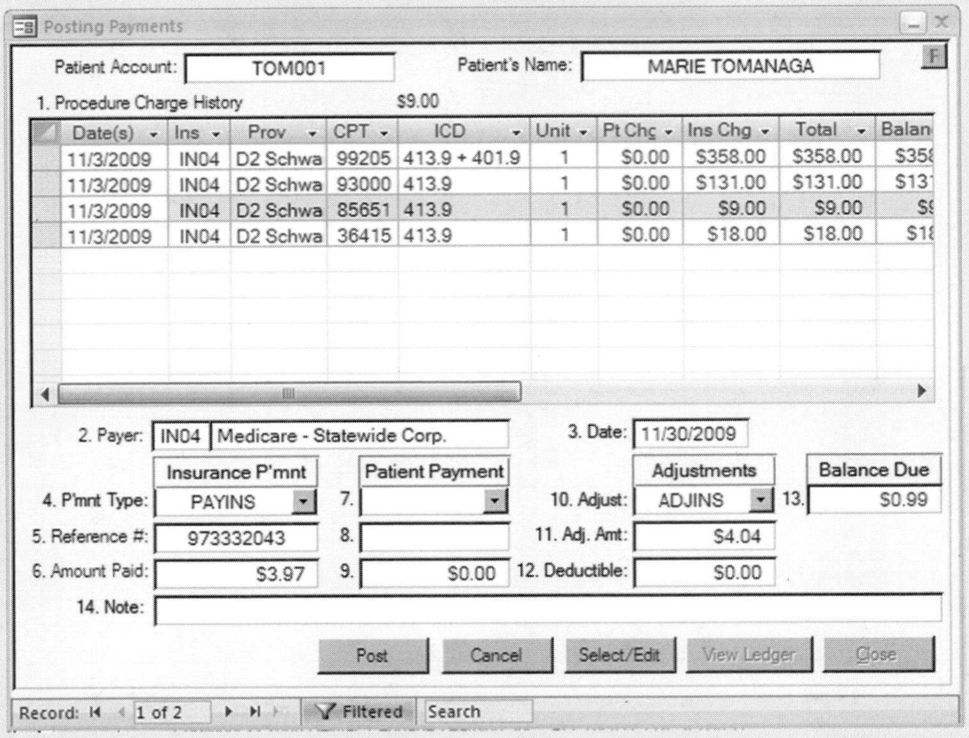

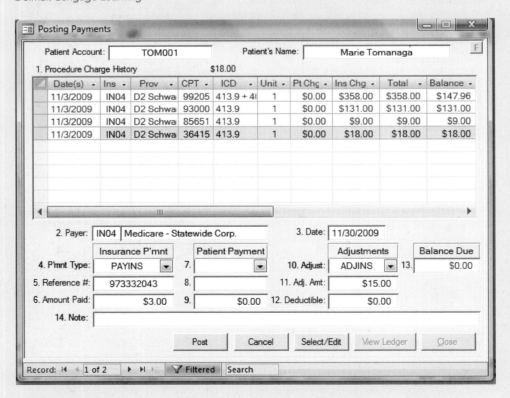

FIGURE 8-39

Delmar/Cengage Learning

FIGURE 8-40

Delmar/Cengage Learning

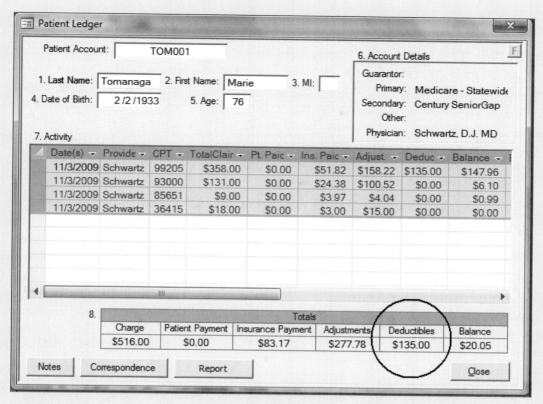

FIGURE 8-41

Delmar/Cengage Learning

STEP 10

Include a note in patient Tomanga's ledger about the $135.00 deductible, as previously learned. Check your work with Figure 8-42. When finished, close all open windows and return to the Main Menu.

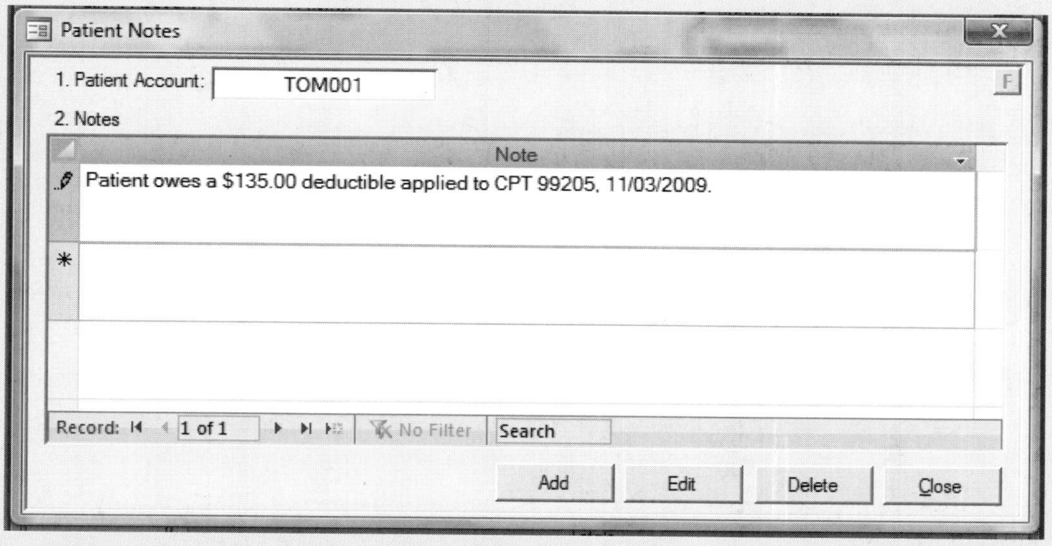

FIGURE 8-42

Delmar/Cengage Learning

READING A GENERAL EXPLANATION OF BENEFITS (EOB)

Now that payments have been posted using Medicare RA notices, the transition to reading general EOBs should be less complicated. The key to reading EOBs from various insurance carriers is being able to recognize nuances with the terminology and headings used. Often, with a little analysis, you soon realize that the same or similar information is being referred to with another word. For instance, on the Medicare RA, the payment made to the physician was in a column called "PROV-PD," meaning "provider paid." However, the EOBs from the FlexiHealth PPO Plan refer to the payment made to the provider in a column called "plan liability." In both instances, each column shows the amount paid on the claim by the insurance.

When posting payments, in general it does help to know some of the guidelines for the health plans your employer accepts. For instance, information regarding whether the provider participates, accepts assignment, and has any contractual obligations, assists in knowing what to write off and what to bill to a secondary plan or to the patient. Health plans the physician participates with provide the medical office with a "provider reference manual." With the convenience of Web sites and the Internet, the trend has been to make provider resources available online, instead of through books that are issued for the office. These resources are easily accessed by visiting the Web site for the health plan, and often include reimbursement and medical policies as well as administrative guides. These resources should be consulted as needed to understand the components of the EOB or RA and other details specific to each plan.

While the EOB guides you to a point, there are hundreds of health plans with differing criteria. Be assured that once you are employed at a particular facility, you will become familiar with the health plans, carriers, regulations, and guidelines that are common in your office and region. You will learn this essential information during orientation to your position, and, of course, through experience by actually using this information in your daily work.

LET'S TRY IT! 8-6 USING A GENERAL EOB TO POST DEDUCTIBLES FOR OUT-OF-NETWORK SERVICES—KRAMER, STANLEY

Objective: The reader posts deductibles applied for services rendered to Stanley Kramer. The information is based on an EOB from the FlexiHealth PPO Plan (Source Document 8-4).

STEP 1

Start MOSS.

STEP 2

Refer to Source Document 8-4 in the Source Document Appendix. Review the information on the EOB, and then answer the following questions. *Cover the answers using the tear-off bookmark from the cover of your book. Check your work before entering data into MOSS to be sure you have correctly interpreted the source documents.*

A.	Who is the insured (policyholder) and who is the covered patient (dependent) for this FlexiHealth PPO plan?	**The insured, and the patient, is Stanley Kramer.**
B.	Who was the provider of services? Is this physician an in-network or out-of-network provider?	**D.J. Schwartz, MD, an out-of-network provider for FlexiHealth PPO**
C.	What were the dates of service as shown on the EOB?	**10/27 through 10/30/2009 (consecutive dates in hospital)**
D.	How much, total, did FlexiHealth pay towards patient Kramer's services? Explain your answer using the benefit determination notes for guidance.	**There was no payment. The covered amounts were applied to the deductible.**
E.	Will the doctor have to write-off any amount for these services?	**No, the patient is responsible for payment of the non-covered amount when services are received from an out-of-network provider.**

STEP 3

Recall that Dr. Heath is an in-network provider for FlexiHealth, and Dr. Schwartz is an out-of-network provider. This changes the reimbursement for services, as shown on the Benefits-at-a-Glance form in Unit 4, Figure 4-5. Out-of-network services provided in the hospital are reimbursed at 50% of the covered amount. However, patient Kramer has still not met his annual deductible. In fact, all of the services were applied towards the deductible, which is why the insurance company did not pay.

STEP 4

Click on the *Posting Payments button* on the Main Menu. The Patient Selection window opens. Open a Payment Entry screen for Stanley Kramer.

STEP 5

Click on the first *line entry*, CPT 99221, in the Procedure Charge History area and then click on the *Select/Edit button*. The Balance field should display $145.00. Enter a posting date of 11/30/2009 in Field 3 and the Reference Number in Field 5. The only item to be posted is the deductible that was applied, which will be entered in Field 12 for $93.00. Enter the data and then compare your screen to Figure 8-43 before clicking on the *Post button*.

continues

USING A GENERAL EOB TO POST DEDUCTIBLES FOR OUT-OF-NETWORK SERVICES—KRAMER, STANLEY *continued*

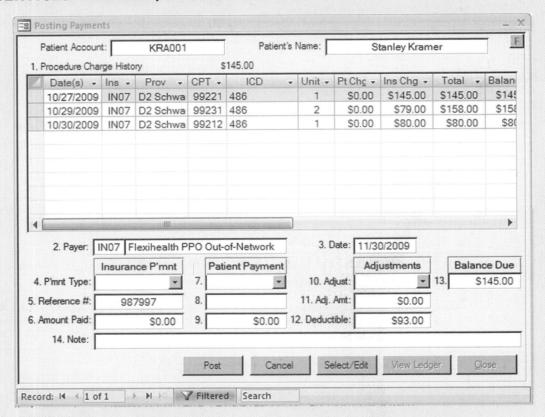

FIGURE 8-43

Delmar/Cengage Learning

NOTE: As indicated by Note B at the bottom of the EOB, there is no adjustment. Since Dr. Schwartz is an out-of-network provider, the patient is also responsible for paying the non-covered amount of $52.00.

STEP 6

Follow the same procedures for posting the amounts applied to the deductible for the remaining services on patient Kramer. Check your work with Figure 8-44 through Figure 8-46 before clicking the *Post button* for each entry.

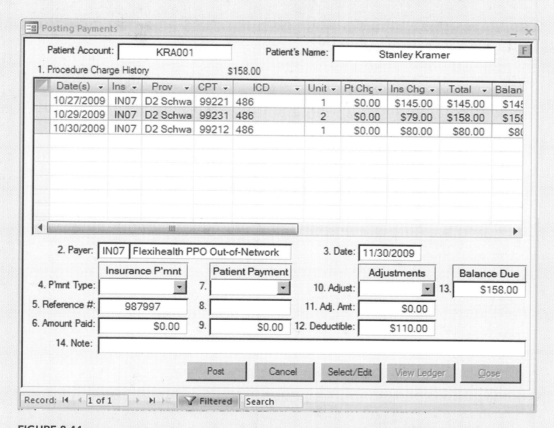

FIGURE 8-44

Delmar/Cengage Learning

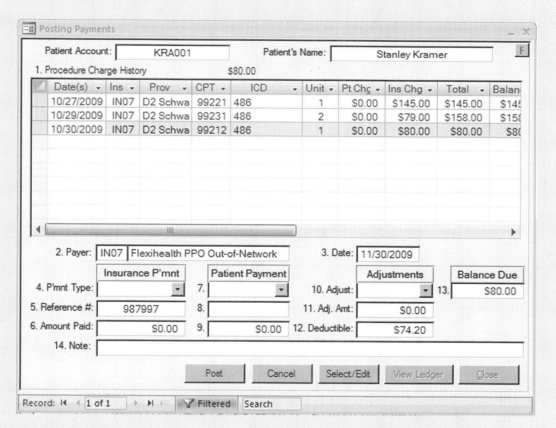

FIGURE 8-45

Delmar/Cengage Learning

continues

USING A GENERAL EOB TO POST DEDUCTIBLES FOR OUT-OF-NETWORK SERVICES—KRAMER, STANLEY *continued*

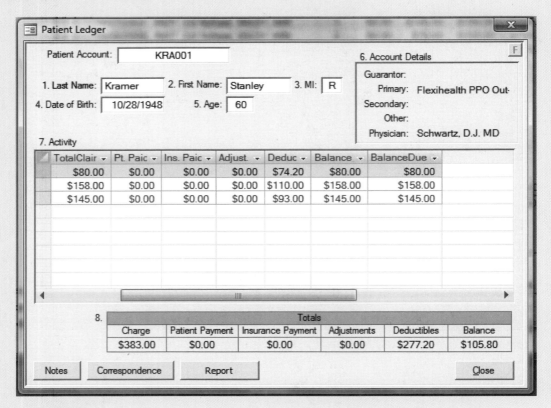

FIGURE 8-46

Delmar/Cengage Learning

STEP 7

As done before, write a note in the "Notes" area of the Patient Ledger, indicating patient Kramer owes not only the deductible, but also the non-covered portion of his charges. In this case, it is especially useful to have these notes to remind the staff of special circumstances regarding the patient account.

   With patient Kramer's Patient Ledger still open, click on the *Notes button*. Then, on the Patient Notes window, click on the *Add button* and click *inside the note box*. Type the following: "Patient owes the deductible and non-covered portion of charges since Dr. Schwartz is an out-of-network physician with FlexiHealth PPO."

   Check your work with Figure 8-47 before closing the Patient Notes window.

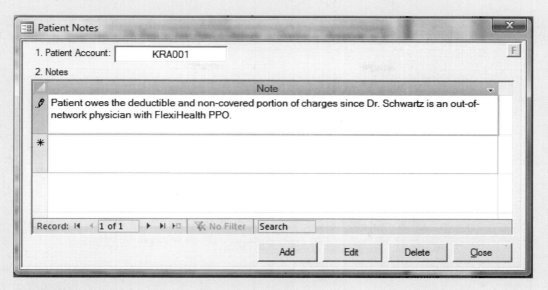

FIGURE 8-47

Delmar/Cengage Learning

STEP 8

When finished, close all windows and return to the Main Menu.

LET'S TRY IT! 8-7 USING A GENERAL EOB TO POST AN IN-NETWORK FLEXIHEALTH PPO PAYMENT—KINZLER, LINDA

Objective: The reader posts a payment for Linda Kinzler based on information contained on an EOB from FlexiHealth PPO Plan (Source Document 8-5).

STEP 1

Start MOSS.

STEP 2

Refer to the EOB in Source Document 8-5 in the Source Document Appendix. Review the information on the EOB, then answer the following questions.

continues

A.	Who is the insured (policyholder) and who is the covered patient (dependent) for this FlexiHealth PPO plan?	**The insured is Jennifer Wade and the patient is Linda Kinzler.**
B.	Who was the provider of services? Is this physician an in-network or out-of-network provider?	**L.D. Heath, MD, an in-network provider**
C.	What were the dates of service as shown on the EOB?	**11/09/2009**
D.	How much, total, did FlexiHealth pay towards patient Kinzler's services? Explain your answer using the benefit determination notes for guidance.	**$160.00. The flu vaccination was not covered, and there was a $20.00 preferred provider discount applied.**
E.	Will the doctor have to write off any amount for these services?	**Yes, the doctor will have to write off the $20.00 in-network provider discount.**

STEP 3

Recall that Dr. Heath is an in-network provider for FlexiHealth. As shown on the FlexiHealth PPO Plan Benefits-at-a-Glance chart in Unit 4, Figure 4-5, the patient has a $20.00 co-payment due at each office visit. Because she uses an in-network provider, she gets a discount, which is a write-off. As indicated by the benefit determination note, the flu vaccination is not covered by this health plan. That remains the patient's responsibility to pay.

STEP 4

Click on the *Posting Payments button* from the Main Menu. The Patient Selection window opens. Open the Payment Entry screen for Linda Kinzler.

STEP 5

HINT: A payment made on the date of service, 11/09/2009, was previously recorded.

Single click on the *line entry* for CPT code 99203 and click the ***Select/ Edit button***. In Field 3, enter a date of 11/30/2009. Recall that the patient made a $20.00 co-payment at the time of the visit. The remaining Balance Due should read $180.00 in Field 13.

STEP 6

As shown on the EOB, out of the $200.00 in charges, $20.00 is an insurance adjustment and the insurance paid $160.00. Enter the data, using the reference number on the EOB for Field 5. Compare your screen to Figure 8-48 before clicking on the *Post button*.

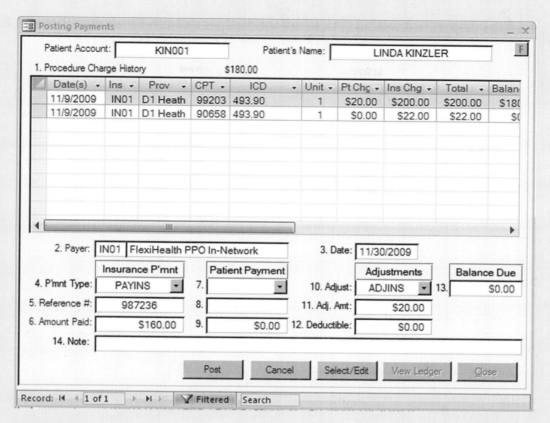

FIGURE 8-48

Delmar/Cengage Learning

STEP 7

Next, view the Patient's Ledger. Note that the patient paid for the flu vaccination at the time of her visit. Because the patient paid for this non-covered service at the time of her visit, no further posting is required. Click on the *Close button*.

STEP 8

When finished, close all open windows and return to the Main Menu.

LET'S TRY IT! 8-8 POSTING PAYMENTS FOR MULTIPLE PATIENTS LISTED ON ONE EOB FOR FLEXIHEALTH PPO

Objective: The reader posts payments for select patients that have the FlexiHealth PPO plan.

NOTE: FlexiHealth PPO typically sends one check and one EOB with several patients listed on it. There are three patients on the EOB in Source Document 8-6 in the Source Document Appendix. The insurance sent one check for $476.44. A portion of this payment pertains to each patient. Using the methods just learned, post payments for each patient as indicated on the EOB.

STEP 1
Start MOSS.

STEP 2
Refer to the EOB in Source Document 8-6. Review the information on the EOB, then answer the following questions. *Cover the answers using the tear-off bookmark from the cover of your book. Check your work before entering data into MOSS to be sure you have correctly interpreted the source documents.*

A.	What are the names of the insured (policyholders) and what are the names of the patients (dependents)?	**Insured: Michael Mallory; Patient: Christina Mallory** **Insured: Richard Manaly; Patient: Richard Manaly** **Insured: Robert Ruhl; Patient: Mary Ruhl**
B.	For each patient, identify the provider and whether he or she is in-network or out-of-network.	**Mallory: Dr. Heath, an in-network provider** **Manaly: Dr. Schwartz, an out-of-network provider** **Ruhl: Dr. Heath, an in-network provider**

Now review each service and charge. Analyze each column, using the benefit determination notes to assist you with the information. Write down service date, CPT code(s), charge(s) submitted, the non-covered or discount amount, the amount covered, the co-insurance amount, and the covered balance or plan liability for each patient that will be used for posting the payment. *Cover the answers below using the tear-off bookmark from the cover of your book.*

Mallory

Service date:	CPT code	Charge submitted:	Discount:	Amount covered:	Plan liability:	Co-insurance

Manaly

Service date:	CPT code	Charge submitted:	Amount not covered:	Amount covered:	Plan liability:	Co-insurance

Ruhl

Service date:	CPT code	Charge submitted:	Discount:	Amount covered:	Plan liability:	Co-insurance

Mallory

Service date:	CPT code	Charge submitted:	Discount:	Amount covered:	Plan liability:	Co-insurance
11/14/2009	99221	$145.00	$52.00	$93.00	$74.40	$18.60
11/15/2009	99238	$145.00	$86.60	$58.20	$46.56	$11.64

Manaly

Service date:	CPT code	Charge submitted:	Amount not covered:	Amount covered:	Plan liability:	Co-insurance
10/21/2009	99213	$111.00	$28.60	$82.40	$65.92	$16.48

Ruhl

Service date:	CPT code	Charge submitted:	Discount:	Amount covered:	Plan liability:	Co-insurance
11/5/2009	99221	$145.00	$52.00	$93.00	$74.40	$18.60
11/6 through 11/9/2009	99231	$316.00	$104.00	$212.00	$169.60	$42.40
11/10/2009	99238	$145.00	$86.80	$58.20	$46.56	$11.64

STEP 3

Click on the *Posting Payments button* from the Main Menu. The Patient Selection window opens. Open a Payment Entry screen for Christina Mallory.

STEP 4

HINT: Use 11/30/2009 as the posting date and use Field 5 to record the reference number.

Post the two payments for patient Mallory using the information you read from the EOB in Step 2. Before clicking the *Post button*, check your work with Figure 8-49 through Figure 8-50. Last, view the Patient Ledger and compare to Figure 8-51.

continues

POSTING PAYMENTS FOR MULTIPLE PATIENTS LISTED ON ONE EOB FOR FLEXIHEALTH PPO *continued*

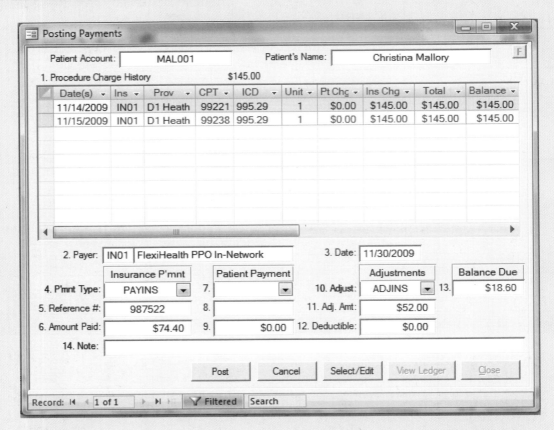

FIGURE 8-49

Delmar/Cengage Learning

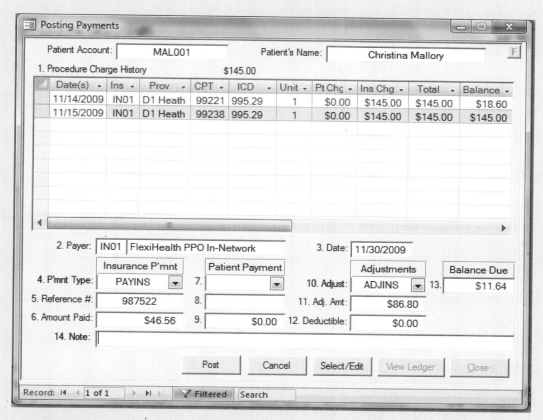

FIGURE 8-50

Delmar/Cengage Learning

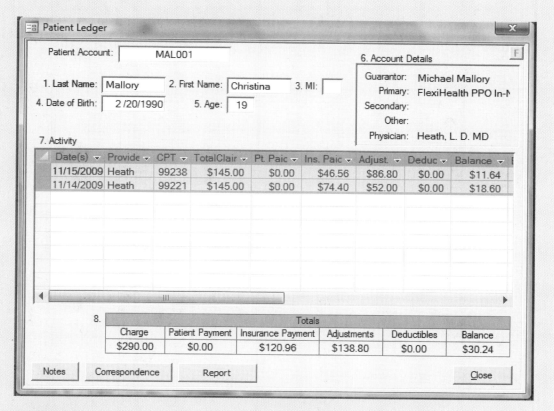

FIGURE 8-51

Delmar/Cengage Learning

continues

POSTING PAYMENTS FOR MULTIPLE PATIENTS LISTED ON ONE EOB FOR FLEXIHEALTH PPO *continued*

STEP 5

When finished, and the Patient Ledger has been viewed (Figure 8-51), close any open windows and return to the Main Menu of MOSS.

STEP 6

Click on the *Posting Payments button* from the Main Menu. The Patient Selection window opens. Open a Payment Entry screen for Richard Manaly.

HINT: Use 11/30/2009 as the posting date and use Field 5 to record the reference number.

STEP 7

Post the payment for patient Manaly using the information you read from the EOB in Step 2. Before clicking the *Post button*, check your work with Figure 8-52.

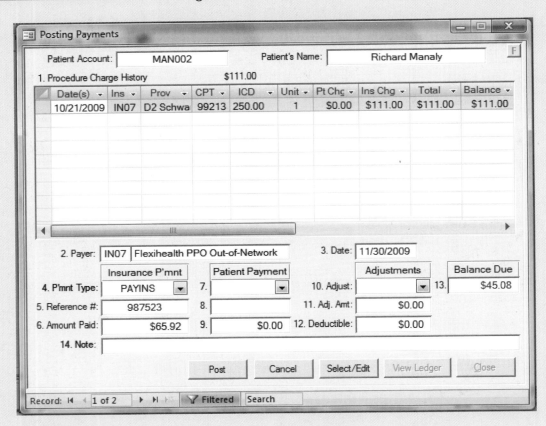

FIGURE 8-52

Delmar/Cengage Learning

STEP 8

Last, open the Patient Ledger for patient Manaly and check your work with Figure 8-53. Add a note to the ledger, as previously learned, that reads: "Patient owes the non-covered portion of the charges; Dr. Schwartz is an out-of-network physician for FlexiHealth PPO."

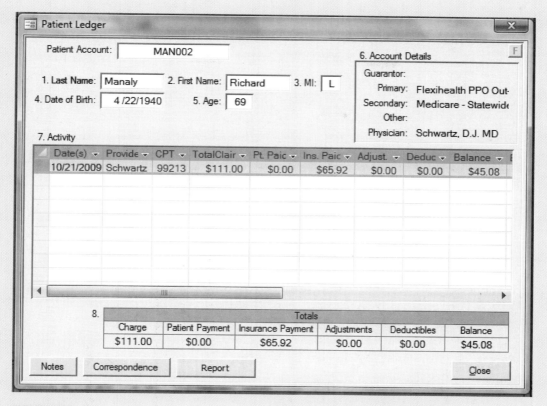

FIGURE 8-53

Delmar/Cengage Learning

STEP 9

When finished and the Patient Ledger has been viewed (Figure 8-53) and the note added, close any open windows and return to the Main Menu of MOSS.

STEP 10

Click on the *Posting Payments button* from the Main Menu. The Patient Selection window opens. Open a Payment Entry screen for Mary Ruhl.

NT: Use 11/30/2009 as the sting date and use Field 5 to ord the reference number.

STEP 11

Post the three payments for patient Ruhl using the information you read from the EOB in Step 2. Before clicking the *Post button*, check your work with Figure 8-54 through Figure 8-56. Last, view the Patient Ledger and compare with Figure 8-57.

continues

POSTING PAYMENTS FOR MULTIPLE PATIENTS LISTED ON ONE EOB FOR FLEXIHEALTH PPO *continued*

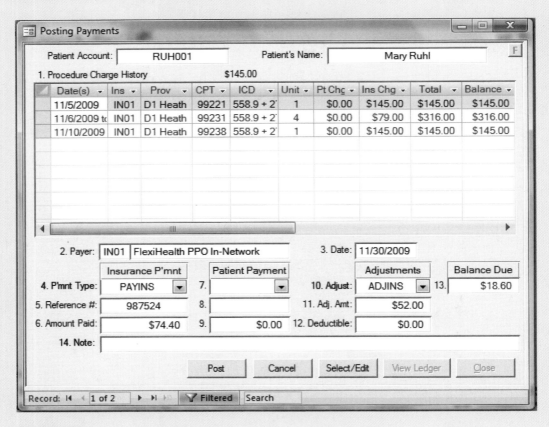

FIGURE 8-54

Delmar/Cengage Learning

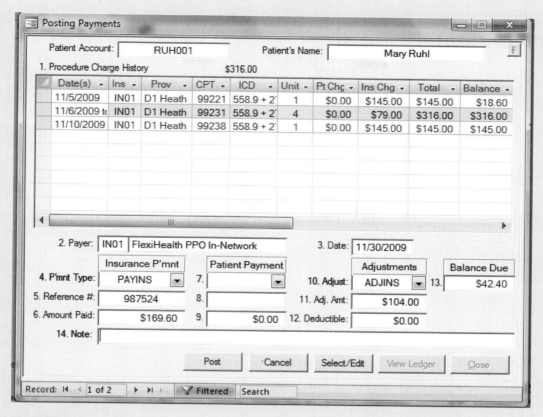

FIGURE 8-55

Delmar/Cengage Learning

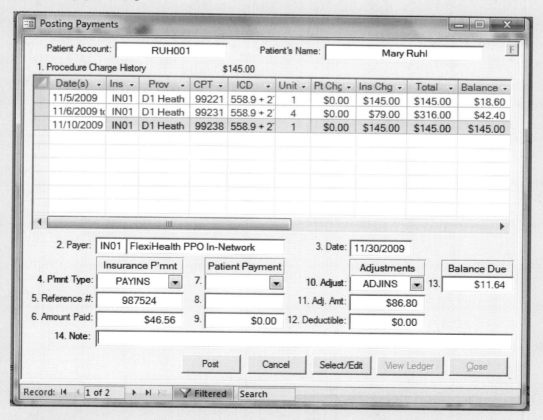

FIGURE 8-56

Delmar/Cengage Learning

continues

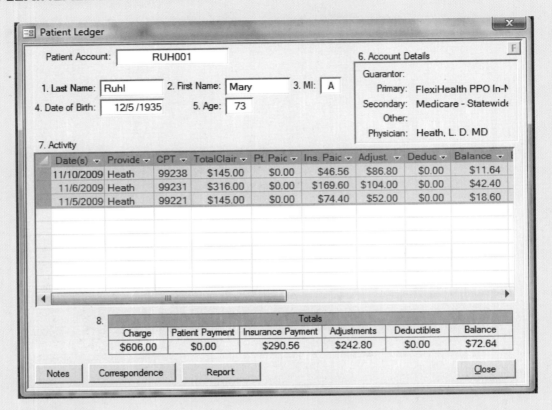

FIGURE 8-57

Delmar/Cengage Learning

STEP 12

When finished, and the Patient Ledger has been viewed (Figure 8-57), close any open windows and return to the Main Menu of MOSS.

LET'S TRY IT! 8-9 POSTING PAYMENTS FOR MULTIPLE PATIENTS LISTED ON ONE EOB FOR FLEXIHEALTH PPO

Objective: The reader posts payments for select patients who have the FlexiHealth PPO plan (Source Document 8-7). This is another EOB with several patients listed on it. The insurance sent one check for $555.60. A portion of this payment pertains to each patient. Post payments for each patient as indicated on the EOB.

STEP 1
Start MOSS.

STEP 2
Refer to the EOB in Source Document 8-7 in the Source Document Appendix. Review the information on the EOB, then answer the following questions. *Cover the answers using the tear-off bookmark from the cover of your book. Check your work before entering data into MOSS to be sure you have correctly interpreted the source documents.*

A.	What are the names of the insured (policyholders) and what are the names of the patients (dependents)?	Insured: **Cynthia Worthington**; Patient: **Cynthia Worthington** Insured: **Ross Ybarra**; Patient: **Elane Ybarra** Insured: **Jason Tate**; Patient: **Jason Tate**
B.	For each patient, identify the provider and whether he or she is in-network or out-of-network.	**Worthington: Dr. Heath, an in-network provider** **Ybarra: Dr. Schwartz, an out-of-network provider** **Tate: Dr. Heath, an in-network provider**

Review each service and charge. Analyze each column, using the benefit determination notes to assist you with the information. Write down service date, CPT code(s), charge(s) submitted, the non-covered or discount amount, the amount covered, the co-insurance amount, and the covered balance and plan liability for each patient that will be used for posting the payment. *Cover the answers below using the tear-off bookmark from the cover of your book.*

Worthington

Service date:	CPT code	Charge submitted:	Discount:	Amount covered:	Plan liability:	Co-insurance

Ybarra

Service date:	CPT code	Charge submitted:	Amount not covered:	Amount covered:	Plan liability:	Co-insurance

continues

POSTING PAYMENTS FOR MULTIPLE PATIENTS LISTED ON ONE EOB FOR FLEXIHEALTH PPO *continued*

Tate

Service date:	CPT code	Charge submitted:	Discount:	Amount covered:	Plan liability:	Co-insurance

Worthington

Service date:	CPT code	Charge submitted:	Discount:	Amount covered:	Plan liability:	Co-insurance
10/30/2009	99213	$111.00	$28.60	$82.40	$62.40	$20.00

Ybarra

Service date:	CPT code	Charge submitted:	Amount not covered:	Amount covered:	Plan liability:	Co-insurance
10/16/2009	99214	$180.00	$11.50	$168.50	$134.80	$33.70
10/16/2009	87081	$16.00	$0.00	$16.00	$12.80	$3.20
11/6/2009	99215	$249.00	$33.20	$215.80	$172.64	$43.16
11/6/2009	81000	$12.00	$0.00	$12.00	$9.60	$2.40

Tate

Service date:	CPT code	Charge submitted:	Discount:	Amount covered:	Plan liability:	Co-insurance
11/3/2009	99221	$145.00	$52.00	$93.00	$74.40	$18.60
11/4/2009	99231	$79.00	$26.00	$53.00	$42.40	$10.60
11/6/2009	99238	$145.00	$86.80	$58.20	$46.56	$11.64

STEP 3

Click on the *Posting Payments button* from the Main Menu. The Patient Selection window opens. Open a Payment Entry screen for Cynthia Worthington.

HINT: Use 11/30/2009 as the posting date and use Field 5 to record the reference number.

STEP 4

Post the payment for patient Worthington using the information you read from the EOB in Step 2. Before clicking the *Post button*, check your work with Figure 8-58. Last, view the Patient Ledger and compare to Figure 8-59.

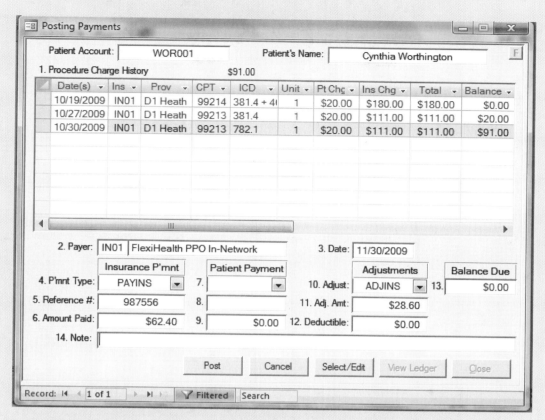

FIGURE 8-58

Delmar/Cengage Learning

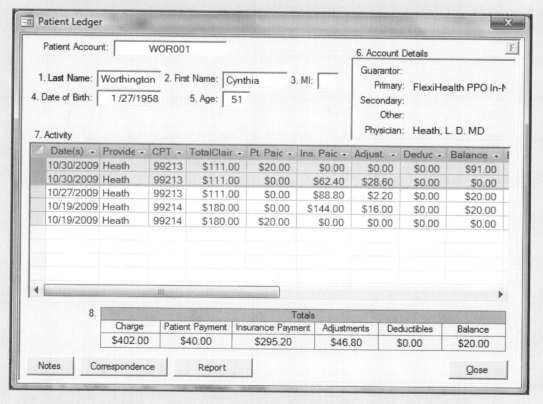

FIGURE 8-59

Delmar/Cengage Learning

continues

POSTING PAYMENTS FOR MULTIPLE PATIENTS LISTED ON ONE EOB FOR FLEXIHEALTH PPO *continued*

STEP 5

When finished, and the Patient Ledger has been viewed (Figure 8-59), close any open windows and return to Main Menu of MOSS.

STEP 6

Click on the *Posting Payments button* from the Main Menu. The Patient Selection window opens. Open a Payment Entry screen for Elane Ybarra.

HINT: Use 11/30/2009 as the posting date and use Field 5 to record the reference number.

STEP 7

Post the payment for services on 10/16/2009 for patient Ybarra using the information you read from the EOB in Step 2. Before clicking the *Post button*, check your work with Figure 8-60 and Figure 8-61.

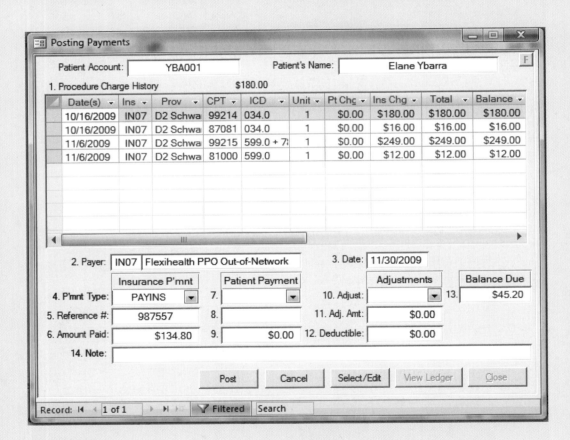

FIGURE 8-60

Delmar/Cengage Learning

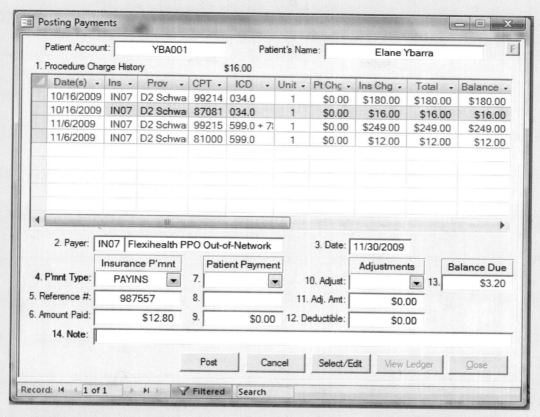

FIGURE 8-61

Delmar/Cengage Learning

STEP 8

Open the Patient Ledger for patient Ybarra and check your work with Figure 8-62. Add a note to the ledger, as previously learned, that reads: "Patient owes the non-covered portion of the charges; Dr. Schwartz is an out-of-network physician for FlexiHealth PPO."

continues

POSTING PAYMENTS FOR MULTIPLE PATIENTS LISTED ON ONE EOB FOR FLEXIHEALTH PPO *continued*

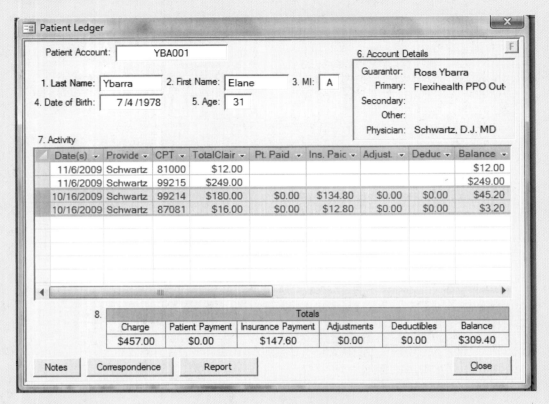

FIGURE 8-62

Delmar/Cengage Learning

STEP 9

When finished, close the Patient Ledger and continue posting payments for procedures on 11/6/2009 for patient Ybarra, using the information you read from the EOB in Step 2. Continue using 11/30/2009 as the posting date and the reference number from the EOB in Field 5. Check your work with Figure 8-63 and Figure 8-64.

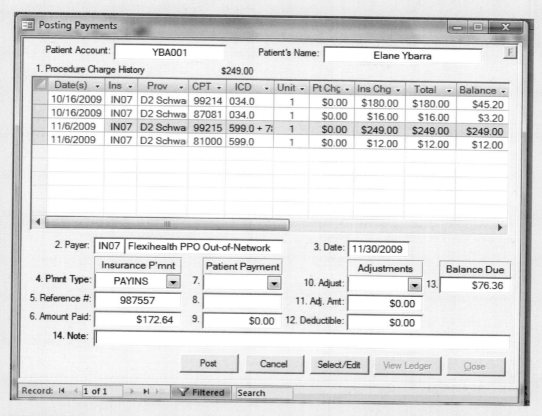

FIGURE 8-63

Delmar/Cengage Learning

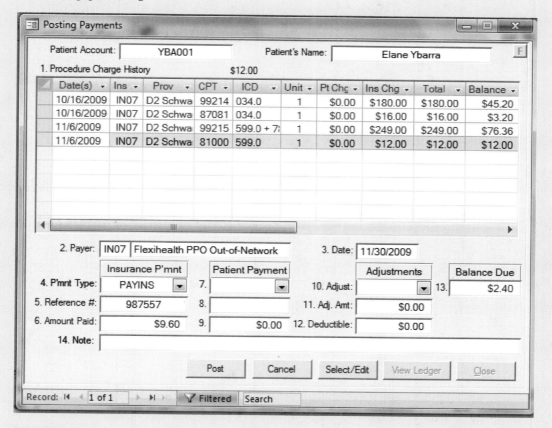

FIGURE 8-64

Delmar/Cengage Learning

continues

POSTING PAYMENTS FOR MULTIPLE PATIENTS LISTED ON ONE EOB FOR FLEXIHEALTH PPO *continued*

STEP 10

View the ledger for Patient Ybarra and check your work with Figure 8-65. When finished, closed all open windows and return to the Main Menu.

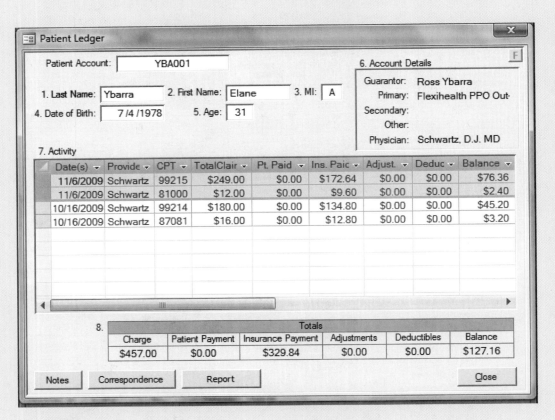

FIGURE 8-65

Delmar/Cengage Learning

STEP 11

Click on the *Posting Payments button* from the Main Menu. The Patient Selection window opens. Open a Payment Entry screen for Jason Tate.

HINT: Use 11/30/2009 as the posting date, and use Field 5 to record the reference number.

STEP 12

Post the three payments for patient Tate using the information you read from the EOB in Step 2. Before clicking the *Post button*, check your work with Figure 8-66 through Figure 8-68. Last, view the Patient Ledger and compare with Figure 8-69.

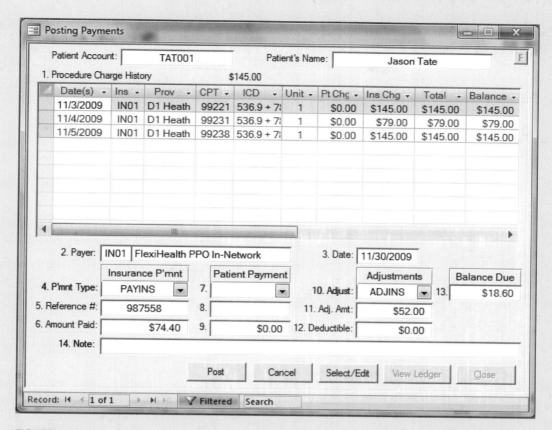

FIGURE 8-66

Delmar/Cengage Learning

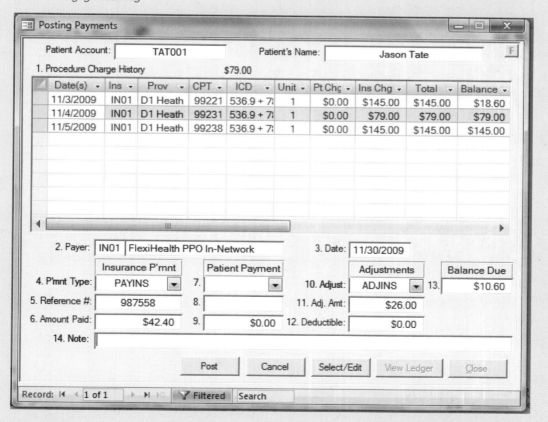

FIGURE 8-67

Delmar/Cengage Learning

continues

POSTING PAYMENTS FOR MULTIPLE PATIENTS LISTED ON ONE EOB FOR FLEXIHEALTH PPO *continued*

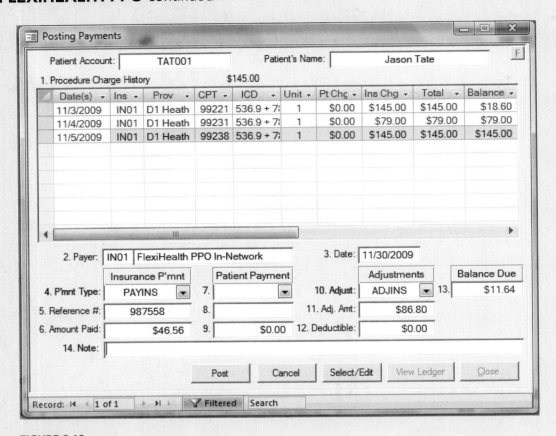

FIGURE 8-68

Delmar/Cengage Learning

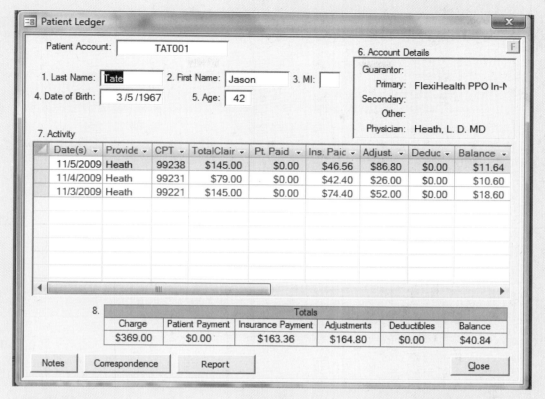

FIGURE 8-69

Delmar/Cengage Learning

STEP 13

When finished, and the Patient Ledger has been viewed (Figure 8-69), close any open windows and return to the Main Menu of MOSS.

LET'S TRY IT! 8-10 POSTING PAYMENTS FROM HRA PLANS

Objective: The reader posts payments for select patients who have ConsumerONE HRA plans, as indicated on the EOB (Source Document 8-8).

> **NOTE:** As you have studied previously, a Health Reimbursement Arrangement (HRA) is an employer-funded account that repays the medical expenses of employees. There is usually a certain amount of funds available. An HRA is accompanied by a major medical insurance plan, which is used if the employer-contributed funds and patient responsibility portions are used completely. The ConsumerONE HRA plan has three levels, which were discussed in Unit 4. Refer to Figure 4-7 on page 163. The following exercises use an EOB to post payments as they relate to these levels.

continues

STEP 1

Start MOSS.

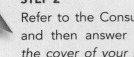

STEP 2

Refer to the ConsumerONE EOB in Source Document 8-8. Review the information on the EOB, and then answer the questions below. *Cover the answers using the tear-off bookmark from the cover of your book. Check your work before entering data into MOSS to be sure you have correctly interpreted the source documents.*

A.	Using the remark codes, identify the patient(s) who is/are in level one, level two, or level three of his or her HRA plan.	John Conway: level one Leona Goodnow: level three Eric Gordon: level two Kabin Pradhan: level one
B.	Both Drs. Heath and Schwartz are ConsumerONE in-network providers. Will there be write-offs for any of the patients on the EOB? If yes, which patients have write-offs and what is the amount of each one?	John Conway: $11.30 Leona Goodnow: None Eric Gordon: $11.30 and $23.00 Kabin Pradhan: $5.40
C.	Which patients on the EOB have exhausted their Employee Personal Account (EPA)? Up to what dollar limit will these patients have to pay for medical expenses out-of-pocket before proceeding to level three?	Eric Gordon has exhausted his EPA, and will need to pay up to $500.00 out-of-pocket in level two, before proceeding to level three (the 80/20 part of the plan).

STEP 3

Click on the *Posting Payments button* on the Main Menu. The Patient Selection window opens. Open a Payment Entry screen for John Conway.

STEP 4

Patient Conway is in level one of his plan. Funds from the EPA are used to pay for his medical expenses. Post the payment as indicated on the EOB for the $180.00 charge. Use 11/30/2009 as the posting date and the claim number in the reference field. Be sure to adjust the write-off. Check your screen with Figure 8-70 before clicking on the *Post button*.

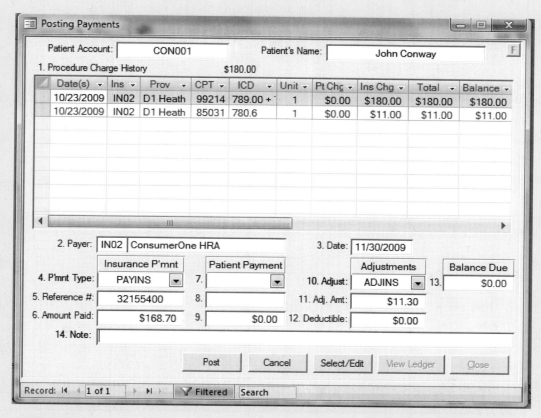

FIGURE 8-70

Delmar/Cengage Learning

STEP 5

Next, apply the payment for the $11.00 charge in the same manner. Check your work with Figure 8-71 before clicking on the *Post button*. When finished, click on *View Ledger* and compare your screen to Figure 8-72. Close any open windows and return to the Patient Selection screen for payment posting.

continues

POSTING PAYMENTS FROM HRA PLANS *continued*

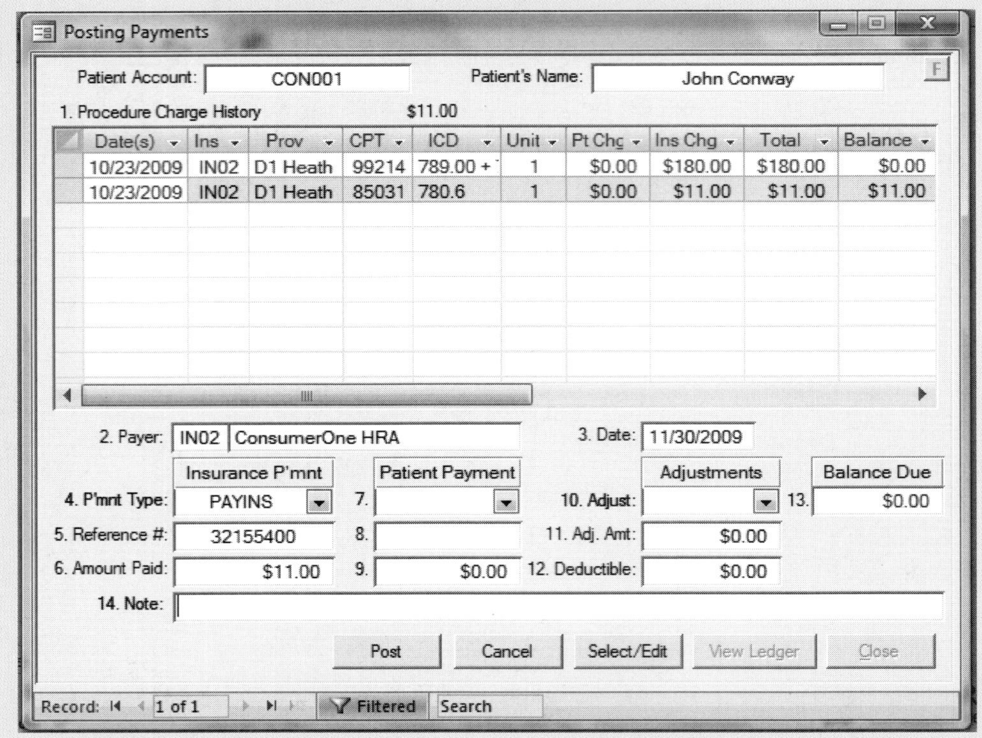

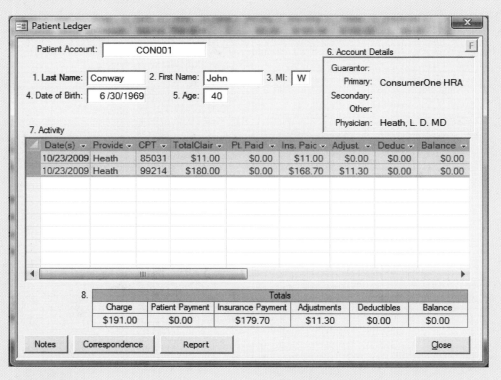

FIGURE 8-71

Delmar/Cengage Learning

FIGURE 8-72

Delmar/Cengage Learning

STEP 6

Refer to Source Document 8-8 and locate patient Goodnow. The remark code indicates she is in level three of her plan. This means that she has exhausted the funds in her EPA, and she has paid for her medical expenses out-of-pocket in level two, up to $500.00. She is now using the HRA in the major medical plan and is responsible for a co-insurance. At the start of the coming year, she will be back to level one, when her employer contributes funds into her account for medical expenses for the coming year.

Post the payment for patient Goodnow, using 11/30/2009 as the posting date and the claim number in the reference field. Check your work with Figure 8-73 before posting. After you have posted the payment, compare the Patient's Ledger screen to Figure 8-74. Close any open windows and return to the Patient Selection screen for payment posting.

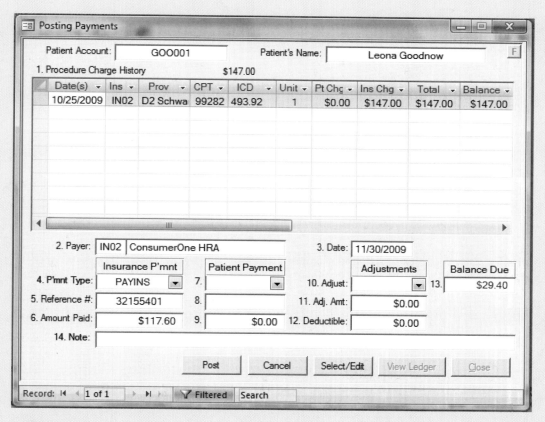

FIGURE 8-73

Delmar/Cengage Learning

continues

POSTING PAYMENTS FROM HRA PLANS *continued*

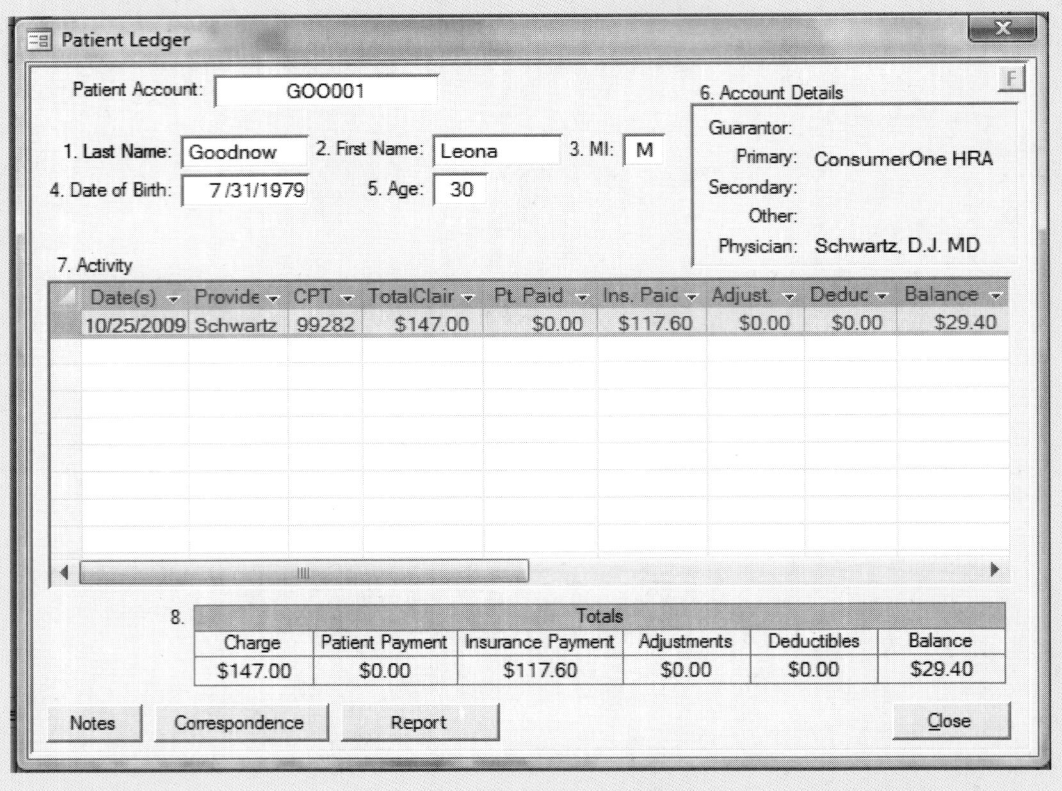

```
┌─────────────────────────────────────────────────────────────────────────┐
│ ▣ Patient Ledger                                                      ✕  │
├─────────────────────────────────────────────────────────────────────────┤
│                                                                      F    │
│   Patient Account:        GOO001              6. Account Details          │
│                                                                           │
│                                              Guarantor:                   │
│  1. Last Name: Goodnow  2. First Name: Leona  3. MI: M   Primary: ConsumerOne HRA │
│  4. Date of Birth:  7/31/1979   5. Age:  30   Secondary:                  │
│                                                  Other:                   │
│                                              Physician: Schwartz, D.J. MD │
│                                                                           │
│  7. Activity                                                              │
│  ┌──────────┬─────────┬──────┬──────────┬─────────┬─────────┬────────┬───────┬─────────┐ │
│  │ Date(s) ▾│Provide ▾│CPT ▾│TotalClair▾│Pt. Paid▾│Ins. Paic▾│Adjust.▾│Deduc ▾│Balance ▾│ │
│  │10/25/2009│Schwartz │99282│  $147.00 │  $0.00  │ $117.60 │ $0.00 │ $0.00 │ $29.40 │ │
│  │          │         │      │          │         │         │        │       │         │ │
│  └──────────┴─────────┴──────┴──────────┴─────────┴─────────┴────────┴───────┴─────────┘ │
│  ◀ ▌▌▌▌▌▌                                                              ▶  │
│                                                                           │
│      8. ┌──────────────────────────── Totals ─────────────────────────┐  │
│         │ Charge │Patient Payment│Insurance Payment│Adjustments│Deductibles│Balance │ │
│         │$147.00 │    $0.00      │    $117.60      │   $0.00   │  $0.00   │ $29.40 │ │
│                                                                           │
│  ┌────────┐ ┌──────────────┐ ┌────────┐                      ┌────────┐  │
│  │ Notes  │ │Correspondence│ │ Report │                      │ Close  │  │
│  └────────┘ └──────────────┘ └────────┘                      └────────┘  │
└─────────────────────────────────────────────────────────────────────────┘
```

FIGURE 8-74

Delmar/Cengage Learning

STEP 7

Patient Gordon is in level two of his plan, meaning that he has to pay up to $500.00 in medical expenses out-of-pocket before major medical benefits begin in level three. The allowed charges are applied as a deductible. Post the deductible and the corresponding in-network write-off (the amount disallowed). A statement will be sent to this patient later for payment. Check your screen with Figure 8-75 before clicking on the *Post button*.

STEP 8

Next, view the Patient Ledger and compare your work to Figure 8-76. Type a note in the Patient Ledger that reads: "Patient in level 2; owes balance $168.70 as deductible."

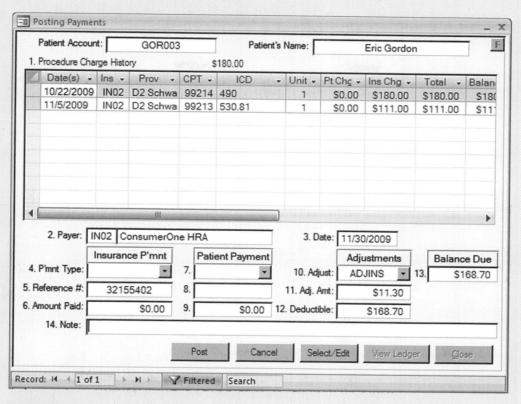

FIGURE 8-75

Delmar/Cengage Learning

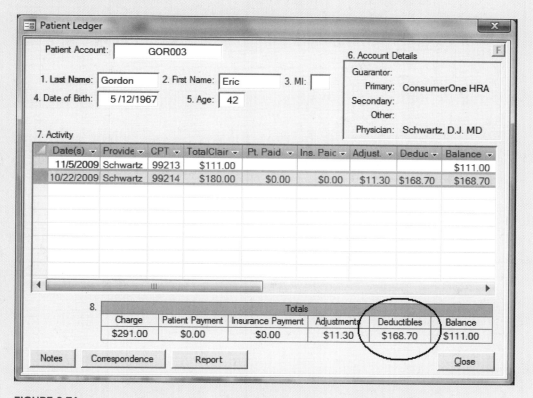

FIGURE 8-76

Delmar/Cengage Learning

continues

POSTING PAYMENTS FROM HRA PLANS *continued*

> **HINT:** Remember to make a note on the Patient Ledger to remind the staff about the deductible amount due of $88.00.

STEP 9

Enter the 11/05/09 EOB data and check your work with Figure 8-77 before posting. Next, view the Patient Ledger and compare your work to Figure 8-78. Close any open windows and return to the Patient Selection screen for payment posting.

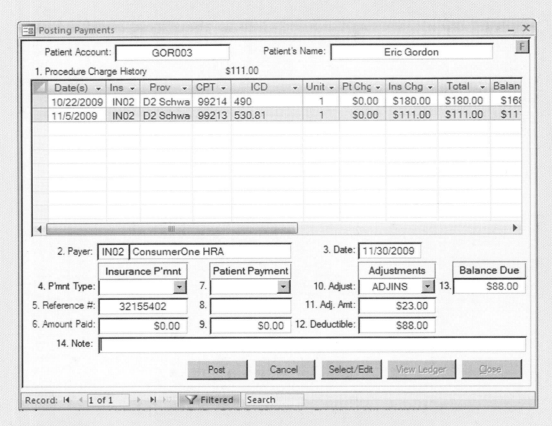

FIGURE 8-77

Delmar/Cengage Learning

STEP 10

Post the payment as indicated on the EOB for patient Pradhan. Use 11/30/2009 as the posting date and the claim number in the reference field. Check your work with Figure 8-79 before clicking on the *Post button*, and the Patient Ledger in Figure 8-80 when you have completed the posting.

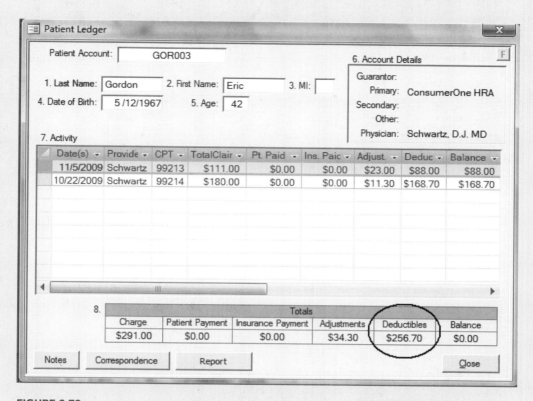

FIGURE 8-78

Delmar/Cengage Learning

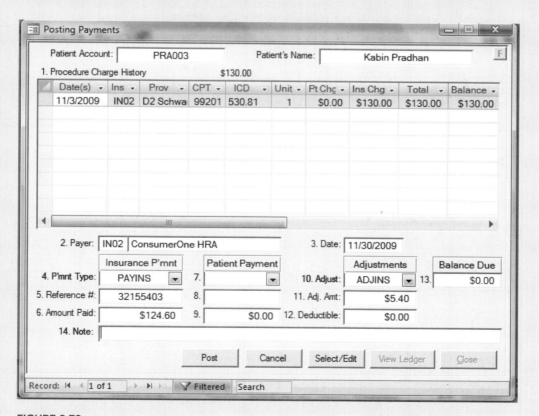

FIGURE 8-79

Delmar/Cengage Learning

continues

POSTING PAYMENTS FROM HRA PLANS *continued*

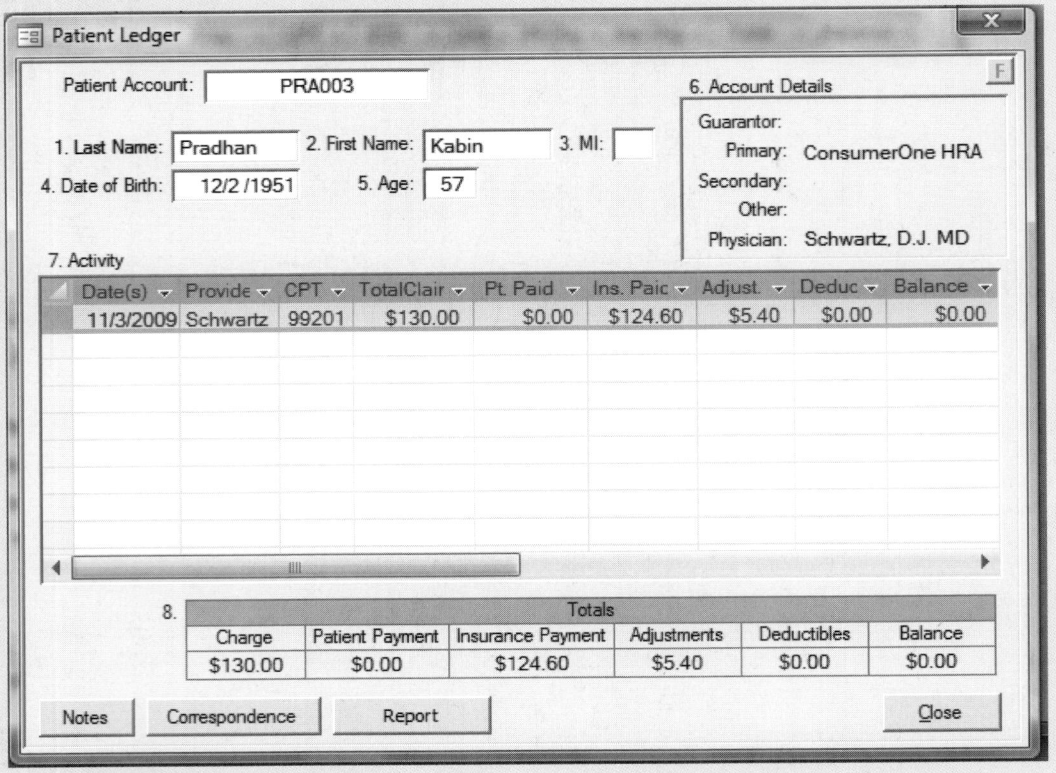

Patient Ledger									X

Patient Account: PRA003

6. Account Details

1. Last Name: Pradhan **2. First Name:** Kabin **3. MI:**

4. Date of Birth: 12/2/1951 **5. Age:** 57

Guarantor:
Primary: ConsumerOne HRA
Secondary:
Other:
Physician: Schwartz, D.J. MD

7. Activity

Date(s) ▾	Provide ▾	CPT ▾	TotalClair ▾	Pt. Paid ▾	Ins. Paic ▾	Adjust. ▾	Deduc ▾	Balance ▾
11/3/2009	Schwartz	99201	$130.00	$0.00	$124.60	$5.40	$0.00	$0.00

8.

	Totals				
Charge	Patient Payment	Insurance Payment	Adjustments	Deductibles	Balance
$130.00	$0.00	$124.60	$5.40	$0.00	$0.00

Notes | Correspondence | Report | Close

FIGURE 8-80

Delmar/Cengage Learning

STEP 11

Close any open windows and return to the Main Menu.

COORDINATION OF BENEFITS AND SECONDARY BILLING

Many of the patients in this book have dual insurance, a primary and secondary health plan that pays for medical expenses. The expression **Coordination of Benefits (COB)** means that benefits are paid so that no more than 100% of **usual, customary, and reasonable (UCR)** expenses are covered under the combined benefits of all plans. COB applies when a patient is covered by more than one plan. In Unit 4, Medigap was discussed as coverage that supplements Medicare, and is therefore a secondary payer. This is also true of a health plan a patient had while employed that converts to a supplemental policy to Medicare after retirement (although this conversion is not available to all workers). Additionally, some patients qualify for both Medicare and Medicaid, and in those cases, Medicaid is most likely the secondary payer. These situations have been discussed previously.

For commercial plans, where the patient has dual coverage, the order of payment is determined by certain rules. Before preparing claims for secondary billing, these rules will be discussed for the purpose of review and to better familiarize you with common situations that determine when a health plan is primary or secondary.

DETERMINING PRIMARY AND SECONDARY PAYER

At the time of patient registration, or whenever a patient is covered by two or more health plans, determining which plan pays first is key for insurance billing. In some cases, the insured, or even the patient, may not know which plan is primary. In other cases, the process may not be understood well by the patient, or the existence of another plan may even be withheld from the medical office.

The patient will usually indicate when two plans exist and which is primary. All medical staff should have an understanding of the general rules for coordinating dual insurance in order to verify the information given by the patient. This information then can be confirmed with the insurance company at the time verification or benefits eligibility is done.

Rule One: Employees and Group Health Plans (GHP)

If an employee is covered by a group health plan (GHP), and also by a spouse's plan, the employee's own plan is primary. Example: Mrs. Vera Diggs is covered by a GHP through her employer. She is also covered by her husband's GHP through his employer. When she receives medical services, her own insurance plan is billed first and the husband's plan is secondary.

If an employee is covered by two GHPs (both belonging to the employee), the plan with the earliest effective date is considered the primary plan.

Rule Two: Dependent Children and the Birthday Rule

The **Birthday Rule** is an informal procedure used by insurers to help determine which health plan pays first when children are dependents on more than one health plan. This situation is more common with divorced parents. In some cases, including children on each parent's insurance plan maximizes coverage.

The Birthday Rule states that the health plan of the parent whose birthday comes first in the calendar year will be considered the primary plan. The year of birth and the age of the parents are disregarded. If the parents have the same birthday, the one who has had their plan longer is primary.

Example 1: In the Johnson family, the mother's birthday is 12/5/1964. The father's birthday is 4/11/1967. The father's plan is primary for the children since April precedes December.

Example 2: In the Rogers family, the mother's birthday is 6/9/1955 and the father's birthday is 6/11/1962. The mother's plan is primary for the children since 6/9 precedes 6/11 on the calendar.

One important exception to this rule applies when the parents are either divorced or separated. The plan of the parent who has legal custody is considered primary. If the custodial parent remarries, the new spouse's plan is considered secondary. The plan of the parent without custody pays last. Additionally, group plans are considered primary over individual plans.

Rule Three: Medicare as Secondary Payer (MSP)

There are certain circumstances under which Medicare may be the secondary payer and should be billed second. The following list reviews some of the more common examples:

1. **Large Group Health Plan (LGHP).** If the patient is age 65 or over and covered by an LGHP because he or she is currently employed, or has coverage through the employment of a spouse, Medicare is the secondary payer. A **large group health plan (LGHP)** is one provided by an employer with more than 100 employees.

This means that LGHPs are the primary payers for hospital and medical expenses. If the LGHP does not pay all of the expenses, Medicare is billed second. However, upon review of the claim, Medicare considers only Medicare-covered health care services, and pays only up to the Medicare-approved amounts.

If the group health plan is provided by an employer with fewer than 20 employees, Medicare is the primary payer. In addition, the patient may choose to decline the group plan from his own or the spouse's employer. In this case, Medicare is the primary payer (and will probably be the only insurance the patient has).

2. **No-fault and Liability Insurance.** Medicare is the secondary payer where no-fault or liability insurance is applicable. **No-fault** is insurance that pays for health care services resulting from injury to the patient, or damage to property, regardless of who is at fault for causing the accident. Examples of no-fault insurance include, but are not limited to, automobile insurance, commercial insurance plans, and homeowner's insurance.

Liability insurance is coverage that protects against claims based on negligence, inappropriate action, or inaction that results in injury to someone or damage to property. Examples of liability insurance include, but are not limited to, homeowner's liability insurance, product liability insurance, automobile liability insurance, malpractice liability insurance, and underinsured motorist liability insurance.

3. **Workers' Compensation Insurance. Workers' compensation** is insurance that employers are required to carry for employees who may get sick or injured on the job. Workers' compensation pays first on the bills for health care items or services received because of work-related illness or injury.

If payment is denied by the state workers' compensation insurance, Medicare pays only for Medicare-covered items and services. Medicare should be billed only if the claim is denied or contested by the employer, or if the provider is not required to accept workers' compensation payment as payment in full. If the claim is contested, a statement for benefits contested must be provided so that Medicare will consider making conditional payment.

SECONDARY INSURANCE BILLING ROUTINES

The secondary health plan is never billed until payment from the primary plan has been received. Most health plans that pay second on a claim require a copy of the EOB (or RA) from the primary plan to accompany the claim. In some cases, after making payment, the primary insurance may "crossover" the claim to the secondary insurance. This means the payment information is automatically sent to the secondary payer by the primary insurance. The secondary payer will then make payments according to the COB criteria. This is common with Medicare when Medigap plans or Medicaid are secondary.

PROCESSING SECONDARY INSURANCE CLAIMS

Earlier in this unit, a number of payments from various insurance plans were posted to patient accounts. Some of those patients have a secondary insurance plan that must be billed for any remaining co-insurance or other eligible balances due. Secondary claims are created in the same manner that the primary claims were in Unit 7, with the exception of one setting change.

If the *Let's Try It!* exercises from earlier in this unit have not been completed, **do not proceed.** Go back and finish them now before proceeding to secondary billing.

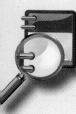

LET'S TRY IT! 8-11 SENDING SECONDARY CLAIMS TO CENTURY SENIORGAP

Objective: The reader selects patients and processes paper claims to be sent to secondary insurance companies.

STEP 1

Start MOSS.

STEP 2

On the Main Menu, click on the *Insurance Billing button*. Select the following:

A. Sort Order: Patient Name

B. Provider: ALL

C. Service Dates: 10/01/2009 through 11/30/2009

D. Patient Name: All

E. Transmit Type: Paper

F. Billing Options: Check *Secondary*. Be sure the other two selections are unchecked.

G. Payer: Century SeniorGap

STEP 3

Check your screen with Figure 8-81 before proceeding. Make corrections if needed, and then click on the *Prebilling Worksheet button*. The report shown in Figure 8-82 will display with data for patients Muñoz, Ramirez, and Tomanaga. Print the report by clicking on the *Printer icon* at the top left of the window.

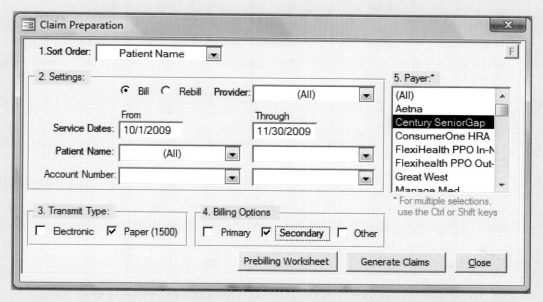

FIGURE 8-81

Delmar/Cengage Learning

continues

INSURANCE PREBILLING WORKSHEET
Student1

Dates of Service	Diag Code	Proc Code	POS	Units	Dr	As	Bill Amt	Receipts	Net
Century SeniorGap									
Munoz, Geraldo									
11/6/2009	427.31	99221	21	1.00	D1	Y	$18.47	$0.00	$18.47
11/7/2009	427.31	99231	21	2.00	D1	Y	$15.63	$0.00	$15.63
11/9/2009	427.31	99238	21	1.00	D1	Y	$14.63	$0.00	$14.63
					Totals		$48.73	$0.00	$48.73
Ramirez, Manuel									
10/19/2009	536.9	99213	11	1.00	D1	Y	$13.83	$0.00	$13.83
10/30/2009	536.9	45378	11	1.00	D1	Y	$90.30	$0.00	$90.30
10/30/2009	536.9	99215	11	1.00	D1	Y	$28.06	$0.00	$28.06
					Totals		$132.19	$0.00	$132.19
Tomanaga, Marie									
11/3/2009	413.9	85651	11	1.00	D2	Y	$0.99	$0.00	$0.99
11/3/2009	413.9	93000	11	1.00	D2	Y	$6.10	$0.00	$6.10
11/3/2009	413.9	99205	11	1.00	D2	Y	$147.96	$0.00	$147.96
					Totals		$155.05	$0.00	$155.05
		TOTAL TO BE BILLED FOR Century SeniorGap							$335.97
Grand Total		*Grand Total*							$335.97

FIGURE 8-82

Delmar/Cengage Learning

STEP 4

Use the printout of the Insurance Prebilling Worksheet to compare the results to each Patient's Ledger. When viewing the Patient Ledgers, be sure to scroll to the far right (Field 7, Activity) to compare the "Balance Due" totals to the "Net" column on the report. An example of the ledger balance due column is shown in Figure 8-83. Check the "Balance Due" for patients Muñoz, Ramirez, and Tomanaga from each of their ledgers to the "Net" column on the report.

STEP 5

Close the report (see Figure 8-84) to return to the Claim Preparation window. Next, click on the *Generate Claims button*. Review the CMS-1500 claim forms for each patient, as shown in Figure 8-85 through Figure 8-87. Each claim form should be addressed to Century SeniorGap at the top, and show the respective procedures and balance due amounts at the bottom being billed to the secondary insurance.

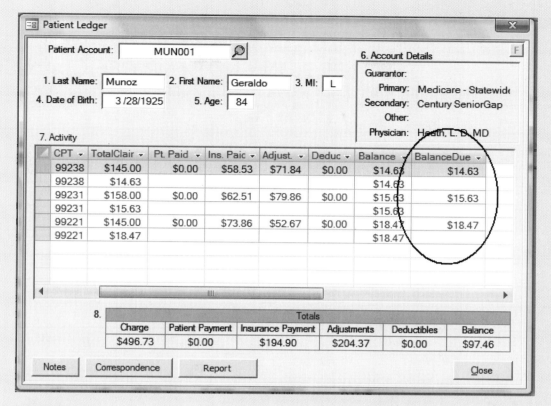

FIGURE 8-83

Delmar/Cengage Learning

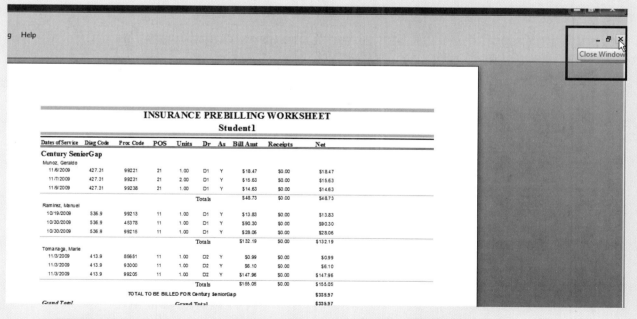

FIGURE 8-84

Delmar/Cengage Learning

continues

1500	TEST VERSION - NOT FOR OFFICIAL USE	

HEALTH INSURANCE CLAIM FORM
APPROVED BY NATIONAL UNIFORM CLAIM COMMITTEE 08/05

Century SeniorGap
4500 Old Town Way
Lowville, NY 01453

Student No: Student1

☐☐☐ PICA

PICA ☐☐☐

| 1. MEDICARE ☐(Medicare #) | MEDICAID ☐(Medicaid #) | TRICARE CHAMPUS ☐(Sponsor's SSN) | CHAMPVA ☐(Member ID) | GROUP HEALTH PLAN ☐(SSN or ID) | FECA BLK LUNG ☐(SSN) | OTHER ☒(ID) | 1a. INSURED'S I.D. NUMBER (FOR PROGRAM IN ITEM 1) 999512136 |

2. PATIENT'S NAME (Last Name, First Name, Middle Initial)
RAMIREZ MANUEL S

3. PATIENT'S BIRTHDATE 03 | 11 | 1935 **SEX** M ☒ F ☐

4. INSURED'S NAME (Last Name, First Name, Middle Initial)
RAMIREZ MANUEL S

5. PATIENT'S ADDRESS (No., Street)
1211 GRAVEL WAY

6. PATIENT'S RELATIONSHIP TO INSURED
Self ☒ Spouse ☐ Child ☐ Other ☐

7. INSURED'S ADDRESS (No., Street)
SAME

CITY DOUGLASVILLE **STATE** NY

8. PATIENT STATUS
Single ☒ Married ☐ Other ☐

CITY **STATE**

ZIP CODE 01234 **TELEPHONE (include Area Code)** (123) 457-1113

Employed ☐ Full-Time Student ☐ Part-Time Student ☐

ZIP CODE **TELEPHONE (include Area Code)**

9. OTHER INSURED'S NAME (Last Name, First Name, Mid. Initial)
RAMIREZ, MANUEL S.

10. IS PATIENT'S CONDITION RELATED TO:

11. INSURED'S POLICY GROUP OR FECA NUMBER

a. OTHER INSURED'S POLICY OR GROUP NUMBER

a. EMPLOYMENT (CURRENT OR PREVIOUS)
☐ YES ☒ NO

a. INSURED'S DATE OF BIRTH **SEX** M ☐ F ☐

b. OTHER INSURED'S BIRTHDATE 03 | 11 | 1935 **SEX** M ☐ F ☐

b. AUTO ACCIDENT? PLACE (State)
☐ YES ☒ NO

b. EMPLOYER NAME OR SCHOOL NAME

c. EMPLOYER NAME OR SCHOOL NAME

c. OTHER ACCIDENT?
☐ YES ☒ NO

c. INSURANCE PLAN NAME OR PROGRAM NAME
CENTURY SENIORGAP

d. INSURANCE PLAN NAME OR PROGRAM NAME
MEDICARE - STATEWIDE CORP.

10d. RESERVED FOR LOCAL USE

d. IS THERE ANOTHER HEALTH BENEFIT PLAN
☒ YES ☐ NO *If yes, return to and complete 9 a-d.*

READ BACK OF FORM BEFORE COMPLETING & SIGNING THIS FORM.
12. PATIENT'S OR AUTHORIZED PERSONS'S SIGNATURE I authorize the release of any medical or other info necessary to process this claim. I also request payment of government benefits either to myself or the party who accepts assignment below.

SIGNED ___ SIGNATURE ON FILE ___ DATE ___ 10302009 ___

13. PATIENT'S OR AUTHORIZED PERSONS'S SIGNATURE I authorize payment of medical benefits to the undersigned physician or supplier for services described below.

SIGNED ___ SIGNATURE ON FILE ___

14. DATE OF CURRENT: ILLNESS (First symptom) OR INJURY (Accident) OR PREGRANCY (LMP)

15. IF PATIENT HAS HAD SAME ILLNESS, GIVE FIRST DATE

16. DATES PATIENT UNABLE TO WORK IN CURRENT OCCUPATION
FROM ___ TO ___

17. NAME OF REFERRING PROVIDER OR OTHER SOURCE
SAMANTHA GREEN

17a.
17b NPI 9995598741

18. HOSPITALIZATION DATES RELATED TO CURRENT SERVICES
FROM ___ TO ___

19. RESERVED FOR LOCAL USE

20. OUTSIDE LAB? ☐ YES ☒ NO **$ CHARGES**

21. DIAGNOSIS OR NATURE OF ILLNESS OR INJURY (RELATE ITEMS 1, 2, 3 OR 4 TO ITEM 24E BY LINE
1. 536.9
2. 783.21
3. 789.00
4. |_____

22. MEDICAID SUBMISSION CODE **ORIGINAL REF. NO.**

23. PRIOR AUTHORIZATION NUMBER

24. A DATE(S) OF SERVICE From MM DD YY	To MM DD YY	B. Place of Service	C. EMG	D. PROCEDURES, SERVICES OR SUPPLIES (Explain Unusual Circumstances) CPT/HCPCS	MODIFIER	E. DIAGNOSIS POINTER	F. $ CHARGES	G. DAYS OR UNITS	H. EPSDT Family Plan	I. ID. QUAL	J. RENDERING PROVIDER ID#
1	10 19 2009		11		99213		1 2	13 83	1		NPI	999501
2	10 30 2009		11		99215		3	28 06	1		NPI	999501
3	10 30 2009		11		45378		3	90 30	1		NPI	999501
4											NPI	
5											NPI	
6											NPI	

25. FEDERAL TAX I.D. NUMBER 00-1234560 SSN ☐ EIN ☒

26. PATIENT'S ACCOUNT NO. RAM001

27. ACCEPT ASSIGNMENT? ☒ YES ☐ NO

28. TOTAL CHARGE $ 132 19

29. AMOUNT PAID $

30. BALANCE DUE $

31. SIGNATURE OF PHYSICIAN OR SUPPLIER INCLUDING DEGREES OR CREDENTIALS (I certify that the statements on the reverse apply to this bill and are made a part thereof.)
10302009
SIGNED L. D. HEATH, MD DAT

32. SERVICE FACILITY LOCATION INFORMATION
NEW YORK COUNTY HOSPITAL
1402 NORTHERN DR.
KING PARK, NY 01238
a. 9997894320 b.

33. BILLING PROVIDER INFO PH # (123) 456-7890
DOUGLASVILLE MEDICINE ASSOCIATES
5076 BRAND BLVD., SUITE 401
DOUGLASVILLE, NY 01234
a. 9995010111 b.

NUCC Instruction Manual available at: www.nucc.org

OMB APPROVAL PENDING

FIGURE 8-85

Courtesy of the Centers for Medicare & Medicaid Services

1500

TEST VERSION - NOT FOR OFFICIAL USE

HEALTH INSURANCE CLAIM FORM
APPROVED BY NATIONAL UNIFORM CLAIM COMMITTEE 08/05

Century SeniorGap
4500 Old Town Way
Lowville, NY 01453

Student No: Student1

☐☐☐ PICA

PICA ☐☐☐

| 1. MEDICARE ☐ (Medicare #) | MEDICAID ☐ (Medicaid #) | TRICARE CHAMPUS ☐ (Sponsor's SSN) | CHAMPVA ☐ (Member ID | GROUP HEALTH PLAN ☒ (SSN or ID) | FECA BLK LUNG ☐ (SSN) | OTHER ☐ (ID) | 1a. INSURED'S I.D. NUMBER   (FOR PROGRAM IN ITEM 1) 999213166 |

| 2. PATIENT'S NAME (Last Name, First Name, Middle Initial) TOMANAGA MARIE | 3. PATIENT'S BIRTHDATE   SEX 02 | 02 | 1933   M ☐ F ☒ | 4. INSURED'S NAME (Last Name, First Name, Middle Initial) TOMANAGA MARIE |

| 5. PATIENT'S ADDRESS (No., Street) 2301 MARBLE WAY | 6. PATIENT'S RELATIONSHIP TO INSURED Self ☒ Spouse ☐ Child ☐ Other ☐ | 7. INSURED'S ADDRESS (No., Street) SAME |

| CITY DOUGLASVILLE | STATE NY | 8. PATIENT STATUS Single ☐   Married ☒   Other ☐ | CITY | STATE |

| ZIP CODE 01234 | TELEPHONE (include Area Code) (123) 457-2110 | Employed ☐ Full-Time Student ☐ Part-Time Student ☐ | ZIP CODE | TELEPHONE (include Area Code) |

| 9. OTHER INSURED'S NAME (Last Name, First Name, Mid. Initial) TOMANAGA, MARIE | 10. IS PATIENT'S CONDITION RELATED TO: | 11. INSURED'S POLICY GROUP OR FECA NUMBER MG612 |

| a. OTHER INSURED'S POLICY OR GROUP NUMBER | a. EMPLOYMENT (CURRENT OR PREVIOUS) ☐ YES ☒ NO | a. INSURED'S DATE OF BIRTH   SEX   M ☐ F ☐ |

| b. OTHER INSURED'S BIRTHDATE   SEX 02 | 02 | 1933   M ☒ F ☐ | b. AUTO ACCIDENT?   PLACE (State) ☐ YES ☒ NO | b. EMPLOYER NAME OR SCHOOL NAME |

| c. EMPLOYER NAME OR SCHOOL NAME | c. OTHER ACCIDENT? ☐ YES ☒ NO | c. INSURANCE PLAN NAME OR PROGRAM NAME CENTURY SENIORGAP |

| d. INSURANCE PLAN NAME OR PROGRAM NAME MEDICARE - STATEWIDE CORP. | 10d. RESERVED FOR LOCAL USE | d. IS THERE ANOTHER HEALTH BENEFIT PLAN ☒ YES ☐ NO   If yes, return to and complete 9 a-d. |

READ BACK OF FORM BEFORE COMPLETING & SIGNING THIS FORM.

12. PATIENT'S OR AUTHORIZED PERSONS'S SIGNATURE I authorize the release of any medical or other info necessary to process this claim. I also request payment of government benefits either to myself or the party who accepts assignment below.

SIGNED   SIGNATURE ON FILE   DATE   11032009

13. PATIENT'S OR AUTHORIZED PERSONS'S SIGNATURE I authorize payment of medical benefits to the undersigned physician or supplier for services described below.

SIGNED   SIGNATURE ON FILE

| 14. DATE OF CURRENT: ◄ ILLNESS (First symptom) OR INJURY (Accident) OR PREGNANCY (LMP) | 15. IF PATIENT HAS HAD SAME ILLNESS, GIVE FIRST DATE | 16. DATES PATIENT UNABLE TO WORK IN CURRENT OCCUPATION FROM   TO |

| 17. NAME OF REFERRING PROVIDER OR OTHER SOURCE | 17a.   17b NPI | 18. HOSPITALIZATION DATES RELATED TO CURRENT SERVICES FROM   TO |

| 19. RESERVED FOR LOCAL USE | 20. OUTSIDE LAB? $ CHARGES ☒ YES ☐ NO |

21. DIAGNOSIS OR NATURE OF ILLNESS OR INJURY (RELATE ITEMS 1, 2, 3 OR 4 TO ITEM 24E BY LINE)

1. | 413.9   3. |
2. | 401.9   4. |

| 22. MEDICAID SUBMISSION CODE   ORIGINAL REF. NO. |
| 23. PRIOR AUTHORIZATION NUMBER |

24. A DATE(S) OF SERVICE			B. Place of Service	C. EMG	D. PROCEDURES, SERVICES OR SUPPLIES (Explain Unusual Circumstances) CPT/HCPCS MODIFIER	E. DIAGNOSIS POINTER	F. $ CHARGES	G. DAYS OR UNITS	H. EPSDT Family Plan	I. ID. QUAL	J. RENDERING PROVIDER ID#
From MM DD YY	To MM DD YY										
1	11 03 2009		11		99205	1 2	147 96	1		NPI	999502
2	11 03 2009		11		93000	1	6 10	1		NPI	999502
3	11 03 2009		11		85651	1	0 99	1		NPI	999502
4										NPI	
5										NPI	
6										NPI	

| 25. FEDERAL TAX I.D. NUMBER   SSN EIN 00-1234560   ☐ ☒ | 26. PATIENT'S ACCOUNT NO. TOM001 | 27. ACCEPT ASSIGNMENT? ☒ YES ☐ NO | 28. TOTAL CHARGE $ 155 05 | 29. AMOUNT PAID $ | 30. BALANCE DUE $ |

| 31. SIGNATURE OF PHYSICIAN OR SUPPLIER INCLUDING DEGREES OR CREDENTIALS (I certify that the statements on the reverse apply to this bill and are made a part thereof.) 11032009 SIGNED   D.J. SCHWARTZ, MD   DAT | 32. SERVICE FACILITY LOCATION INFORMATION BIOPACE LABORATORY 1600 MIDWAY AVE. DOUGLASVILLE, NY 01234 a. 9992849492   b. | 33. BILLING PROVIDER INFO PH #   (123) 456-7892 DOUGLASVILLE MEDICINE ASSOCIATES 5076 BRAND BLVD., SUITE 401 DOUGLASVILLE, NY 01234 a. 9995020212   b. |

NUCC Instruction Manual available at: www.nucc.org

OMB APPROVAL PENDING

FIGURE 8-86

Courtesy of the Centers for Medicare & Medicaid Services

continues

1500	**TEST VERSION - NOT FOR OFFICIAL USE**	

HEALTH INSURANCE CLAIM FORM
APPROVED BY NATIONAL UNIFORM CLAIM COMMITTEE 08/05

Century SeniorGap
4500 Old Town Way
Lowville, NY 01453

Student No: Student1

☐☐☐ PICA   PICA ☐☐☐

1. MEDICARE	MEDICAID	TRICARE CHAMPUS	CHAMPVA	GROUP HEALTH PLAN	FECA BLK LUNG	OTHER	1a. INSURED'S I.D. NUMBER (FOR PROGRAM IN ITEM 1)
☐(Medicare #)	☐(Medicaid #)	☐(Sponsor's SSN)	☐(Member ID	☒(SSN or ID)	☐(SSN)	☐(ID)	999832166

2. PATIENT'S NAME (Last Name, First Name, Middle Initial)	3. PATIENT'S BIRTHDATE SEX	4. INSURED'S NAME (Last Name, First Name, Middle Initial)
MUNOZ GERALDO L	03 | 28 | 1925 M ☒ F ☐	MUNOZ GERALDO L

5. PATIENT'S ADDRESS (No., Street)	6. PATIENT'S RELATIONSHIP TO INSURED	7. INSURED'S ADDRESS (No., Street)
1287 BOULDER COURT	Self ☒ Spouse ☐ Child ☐ Other ☐	SAME

CITY	STATE	8. PATIENT STATUS	CITY	STATE
DOUGLASVILLE	NY	Single ☒ Married ☐ Other ☐		
ZIP CODE TELEPHONE (include Area Code)		Employed ☐ Full-Time Student ☐ Part-Time Student ☐	ZIP CODE TELEPHONE (include Area Code)	
01234 (123) 457-0018				

9. OTHER INSURED'S NAME (Last Name, First Name, Mid. Initial)	10. IS PATIENT'S CONDITION RELATED TO:	11. INSURED'S POLICY GROUP OR FECA NUMBER
MUNOZ, GERALDO L.		MG5121
a. OTHER INSURED'S POLICY OR GROUP NUMBER	a. EMPLOYMENT (CURRENT OR PREVIOUS) ☐YES ☒NO	a. INSURED'S DATE OF BIRTH SEX M ☐ F ☐
b. OTHER INSURED'S BIRTHDATE SEX 03 | 28 | 1925 M ☐ F ☐	b. AUTO ACCIDENT? PLACE (State) ☐YES ☒NO	b. EMPLOYER NAME OR SCHOOL NAME
c. EMPLOYER NAME OR SCHOOL NAME	c. OTHER ACCIDENT? ☐YES ☒NO	c. INSURANCE PLAN NAME OR PROGRAM NAME CENTURY SENIORGAP
d. INSURANCE PLAN NAME OR PROGRAM NAME MEDICARE - STATEWIDE CORP.	10d. RESERVED FOR LOCAL USE	d. IS THERE ANOTHER HEALTH BENEFIT PLAN ☒ YES ☐ NO If yes, return to and complete 9 a-d.

READ BACK OF FORM BEFORE COMPLETING & SIGNING THIS FORM.

12. PATIENT'S OR AUTHORIZED PERSONS'S SIGNATURE I authorize the release of any medical or other info necessary to process this claim. I also request payment of government benefits either to myself or the party who accepts assignment below.	13. PATIENT'S OR AUTHORIZED PERSONS'S SIGNATURE I authorize payment of medical benefits to the undersigned physician or supplier for services described below.
SIGNED _____ SIGNATURE ON FILE _____ DATE ___11092009___	SIGNED _____ SIGNATURE ON FILE _____

14. DATE OF CURRENT: ◄ ILLNESS (First symptom) OR INJURY (Accident) OR PREGRACY (LMP)	15. IF PATIENT HAS HAD SAME ILLNESS, GIVE FIRST DATE	16. DATES PATIENT UNABLE TO WORK IN CURRENT OCCUPATION FROM TO
17. NAME OF REFERRING PROVIDER OR OTHER SOURCE	17a 17b NPI	18. HOSPITALIZATION DATES RELATED TO CURRENT SERVICES FROM 11 | 06 | 2009 TO 11 | 09 | 09
19. RESERVED FOR LOCAL USE		20. OUTSIDE LAB? ☐YES ☒NO $ CHARGES

21. DIAGNOSIS OR NATURE OF ILLNESS OR INJURY (RELATE ITEMS 1, 2, 3 OR 4 TO ITEM 24E BY LINE)	22. MEDICAID SUBMISSION CODE ORIGINAL REF. NO.
1. | 427.31 3. | _____	
2. | _____ 4. | _____	23. PRIOR AUTHORIZATION NUMBER

24. A DATE(S) OF SERVICE From To MM DD YY MM DD YY	B. Place of Service	C. EMG	D. PROCEDURES, SERVICES OR SUPPLIES (Explain Unusual Circumstances) CPT/HCPCS MODIFIER	E. DIAGNOSIS POINTER	F. $ CHARGES	G. DAYS OR UNITS	H. EPSDT Famly Plan	I. ID. QUAL	J. RENDERING PROVIDER ID#
1	11 06 2009		21		99221	1	18 47	1		NPI	999501
2	11 07 2009 11 08 2009		21		99231	1	15 26	2		NPI	999501
3	11 09 2009		21		99238	1	14 63	1		NPI	999501
4										NPI	
5										NPI	
6										NPI	

25. FEDERAL TAX I.D. NUMBER SSN EIN	26. PATIENT'S ACCOUNT NO	27. ACCEPT ASSIGNMENT?	28. TOTAL CHARGE	29. AMOUNT PAID	30. BALANCE DUE
00-1234560 ☐ ☒	MUN001	☒YES ☐NO	$ 48 73	$	$

31. SIGNATURE OF PHYSICIAN OR SUPPLIER INCLUDING DEGREES OR CREDENTIALS (I certify that the statements on the reverse apply to this bill and are made a part thereof.)	32. SERVICE FACILITY LOCATION INFORMATION	33. BILLING PROVIDER INFO PH # (123) 456-7890
11092009 SIGNED L. D. HEATH, MD DAT	NEW YORK COUNTY HOSPITAL 1402 NORTHERN DR. KING PARK, NY 01238 a. 9997894320 b.	DOUGLASVILLE MEDICINE ASSOCIATES 5076 BRAND BLVD., SUITE 401 DOUGLASVILLE, NY 01234 a. 9995010111 b.

NUCC Instruction Manual available at: www.nucc.org   OMB APPROVAL PENDING

FIGURE 8-87
Courtesy of the Centers for Medicare & Medicaid Services

STEP 6

When claims are ready to be printed, click on the *Print Forms button*. In a medical office, the provider, or authorized representative, would sign the claim forms. Then, a copy of the RA from the primary insurance, in this case Medicare, is attached to the claim form and mailed to the secondary payer. Find the source document from the back of your book with the Medicare RA that shows the primary billing and payments made, and attach it to your claim form. Be sure to adhere to HIPAA privacy guidelines and send only EOB information pertinent to the patient. If more than one patient is listed on the EOB, that information must be removed.

HINT: If needed, make copies of the Medicare RA to attach to other secondary patient claims.

STEP 7

Save the hard copies of the claims, or follow the directions of your instructor for turning in your work. Close all open windows in MOSS when finished and return to the Main Menu.

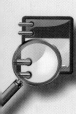

LET'S TRY IT! 8-12 PREPARING AND PROCESSING SECONDARY CLAIMS—MANALY, RICHARD

Objective: The reader selects patients and processes paper claims to be sent to secondary insurance companies. Patient Manaly is an example of a senior who is still working and has an LGHP through his employer. He also has Medicare, which is the secondary plan. Recall the rules that were studied previously for COB for patients with dual insurance.

STEP 1

Start MOSS.

STEP 2

On the Main Menu, click on the *Insurance Billing button*. Select the following:

  A. Sort Order: Patient Name

  B. Provider: ALL

  C. Service Dates: 10/01/2009 through 11/30/2009

  D. Patient Name: Richard Manaly

  E. Transmit Type: Paper

  F. Billing Options: Check *Secondary*. Be sure the other two selections are unchecked.

  G. Payer: ALL

STEP 3

Check your screen with Figure 8-88 before proceeding. Make corrections if needed, and then click on the *Prebilling Worksheet button*. The report shown in Figure 8-89 will display the data for patient Manaly. Print the report by clicking on the *Printer icon* at the top left of the window.

continues

PREPARING AND PROCESSING SECONDARY CLAIMS—MANALY, RICHARD *continued*

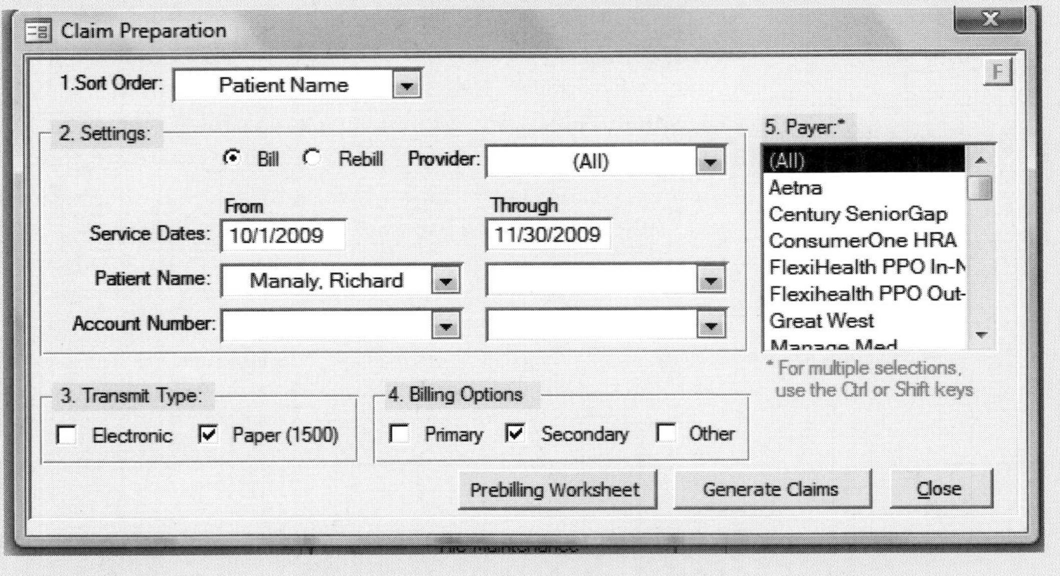

FIGURE 8-88

Delmar/Cengage Learning

INSURANCE PREBILLING WORKSHEET

Student1

Dates of Service	Diag Code	Proc Code	POS	Units	Dr	As	Bill Amt	Receipts	Net
Medicare - Statewide Corp.									
Manaly, Richard									
10/21/2009	250.00	99213	11	1.00	D2	N	$45.08	$0.00	$45.08
				Totals			$45.08	$0.00	$45.08
		TOTAL TO BE BILLED FOR Medicare - Statewide Corp.							**$45.08**
Grand Total			**Grand Total**						**$45.08**

FIGURE 8-89

Delmar/Cengage Learning

STEP 4

Use the printout of the Insurance Prebilling Worksheet to compare the results to patient Manaly's ledger. Remember to scroll to the far right (Field 7, Activity) to compare the "Balance Due" totals to the "Net" column on the report.

STEP 5

Close the report to return to the Claim Preparation window. Next, click on the *Generate Claims button*. Review the CMS-1500 claim form for Richard Manaly, as shown in Figure 8-90. The claim form should be addressed to Medicare–Statewide Corporation at the top, and show the procedure and balance due amount being billed to the secondary insurance.

1500		TEST VERSION - NOT FOR OFFICIAL USE			

HEALTH INSURANCE CLAIM FORM
APPROVED BY NATIONAL UNIFORM CLAIM COMMITTEE 08/05

Medicare - Statewide Corp.
200 Tech Center
Queens City, NY 01135

Student No: Student1

☐☐☐ PICA   PICA ☐☐

1. MEDICARE MEDICAID TRICARE CHAMPVA GROUP FECA OTHER	1a. INSURED'S I.D. NUMBER (FOR PROGRAM IN ITEM 1)

☒ (Medicare #) ☐ (Medicaid #) ☐ CHAMPUS (Sponsor's SSN) ☐ (Member ID) ☐ HEALTH PLAN (SSN or ID) ☐ BLK LUNG (SSN) ☐ (ID)

1a. INSURED'S I.D. NUMBER (FOR PROGRAM IN ITEM 1)
999236189A

2. PATIENT'S NAME (Last Name, First Name, Middle Initial)
MANALY RICHARD L

3. PATIENT'S BIRTHDATE   SEX
04 | 22 | 1940   M ☒ F ☐

4. INSURED'S NAME (Last Name, First Name, Middle Initial)

5. PATIENT'S ADDRESS (No., Street)
116 GRANITE STREET

6. PATIENT'S RELATIONSHIP TO INSURED
Self ☐ Spouse ☐ Child ☐ Other ☐

7. INSURED'S ADDRESS (No., Street)

CITY **DOUGLASVILLE**   STATE **NY**

8. PATIENT STATUS
Single ☒   Married ☐   Other ☐

CITY   STATE

ZIP CODE **01235**   TELEPHONE (include Area Code) **(123) 457-8724**

Employed ☒   Full-Time Student ☐   Part-Time Student ☐

ZIP CODE   TELEPHONE (include Area Code)

9. OTHER INSURED'S NAME (Last Name, First Name, Mid. Initial)

10. IS PATIENT'S CONDITION RELATED TO:

11. INSURED'S POLICY GROUP OR FECA NUMBER
NONE

a. OTHER INSURED'S POLICY OR GROUP NUMBER

a. EMPLOYMENT (CURRENT OR PREVIOUS)
☐ YES ☒ NO

a. INSURED'S DATE OF BIRTH   SEX
M ☐ F ☐

b. OTHER INSURED'S BIRTHDATE   SEX
M ☐ F ☐

b. AUTO ACCIDENT?   PLACE (State)
☐ YES ☒ NO

b. EMPLOYER NAME OR SCHOOL NAME

c. EMPLOYER NAME OR SCHOOL NAME

c. OTHER ACCIDENT?
☐ YES ☒ NO

c. INSURANCE PLAN NAME OR PROGRAM NAME

d. INSURANCE PLAN NAME OR PROGRAM NAME

10d. RESERVED FOR LOCAL USE

d. IS THERE ANOTHER HEALTH BENEFIT PLAN
☐ YES ☐ NO   If yes, return to and complete 9 a-d.

READ BACK OF FORM BEFORE COMPLETING & SIGNING THIS FORM.
12. PATIENT'S OR AUTHORIZED PERSONS'S SIGNATURE I authorize the release of any medical or other info necessary to process this claim. I also request payment of government benefits either to myself or the party who accepts assignment below.

SIGNED ___ SIGNATURE ON FILE ___ DATE **10212009**

13. PATIENT'S OR AUTHORIZED PERSONS'S SIGNATURE I authorize payment of medical benefits to the undersigned physician or supplier for services described below.

SIGNED ___

14. DATE OF CURRENT: ◄ ILLNESS (First symptom) OR INJURY (Accident) OR PREGNANCY (LMP)

15. IF PATIENT HAS HAD SAME ILLNESS, GIVE FIRST DATE

16. DATES PATIENT UNABLE TO WORK IN CURRENT OCCUPATION
FROM   TO

17. NAME OF REFERRING PROVIDER OR OTHER SOURCE
17a
17b NPI

18. HOSPITALIZATION DATES RELATED TO CURRENT SERVICES
FROM   TO

19. RESERVED FOR LOCAL USE

20. OUTSIDE LAB? ☐ YES ☒ NO $ CHARGES

21. DIAGNOSIS OR NATURE OF ILLNESS OR INJURY (RELATE ITEMS 1, 2, 3 OR 4 TO ITEM 24E BY LINE)
1. **250.00**   3. |___
2. |___   4. |___

22. MEDICAID SUBMISSION CODE   ORIGINAL REF. NO.

23. PRIOR AUTHORIZATION NUMBER

24. A DATE(S) OF SERVICE From MM DD YY / To MM DD YY	B. Place of Service	C. EMG	D. PROCEDURES, SERVICES OR SUPPLIES (Explain Unusual Circumstances) CPT/HCPCS / MODIFIER	E. DIAGNOSIS POINTER	F. $ CHARGES	G. DAYS OR UNITS	H. EPSDT Family Plan	I. ID. QUAL	J. RENDERING PROVIDER ID#
1 10 21 2009	11		99213	1	45 08	1		NPI	999502
2								NPI	
3								NPI	
4								NPI	
5								NPI	
6								NPI	

25. FEDERAL TAX I.D. NUMBER   SSN EIN
00-1234560   ☐ ☒

26. PATIENT'S ACCOUNT NO
MAN002

27. ACCEPT ASSIGNMENT?
☐ YES ☒ NO

28. TOTAL CHARGE
$ **45 08**

29. AMOUNT PAID
$

30. BALANCE DUE
$

31. SIGNATURE OF PHYSICIAN OR SUPPLIER INCLUDING DEGREES OR CREDENTIALS (I certify that the statements on the reverse apply to this bill and are made a part thereof.)
10212009
SIGNED **D.J. SCHWARTZ, MD** DAT

32. SERVICE FACILITY LOCATION INFORMATION
DOUGLASVILLE MEDICINE ASSOCIATES
5076 BRAND BLVD., SUITE 401
DOUGLASVILLE, NY 01234
a. **9995020212**   b.

33. BILLING PROVIDER INFO PH # **(123) 456-7892**
DOUGLASVILLE MEDICINE ASSOCIATES
5076 BRAND BLVD., SUITE 401
DOUGLASVILLE, NY 01234
a. **9995020212**   b.

NUCC Instruction Manual available at: www.nucc.org   OMB APPROVAL PENDING

FIGURE 8-90

Courtesy of the Centers for Medicare & Medicaid Services

continues

PREPARING AND PROCESSING SECONDARY CLAIMS—MANALY, RICHARD *continued*

STEP 6

When the claim is ready to be printed, click on the *Print Forms button*. In a medical office, the provider, or authorized representative, would sign the claim forms. Then, a copy of the EOB from the primary insurance, in this case FlexiHealth PPO Out-of-Network, is attached to the claim form and mailed to the secondary payer. Find the source document from the back of your book with the FlexiHealth EOB that shows the primary billing and payments made, and attach it to your claim form. Be sure to adhere to HIPAA privacy guidelines and send only EOB information pertinent to the patient. If more than one patient is listed on the EOB, that information must be removed.

STEP 7

Save the hard copies of the claims, or follow the directions of your instructor for turning in your work. Close all open windows in MOSS when finished and return to the Main Menu.

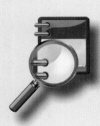

LET'S TRY IT! 8-13 PREPARING AND PROCESSING SECONDARY CLAIMS—RUHL, MARY

Objective: The reader selects patients and processes paper claims to be sent to secondary insurance companies. Patient Ruhl is an example of a senior with Medicare who is covered as a dependent on her spouse's health plan. Since her husband has an LGHP with his employer, the plan is primary for Mary's medical expenses. Medicare is billed second.

STEP 1
Start MOSS.

STEP 2
On the Main Menu, click on the *Insurance Billing button*. Select the following:

A. Sort Order: Patient Name

B. Provider: ALL

C. Service Dates: 10/01/2009 through 11/30/2009

D. Patient Name: Mary Ruhl

E. Transmit Type: Paper

F. Billing Options: Check *Secondary*. Be sure the other two selections are unchecked.

G. Payer: ALL

STEP 3
Check your screen with Figure 8-91 before proceeding. Make corrections if needed, and then click on the *Prebilling Worksheet button*. The report shown in Figure 8-92 will display the data for patient Ruhl. Print the report by clicking on the *Printer icon* at the top left of the window.

STEP 4
Use the printout of the Insurance Prebilling Worksheet to compare the results to patient Ruhl's ledger. Remember to scroll to the far right (Field 7, Activity) to compare the "Balance Due" totals to the "Net" column on the report.

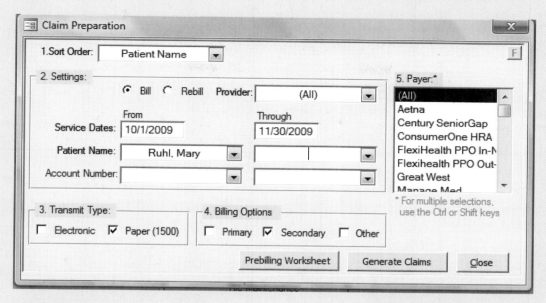

FIGURE 8-91
Delmar/Cengage Learning

INSURANCE PREBILLING WORKSHEET
Student1

Dates of Service	Diag Code	Proc Code	POS	Units	Dr	As	Bill Amt	Receipts	Net
Medicare - Statewide Corp.									
Ruhl, Mary									
11/5/2009	558.9	99221	21	1.00	D1	Y	$18.60	$0.00	$18.60
11/6/2009	558.9	99231	21	4.00	D1	Y	$42.40	$0.00	$42.40
11/10/2009	558.9	99238	21	1.00	D1	Y	$11.64	$0.00	$11.64
						Totals	$72.64	$0.00	$72.64
		TOTAL TO BE BILLED FOR Medicare - Statewide Corp.							$72.64
Grand Total		*Grand Total*							$72.64

FIGURE 8-92
Delmar/Cengage Learning

STEP 5

Close the report to return to the Claim Preparation window. Next, click on the *Generate Claims* button. Review the CMS-1500 claim form for Mary Ruhl, as shown in Figure 8-93. The claim form should be addressed to Medicare – Statewide Corporation at the top, and show the respective procedures and balance due amounts at the bottom being billed to the secondary insurance.

continues

PREPARING AND PROCESSING SECONDARY CLAIMS—RUHL, MARY *continued*

1500	**TEST VERSION - NOT FOR OFFICIAL USE**

HEALTH INSURANCE CLAIM FORM
APPROVED BY NATIONAL UNIFORM CLAIM COMMITTEE 08/05

Medicare - Statewide Corp.
200 Tech Center
Queens City, NY 01135

Student No: Student1

☐☐ PICA   PICA ☐☐☐

1. MEDICARE ☒(Medicare #) MEDICAID ☐(Medicaid #) TRICARE CHAMPUS ☐(Sponsor's SSN) CHAMPVA ☐(Member ID) GROUP HEALTH PLAN ☐(SSN or ID) FECA BLK LUNG ☐(SSN) OTHER ☐(ID)	1a. INSURED'S I.D. NUMBER (FOR PROGRAM IN ITEM 1) 999321168B

2. PATIENT'S NAME (Last Name, First Name, Middle Initial) RUHL MARY A	3. PATIENT'S BIRTHDATE 12 | 05 | 1935 SEX M☐ F☒	4. INSURED'S NAME (Last Name, First Name, Middle Initial)

5. PATIENT'S ADDRESS (No., Street) 1233 GRAVEL WAY	6. PATIENT'S RELATIONSHIP TO INSURED Self☐ Spouse☐ Child☐ Other☐	7. INSURED'S ADDRESS (No., Street)

CITY DOUGLASVILLE STATE NY	8. PATIENT STATUS Single☐ Married☒ Other☐	CITY DOUGLASVILLE STATE NY

ZIP CODE 01234 TELEPHONE (include Area Code) (123) 457-2133	Employed☐ Full-Time Student☐ Part-Time Student☐	ZIP CODE 01234 TELEPHONE (include Area Code) (123) 457-2133

9. OTHER INSURED'S NAME (Last Name, First Name, Mid. Initial)	10. IS PATIENT'S CONDITION RELATED TO:	11. INSURED'S POLICY GROUP OR FECA NUMBER NONE

a. OTHER INSURED'S POLICY OR GROUP NUMBER	a. EMPLOYMENT (CURRENT OR PREVIOUS) ☐YES ☒NO	a. INSURED'S DATE OF BIRTH SEX M☐ F☐

b. OTHER INSURED'S BIRTHDATE SEX M☐ F☐	b. AUTO ACCIDENT? ☐YES ☒NO PLACE (State)	b. EMPLOYER NAME OR SCHOOL NAME

c. EMPLOYER NAME OR SCHOOL NAME	c. OTHER ACCIDENT? ☐YES ☒NO	c. INSURANCE PLAN NAME OR PROGRAM NAME

d. INSURANCE PLAN NAME OR PROGRAM NAME	10d. RESERVED FOR LOCAL USE	d. IS THERE ANOTHER HEALTH BENEFIT PLAN ☐YES ☐NO If yes, return to and complete 9 a-d.

READ BACK OF FORM BEFORE COMPLETING & SIGNING THIS FORM.

12. PATIENT'S OR AUTHORIZED PERSONS'S SIGNATURE I authorize the release of any medical or other info necessary to process this claim. I also request payment of government benefits either to myself or the party who accepts assignment below.

SIGNED ___SIGNATURE ON FILE___   DATE ___11102009___

13. PATIENT'S OR AUTHORIZED PERSONS'S SIGNATURE I authorize payment of medical benefits to the undersigned physician or supplier for services described below.

SIGNED _____

14. DATE OF CURRENT: ◄ ILLNESS (First symptom) OR INJURY (Accident) OR PREGNANCY (LMP)	15. IF PATIENT HAS HAD SAME ILLNESS, GIVE FIRST DATE	16. DATES PATIENT UNABLE TO WORK IN CURRENT OCCUPATION FROM ___ TO ___

17. NAME OF REFERRING PROVIDER OR OTHER SOURCE	17a. 17b. NPI	18. HOSPITALIZATION DATES RELATED TO CURRENT SERVICES FROM 11 | 05 | 2009 TO 11 | 10 | 10

19. RESERVED FOR LOCAL USE		20. OUTSIDE LAB? ☐YES ☒NO $ CHARGES

21. DIAGNOSIS OR NATURE OF ILLNESS OR INJURY (RELATE ITEMS 1, 2, 3 OR 4 TO ITEM 24E BY LINE)

1. 558.9   3. 780.6
2. 276.51   4.

22. MEDICAID SUBMISSION CODE ORIGINAL REF. NO.
23. PRIOR AUTHORIZATION NUMBER 22136950

24. A. DATE(S) OF SERVICE From MM DD YY To MM DD YY	B. Place of Service	C. EMG	D. PROCEDURES, SERVICES OR SUPPLIES (Explain Unusual Circumstances) CPT/HCPCS MODIFIER	E. DIAGNOSIS POINTER	F. $ CHARGES	G. DAYS OR UNITS	H. EPSDT Family Plan	I. ID. QUAL	J. RENDERING PROVIDER ID#
1	11 05 2009	21		99221	1 2 3	18 60	1		NPI	999501
2	11 06 2009 11 09 2009	21		99231	1 2 3	42 60	4		NPI	999501
3	11 10 2009	21		99238	1 2 3	11 64	1		NPI	999501
4									NPI	
5									NPI	
6									NPI	

25. FEDERAL TAX I.D. NUMBER 00-1234560 SSN☐ EIN☒	26. PATIENT'S ACCOUNT NO. RUH001	27. ACCEPT ASSIGNMENT? ☒YES ☐NO	28. TOTAL CHARGE $ 72 64	29. AMOUNT PAID $	30. BALANCE DUE $

31. SIGNATURE OF PHYSICIAN OR SUPPLIER INCLUDING DEGREES OR CREDENTIALS (I certify that the statements on the reverse apply to this bill and are made a part thereof.) SIGNED L. D. HEATH, MD DAT 11102009	32. SERVICE FACILITY LOCATION INFORMATION NEW YORK COUNTY HOSPITAL 1402 NORTHERN DR. KING PARK, NY 01238 a. 9997894320 b.	33. BILLING PROVIDER INFO PH # (123) 456-7890 DOUGLASVILLE MEDICINE ASSOCIATES 5076 BRAND BLVD., SUITE 401 DOUGLASVILLE, NY 01234 a. 9995010111 b.

NUCC Instruction Manual available at: www.nucc.org   OMB APPROVAL PENDING

FIGURE 8-93

Courtesy of the Centers for Medicare & Medicaid Services

STEP 6

When the claim is ready to be printed, click on the *Print Forms button*. In a medical office, the provider, or authorized representative, would sign the claim forms. Then, a copy of the EOB from the primary insurance, in this case FlexiHealth PPO In-Network, is attached to the claim form and mailed to the secondary payer. Find the source document from the back of your book with the FlexiHealth EOB that shows the primary billing and payments made, and attach it to your claim form. Be sure to adhere to HIPAA privacy guidelines and send only EOB information pertinent to the patient. If more than one patient is listed on the EOB, that information must be removed.

STEP 7

Save the hard copies of the claims, or follow the directions of your instructor for turning in your work. Close all open windows in MOSS when finished and return to the Main Menu.

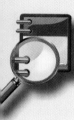

LET'S TRY IT! 8-14 PRINTING SECONDARY CLAIMS FOR THE PATIENT RECORD

Objective: Several patients in this book have Medicare as the primary and Medicaid as the secondary payer. Whenever Medicare is billed, and pays on a claim, Medicare automatically forwards any remaining balances to Medicaid for payment. As discussed earlier, this is an example of a "crossover" claim. This was indicated on the Medicare RA for patients Chang, Pinkston, and Blanc in Source Documents 8-01 and 8-02 in the back of the book. In this exercise, the reader prepares and prints the Medicaid claim forms to be placed in the patient's file for record-keeping purposes only.

STEP 1

Start MOSS.

STEP 2

On the Main Menu, click on the *Insurance Billing button*. Select the following:

A. Sort Order: Patient Name

B. Provider: ALL

C. Service Dates: 10/01/2009 through 11/30/2009

D. Patient Name: ALL

E. Transmit Type: Paper

F. Billing Options: Check *Secondary*. Be sure the other two selections are unchecked.

G. Payer: Medicaid

Check your screen with Figure 8-94 before proceeding. Make corrections if needed, and then click on the *Prebilling Worksheet button*. The report shown in Figure 8-95 will display the data for the patients who have claims being crossed over from Medicare to Medicaid. Print the report by clicking on the *Printer icon* at the top left of the window.

STEP 4

Use the printout of the Insurance Prebilling Worksheet to compare the results to each Patient's Ledger. Remember to scroll to the far right (Field 7, Activity) to compare the "Balance Due" totals to the "Net" column on the report.

continues

PRINTING SECONDARY CLAIMS FOR THE PATIENT RECORD *continued*

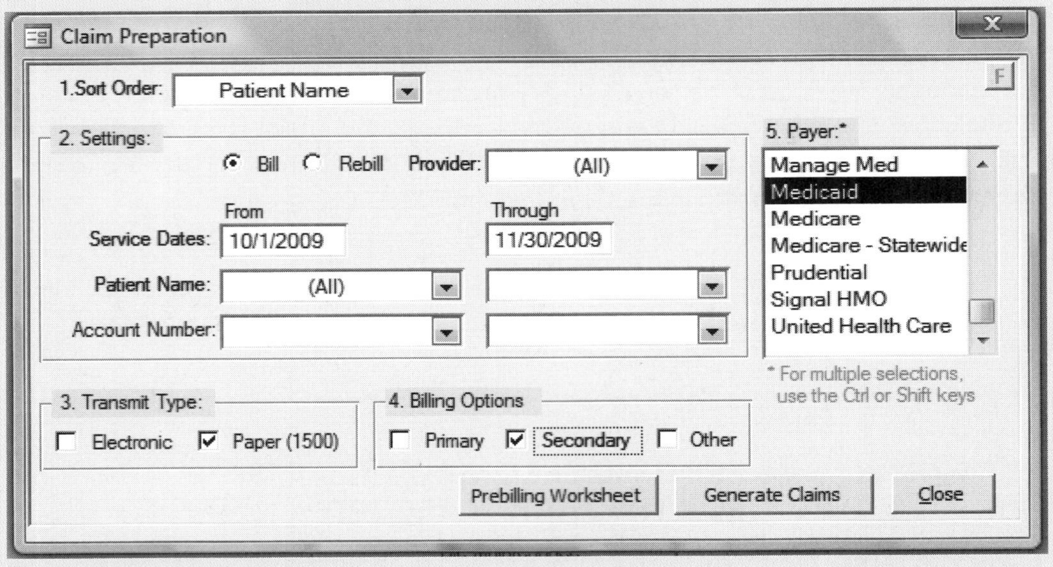

FIGURE 8-94

Delmar/Cengage Learning

INSURANCE PREBILLING WORKSHEET
Student1

Dates of Service	Diag Code	Proc Code	POS	Units	Dr	As	Bill Amt	Receipts	Net
Medicaid									
Blanc, Francois									
10/27/2009	496	99307	31	1.00	D1	Y	$7.12	$0.00	$7.12
11/24/2009	401.9	99307	32	1.00	D1	Y	$7.12	$0.00	$7.12
					Totals		$14.24	$0.00	$14.24
Chang, Xao									
10/16/2009	250.00	99307	31	1.00	D1	Y	$7.12	$0.00	$7.12
11/24/2009	780.39	99307	31	1.00	D1	Y	$7.12	$0.00	$7.12
					Totals		$14.24	$0.00	$14.24
Pinkston, Anna									
10/20/2009	401.9	99308	31	1.00	D1	Y	$14.80	$0.00	$14.80
11/24/2009	443.9	99308	31	1.00	D1	Y	$11.81	$0.00	$11.81
					Totals		$26.61	$0.00	$26.61
		TOTAL TO BE BILLED FOR Medicaid							$55.09
Grand Total					*Grand Total*				$55.09

FIGURE 8-95

Delmar/Cengage Learning

STEP 5

Close the report to return to the Claim Preparation window. Next, click on the *Generate Claims button*. Review the CMS-1500 claim forms for patients Blanc, Chang and Pinkston, as shown in Figure 8-96 through Figure 8-101. Each claim form should be addressed to Medicaid at the top, and show the respective procedures and balance due amounts at the bottom being billed to the secondary insurance.

1500	TEST VERSION - NOT FOR OFFICIAL USE

HEALTH INSURANCE CLAIM FORM
APPROVED BY NATIONAL UNIFORM CLAIM COMMITTEE 08/05

Medicaid
POB 345
Albany, NY

Student No: Student1

☐☐☐ PICA

PICA ☐☐

1. MEDICARE	MEDICAID	TRICARE CHAMPUS	CHAMPVA	GROUP HEALTH PLAN	FECA BLK LUNG	OTHER	1a. INSURED'S I.D. NUMBER (FOR PROGRAM IN ITEM 1)
☐(Medicare #)	☒(Medicaid #)	☐(Sponsor's SSN)	☐(Member ID)	☐(SSN or ID)	☐(SSN)	☐(ID)	99145611

2. PATIENT'S NAME (Last Name, First Name, Middle Initial)
BLANC FRANCOIS

3. PATIENT'S BIRTHDATE   SEX
12 | 25 | 1917   M ☒ F ☐

4. INSURED'S NAME (Last Name, First Name, Middle Initial)

5. PATIENT'S ADDRESS (No., Street)
890 MILLENNIUM WAY

6. PATIENT'S RELATIONSHIP TO INSURED
Self ☐ Spouse ☐ Child ☐ Other ☐

7. INSURED'S ADDRESS (No., Street)
SAME

CITY
DOUGLASVILLE   STATE NY

8. PATIENT STATUS
Single ☒ Married ☐ Other ☐

CITY   STATE

ZIP CODE   TELEPHONE (include Area Code)
01234   (123) 528-0012

Employed ☐ Full-Time Student ☐ Part-Time Student ☐

ZIP CODE   TELEPHONE (include Area Code)

9. OTHER INSURED'S NAME (Last Name, First Name, Mid. Initial)

10. IS PATIENT'S CONDITION RELATED TO:

11. INSURED'S POLICY GROUP OR FECA NUMBER

a. OTHER INSURED'S POLICY OR GROUP NUMBER

a. EMPLOYMENT (CURRENT OR PREVIOUS)
☐ YES ☒ NO

a. INSURED'S DATE OF BIRTH   SEX
M ☐   F ☐

b. OTHER INSURED'S BIRTHDATE   SEX
M ☐ F ☐

b. AUTO ACCIDENT?   PLACE (State)
☐ YES ☒ NO

b. EMPLOYER NAME OR SCHOOL NAME

c. EMPLOYER NAME OR SCHOOL NAME

c. OTHER ACCIDENT?
☐ YES ☒ NO

c. INSURANCE PLAN NAME OR PROGRAM NAME

d. INSURANCE PLAN NAME OR PROGRAM NAME

10d. RESERVED FOR LOCAL USE
MCD 99145611

d. IS THERE ANOTHER HEALTH BENEFIT PLAN
☐ YES   ☐ NO   If yes, return to and complete 9 a-d.

READ BACK OF FORM BEFORE COMPLETING & SIGNING THIS FORM.

12. PATIENT'S OR AUTHORIZED PERSON'S SIGNATURE I authorize the release of any medical or other info necessary to process this claim. I also request payment of government benefits either to myself or the party who accepts assignment below.

SIGNED _____ SIGNATURE ON FILE _____   DATE _____ 10272009 _____

13. PATIENT'S OR AUTHORIZED PERSON'S SIGNATURE I authorize payment of medical benefits to the undersigned physician or supplier for services described below.

SIGNED _____

14. DATE OF CURRENT: ILLNESS (First symptom) OR INJURY (Accident) OR PREGNACY (LMP)

15. IF PATIENT HAS HAD SAME ILLNESS, GIVE FIRST DATE

16. DATES PATIENT UNABLE TO WORK IN CURRENT OCCUPATION
FROM _____ TO _____

17. NAME OF REFERRING PROVIDER OR OTHER SOURCE
17a
17b NPI

18. HOSPITALIZATION DATES RELATED TO CURRENT SERVICES
FROM _____ TO _____

19. RESERVED FOR LOCAL USE

20. OUTSIDE LAB?   ☐ YES ☒ NO $ CHARGES

21. DIAGNOSIS OR NATURE OF ILLNESS OR INJURY (RELATE ITEMS 1, 2, 3 OR 4 TO ITEM 24E BY LINE)
1. 496   3.
2. 276.5   4.

22. MEDICAID SUBMISSION CODE   ORIGINAL REF. NO.

23. PRIOR AUTHORIZATION NUMBER

24. A DATE(S) OF SERVICE						B. Place of Service	C. EMG	D. PROCEDURES, SERVICES OR SUPPLIES (Explain Unusual Circumstances)		E. DIAGNOSIS POINTER	F. $ CHARGES		G. DAYS OR UNITS	H. EPSDT Family Plan	I. ID. QUAL	J. RENDERING PROVIDER ID#
From MM	DD	YY	To MM	DD	YY			CPT/HCPCS	MODIFIER							
10	27	2009				31		99307		1 2	7	12	1		NPI	999501
														NPI	
														NPI	
														NPI	
														NPI	
														NPI	

25. FEDERAL TAX I.D. NUMBER   SSN ☐ EIN ☒
00-1234560

26. PATIENT'S ACCOUNT NO
BLA001

27. ACCEPT ASSIGNMENT?
☒ YES ☐ NO

28. TOTAL CHARGE
$ 7 12

29. AMOUNT PAID
$

30. BALANCE DUE
$

31. SIGNATURE OF PHYSICIAN OR SUPPLIER INCLUDING DEGREES OR CREDENTIALS
(I certify that the statements on the reverse apply to this bill and are made a part thereof.)
10272009
SIGNED L. D. HEATH, MD   DAT

32. SERVICE FACILITY LOCATION INFORMATION
RETIREMENT INN NURSING HOME
890 MILLENNIUM WAY
DOUGLASVILLE, NY 01234
a. 9990928531   b.

33. BILLING PROVIDER INFO PH #   (123) 456-7890
DOUGLASVILLE MEDICINE ASSOCIATES
5076 BRAND BLVD., SUITE 401
DOUGLASVILLE, NY 01234
a. 9995010111   b.

NUCC Instruction Manual available at: www.nucc.org

OMB APPROVAL PENDING

FIGURE 8-96

Courtesy of the Centers for Medicare & Medicaid Services

continues

PRINTING SECONDARY CLAIMS FOR THE PATIENT RECORD *continued*

1500	**TEST VERSION - NOT FOR OFFICIAL USE**	
HEALTH INSURANCE CLAIM FORM	**Medicaid**	**Student No: Student1**
APPROVED BY NATIONAL UNIFORM CLAIM COMMITTEE 08/05	POB 345 Albany, NY	

[ ][ ][ ] PICA   PICA [ ][ ][ ]

1. MEDICARE ☐ (Medicare #)	MEDICAID ☒ (Medicaid #)	TRICARE CHAMPUS ☐ (Sponsor's SSN)	CHAMPVA ☐ (Member ID)	GROUP HEALTH PLAN ☐ (SSN or ID)	FECA BLK LUNG ☐ (SSN)	OTHER ☐ (ID)	1a. INSURED'S I.D. NUMBER (FOR PROGRAM IN ITEM 1) 99145611

2. PATIENT'S NAME (Last Name, First Name, Middle Initial) BLANC FRANCOIS	3. PATIENT'S BIRTHDATE 12 | 25 | 1917 SEX M ☒ F ☐	4. INSURED'S NAME (Last Name, First Name, Middle Initial)

5. PATIENT'S ADDRESS (No., Street) 890 MILLENNIUM WAY	6. PATIENT'S RELATIONSHIP TO INSURED Self ☐ Spouse ☐ Child ☐ Other ☐	7. INSURED'S ADDRESS (No., Street) SAME

CITY DOUGLASVILLE	STATE NY	8. PATIENT STATUS Single ☒ Married ☐ Other ☐	CITY	STATE

ZIP CODE 01234	TELEPHONE (include Area Code) (123) 528-0012	Employed ☐ Full-Time Student ☐ Part-Time Student ☐	ZIP CODE	TELEPHONE (include Area Code)

9. OTHER INSURED'S NAME (Last Name, First Name, Mid. Initial)	10. IS PATIENT'S CONDITION RELATED TO:	11. INSURED'S POLICY GROUP OR FECA NUMBER

a. OTHER INSURED'S POLICY OR GROUP NUMBER	a. EMPLOYMENT (CURRENT OR PREVIOUS) ☐ YES ☒ NO	a. INSURED'S DATE OF BIRTH SEX M ☐ F ☐

b. OTHER INSURED'S BIRTHDATE SEX M ☐ F ☐	b. AUTO ACCIDENT? ☐ YES ☒ NO PLACE (State)	b. EMPLOYER NAME OR SCHOOL NAME

c. EMPLOYER NAME OR SCHOOL NAME	c. OTHER ACCIDENT? ☐ YES ☒ NO	c. INSURANCE PLAN NAME OR PROGRAM NAME

d. INSURANCE PLAN NAME OR PROGRAM NAME	10d. RESERVED FOR LOCAL USE MCD 99145611	d. IS THERE ANOTHER HEALTH BENEFIT PLAN ☐ YES ☐ NO If yes, return to and complete 9 a-d.

READ BACK OF FORM BEFORE COMPLETING & SIGNING THIS FORM.

12. PATIENT'S OR AUTHORIZED PERSONS'S SIGNATURE I authorize the release of any medical or other info necessary to process this claim. I also request payment of government benefits either to myself or the party who accepts assignment below. SIGNED _SIGNATURE ON FILE_ DATE _11242009_	13. PATIENT'S OR AUTHORIZED PERSONS'S SIGNATURE I authorize payment of medical benefits to the undersigned physician or supplier for services described below. SIGNED _____

14. DATE OF CURRENT: ILLNESS (First symptom) OR INJURY (Accident) OR PREGNANCY (LMP)	15. IF PATIENT HAS HAD SAME ILLNESS, GIVE FIRST DATE	16. DATES PATIENT UNABLE TO WORK IN CURRENT OCCUPATION FROM TO

17. NAME OF REFERRING PROVIDER OR OTHER SOURCE	17a	18. HOSPITALIZATION DATES RELATED TO CURRENT SERVICES
	17b NPI	FROM TO

19. RESERVED FOR LOCAL USE	20. OUTSIDE LAB? ☐ YES ☒ NO $ CHARGES

21. DIAGNOSIS OR NATURE OF ILLNESS OR INJURY (RELATE ITEMS 1, 2, 3 OR 4 TO ITEM 24E BY LINE) 1. 401.9 3. 2. 250.02 4.	22. MEDICAID SUBMISSION CODE ORIGINAL REF. NO.
	23. PRIOR AUTHORIZATION NUMBER

24. A. DATE(S) OF SERVICE From MM DD YY — To MM DD YY	B. Place of Service	C. EMG	D. PROCEDURES, SERVICES OR SUPPLIES (Explain Unusual Circumstances) CPT/HCPCS	MODIFIER	E. DIAGNOSIS POINTER	F. $ CHARGES	G. DAYS OR UNITS	H. EPSDT Family Plan	I. ID. QUAL	J. RENDERING PROVIDER ID#
1	11 24 2009	31		99307		1 2	7 12	1		NPI	999501
2										NPI	
3										NPI	
4										NPI	
5										NPI	
6										NPI	

25. FEDERAL TAX I.D. NUMBER SSN EIN 00-1234560 ☐ ☒	26. PATIENT'S ACCOUNT NO BLA001	27. ACCEPT ASSIGNMENT? ☒ YES ☐ NO	28. TOTAL CHARGE $ 7 12	29. AMOUNT PAID $	30. BALANCE DUE $

31. SIGNATURE OF PHYSICIAN OR SUPPLIER INCLUDING DEGREES OR CREDENTIALS (I certify that the statements on the reverse apply to this bill and are made a part thereof.) SIGNED L. D. HEATH, MD DAT 11242009	32. SERVICE FACILITY LOCATION INFORMATION RETIREMENT INN NURSING HOME 890 MILLENNIUM WAY DOUGLASVILLE, NY 01234 a. 9990928531 b.	33. BILLING PROVIDER INFO PH # (123) 456-7890 DOUGLASVILLE MEDICINE ASSOCIATES 5076 BRAND BLVD., SUITE 401 DOUGLASVILLE, NY 01234 a. 9995010111 b.

NUCC Instruction Manual available at: www.nucc.org   OMB APPROVAL PENDING

FIGURE 8-97

Courtesy of the Centers for Medicare & Medicaid Services

1500	TEST VERSION - NOT FOR OFFICIAL USE

HEALTH INSURANCE CLAIM FORM
APPROVED BY NATIONAL UNIFORM CLAIM COMMITTEE 08/05

Medicaid
POB 345
Albany, NY

[ ][ ][ ] PICA

PICA [ ][ ][ ]

1. MEDICARE	MEDICAID	TRICARE CHAMPUS	CHAMPVA	GROUP HEALTH PLAN	FECA BLK LUNG	OTHER	1a. INSURED'S I.D. NUMBER (FOR PROGRAM IN ITEM 1)
[ ] (Medicare #)	[X] (Medicaid #)	[ ] (Sponsor's SSN)	[ ] (Member ID)	[ ] (SSN or ID)	[ ] (SSN)	[ ] (ID)	999599844

2. PATIENT'S NAME (Last Name, First Name, Middle Initial)
PINKSTON ANNA

3. PATIENT'S BIRTHDATE   SEX
07 | 28 | 1922   M [ ]   F [X]

4. INSURED'S NAME (Last Name, First Name, Middle Initial)

5. PATIENT'S ADDRESS (No., Street)
690 PARK ROSE AVE

6. PATIENT'S RELATIONSHIP TO INSURED
Self [ ] Spouse [ ] Child [ ] Other [ ]

7. INSURED'S ADDRESS (No., Street)
SAME

CITY
DOUGLASVILLE

STATE
NY

8. PATIENT STATUS
Single [X]   Married [ ]   Other [ ]

CITY

STATE

ZIP CODE
01235

TELEPHONE (include Area Code)
(123) 528-0112

Employed [ ]   Full-Time Student [ ]   Part-Time Student [ ]

ZIP CODE

TELEPHONE (include Area Code)

9. OTHER INSURED'S NAME (Last Name, First Name, Mid. Initial)

10. IS PATIENT'S CONDITION RELATED TO:

11. INSURED'S POLICY GROUP OR FECA NUMBER

a. OTHER INSURED'S POLICY OR GROUP NUMBER

a. EMPLOYMENT (CURRENT OR PREVIOUS)
[ ] YES [X] NO

a. INSURED'S DATE OF BIRTH   SEX
M [ ]   F [ ]

b. OTHER INSURED'S BIRTHDATE   SEX
M [ ]   F [ ]

b. AUTO ACCIDENT?   PLACE (State)
[ ] YES [X] NO

b. EMPLOYER NAME OR SCHOOL NAME

c. EMPLOYER NAME OR SCHOOL NAME

c. OTHER ACCIDENT?
[ ] YES [X] NO

c. INSURANCE PLAN NAME OR PROGRAM NAME

d. INSURANCE PLAN NAME OR PROGRAM NAME

10d. RESERVED FOR LOCAL USE
MCD 999599844

d. IS THERE ANOTHER HEALTH BENEFIT PLAN
[ ] YES   [ ] NO   If yes, return to and complete 9 a-d.

READ BACK OF FORM BEFORE COMPLETING & SIGNING THIS FORM.

12. PATIENT'S OR AUTHORIZED PERSONS'S SIGNATURE I authorize the release of any medical or other info necessary to process this claim. I also request payment of government benefits either to myself or the party who accepts assignment below.

SIGNED SIGNATURE ON FILE   DATE 10202009

13. PATIENT'S OR AUTHORIZED PERSONS'S SIGNATURE I authorize payment of medical benefits to the undersigned physician or supplier for services described below.

SIGNED

14. DATE OF CURRENT: ILLNESS (First symptom) OR INJURY (Accident) OR PREGNANCY (LMP)

15. IF PATIENT HAS HAD SAME ILLNESS, GIVE FIRST DATE

16. DATES PATIENT UNABLE TO WORK IN CURRENT OCCUPATION
FROM   TO

17. NAME OF REFERRING PROVIDER OR OTHER SOURCE

17a
17b NPI

18. HOSPITALIZATION DATES RELATED TO CURRENT SERVICES
FROM   TO

19. RESERVED FOR LOCAL USE

20. OUTSIDE LAB?   [ ] YES [X] NO $ CHARGES

21. DIAGNOSIS OR NATURE OF ILLNESS OR INJURY (RELATE ITEMS 1, 2, 3 OR 4 TO ITEM 24E BY LINE)
1. 401.9   3. |
2. 428.0   4. |

22. MEDICAID SUBMISSION CODE   ORIGINAL REF. NO.

23. PRIOR AUTHORIZATION NUMBER

24. A DATE(S) OF SERVICE						B. Place of Service	C. EMG	D. PROCEDURES, SERVICES OR SUPPLIES (Explain Unusual Circumstances)		E. DIAGNOSIS POINTER	F. $ CHARGES		G. DAYS OR UNITS	H. EPSDT Family Plan	I. ID. QUAL	J. RENDERING PROVIDER ID#
From MM	DD	YY	To MM	DD	YY			CPT/HCPCS	MODIFIER							
1	10	20	2009				31		99308		1 2	14	80	1		NPI	999501
2															NPI	
3															NPI	
4															NPI	
5															NPI	
6															NPI	

25. FEDERAL TAX I.D. NUMBER   SSN EIN
00-1234560   [ ] [X]

26. PATIENT'S ACCOUNT NO
PIN001

27. ACCEPT ASSIGNMENT?
[X] YES   [ ] NO

28. TOTAL CHARGE
$ 14 80

29. AMOUNT PAID
$

30. BALANCE DUE
$

31. SIGNATURE OF PHYSICIAN OR SUPPLIER INCLUDING DEGREES OR CREDENTIALS (I certify that the statements on the reverse apply to this bill and are made a part thereof.)
10202009
SIGNED L. D. HEATH, MD   DAT

32. SERVICE FACILITY LOCATION INFORMATION
RETIREMENT INN NURSING HOME
890 MILLENNIUM WAY
DOUGLASVILLE, NY 01234
a. 9990928531   b.

33. BILLING PROVIDER INFO PH #   (123) 456-7890
DOUGLASVILLE MEDICINE ASSOCIATES
5076 BRAND BLVD., SUITE 401
DOUGLASVILLE, NY 01234
a. 9995010111   b.

NUCC Instruction Manual available at: www.nucc.org

OMB APPROVAL PENDING

FIGURE 8-98

Courtesy of the Centers for Medicare & Medicaid Services

continues

PRINTING SECONDARY CLAIMS FOR THE PATIENT RECORD *continued*

1500	TEST VERSION - NOT FOR OFFICIAL USE	

HEALTH INSURANCE CLAIM FORM
APPROVED BY NATIONAL UNIFORM CLAIM COMMITTEE 08/05

Medicaid
POB 345
Albany, NY

Student No: Student1

☐☐☐ PICA / PICA ☐☐☐

1. MEDICARE ☐ (Medicare #) MEDICAID ☒ (Medicaid #) TRICARE CHAMPUS ☐ (Sponsor's SSN) CHAMPVA ☐ (Member ID) GROUP HEALTH PLAN ☐ (SSN or ID) FECA BLK LUNG ☐ (SSN) OTHER ☐ (ID)	1a. INSURED'S I.D. NUMBER (FOR PROGRAM IN ITEM 1) 999599844

2. PATIENT'S NAME (Last Name, First Name, Middle Initial) PINKSTON ANNA	3. PATIENT'S BIRTHDATE 07 | 28 | 1922 SEX M ☐ F ☒	4. INSURED'S NAME (Last Name, First Name, Middle Initial)

5. PATIENT'S ADDRESS (No., Street) 690 PARK ROSE AVE	6. PATIENT'S RELATIONSHIP TO INSURED Self ☐ Spouse ☐ Child ☐ Other ☐	7. INSURED'S ADDRESS (No., Street) SAME

CITY DOUGLASVILLE	STATE NY	8. PATIENT STATUS Single ☒ Married ☐ Other ☐	CITY	STATE

ZIP CODE 01235	TELEPHONE (include Area Code) (123) 528-0112	Employed ☐ Full-Time Student ☐ Part-Time Student ☐	ZIP CODE	TELEPHONE (include Area Code)

9. OTHER INSURED'S NAME (Last Name, First Name, Mid. Initial)	10. IS PATIENT'S CONDITION RELATED TO:	11. INSURED'S POLICY GROUP OR FECA NUMBER
a. OTHER INSURED'S POLICY OR GROUP NUMBER	a. EMPLOYMENT (CURRENT OR PREVIOUS) ☐ YES ☒ NO	a. INSURED'S DATE OF BIRTH SEX M ☐ F ☐
b. OTHER INSURED'S BIRTHDATE SEX M ☐ F ☐	b. AUTO ACCIDENT? ☐ YES ☒ NO PLACE (State)	b. EMPLOYER NAME OR SCHOOL NAME
c. EMPLOYER NAME OR SCHOOL NAME	c. OTHER ACCIDENT? ☐ YES ☒ NO	c. INSURANCE PLAN NAME OR PROGRAM NAME
d. INSURANCE PLAN NAME OR PROGRAM NAME	10d. RESERVED FOR LOCAL USE MCD 999599844	d. IS THERE ANOTHER HEALTH BENEFIT PLAN ☐ YES ☐ NO *If yes, return to and complete 9 a-d.*

READ BACK OF FORM BEFORE COMPLETING & SIGNING THIS FORM.
12. PATIENT'S OR AUTHORIZED PERSONS'S SIGNATURE I authorize the release of any medical or other info necessary to process this claim. I also request payment of government benefits either to myself or the party who accepts assignment below.

SIGNED _SIGNATURE ON FILE_ DATE _11242009_

13. PATIENT'S OR AUTHORIZED PERSONS'S SIGNATURE I authorize payment of medical benefits to the undersigned physician or supplier for services described below.

SIGNED _____

14. DATE OF CURRENT: ◄ ILLNESS (First symptom) OR INJURY (Accident) OR PREGNANCY (LMP)	15. IF PATIENT HAS HAD SAME ILLNESS, GIVE FIRST DATE	16. DATES PATIENT UNABLE TO WORK IN CURRENT OCCUPATION FROM TO
17. NAME OF REFERRING PROVIDER OR OTHER SOURCE 17a 17b NPI		18. HOSPITALIZATION DATES RELATED TO CURRENT SERVICES FROM TO
19. RESERVED FOR LOCAL USE		20. OUTSIDE LAB? ☐ YES ☒ NO $ CHARGES

21. DIAGNOSIS OR NATURE OF ILLNESS OR INJURY (RELATE ITEMS 1, 2, 3 OR 4 TO ITEM 24E BY LINE)
1. | 443.9
2. |
3. |
4. |

22. MEDICAID SUBMISSION CODE ORIGINAL REF. NO.
23. PRIOR AUTHORIZATION NUMBER

24. A DATE(S) OF SERVICE From MM DD YY To MM DD YY	B. Place of Service	C. EMG	D. PROCEDURES, SERVICES OR SUPPLIES (Explain Unusual Circumstances) CPT/HCPCS MODIFIER	E. DIAGNOSIS POINTER	F. $ CHARGES	G. DAYS OR UNITS	H. EPSDT Famly Plan	I. ID. QUAL	J. RENDERING PROVIDER ID#
1 11 24 2009	31		99308	1	11 81	1		NPI	999501
2								NPI	
3								NPI	
4								NPI	
5								NPI	
6								NPI	

25. FEDERAL TAX I.D. NUMBER 00-1234560 SSN ☐ EIN ☒	26. PATIENT'S ACCOUNT NO. PIN001	27. ACCEPT ASSIGNMENT? ☒ YES ☐ NO	28. TOTAL CHARGE $ 11 81	29. AMOUNT PAID $	30. BALANCE DUE $

31. SIGNATURE OF PHYSICIAN OR SUPPLIER INCLUDING DEGREES OR CREDENTIALS (I certify that the statements on the reverse apply to this bill and are made a part thereof.) SIGNED L. D. HEATH, MD DAT 11242009	32. SERVICE FACILITY LOCATION INFORMATION RETIREMENT INN NURSING HOME 890 MILLENNIUM WAY DOUGLASVILLE, NY 01234 a. 9990928531 b.	33. BILLING PROVIDER INFO PH # (123) 456-7890 DOUGLASVILLE MEDICINE ASSOCIATES 5076 BRAND BLVD., SUITE 401 DOUGLASVILLE, NY 01234 a. 9995010111 b.

NUCC Instruction Manual available at: www.nucc.org OMB APPROVAL PENDING

FIGURE 8-99

Courtesy of the Centers for Medicare & Medicaid Services

1500	**TEST VERSION - NOT FOR OFFICIAL USE**

HEALTH INSURANCE CLAIM FORM
APPROVED BY NATIONAL UNIFORM CLAIM COMMITTEE 08/05

Medicaid
POB 345
Albany, NY

Student No: Student1

☐☐☐ PICA   PICA ☐☐☐

1. MEDICARE MEDICAID TRICARE CHAMPVA GROUP FECA OTHER	1a. INSURED'S I.D. NUMBER (FOR PROGRAM IN ITEM 1)
☐(Medicare #) ☒(Medicaid #) ☐(Sponsor's SSN) ☐(Member ID) ☐HEALTH PLAN(SSN or ID) ☐BLK LUNG(SSN) ☐(ID)	999321156

2. PATIENT'S NAME (Last Name, First Name, Middle Initial)	3. PATIENT'S BIRTHDATE SEX	4. INSURED'S NAME (Last Name, First Name, Middle Initial)
CHANG XAO	11 | 13 | 1926 M ☒ F ☐	

5. PATIENT'S ADDRESS (No., Street)	6. PATIENT'S RELATIONSHIP TO INSURED	7. INSURED'S ADDRESS (No., Street)
890 MILLENNIUM WAY	Self ☐ Spouse ☐ Child ☐ Other ☐	SAME

CITY	STATE	8. PATIENT STATUS	CITY	STATE
DOUGLASVILLE	NY	Single ☒ Married ☐ Other ☐		

ZIP CODE	TELEPHONE (include Area Code)		ZIP CODE	TELEPHONE (include Area Code)
01234	(123) 528-0112	Employed ☐ Full-Time Student ☐ Part-Time Student ☐		

9. OTHER INSURED'S NAME (Last Name, First Name, Mid. Initial)	10. IS PATIENT'S CONDITION RELATED TO:	11. INSURED'S POLICY GROUP OR FECA NUMBER
a. OTHER INSURED'S POLICY OR GROUP NUMBER	a. EMPLOYMENT (CURRENT OR PREVIOUS) ☐YES ☒NO	a. INSURED'S DATE OF BIRTH SEX M ☐ F ☐
b. OTHER INSURED'S BIRTHDATE SEX M ☐ F ☐	b. AUTO ACCIDENT? PLACE (State) ☐YES ☒NO	b. EMPLOYER NAME OR SCHOOL NAME
c. EMPLOYER NAME OR SCHOOL NAME	c. OTHER ACCIDENT? ☐YES ☒NO	c. INSURANCE PLAN NAME OR PROGRAM NAME
d. INSURANCE PLAN NAME OR PROGRAM NAME	10d. RESERVED FOR LOCAL USE MCD 999321156	d. IS THERE ANOTHER HEALTH BENEFIT PLAN ☐YES ☐NO If yes, return to and complete 9 a-d.

READ BACK OF FORM BEFORE COMPLETING & SIGNING THIS FORM.

12. PATIENT'S OR AUTHORIZED PERSONS'S SIGNATURE I authorize the release of any medical or other info necessary to process this claim. I also request payment of government benefits either to myself or the party who accepts assignment below.

SIGNED _____ SIGNATURE ON FILE _____ DATE ___ 10162009 ___

13. PATIENT'S OR AUTHORIZED PERSONS'S SIGNATURE I authorize payment of medical benefits to the undersigned physician or supplier for services described below.

SIGNED _____

14. DATE OF CURRENT: ◄ ILLNESS (First symptom) OR INJURY (Accident) OR PREGNANCY (LMP)	15. IF PATIENT HAS HAD SAME ILLNESS, GIVE FIRST DATE	16. DATES PATIENT UNABLE TO WORK IN CURRENT OCCUPATION FROM ___ TO ___
17. NAME OF REFERRING PROVIDER OR OTHER SOURCE	17a 17b NPI	18. HOSPITALIZATION DATES RELATED TO CURRENT SERVICES FROM ___ TO ___
19. RESERVED FOR LOCAL USE		20. OUTSIDE LAB? $ CHARGES ☐YES ☒NO

21. DIAGNOSIS OR NATURE OF ILLNESS OR INJURY (RELATE ITEMS 1, 2, 3 OR 4 TO ITEM 24E BY LINE	22. MEDICAID SUBMISSION CODE ORIGINAL REF. NO.
1. | 250.00 3. |_____	
2. |_____ 4. |_____	23. PRIOR AUTHORIZATION NUMBER

24. A DATE(S) OF SERVICE From — To MM DD YY MM DD YY	B. Place of Service	C. EMG	D. PROCEDURES, SERVICES OR SUPPLIES (Explain Unusual Circumstances) CPT/HCPCS MODIFIER	E. DIAGNOSIS POINTER	F. $ CHARGES	G. DAYS OR UNITS	H. EPSDT Family Plan	I. ID. QUAL	J. RENDERING PROVIDER ID#
1 10 16 2009	31		99307	1	7 12	1		NPI	999501
2								NPI	
3								NPI	
4								NPI	
5								NPI	
6								NPI	

25. FEDERAL TAX I.D. NUMBER SSN EIN	26. PATIENT'S ACCOUNT NO	27. ACCEPT ASSIGNMENT?	28. TOTAL CHARGE	29. AMOUNT PAID	30. BALANCE DUE
00-1234560 ☐ ☒	CHA001	☒ YES ☐ NO	$ 7 12	$	$

31. SIGNATURE OF PHYSICIAN OR SUPPLIER INCLUDING DEGREES OR CREDENTIALS (I certify that the statements on the reverse apply to this bill and are made a part thereof.) 10162009 SIGNED L. D. HEATH, MD DAT	32. SERVICE FACILITY LOCATION INFORMATION RETIREMENT INN NURSING HOME 890 MILLENNIUM WAY DOUGLASVILLE, NY 01234 a. 9990928531 b.	33. BILLING PROVIDER INFO PH # (123) 456-7890 DOUGLASVILLE MEDICINE ASSOCIATES 5076 BRAND BLVD., SUITE 401 DOUGLASVILLE, NY 01234 a. 9995010111 b.

NUCC Instruction Manual available at: www.nucc.org

OMB APPROVAL PENDING

FIGURE 8-100

Courtesy of the Centers for Medicare & Medicaid Services

continues

| 1500 | TEST VERSION - NOT FOR OFFICIAL USE |

HEALTH INSURANCE CLAIM FORM
APPROVED BY NATIONAL UNIFORM CLAIM COMMITTEE 08/05

Medicaid
POB 345
Albany, NY

Student No: Student1

☐☐☐ PICA

PICA ☐☐☐

1. MEDICARE	MEDICAID	TRICARE CHAMPUS	CHAMPVA	GROUP HEALTH PLAN	FECA BLK LUNG	OTHER	1a. INSURED'S I.D. NUMBER	(FOR PROGRAM IN ITEM 1)
☐ *(Medicare #)*	☒ *(Medicaid #)*	☐ *(Sponsor's SSN)*	☐ *(Member ID)*	☐ *(SSN or ID)*	☐ *(SSN)*	☐ *(ID)*	999321156	

2. PATIENT'S NAME (Last Name, First Name, Middle Initial)
CHANG XAO

3. PATIENT'S BIRTHDATE   SEX
11 | 13 | 1926   M ☒   F ☐

4. INSURED'S NAME (Last Name, First Name, Middle Initial)

5. PATIENT'S ADDRESS (No., Street)
890 MILLENNIUM WAY

6. PATIENT'S RELATIONSHIP TO INSURED
Self ☐ Spouse ☐ Child ☐ Other ☐

7. INSURED'S ADDRESS (No., Street)
SAME

CITY
DOUGLASVILLE

STATE
NY

8. PATIENT STATUS
Single ☒   Married ☐   Other ☐

CITY

STATE

ZIP CODE
01234

TELEPHONE (include Area Code)
(123) 528-0112

Employed ☐ Full-Time Student ☐ Part-Time Student ☐

ZIP CODE

TELEPHONE (include Area Code)

9. OTHER INSURED'S NAME (Last Name, First Name, Mid. Initial)

10. IS PATIENT'S CONDITION RELATED TO:

11. INSURED'S POLICY GROUP OR FECA NUMBER

a. OTHER INSURED'S POLICY OR GROUP NUMBER

a. EMPLOYMENT (CURRENT OR PREVIOUS)
☐ YES ☒ NO

a. INSURED'S DATE OF BIRTH   SEX
M ☐   F ☐

b. OTHER INSURED'S BIRTHDATE   SEX
M ☐   F ☐

b. AUTO ACCIDENT?   PLACE (State)
☐ YES ☒ NO

b. EMPLOYER NAME OR SCHOOL NAME

c. EMPLOYER NAME OR SCHOOL NAME

c. OTHER ACCIDENT?
☐ YES ☒ NO

c. INSURANCE PLAN NAME OR PROGRAM NAME

d. INSURANCE PLAN NAME OR PROGRAM NAME

10d. RESERVED FOR LOCAL USE
MCD 999321156

d. IS THERE ANOTHER HEALTH BENEFIT PLAN
☐ YES   ☐ NO   *If yes, return to and complete 9 a-d.*

READ BACK OF FORM BEFORE COMPLETING & SIGNING THIS FORM.
12. PATIENT'S OR AUTHORIZED PERSONS'S SIGNATURE I authorize the release of any medical or other info necessary to process this claim. I also request payment of government benefits either to myself or the party who accepts assignment below.

SIGNED ___SIGNATURE ON FILE___   DATE ___11242009___

13. PATIENT'S OR AUTHORIZED PERSONS'S SIGNATURE I authorize payment of medical benefits to the undersigned physician or supplier for services described below.

SIGNED _____

14. DATE OF CURRENT: ◄ ILLNESS (First symptom) OR INJURY (Accident) OR PREGRANCY (LMP)

15. IF PATIENT HAS HAD SAME ILLNESS, GIVE FIRST DATE

16. DATES PATIENT UNABLE TO WORK IN CURRENT OCCUPATION
FROM   TO

17. NAME OF REFERRING PROVIDER OR OTHER SOURCE

17a.
17b. NPI

18. HOSPITALIZATION DATES RELATED TO CURRENT SERVICES
FROM   TO

19. RESERVED FOR LOCAL USE

20. OUTSIDE LAB? $ CHARGES
☐ YES ☒ NO

21. DIAGNOSIS OR NATURE OF ILLNESS OR INJURY (RELATE ITEMS 1, 2, 3 OR 4 TO ITEM 24E BY LINE

1. | 780.39
2. |

3. |
4. |

22. MEDICAID SUBMISSION CODE   ORIGINAL REF. NO.

23. PRIOR AUTHORIZATION NUMBER

24. A. DATE(S) OF SERVICE From MM DD YY	To MM DD YY	B. Place of Service	C. EMG	D. PROCEDURES, SERVICES OR SUPPLIES (Explain Unusual Circumstances) CPT/HCPCS MODIFIER	E. DIAGNOSIS POINTER	F. $ CHARGES	G. DAYS OR UNITS	H. EPSDT Famly Plan	I. ID. QUAL	J. RENDERING PROVIDER ID#
1	11 24 2009		31		99307	1	7 12	1		NPI	999501
2										NPI	
3										NPI	
4										NPI	
5										NPI	
6										NPI	

25. FEDERAL TAX I.D. NUMBER   SSN EIN
00-1234560   ☐ ☒

26. PATIENT'S ACCOUNT NO.
CHA001

27. ACCEPT ASSIGNMENT?
☒ YES ☐ NO

28. TOTAL CHARGE
$ 7 12

29. AMOUNT PAID
$

30. BALANCE DUE
$

31. SIGNATURE OF PHYSICIAN OR SUPPLIER INCLUDING DEGREES OR CREDENTIALS
(I certify that the statements on the reverse apply to this bill and are made a part thereof.)
11242009
SIGNED   L. D. HEATH, MD   DAT

32. SERVICE FACILITY LOCATION INFORMATION
RETIREMENT INN NURSING HOME
890 MILLENNIUM WAY
DOUGLASVILLE, NY 01234
a. 9990928531   b.

33. BILLING PROVIDER INFO PH #   (123) 456-7890
DOUGLASVILLE MEDICINE ASSOCIATES
5076 BRAND BLVD., SUITE 401
DOUGLASVILLE, NY 01234
a. 9995010111   b.

NUCC Instruction Manual available at: www.nucc.org

OMB APPROVAL PENDING

FIGURE 8-101

Courtesy of the Centers for Medicare & Medicaid Services

STEP 6

When the claims are ready to be printed, click on the *Print Forms button*. Since Medicare will automatically crossover the claim (forward it) to Medicaid, the forms simply need to be filed as a reference either in the patient file, or in the place designated by the medical office.

STEP 7

Save the hard copies of the claims, or follow the directions of your instructor for turning in your work. Close all open windows in MOSS when finished and return to the Main Menu.

FINAL NOTES

As illustrated in this unit, proper medical billing of the primary health plans is essential in order for accurate payment posting and secondary insurance billing to follow. Also, the ability to read EOBs from insurance companies can be a challenging task that in itself requires an understanding of the details of many health plans!

Bear in mind that the tasks you have learned thus far may be divided among the medical staff. This depends on how small or large the facility is, and how the work is distributed. As mentioned previously, billers and coders may be responsible for all billing, or only the billing for select health plans. Others exclusively sort and analyze EOBs, and yet others post payments. There are medical collectors for both tracing slow or denied insurance claims, as well as collecting from patients whose accounts become delinquent. In a very small one- or two-physician practice, one or two staff members may very well be responsible for the entire array of tasks.

Using what you have learned in this unit, the next and final steps in the reimbursement cycle are made possible. In the units that follow, sending statements to patients for any remaining balances due from them, as well as tracing and following up with insurance claims that have not been paid, will be covered.

CHECK YOUR KNOWLEDGE

1. Explain the purpose of the RA or EOB.

   _____

   _____

   _____

2. Describe the main components of an EOB from a medical insurance company.

   _____

   _____

   _____

3. Describe what the explanation "Claim Information Forwarded To:" means on a Medicare RA.

_____

_____

_____

4. How will posting an amount applied to a deductible affect the balance due on a patient account?

_____

_____

_____

5. Explain why there might be a write-off, or adjustment, for patients who have a health plan in which the physician participates.

_____

_____

_____

6. Describe some ways reimbursement may be affected by a patient who receives services from an out-of-network provider.

_____

_____

_____

7. Define COB as it relates to a patient who has dual insurance coverage.

_____

_____

_____

8. Selma is retired and has Medicare coverage. Her husband is still working and has a LGHP through his employer. Selma is an eligible dependent on her husband's plan. Which insurance is billed as primary for Selma's medical charges? Explain your answer.

   A. Medicare

   B. The husband's group policy

_____

_____

_____

9. Laura and Paul both have medical benefits, which are group plans, through their respective employers. They are dependents on each other's policies, too. If Paul receives medical services today, which plan is billed as primary? Explain your answer.

   A. Laura's plan

   B. Paul's plan

   _____

   _____

   _____

10. Stanley has been working at the same store for 48 years and has Medicare coverage. He has a LGHP through his employer, which is in effect. Which plan is billed as primary for today's services? Explain your answer.

   A. Medicare

   B. Employer LGHP

   _____

   _____

   _____

11. The Labrelle family consists of John and Mary, a married couple, and their two children, Brandon and Taylor. Both parents have medical insurance through their respective employers. The children are dependents on both plans. How is the primary insurance determined for the children if one of them receives services? How is the primary insurance determined for the parents if one of them receives services?

   _____

   _____

   _____

12. A patient with Medicare is working at a small business with fewer than 20 employees. She has a group plan with this employer. Which insurance is primary for services? Explain your answer.

   A. Medicare

   B. Employer group plan

   _____

   _____

   _____

13. Give examples of times when Medicare is the secondary payer (MSP).

   _____

   _____

   _____

Patient Billing and Collections

OBJECTIVES

Upon completion of this unit, the reader should be able to:

- **Describe techniques for effectively discussing financial matters with patients**

- **Explain common billing cycles used in the medical office, including the drawbacks and benefits of each**

- **Generate and analyze reports for preparation of patient statements and dunning messages**

- **Produce patient statements and print them for mailing using MOSS**

- **Inspect payments made by patients in the form of personal checks and cash, and then post them to patient accounts**

- **Age patient accounts using MOSS and prepare written collection letters for delinquent patients**

- **Describe techniques for proper collections when using the telephone to contact patients about delinquent accounts.**

KEY TERMS

Aging

Bill pay system

Billing cycle

Cancelled check

Current

Cyclic billing

Dun

Dunning message

Restrictive endorsement

Statement

When a patient seeks medical services from a physician, a contract is created. This contract implies that the physician will treat the patient to the best of his or her ability and judgment, and that the patient will adhere to the treatment plan and recommendations of the physician. In return, the patient will pay for such services, whether it is with insurance coverage, out-of-pocket payments, or both.

New patients should always be apprised of fees for services and when co-payments must be paid. Special details that concern their insurance and reimbursement help patients better understand their financial responsibility for the care they receive, regardless of which insurance plan they have. Established patients should be informed regarding any fee changes or insurance issues that may affect them.

Most medical offices offer payment arrangements, often without finance charges. Many accept credit cards. Patients need to be made aware of payment alternatives available to them. Allowing weeks or months to pass before attempting to collect at least part of a bill will decrease the ability to collect it at all.

Discussing fees, and especially delinquent payments, can be uncomfortable and frustrating for the medical staff. It is unavoidable that some patients require collection activity. However, proper communication from the time a new patient calls the office reduces delinquencies and creates greater control over accounts receivable. By the same token, cooperation from patients cannot be expected if the staff does not follow specific payment protocols, such as requesting payment at the time of service. Additionally, medical billing that is continuously backlogged, and delays in sending bills to patients, adversely affect collections efforts.

DISCUSSING FINANCIALS WITH PATIENTS

Patients, and anyone who visits the medical office, deserve courtesy and respect. The tone and attitude displayed towards a patient regarding financial matters will most likely determine the level of success to be achieved with collecting payments. Maintaining a courteous and professional demeanor allows for effective communication; yet, the medical staff should be careful not to project an image that confuses priorities. Much has been said regarding health care facilities seemingly being more interested in the patient's ability to pay, rather than in his or her health and well-being. Avoid this by using care in what is said, and when.

After working in a medical office for some time and interacting with hundreds of patients, it is easy to fall into what may appear to be an impersonal routine. This can alienate patients and unintentionally give the wrong impression. Always practice good manners, including frequent use of "please" and "thank you." Give each patient a few minutes to be greeted upon arriving at the office. This can go a long way before starting actual discussion regarding financial matters, or asking for an insurance card immediately. Remember, patients are more concerned about the health matters that have brought them to the doctor than how they will pay for the services. While financial matters are important, the medical staff's approach should not place insurance coverage and compensation as the first order of business.

As a general rule, it is best to discuss fees, insurance, and payment issues with patients in private. If possible, a separate area that can be used to interview new patients, away from those in the waiting room, is best. Ideally, new patients can be given a brochure or pamphlet that explains office policies, accepted insurance plans, and fees. In fact, these topics can be discussed on the telephone at the time an appointment is scheduled for a new patient.

Any patient who is experiencing family problems, a loss of employment, or other hardship, will be more comfortable discussing their issues in a place where it is less embarrassing. These types of problems, or the loss of insurance coverage, are often the reasons a patient is having difficulty paying for services. Extend the courtesy of taking these matters to a private area for discussion.

Clear and specific language is best when discussing fees, co-payments, or other financial issues. Ambiguous or open-ended statements often cause the patient to make decisions that defeat the purpose of collections. For example, consider the following interaction when a patient is asked, "Mr. Jones, will you be paying your $20.00 co-payment today?" as opposed to, "Your co-payment today is $20.00; will you be paying with a check?" It is clear how the first approach offers a question that puts the patient in control—yes, he will; or no, he will not make a payment—there is a clear choice. The second approach offers direction to the desired action—Mr. Jones is expected to make a payment.

Consider the following examples, and discuss how direct language can affect the outcome:

"Mr. Jones, your account is now 60 days past due. Can you make a payment towards the balance today?"

"Mr. Jones, your account is now 60 days past due. We require a payment of $120.00 today in order to bring your account current."

"Mrs. Smith, your insurance plan applied $250.00 towards your deductible. Would you like to take care of the remaining balance today?"

"Mrs. Smith, your insurance plan applied $250.00 towards your deductible. As you know, deductibles are payable by the policyholder every year. Will you be paying by check or credit card for this today?"

Whenever discussing any business with patients, including financials, use a tone that is friendly, yet professional and unemotional. There is no need to apologize, feel uncomfortable, or guilty regarding fees or the office payment policies. It is always inappropriate to express a derogatory opinion to the patient about his or her insurance plan, especially regarding quality, how long it takes for the plan to pay, or how much (or how little) it pays for services. The objective for the administrative medical staff is to communicate to the patient his or her payment responsibility, and any alternatives, such as a payment plan.

There may be occasions when a patient becomes upset over the discussion of financial matters. It is important to not also get angry and create an inflammatory situation. Rude behavior, intimidating the patient, giving ultimatums, or saying something that jeopardizes the patient's dignity must always be avoided, regardless of whether the patient shows the same courtesy in return. Remaining calm and using tact help keep the situation in control. Offer the patient an explanation of fees or the payment requirements. Never tell a patient you cannot help or do not know an answer without first seeking assistance from a coworker or supervisor, even if you must follow up with the patient at a later time.

Every office has different policies regarding who has authority and who makes final decisions about financial matters. Some offices rely on the business or office manager (or other appropriate supervisor) to handle payment disputes, collections problems, or even make decisions when assigning accounts to collections agencies, or when balances are written off as bad debts. Other offices rely solely on designated administrative staff members for these tasks. However, some physicians prefer to be apprised of these circumstances, and will have the final word on which action to take where financial matters are concerned. Be sure to follow your employer's office policy accordingly.

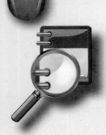

LET'S TRY IT! 9-1 ROLE-PLAY FINANCIAL DISCUSSIONS WITH PATIENT

CASE STUDY 9-A: THE NEW PATIENT—WELCH, STEPHEN

Objective: Mr. Welch is a new patient who has just arrived for his first visit at the office. He needs to be informed of the office policy regarding collecting co-payments at the time of service. Practice the dialogue below with a classmate or study partner.

Front-desk staff: Good morning (afternoon), Mr. Welch. Welcome to our office. Please complete these forms and sign where indicated. We will also need to make copies of your insurance card. Do you have your card with you?

New patient: Yes, I have it here.

Front-desk staff: Thank you. I will return this to you in just a moment. You may have a seat and begin filling out the forms.

New patient: (Patient returns to desk with completed forms a short time later.)

Front-desk staff: Mr. Welch, here is your insurance card. As a Signal HMO patient, you have a co-payment of $10.00 for each visit to the doctor. Our office policy is to collect the co-payment upon arrival for your visit. We would like to collect your co-payment now. Will you be paying with a check or cash?

New patient: I'll pay with a check. (Patient writes out the payment.)

Front-desk staff: Thank you for your payment, Mr. Welch. Please have a seat. You will be called in to see the doctor shortly.

CASE STUDY 9-B: THE ESTABLISHED PATIENT WITH A BALANCE— HOLLIDAY, TRACY

Objective: Ms. Holliday has returned to the front desk after visiting the doctor. She is ready to check out, but has a balance due on her account. Practice the dialogue below with a classmate or study partner.

Front-desk staff: Ms. Holliday, the doctor has indicated that she would like to see you again in one month. Would you like to make that appointment today?

Patient: No, I will have to check my calendar and call you back.

Front-desk staff: That would be fine. Our records indicate that a payment is required today for a balance of $120.00 on your account. Would you like to pay with a check or cash?

Patient: I have a balance on my account? I don't understand.

Front-desk staff: The balance is for the outpatient service on March 5 at Community Hospital. A portion of the doctor's fee, $120.00, was applied to your annual deductible. As you know, charges applied to your deductible are the patient's responsibility to pay.

Patient: I see. I cannot pay $120.00 today.

Front-desk staff: Ms. Holliday, the doctor would be happy to accept a partial payment of $60.00 today. I can let the doctor know that you will pay the remainder next month. Is that acceptable?

Patient: Yes, thank you.

Front-desk staff: I will prepare a written payment agreement for your signature. Your payment today of $60.00 will be applied to your account immediately.

The best way to prepare for discussing fees and policies with patients is to actually practice the dialogue. Much like an actor rehearses lines for a movie or play, practicing how and what will be said to patients in different scenarios makes you feel more comfortable and prepared for this type of discussion.

PREPARING PATIENT STATEMENTS

As you have already learned, the medical office usually does the insurance billing of the primary and secondary plans. Then, payments from insurance companies, and any applicable adjustments, are posted and applied to patient accounts. If any amounts remain that are the patient's responsibility, a statement is prepared as a means to notify patients so they can send in their payment. A **statement** is an itemized bill that specifies the balance due on a patient's account. Figure 9-1 illustrates a sample statement, as produced by MOSS.

Douglasville Medicine Associates
5076 Brand Blvd., Suite 401
Douglasville, NY 01234
Ph: (123) 456-7890
Fax: (123) 456-7891
Email: admin@dfma.com
Website: www.dfma.com

REMAINDER STATEMENT

JASON TATE
8812 MARBLE WAY
DOUGLASVILLE, NY 01234

Date:
Account No: TAT001
Student No: Student1

Date	Patient	Procedure	Total Charges	Patient Co-Pay	Insurance Payment	Adjust- ments	Deduct- ibles	Current Balance
03-Nov-09	JASON TATE	99221	$145.00	$0.00	$74.40	$52.00	$0	$18.60
04-Nov-09	JASON TATE	99231	$79.00	$0.00	$42.40	$26.00	$0	$10.60
05-Nov-09	JASON TATE	99238	$145.00	$0.00	$46.56	$86.80	$0	$11.64
		Totals:	$369.00	$0.00	$163.36	$164.80	$0	$40.84

Please make checks payable to:
Douglasville Medicine Associates

BALANCE DUE $40.84

Important Note:
Your insurance has paid its portion. Please remit the balance due.
Starting November 2009, Douglasville Associates will accept all major credit cards!

Printed On: Tuesday, January 12, 2010 5:25:25 PM   Page 1 of 1   Printed By: Admin

FIGURE 9-1

A sample patient statement, as produced by MOSS. *Delmar/Cengage Learning*

THE BILLING CYCLE

The **billing cycle** refers to the time that elapses between statements being mailed to patients. At a minimum, offices typically send statements monthly. The time of the month that statements are prepared and mailed can be critical to good collections. For instance, employers pay most people on the first and fifteenth of the month. Given this fact, it is ideal to time the arrival of statements to the patient's address approximately five days before a payday. The administrative staff needs to plan the preparation of monthly statements accordingly to meet these dates. One of the drawbacks to billing patients monthly is a tendency to have a surge of payments at one time of the month, then a wane until the next billing cycle. Even phone calls from patients with questions about their bill can become a monumental task in the few days following the arrival of statements.

A good technique that spreads out the flow of income and telephone work throughout the month is referred to as **cyclic billing**. With cyclic billing, patient accounts are split up into smaller segments, which are billed at different times of the month. For example, statements are sent to patients whose last names begin with "A" through "G" the first week of the month, referred to as Cycle 1. In Cycle 2, patients with last names "H" through "L" are sent bills the second week of the month. Then, "M" through "Q" bills are sent as Cycle 3 in the third week, while bills for "R" through "Z" are sent the last week, or Cycle 4. This system works especially well for medical offices with very large volumes of patients. One of the obvious drawbacks to cyclic billing is that not all patients receive statements before a payday. However, with very large practices, the benefit of cash flow throughout the entire month, as well as spreading the work out, far outweighs this problem.

DUNNING MESSAGES

There is a story that dates to the reign of King Henry VII, where it is believed a man called Mr. Joe Dun was assigned the task of collecting debts. Apparently, Mr. Dun had great skill and success collecting taxes for the king, so much so that, when anyone was slow to pay a debt, the creditor was told to "dun him." Although the methods of collections often resorted to harsh treatment, or even prison, the word **dun** became part of the English language, meaning a demand for payment. Today, dunning messages can be included with patient statements to explain balances and encourage payment, and at times, to warn about impending collections action.

Dunning messages help clarify for the patient whether their insurance has been billed, and whether any payment is due from them. The fact remains that a patient who knows what is expected from him or her is more apt to pay than a patient who is unclear about his or her account status. For instance, a patient with a $250.00 balance might receive a dunning message that states "your insurance company has been billed; please remit $50.00 for your co-insurance." Most likely, the other $200.00 is still pending payment from the insurance company. For the patient, it is easier to pay the $50.00 requested of him, rather than wonder about $250.00, and ignore or trash the entire bill. Very few patients, especially those with insurance coverage, will send a payment for the entire balance without first knowing if their insurance company has paid.

Dunning messages also can alert patients to past due amounts. Messages such as, "Have you forgotten to send your payment? A $50.00 payment is now due." are gentle reminders that may prompt a payment. Stronger reminders can accompany seriously overdue accounts and give the patient an opportunity to respond, such as "Your account is now 120 days overdue. Please remit payment by (date) to avoid assignment to our collections agency."

Some medical offices also use dunning messages as a means to make announcements to all patients who receive statements. Examples include an office that has started to accept credit card payments or a new clinic location that is now open. Even holiday or birthday greetings can be included, adding a personalized touch to the patient's statement. You will be instructed during orientation and training regarding your employer's preferences for using dunning messages.

REPORTS AS TOOLS FOR PREPARING STATEMENTS

In general, reports have many uses in the medical office, such as providing data for practice analysis and financial information. Statistical data also can be gleaned from reports that become useful for comparisons and evaluations of income, whether by insurance carrier, or from referral sources, or even generated by medical equipment and its use in the office. For example, a new laboratory machine purchased for the office can be monitored by report, to track the procedures performed, and the billing and revenues received. This can assist managers and physicians in assessing when the machine has paid for itself, and if the equipment is practical in the long run, compared to the cost of maintenance and supplies.

As another example, physicians of a group practice may want to know what portion of total revenues each individual physician has produced. Or, if a physician has joined a health plan as a participating provider, tracking revenue versus volume of patients and types of procedures can be useful on a periodic or annual basis. This data may reveal whether the physician's effort and time investment is being appropriately used, and whether continuing as a participating provider for a particular health plan is feasible.

Practice management software comes with a number of standard reports, and many have customization capabilities. For medical office staff responsible for medical billing and patient accounts, reports can provide information about medical billing activity and past due balances. These reports can provide important assistance with preparing statements, insurance tracking, and the collections process.

Many busy medical offices have hundreds and hundreds of patients who require statements each month. If certain accounts need dunning messages, the task can be quite difficult and time-consuming. Some offices simply generate a statement to all patients who have balances, regardless of whether an insurance payment is pending, or only a portion of the balance is due from the patient. Other offices will be more meticulous about evaluating patient accounts, and will prepare statements that produce the best return of payments to the office. Some offices provide dunning messages only on accounts identified as collections problems, such as those over 60 days past due. Again, you will need to follow the office policy of your employer regarding the preparation of patient statements.

The simulated exercises in this book for Drs. Heath and Schwartz require a more detailed approach to patient statements. Report generation is used as a tool in order to pinpoint accounts that require dunning messages. This improves overall payment collection from patients. If you have not finished the *Let's Try It!* exercises from Unit 8, go back and complete them before proceeding.

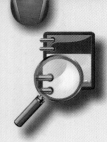

LET'S TRY IT! 9-2 GENERATING REPORTS FOR EVALUATING PATIENT ACCOUNTS

Objective: The reader generates a report that provides data regarding insurance billing and payments. After printing the report, the reader evaluates select data from the report to prepare patient statements.

STEP 1

Start MOSS.

STEP 2

Click on the *Report Generation button* on the Main Menu. This opens the Reports Panel shown in Figure 9-2.

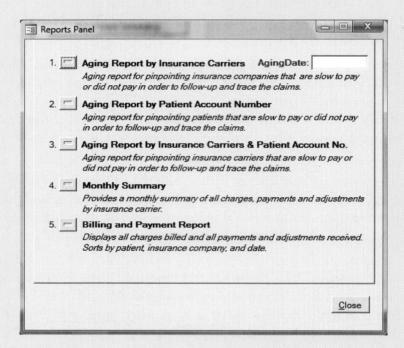

FIGURE 9-2

Delmar/Cengage Learning

STEP 3

The Reports Panel displays five different reports that come standard with MOSS. Select the Billing and Payment Report by clicking on the *box directly to the right of the number 5.* See Figure 9-3 for guidance.

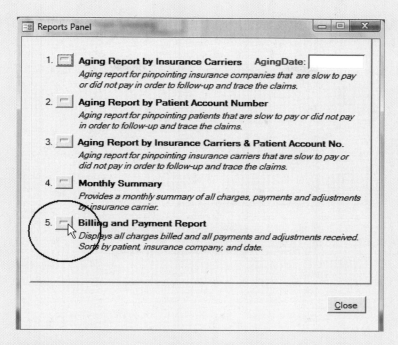

FIGURE 9-3

Delmar/Cengage Learning

STEP 4

Next, enter the start date for the report. For this simulation, enter "10/01/2009." Check your work with Figure 9-4 before clicking OK.

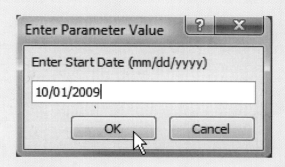

FIGURE 9-4

Delmar/Cengage Learning

continues

GENERATING REPORTS FOR EVALUATING PATIENT ACCOUNTS *continued*

STEP 5

Enter the end date for the report. For this simulation, enter "11/30/2009." Check your work with Figure 9-5 before clicking *OK*.

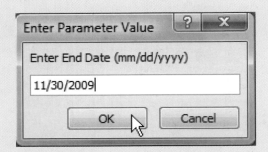

FIGURE 9-5

Delmar/Cengage Learning

STEP 6

A report with the heading Billing & Payments opens. Be sure to maximize the window so the entire page can be viewed. There are several pages to this report. View each page by clicking on the *bar on the lower left corner of the screen*, as shown in Figure 9-6.

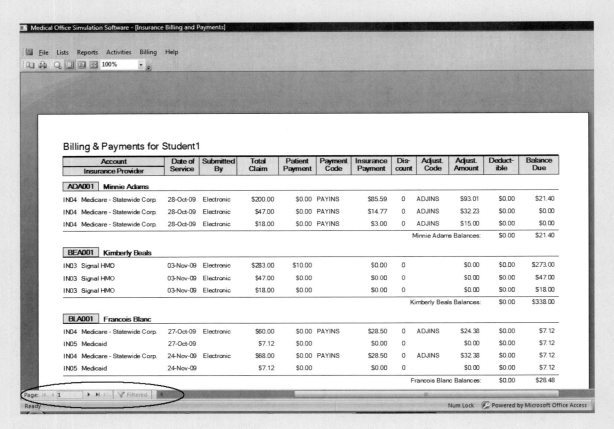

FIGURE 9-6

Delmar/Cengage Learning

STEP 7

Print this report by clicking on the *Printer icon* at the top left corner of the window. Your own student number should appear at the top of the report for easy identification. See Figure 9-7.

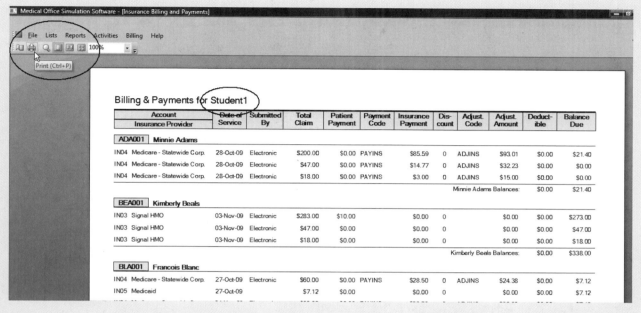

FIGURE 9-7

Delmar/Cengage Learning

STEP 8

Using the hard copy of the report you just printed, locate the first patient, Minnie Adams. Note that by reading across, each header contains data for each service. On the first line, a claim for $200.00 was submitted electronically. An insurance payment is also shown for $85.59 towards that service. Continuing across, a Medicare adjustment of $93.01 is shown. On the next line, a claim for $47.00 was submitted electronically. A $14.77 payment is shown. The $18.00 charge on the next line, also submitted electronically, shows a payment of $3.00. Refer to Figure 9-8.

Billing & Payments for Student1

Account / Insurance Provider	Date of Service	Submitted By	Total Claim	Patient Payment	Payment Code	Insurance Payment	Dis-count	Adjust. Code	Adjust. Amount	Deduct-ible	Balance Due
ADA001 Minnie Adams											
IN04 Medicare - Statewide Corp.	28-Oct-09	Electronic	$200.00	$0.00	PAYINS	$85.59	0	ADJINS	$93.01	$0.00	$21.40
IN04 Medicare - Statewide Corp.	28-Oct-09	Electronic	$47.00	$0.00	PAYINS	$14.77	0	ADJINS	$32.23	$0.00	$0.00
IN04 Medicare - Statewide Corp.	28-Oct-09	Electronic	$18.00	$0.00	PAYINS	$3.00	0	ADJINS	$15.00	$0.00	$0.00
								Minnie Adams Balances:		$0.00	$21.40

FIGURE 9-8

Delmar/Cengage Learning

continues

GENERATING REPORTS FOR EVALUATING PATIENT ACCOUNTS *continued*

STEP 9

The data shown for Minnie Adams on this report can be confirmed by viewing her Patient Ledger. The ledger can be viewed while the report is visible on the screen. Use the pull-down menu called Billing and select Patient Ledger as illustrated in Figure 9-9. Select Minnie Adams using the *Search icon*, shown in Figure 9-10, then select her name and click on *View*.

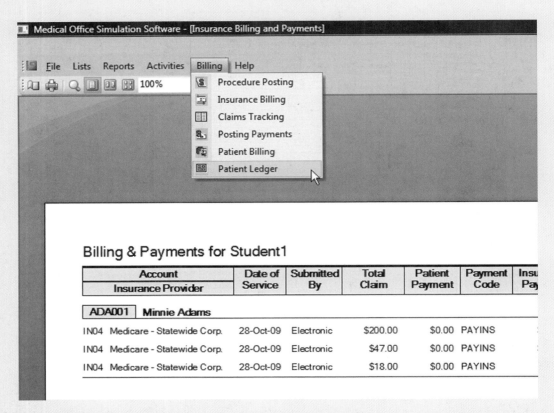

FIGURE 9-9

Delmar/Cengage Learning

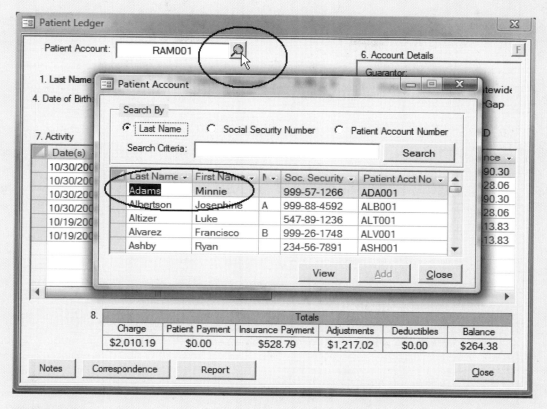

FIGURE 9-10

Delmar/Cengage Learning

STEP 10

Compare the information and Balance Due on patient Adams's ledger to the information and Balance Due column on the Billing & Payments report.

STEP 11

Look at the insurance information in Field 6 of patient Adams's ledger. It indicates that the patient has one insurance, Medicare. The remaining balance of $21.40 will be collected from the patient. Since all insurance claims have been paid, there is no secondary to bill. Make a note on the report in the margin so you will remember the details later.

STEP 12

Next, locate patient Francois Blanc on the report. Notice that there is an entry for a $60.00 charge on 10/27/2009 and another charge of $68.00 on 11/24/2009. These show that Medicare paid $28.50 for each procedure.

When viewing patient Blanc's ledger, note that his secondary insurance is Medicaid. Recall that Medicare, the primary insurance, will crossover the claim to Medicaid. On the report, a balance due of $7.12 from both Medicare and Medicaid appears for each service that was billed. This represents the balance left over after Medicare paid, and the same balance that was billed to Medicaid. As such, for the moment, the total balance due shows as $28.48 (although the actual total balance due from Medicaid is $14.24, or $7.12 for each service that was billed to the secondary).

continues

GENERATING REPORTS FOR EVALUATING PATIENT ACCOUNTS *continued*

STEP 13

Continue analyzing the Billing and Payments report, checking each patient who has a balance against the ledger, as learned in Step 8. and Step 12. As each patient is reviewed, answer the following questions:

    A. What is the total balance due?

    B. Is the balance pending payment from an insurance plan? If yes, which insurance plan?

    C. Is the balance due from the patient? Why or why not?

    D. If you were to create a dunning message for the patient, make a note of how it might read, as applied to the financial situation.

Compare your findings with the table in Figure 9-11.

PATIENT NAME	BALANCE DUE	DUE FROM INSURANCE	DUE FROM PATIENT	SUGGESTED DUNNING MESSAGE
Check the information below with each patient's ledger.				
Adams, Minnie*	$21.40	No	Yes	Your insurance has paid. Balance due from patient.
Beals, Kimberly	$338.00	Yes	No	Still waiting for HMO payment from insurance plan.
Blanc, Francois*	$14.24 (Balance left after Medicare paid)	Yes, Medicaid	No	Medicare has crossed over the claim to Medicaid, office is waiting for payment.
Chang, Xao*	$14.24 (Balance left after Medicare paid)	Yes, Medicaid	No	Medicare has crossed over the claim to Medicaid, office is waiting for payment.
Goodnow, Leona	$29.40	No, ConsumerOne has paid its portion.	Yes, there is no secondary insurance.	Balance due from patient.
Gordon, Eric*	$256.70	No, balance due was applied to the patient's deductible.	Yes.	Amount applied to deductible is due from patient.
James, David	$118.00	Yes	No	Still waiting for HMO payment from insurance plan.

FIGURE 9-11

PATIENT NAME	BALANCE DUE	DUE FROM INSURANCE	DUE FROM PATIENT	SUGGESTED DUNNING MESSAGE
Check the information below with each patient's ledger.				
Kramer, Stanley*	$383.00	No, balance due was applied to the patient's deductible.	Yes. Patient also owes the non-allowed because he uses an out-of-network physician.	Amount applied to deductible and non-covered amounts are due from patient.
Mallory, Christina*	$30.24	No, FlexiHealth has paid its portion.	Yes, there is no secondary insurance.	Patient is responsible for co-insurance for services provided as an inpatient.
Mangano, Vito*	$81.78	No, Medicare paid its portion, and applied part of the charges to the patient's deductible.	Yes, there is no secondary insurance.	Patient is responsible for co-insurance and the portion applied to deductible.
Manaly, Richard	$45.08	Yes, the secondary insurance, Medicare, has been billed for the balance due.	No, waiting for secondary insurance to pay on balance.	Insurance has been billed, waiting for insurance payment.
Montner, Martin	$289.00	Yes	No	Still waiting for HMO payment from insurance plan.
Munoz, Geraldo	$48.73	Yes, the secondary insurance, Century SeniorGap, has been billed for the balance due.	No, waiting for secondary insurance to pay on balance.	Insurance has been billed, waiting for insurance payment.
Pinkston, Anna*	$26.61	Yes, Medicaid	No	Medicare has crossed over the claim to Medicaid, office is waiting for payment.
Practice, Patty	$91.00	Yes, FlexiHealth In-Network	No	Pending insurance payment.
Ramirez, Manuel	$132.19	Yes, the secondary insurance, Century SeniorGap, has been billed for the balance due.	No, waiting for secondary insurance to pay on balance.	Insurance has been billed, waiting for insurance payment.
Ruhl, Mary	$72.64	Yes, the secondary insurance, Medicare, has been billed for the balance due.	No, waiting for secondary insurance to pay on balance.	Insurance has been billed, waiting for insurance payment.

FIGURE 9-11 *Continues*

continues

GENERATING REPORTS FOR EVALUATING PATIENT ACCOUNTS *continued*

PATIENT NAME	BALANCE DUE	DUE FROM INSURANCE	DUE FROM PATIENT	SUGGESTED DUNNING MESSAGE
Check the information below with each patient's ledger.				
Shektar, Paula	$180.00	Yes, Medicare. This report reveals that Medicare has been billed, but no payment has been received yet.	No, Medicare payment needs to be traced.	Insurance has been billed, waiting for insurance payment.
Shinn, Robert	$282.00	Yes	No	Still waiting for HMO payment from insurance plan.
Stearn, Wilma	$14.49	No, Medicare paid its portion.	Yes, there is no secondary insurance.	Patient is responsible for co-insurance.
Sykes, Eugene	$320.00	Yes	No	Still waiting for HMO payment from insurance plan
Tate, Jason*	$40.84	No, FlexiHealth has paid its portion.	Yes, there is no secondary insurance.	Patient is responsible for co-insurance for services provided as an inpatient.
Tomanaga, Marie	$155.05	Yes, the secondary insurance, Century SeniorGap, has been billed for the balance due, including a portion applied to the patient's dedutible.	No, waiting for secondary insurance to pay on balance.	Insurance has been billed, waiting for insurance payment.
Villanova, Ricky	$139.00	Yes	No	Still waiting for HMO payment from insurance plan
Worthington, Cynthia	$20.00	No, FlexiHealth has paid it portion.	Yes. This report reveals that the patient did not pay the required co-payment at the time of visit on 10/27/2009.	Co-payment due from patient.
Ybarra, Elane*	$127.16	No, FlexiHealth Out-of-Network has paid its portion.	Yes, there is no secondary insurance.	Patient is responsible for non-covered portion and co-insurance when using an out-of-network physician.
* It is helpful to look at the EOB/RA for the payments of the starred patients.				

FIGURE 9-11 *Continues*

STEP 14

When completed, close all open windows and return to the Main Menu.

LET'S TRY IT! 9-3 **PREPARING PATIENT STATEMENTS WITH DUNNING MESSAGES**

Objective: The reader uses the Billing and Payments report and Figure 9-11 to prepare patient statements with dunning messages. When completed, the statements are printed for mailing.

STEP 1
Start MOSS.

STEP 2
Click on the *Patient Billing button* on the Main Menu. This opens the Patient Billing window, ready to input settings.

STEP 3
Select the following settings as shown below:

A. Field 1, Remainder Statement. Click on *Remainder Statement* to produce statements that show only the remaining balances due.

B. Field 2, Provider. Drop down the selections and click on *All* for all physicians.

C. Field 3, Settings. In the "From/To" fields for the service dates, enter "10/01/2009" through "11/30/2009." The statements will be mailed by 11/20/2009 so that patients receive them shortly before the usual payday.

D. Field 3, Settings. In the Patient Name field, drop down the selections and click on *All* for all patients with balances.

> **TIP:** If the statements are to rectly to the printer, *Print* e checked. However, it is nmended that the state- s be previewed first.

E. Field 4, Process Type. The Preview on Screen selection should be checked.

F. Field 5, Global Dunning Message. Any message typed in this field appears on all patient statements. Type the following message: "We are proud to announce that Dr. G. A. Patel will be joining our practice on January 1, 2010. Dr. Patel specializes in asthma, allergy, and immunology."

G. Field 6, Account Dunning Message. This field is used to type in a dunning message that appears only on specific patient accounts. Figure 9-11 shows 10 patients who owe balances after their insurance plans were billed and paid. They will receive a unique dunning message that appears only on their statements. Type the following message: "Your insurance has been billed. The balance shown is your responsibility. Thank you for your prompt payment."

> **TIP:** Do not let go of the ey until you have clicked ch patient's *name.*

H. Next, select the individual patients who will receive this dunning message by holding down the *Ctrl (Control)* key on the keyboard, and clicking on each patient's *name* from the list in Field 7. The patients are:
Adams, Minnie
Goodnow, Leona
Gordon, Eric
Kramer, Stanley

continues

Mallory, Christina

Mangano, Vito

Stearn, Wilma

Tate, Jason

Worthington, Cynthia

Ybarra, Elaine

l. Check your patient billing screen with Figure 9-12 for accuracy.

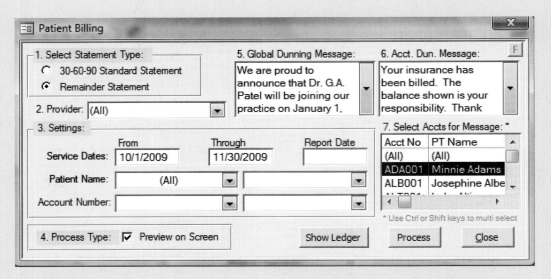

FIGURE 9-12

Delmar/Cengage Learning

STEP 4

Click on the *Process button* to create the statements. Review the statements on the Preview screen by using the *Record bar* on the lower left corner of the screen. Note the patient's name at the top of each statement and the statement information. Check the bottom of each statement and note the dunning messages. Each statement should have the global message announcing Dr. Patel. The 10 patients who were selected for an individual dunning message should also have the special note. See Figure 9-13 as an example.

Douglasville Medicine Associates
5076 Brand Blvd., Suite 401
Douglasville, NY 01234
Ph: (123) 456-7890
Fax: (123) 456-7891
Email: admin@dfma.com
Website: www.dfma.com

REMAINDER STATEMENT

ANNA PINKSTON
690 Park Rose Ave
Douglasville, NY 01235

Date: 11/20/2009
Account No: PIN001
Student No: Student1

Date	Patient	Procedure	Total Charges	Patient Co-Pay	Insurance Payment	Adjust-ments	Deduct-ibles	Current Balance
20-Oct-09	Anna Pinkston	99308	$78.00	$0.00	$59.20	$4.00	$0	$29.60
24-Nov-09	Anna Pinkston	99308	$113.00	$0.00	$47.25	$53.94	$0	$23.62
		Totals:	$191.00	$0.00	$106.45	$57.94	$0	$53.22

Please make checks payable to:
Douglasville Medicine Associates

BALANCE DUE $53.22

Important Note:

We are proud to announce that Dr. G.A. Patel will be joining our practice on January 1, 2010. Dr. Patel specializes in asthma, allergy, and immunology.

Printed On: Tuesday, June 08, 2010 10:09:32 AM   *Page 14 of 26*   *Printed By: Admin*

FIGURE 9-13

A sample patient statement with two dunning messages in the Important Note section.
Delmar/Cengage Learning

NOTE: Remember that a co-payment and a co-insurance are two different items. Co-insurance amounts are not shown on these statements, but they are included in the current balance column. For example, Jason Tate has a balance of $40.84 (see Figure 9-1). This represents the insurance payments applied as well as the adjustments that were made since he sees an in-network physician. The current balance due is the *co-insurance* for which he is responsible to pay.

continues

PREPARING PATIENT STATEMENTS WITH DUNNING MESSAGES *continued*

STEP 5

Next, print the statements for your records, or check if they are to be turned in to your instructor. Figure 9-14 shows the location of the print button. In an actual office, these statements would be ready to be mailed out to the patients.

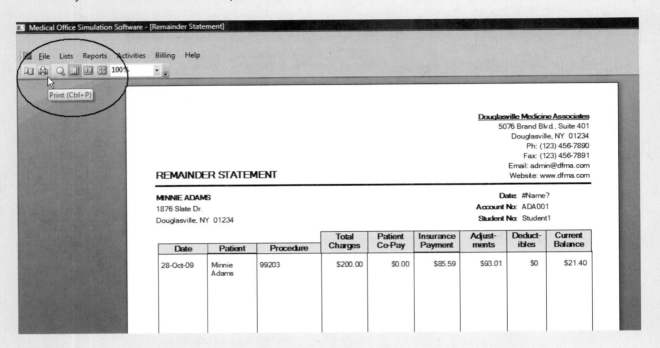

FIGURE 9-14

Delmar/Cengage Learning

STEP 6

Close all open windows and return to the Main Menu.

PATIENT PAYMENTS BY MAIL

Shortly after patient billing is completed and statements have been sent, payments will begin to arrive at the office. Some patients may wait until their next office visit to pay; others will personally stop by the office specifically to make a payment. The majority will send a payment by mail in the form of a personal check or money order. It is also popular to send payment through a **bill pay system** with their bank or a service that provides billing management. A bill pay system is a service that allows users to manage and pay bills online through a secure Web site. Funds are typically taken directly from a bank account. The bank or service will often send the funds to the recipient or payee by paper check or electronically.

Each office handles the posting of payments received in the mail differently. An office can apply payments daily, as received, or put aside these payments for several days, then post them all together on a specified date. It is best not to hold on to payments by personal check for an excessive amount of time, because after a while the money may no longer be available in the patient's account.

In addition to personal checks, patients may also make payments with money orders, cashier's checks, credit cards, or, of course, with cash. Whenever a patient pays with a check, money order, or cashier's check, it is important to immediately endorse the payment with a restrictive endorsement. **Restrictive endorsements** are normally placed on the back, left side of a check or money order, and contain information that identifies the party cashing the check. By adding the words "For deposit only," a restriction is placed on the check, indicating it is to be used for that purpose only. In a medical office, the practice or physician name, bank account number to be deposited to, and the bank name are included on a restrictive endorsement. A rubber stamp is typically made available to the staff for endorsing payments received at the office.

By immediately endorsing each payment when it is received or taken out of an envelope, the payment is safeguarded from being improperly used or cashed by any other party. Patients who make payments with cash should always be given a receipt. Despite the fact that cancelled checks are often used as proof of payment, it is not uncommon for medical offices to give patients a receipt every time a payment is made in person, regardless of the method of payment. A **cancelled check** is one that has already been paid to the payee. The actual check can be returned to the payer (person who wrote the check) or viewed as a digital document on many online banking Web sites.

INSPECTING PAYMENTS

When checks, money orders, or cashier's checks are accepted for payment, a quick inspection for key components is necessary before posting them to the patient's account. Any discrepancies need to be rectified, especially for items the bank may not accept as valid for deposit. The following list outlines the items to be inspected. Refer to Figure 9-15 while reviewing this list.

1. Payee information. Be certain that the payment correctly shows to whom the payment should be made. This could be made out to the provider/physician name, facility name, or group practice name. If there are gross misspellings, the bank may not accept the payment.

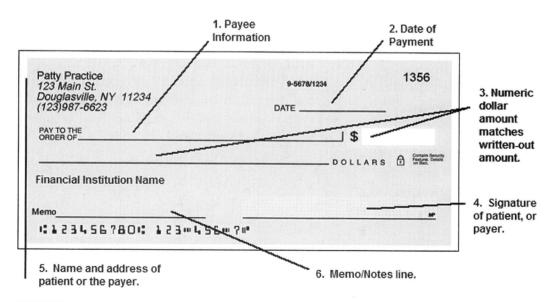

FIGURE 9-15

Components of a personal check. *Delmar/Cengage Learning*

2. Check the date, and follow any instructions from the patient or payer, if provided. For instance, if a patient asks that a check not be cashed until a certain date, or postdates a payment, it is best to check with the patient first before making a deposit on an earlier date. This reduces the risk of the check being bounced for non-sufficient funds (NSF) to cover the check.

   It is important to be aware of some points regarding the Uniform Commercial Codes and the Fair Debt Collection Practices Act as they apply to postdated checks. Most states have adopted the Uniform Commercial Codes, which permits banks to either pay or return a post-dated check, unless the check writer specifically notifies the bank about the check, similar to placing a stop payment. The Fair Debt Collection Practices Act actually prohibits creditors from depositing a postdated check before the check's date. However, there are risks involved, since the bank is not required to adhere to the check's date in order to put it through for payment. The bottom line is that the person or business who accepts a postdated check for payment is in effect extending credit, and is the one the check writer relies on to hold the check until the agreed upon date. Should the check be presented at the bank prior to the written date, the bank is really under no obligation to not accept it.

3. Check to make sure that the numeric dollar amount matches the amount that was written or spelled out. If it does not, the bank will not accept the payment.

4. Checks must be signed. Money orders and cashier's checks also provide information regarding the payer, usually on the face of the document. A missing signature from the payer causes the payment not to be accepted by the bank. Contact the patient or payer and inform them that another payment with proper signature needs to be made.

5. All checks should have the payer's complete name, address, and phone number written in the top left corner on the face of the check. If the payer has a new account, checks may be blank. Blank checks are only used temporarily when a checking account is first opened; therefore, there is no preprinted information on the check. Check with your employer regarding policies for accepting such checks. At a minimum, the name, address, and phone number of the payer need to be filled in by hand in the upper left-hand space.

6. Be alert for any notations the patient or payer may have written on the check, especially on the Memo line. Notes may indicate what the patient is paying for, provide a patient account number, or other useful information. Take care with notations that read "paid in full" when the payment is less than the balance due on the account. The check should not be accepted "as is," as this may legally accept the payment as payment in full. Instead of crossing out the notation, mark the payment as follows: "Received as payment on account, balance due: $(fill in amount)." It is advisable to contact the patient or payer to discuss this further.

7. Check with your employer's policies before accepting out-of-state checks. Whenever in doubt about any payment, consult your manager or the physician for direction.

LET'S TRY IT! 9-4 POST A SINGLE PAYMENT MADE WITH A PERSONAL CHECK—ADAMS, MINNIE

Objective: Payments have arrived at the office by mail over the past several days after statements were mailed before the end of the month in November. Checks were batched together, endorsed with the office stamp, and will be posted to patients' accounts today. The reader posts a payment received from patient Adams. Today's date is 12/04/2009.

STEP 1

Start MOSS.

STEP 2

Refer to the Source Document 9-1 in the Source Document Appendix. This is a personal check from Minnie Adams. Inspect the check to be sure all of the information is accurate.

> **T:** Checks made out to the [off]ice, or the physicians, are [accep]table.

Next, starting from the Main Menu, click on the *Posting Payments button* and select patient Adams from the list in order to apply a payment.

STEP 3

There is one procedure for service date 10/28/2009 with a balance due of $21.40. Select procedure 99203 by clicking on the *line item*, and then click the *Select/Edit button* along the bottom of the screen. This displays the $21.40 balance due amount in Field 13, indicating you are ready to post the payment, as shown in Figure 9-16.

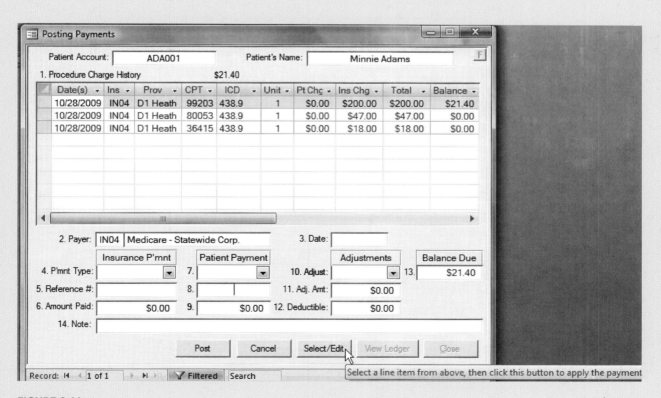

FIGURE 9-16
Delmar/Cengage Learning

continues

POST A SINGLE PAYMENT MADE WITH A PERSONAL CHECK— ADAMS, MINNIE *continued*

STEP 4

Enter the posting date, which is 12/04/2009, in Field 3. Click or tab down to Field 7, under Patient Payment, and drop down the box of selections. Click on *PATCHECK*, indicating a check payment from the patient. As a reference, enter the check number in Field 8. In Field 9, enter the amount of the payment that pertains to this service, which is $21.40. Upon pressing the *Enter key*, the Balance Due in Field 13 should display zero. Check your work with Figure 9-17.

HINT: The check number is located in the upper right corner of a personal check.

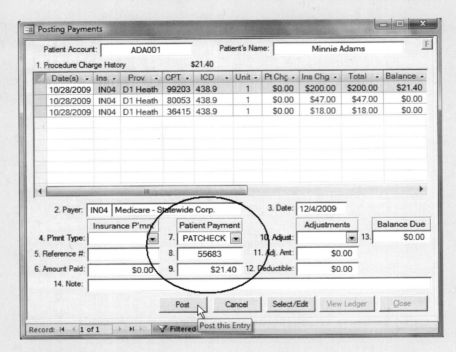

FIGURE 9-17

Delmar/Cengage Learning

STEP 5

Click on the *Post button* to apply the payment. Check your work by clicking on the *Patient Ledger button* to view the entry. Compare your screen to Figure 9-18.

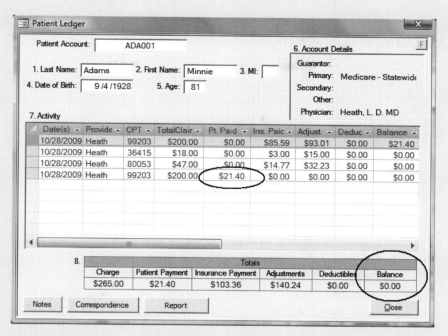

FIGURE 9-18

Delmar/Cengage Learning

STEP 6

When finished, close all open windows and return to the Main Menu.

LET'S TRY IT! 9-5 POST A SINGLE PAYMENT AND APPLY TO THE DEDUCTIBLES FOR TWO PROCEDURES—GORDON, ERIC

Objective: Payments have arrived at the office by mail over the past several days after statements were mailed before the end of the month in November. Checks were batched together, endorsed with the office stamp, and will be posted to patients' accounts today. The reader posts a payment received from patient Gordon. Today's date is 12/04/2009.

STEP 1

Start MOSS.

continues

POST A SINGLE PAYMENT AND APPLY TO THE DEDUCTIBLES FOR TWO PROCEDURES—GORDON, ERIC *continued*

STEP 2

HINT: Checks made out to the practice, or the physicians, are acceptable.

Refer to the Source Document 9-2 in the Source Document Appendix. This is a personal check from Eric Gordon. Inspect the check to be sure all of the information is accurate.

Next, starting from the Main Menu, click on the *Posting Payments button* and select patient Gordon from the list in order to apply a payment.

STEP 3

There are two procedures, one for service date 10/22/2009 and another for service date 11/5/2009. The insurance applied both covered amounts to the patient's deductible. The balance due is $256.70, and was paid with one personal check. The payment will need to be applied to each procedure separately.

Select procedure 99214 by clicking on the *line item*, and then click the *Select/Edit button* along the bottom of the screen. This displays the $168.70 Balance Due amount in Field 13, indicating you are ready to post the payment, as shown in Figure 9-19.

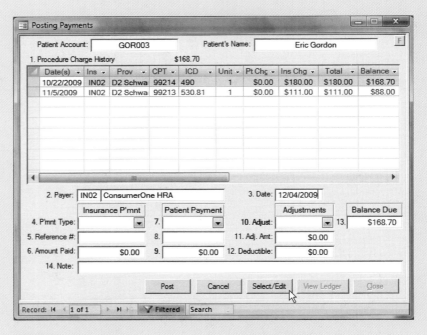

FIGURE 9-19

Delmar/Cengage Learning

STEP 4

Enter the posting date, which is 12/04/2009, in Field 3. Click or tab down to Field 7, under Patient Payment, and drop down the box of selections. Click on *PATCHECK*, indicating a check payment from the patient. As a reference, enter the check number in Field 8. In Field 9, enter the amount of the payment that pertains to this service, which is $168.70. Upon pressing the *Enter key*, the Balance Due in Field 13 should display zero. Check your work with Figure 9-20.

T: The check number ated in the upper right er of a personal check.

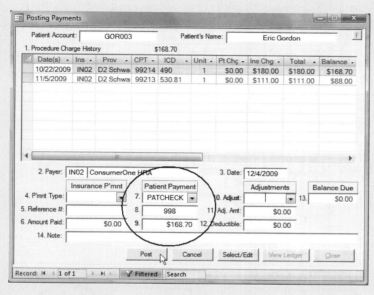

FIGURE 9-20

Delmar/Cengage Learning

STEP 5

Click on the *Post button* to apply the payment. Check your work by clicking on the *Patient Ledger button* to view the entry. Compare your screen to Figure 9-21.

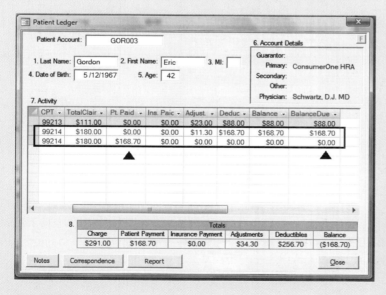

FIGURE 9-21

Delmar/Cengage Learning

continues

POST A SINGLE PAYMENT AND APPLY TO THE DEDUCTIBLES FOR TWO PROCEDURES—GORDON, ERIC *continued*

STEP 6

When finished, close the Patient Ledger and return to the Payment Posting window.

STEP 7

Next, post the rest of the payment to procedure 99213 on 11/5/2009. Select procedure 99213 by clicking on the *line item*, and then click the *Select/Edit button* along the bottom of the screen. This displays the $88.00 Balance Due amount in Field 13, indicating you are ready to post the payment, as shown in Figure 9-22.

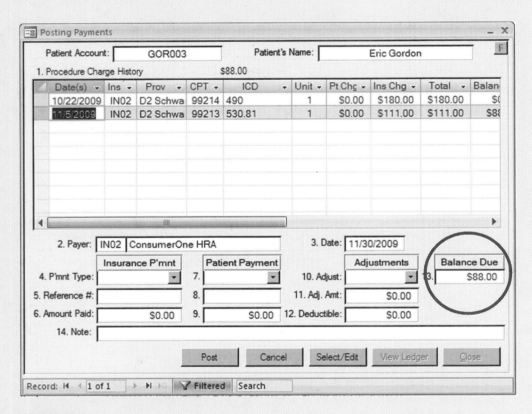

FIGURE 9-22

Delmar/Cengage Learning

STEP 8

Enter the posting date, which is 12/04/2009, in Field 3. Click or tab down to Field 7, under Patient Payment, and drop down the box of selections. Click on *PATCHECK*, indicating a check payment from the patient. As a reference, enter the check number in Field 8. In Field 9, enter the amount of the payment that pertains to this service, which is $88.00. Upon pressing the *Enter key*, the Balance Due in Field 13 should display zero. Check your work with Figure 9-23.

HINT: The check number is located in the upper right corner of a personal check.

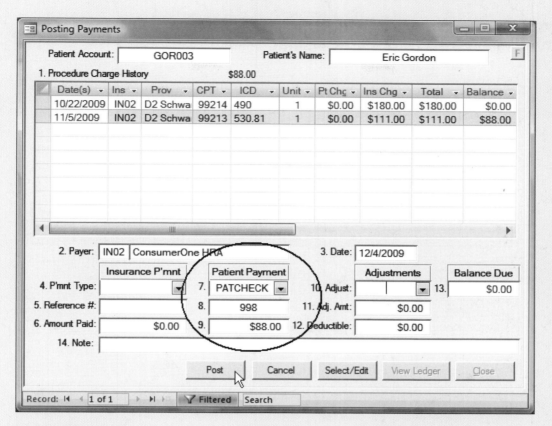

FIGURE 9-23

Delmar/Cengage Learning

STEP 9

Click on the *Post button* to apply the payment. Check your work by clicking on the *Patient Ledger button* to view the entry. Compare your screen to Figure 9-24.

continues

POST A SINGLE PAYMENT AND APPLY TO THE DEDUCTIBLES FOR TWO PROCEDURES—GORDON, ERIC *continued*

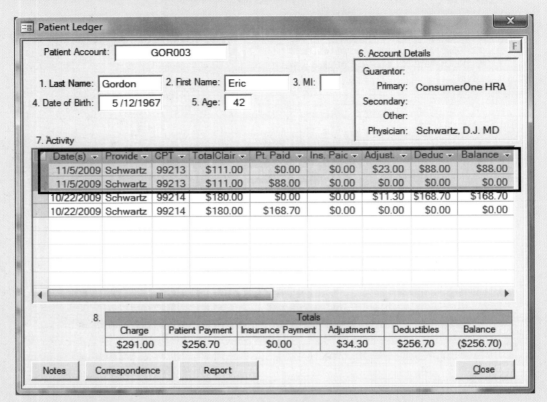

FIGURE 9-24

Delmar/Cengage Learning

STEP 10

When finished, close all open windows and return to the Main Menu.

LET'S TRY IT! 9-6 POST A SINGLE PAYMENT AND APPLY TO DEDUCTIBLES, CO-INSURANCE, AND NON-ALLOWED BALANCES— KRAMER, STANLEY

Objective: Payments have arrived at the office by mail over the past several days after statements were mailed before the end of the month in November. Checks were batched together, endorsed with the office stamp, and will be posted to patients' accounts today. The reader posts a payment received from Stanley Kramer. Today's date is 12/04/2009.

STEP 1

Start MOSS.

STEP 2

Refer to the Source Document 9-3 in the Source Document Appendix. This is a personal check from Stanley Kramer. Inspect the check to be sure all of the information is accurate.

Next, starting from the Main Menu, click on the Posting Payments button and select patient Kramer from the list in order to apply a payment.

STEP 3

There are three procedure line entries for service dates 10/27/2009, 10/29/2009, and 10/30/2009. The insurance applied covered amounts to the patient's deductible. In addition, because Dr. Schwartz is an out-of-network physician with the patient's insurance company, patient Kramer is responsible for the non-allowed portions of the charges as well. The balance due is $383.00, and was paid with one personal check. The payment will need to be applied to each procedure line separately.

Select procedure 99221 by clicking on the *line item*, and then click the *Select/Edit button* along the bottom of the screen. This displays the $145.00 Balance Due amount in Field 13, indicating you are ready to post the payment, as shown in Figure 9-25.

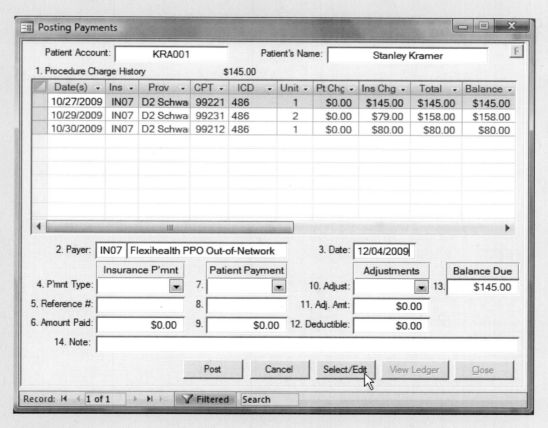

FIGURE 9-25

Delmar/Cengage Learning

continues

POST A SINGLE PAYMENT AND APPLY TO DEDUCTIBLES, CO-INSURANCE, AND NON-ALLOWED BALANCES—KRAMER, STANLEY *continued*

STEP 4

Enter the posting date, which is 12/04/2009, in Field 3. Click or tab down to Field 7, under Patient Payment, and drop down the box of selections. Click on *PATCHECK*, indicating a check payment from the patient. As a reference, enter the check number in Field 8. In Field 9, enter the amount of the payment that pertains to this service, which is $145.00. Upon pressing the *Enter key*, the Balance Due in Field 13 should display zero. Check your work with Figure 9-26.

HINT: The check number is located in the upper right corner of a personal check.

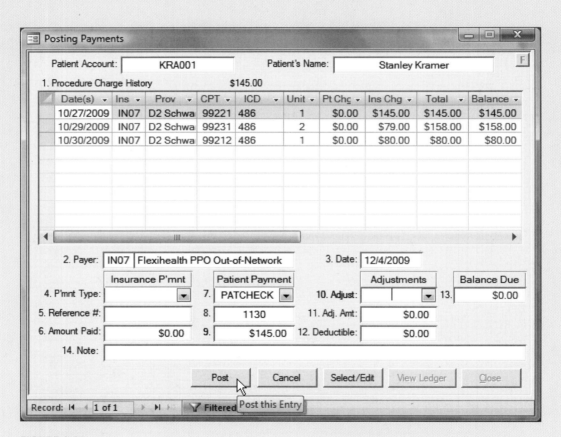

FIGURE 9-26

Delmar/Cengage Learning

STEP 5

Click on the *Post button* to apply the payment. Check your work by clicking on the *Patient Ledger button* to view the entry. Compare your screen to Figure 9-27.

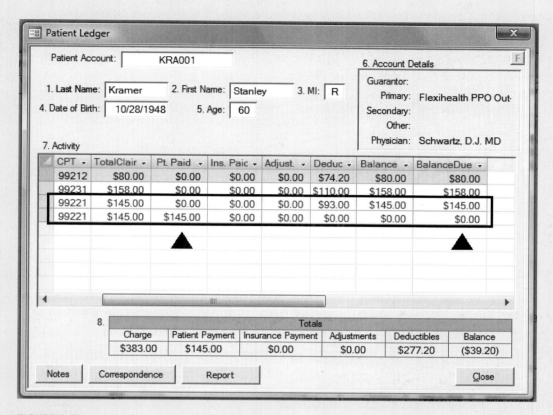

FIGURE 9-27

Delmar/Cengage Learning

continues

POST A SINGLE PAYMENT AND APPLY TO DEDUCTIBLES, CO-INSURANCE, AND NON-ALLOWED BALANCES—KRAMER, STANLEY *continued*

STEP 6

When finished, close the Patient Ledger and return to the Payment Posting window.

STEP 7

Next, post a payment to procedure 99231 on 10/29/2009. Select procedure 99231 by clicking on the *line item*, and then click the *Select/Edit button* along the bottom of the screen. This displays the $158.00 Balance Due amount in Field 13, indicating you are ready to post the payment, as shown in Figure 9-28.

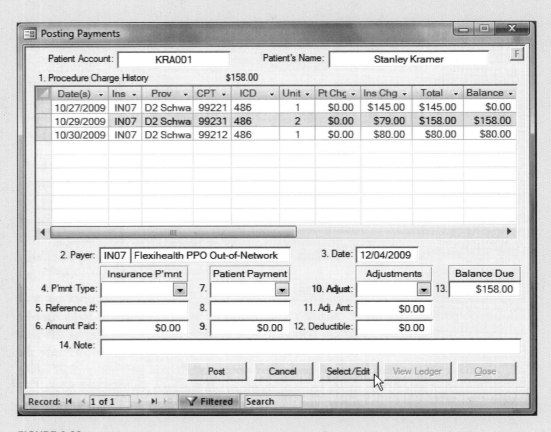

FIGURE 9-28

Delmar/Cengage Learning

STEP 8

Enter the posting date, which is 12/04/2009, in Field 3. Click or tab down to Field 7, under Patient Payment, and drop down the box of selections. Click on *PATCHECK*, indicating a check payment from the patient. As a reference, enter the check number in Field 8. In Field 9, enter the amount of the payment that pertains to this service, which is $158.00. Upon pressing the *Enter key*, the Balance Due in Field 13 should display zero. Check your work with Figure 9-29.

T: The check number cated in the upper right er of a personal check.

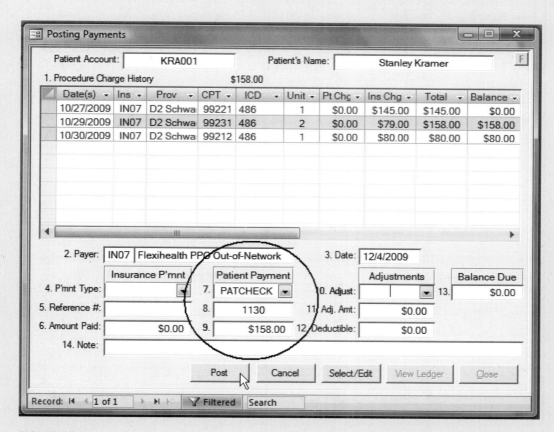

FIGURE 9-29

Delmar/Cengage Learning

continues

POST A SINGLE PAYMENT AND APPLY TO DEDUCTIBLES, CO-INSURANCE, AND NON-ALLOWED BALANCES—KRAMER, STANLEY *continued*

STEP 9

Click on the *Post button* to apply the payment. Check your work by clicking on the *Patient Ledger button* to view the entry. Compare your screen to Figure 9-30.

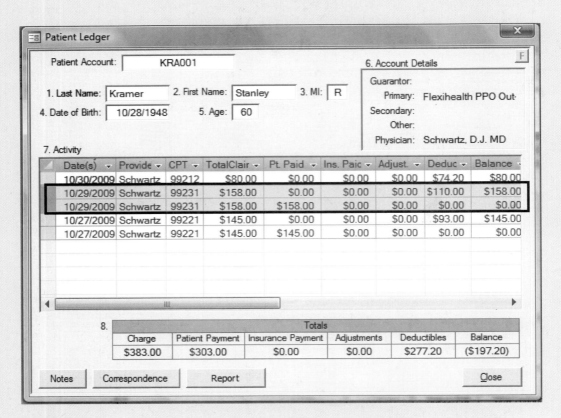

FIGURE 9-30

Delmar/Cengage Learning

STEP 10

When finished, close the Patient Ledger and return to the Payment Posting window.

STEP 11

Next, post a payment to procedure 99212 on 10/29/2009. Select procedure 99212 by clicking on the *line item*, and then click the *Select/Edit button* along the bottom of the screen. This displays the $80.00 Balance Due amount in Field 13, indicating you are ready to post the payment, as shown in Figure 9-31.

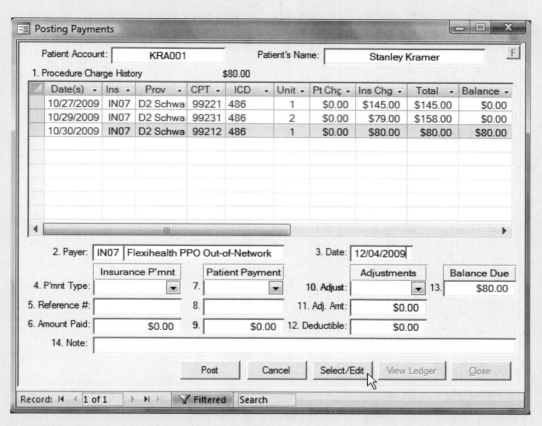

FIGURE 9-31

Delmar/Cengage Learning

continues

POST A SINGLE PAYMENT AND APPLY TO DEDUCTIBLES, CO-INSURANCE, AND NON-ALLOWED BALANCES—KRAMER, STANLEY *continued*

STEP 12

Enter the posting date, which is 12/04/2009, in Field 3. Click or tab down to Field 7, under Patient Payment, and drop down the box of selections. Click on *PATCHECK*, indicating a check payment from the patient. As a reference, enter the check number in Field 8. In Field 9, enter the amount of the payment that pertains to this service, which is $80.00. Upon pressing the *Enter key*, the Balance Due in Field 13 should display zero. Check your work with Figure 9-32.

HINT: The check number is located in the upper right corner of a personal check.

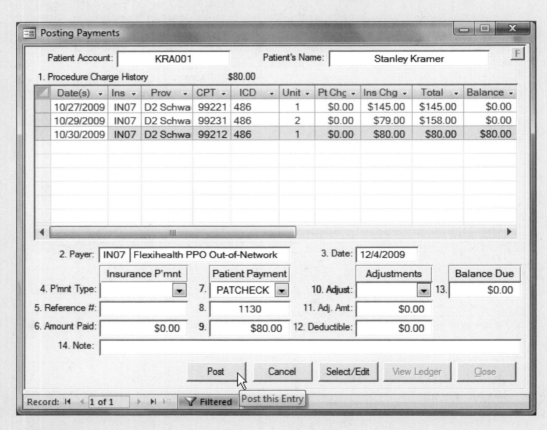

FIGURE 9-32

Delmar/Cengage Learning

STEP 13

Click on the *Post button* to apply the payment. Check your work by clicking on the *Patient Ledger button* to view the entry. Compare your screen to Figure 9-33.

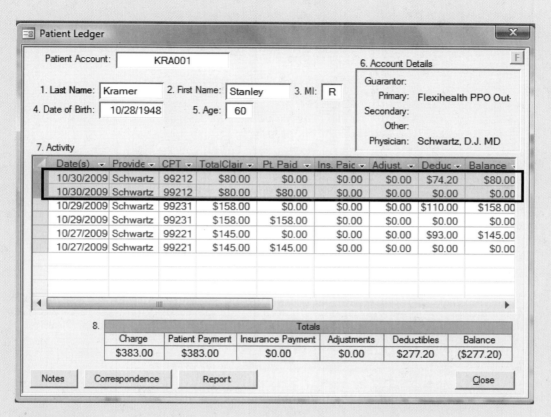

FIGURE 9-33

Delmar/Cengage Learning

STEP 14

When finished, close all open windows and return to the Main Menu.

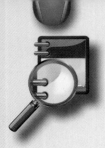

LET'S TRY IT! 9-7 POST A SINGLE PAYMENT AND APPLY TO THE BALANCE DUE AFTER THE INSURANCE HAS PAID ITS PORTION—MALLORY, CHRISTINA

Objective: Payments have arrived at the office by mail over the past several days after statements were mailed before the end of the month in November. Checks were batched together, endorsed with the office stamp, and will be posted to patients' accounts today. The reader posts a payment received from Christina Mallory. Today's date is 12/04/2009.

STEP 1
Start MOSS.

STEP 2
Refer to the Source Document 9-4 in the Source Document Appendix. This is a personal check from Michael Mallory, Christina's father. Inspect the check to be sure all of the information is accurate.

> **HINT:** Checks made out to the practice, or the physicians, are acceptable.

Next, starting from the Main Menu, click on the *Posting Payments button* and select patient Mallory from the list in order to apply a payment.

STEP 3
There are two procedure line entries for service dates 11/14/2009 and 11/15/2009. The insurance has paid its portion and all applicable adjustments have been made. The balance due is the co-insurance due from the patient. The payment will need to be applied to each procedure line separately.

Select procedure 99221 by clicking on the *line item*, and then click the *Select/Edit button* along the bottom of the screen. This displays the $18.60 Balance Due amount in Field 13, indicating you are ready to post the payment, as shown in Figure 9-34.

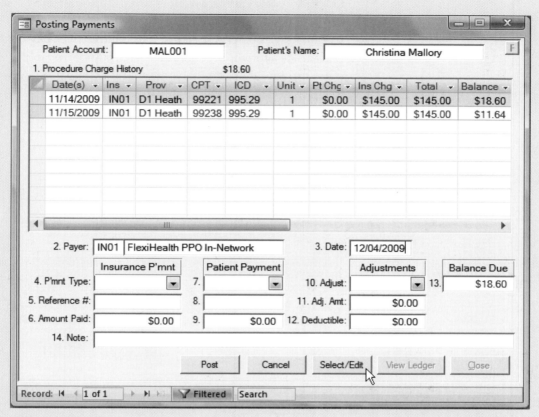

FIGURE 9-34

Delmar/Cengage Learning

continues

POST A SINGLE PAYMENT AND APPLY TO THE BALANCE DUE AFTER THE INSURANCE HAS PAID ITS PORTION—MALLORY, CHRISTINA *continued*

STEP 4

Enter the posting date, which is 12/04/2009, in Field 3. Click or tab down to Field 7, under Patient Payment, and drop down the box of selections. Click on *PATCHECK*, indicating a check payment from the patient. As a reference, enter the check number in Field 8. In Field 9, enter the amount of the payment that pertains to this service, which is $18.60. Upon pressing the *Enter key*, the Balance Due in Field 13 should display zero. Check your work with Figure 9-35.

HINT: The check number is located in the upper right corner of a personal check.

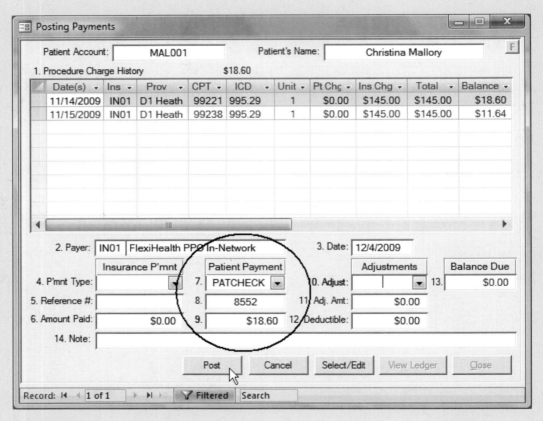

FIGURE 9-35

Delmar/Cengage Learning

STEP 5

Click on the *Post button* to apply the payment. Check your work by clicking on the *Patient Ledger button* to view the entry. Compare your screen to Figure 9-36. Close the ledger to return to the Posting Payments screen.

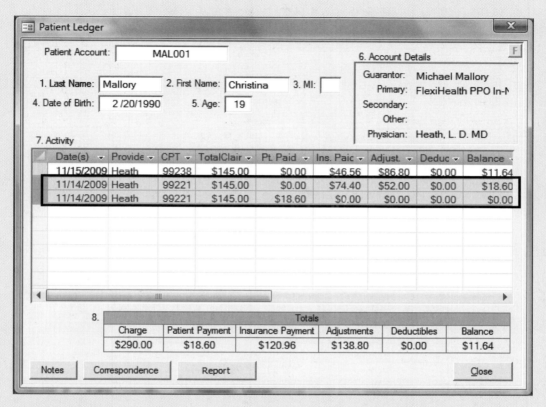

FIGURE 9-36

Delmar/Cengage Learning

continues

POST A SINGLE PAYMENT AND APPLY TO THE BALANCE DUE AFTER THE INSURANCE HAS PAID ITS PORTION—MALLORY, CHRISTINA *continued*

STEP 6

Select procedure 99238 by clicking on the *line item*, and then click the *Select/Edit button* along the bottom of the screen. This displays the $11.64 Balance Due amount in Field 13, indicating you are ready to post the payment, as shown in Figure 9-37.

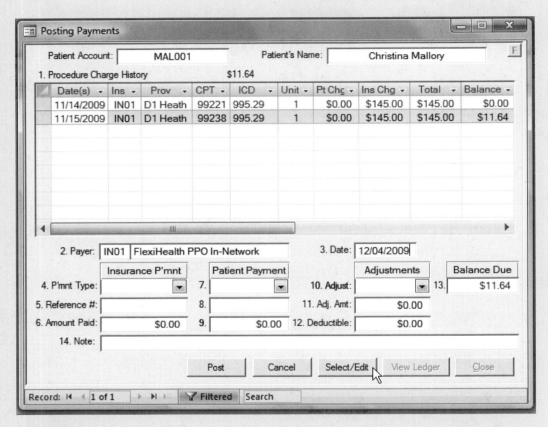

FIGURE 9-37

Delmar/Cengage Learning

STEP 7

Enter the posting date, which is 12/04/2009, in Field 3. Click or tab down to Field 7, under Patient Payment, and drop down the box of selections. Click on *PATCHECK*, indicating a check payment from the patient. As a reference, enter the check number in Field 8. In Field 9, enter the amount of the payment that pertains to this service, which is $11.64. Upon pressing the *Enter key*, the Balance Due in Field 13 should display zero. Check your work with Figure 9-38.

IT: The check number cated in the upper right er of a personal check.

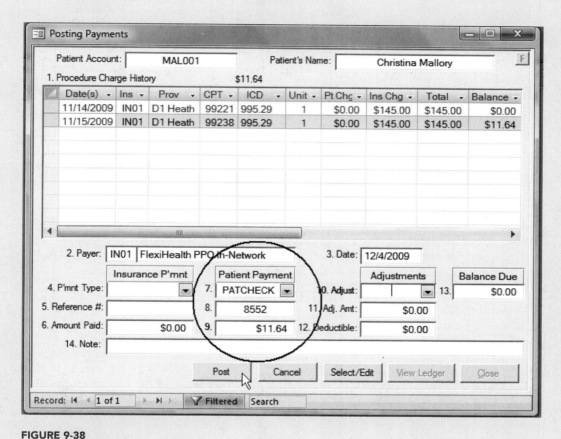

FIGURE 9-38

Delmar/Cengage Learning

continues

POST A SINGLE PAYMENT AND APPLY TO THE BALANCE DUE AFTER THE INSURANCE HAS PAID ITS PORTION—MALLORY, CHRISTINA *continued*

STEP 8

Click on the *Post button* to apply the payment. Check your work by clicking on the *Patient Ledger button* to view the entry. Compare your screen to Figure 9-39.

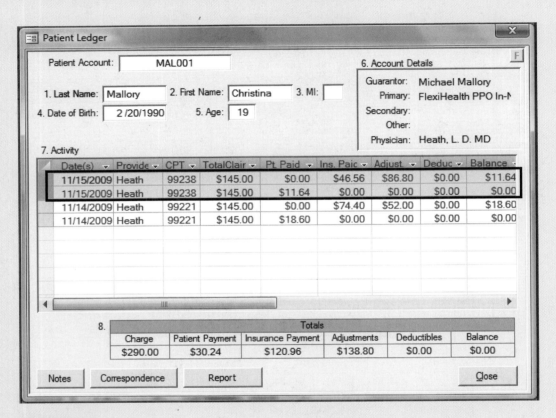

FIGURE 9-39

Delmar/Cengage Learning

STEP 9

When finished, close all open windows and return to the Main Menu.

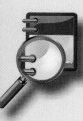

LET'S TRY IT! 9-8 POSTING PAYMENTS—ALL REMAINING PATIENTS

Objective: Using the skills just learned for posting payments from patients, the reader will apply the remaining payments to each patient account as applicable. Today's date is 12/04/2009, and will continue to be used as the posting date.

CASE STUDY 9-C: MANGANO, VITO

STEP 1

Refer to the personal check in Source Document 9-5 in the Source Document Appendix and inspect the check information. Select patient Mangano from the Posting Payments area.

STEP 2

The patient has paid the deductible of $75.00 and co-insurance amount of $0.89. Post the payment to each date of service, and then check your work with Figure 9-40 and Figure 9-41 before posting each one. Continue to use 12/04/2009 as the date of posting.

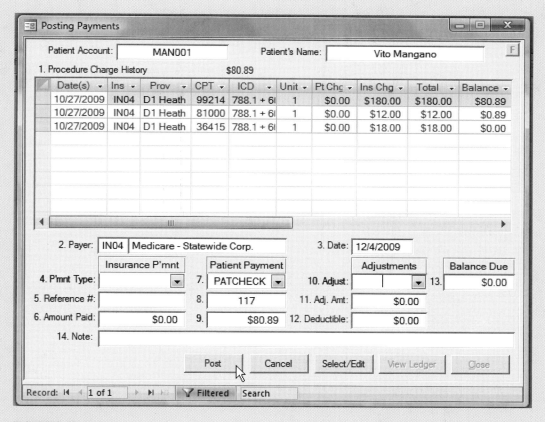

FIGURE 9-40

Delmar/Cengage Learning

Case Study 9-C Continues >>

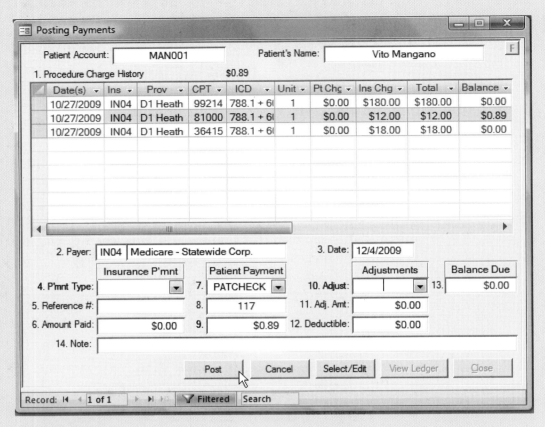

FIGURE 9-41

Delmar/Cengage Learning

STEP 3

When each payment posting has been completed, check the Patient Ledger with Figure 9-42.

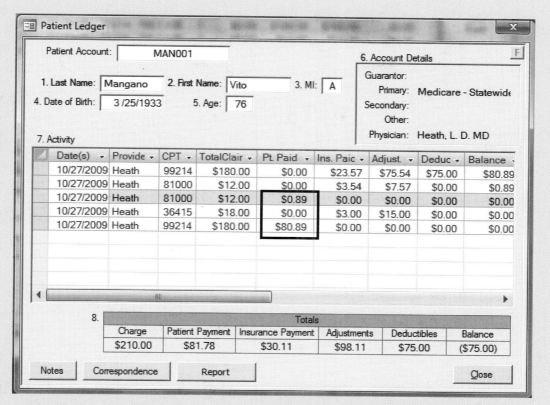

FIGURE 9-42

Delmar/Cengage Learning

STEP 4

When finished, close the Patient Ledger and Payment Posting windows. The Patient Selection window for posting payments should be available to select the next patient. If not, click on the *Posting Payments button* on the Main Menu.

CASE STUDY 9-D: TATE, JASON

STEP 1
Refer to the personal check in Source Document 9-6 in the Source Document Appendix. Inspect the check information. Select patient Tate from the Posting Payments area.

STEP 2
The patient has paid the remainder balance of $40.84. Post the payment to each date of service, and then check your work with Figure 9-43 through Figure 9-45 before posting each one. Continue to use 12/04/2009 as the date of posting.

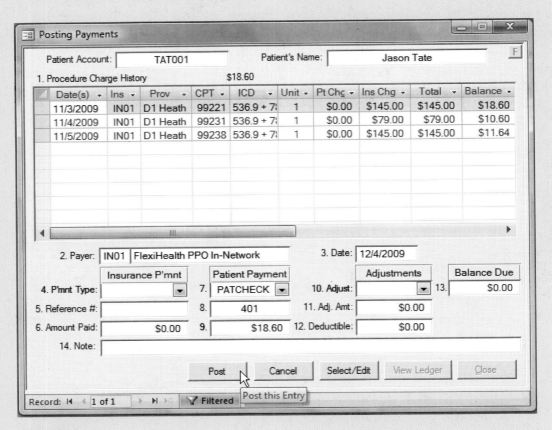

FIGURE 9-43

Delmar/Cengage Learning

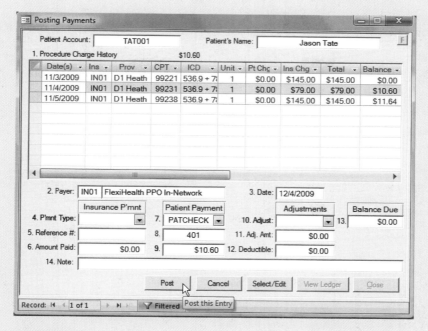

FIGURE 9-44

Delmar/Cengage Learning

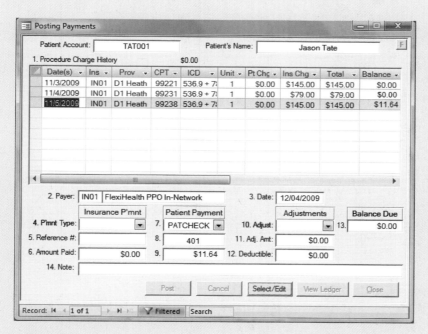

FIGURE 9-45

Delmar/Cengage Learning

STEP 3

When each payment posting has been completed, check the Patient Ledger with Figure 9-46.

Case Study 9-D Continues >>

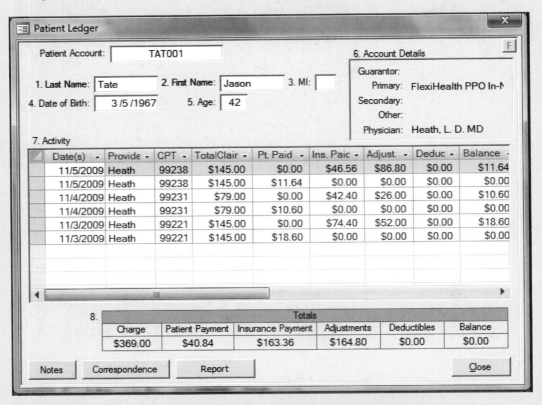

FIGURE 9-46

Delmar/Cengage Learning

STEP 4

When finished, close the Patient Ledger and Payment Posting windows. The patient selection window for posting payments should be available to select the next patient. If not, click on the *Posting Payments button* on the Main Menu.

CASE STUDY 9-E: WORTHINGTON, CYNTHIA

STEP 1

Refer to the personal check in Source Document 9-7 in the Source Document Appendix from Cynthia Worthington. Inspect the check information. How does the information in the memo line assist with posting this payment? Select patient Worthington from the list in order to apply a payment.

STEP 2

The patient has paid the co-payment amount of $20.00. Post the payment to the service date 10/27/2009, and then check your work with Figure 9-47 before clicking the *Post button*.

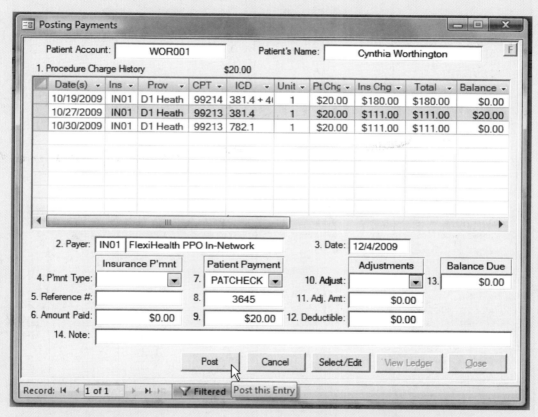

FIGURE 9-47

Delmar/Cengage Learning

Case Study 9-E Continues >>

Case Study 9-E Continued

STEP 3

When the payment posting has been completed, check the Patient Ledger with Figure 9-48.

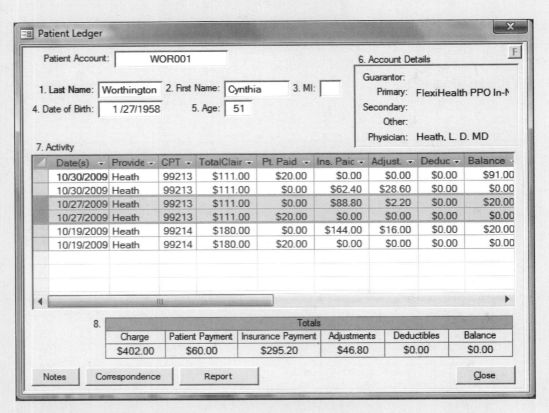

FIGURE 9-48

Delmar/Cengage Learning

STEP 4

When finished, close the Patient Ledger and Payment Posting windows. The Patient Selection window for posting payments should be available to select the next patient. If not, click on the *Posting Payments button* on the Main Menu.

CASE STUDY 9-F: GOODNOW, LEONA

STEP 1

Refer to the personal check in Source Document 9-8 in the Source Document Appendix from Thomas Goodnow. Inspect the check information. Select patient Goodnow from the list in order to apply a payment.

STEP 2

The patient has paid the remainder balance of $29.40. Post the payment to the service date 10/25/2009, and then check your work with Figure 9-49 before clicking the *Post button*.

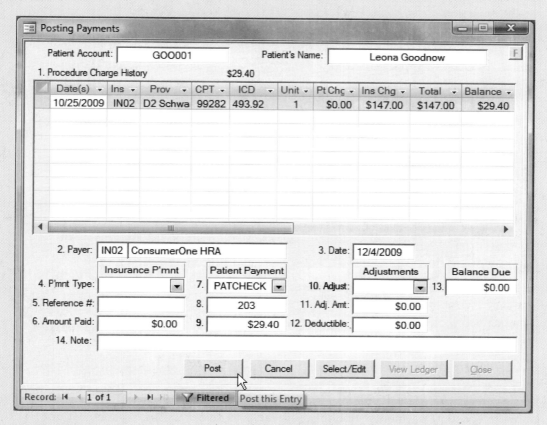

FIGURE 9-49

Delmar/Cengage Learning

Case Study 9-F Continues >>

STEP 3

When the payment posting has been completed, check the Patient Ledger with Figure 9-50.

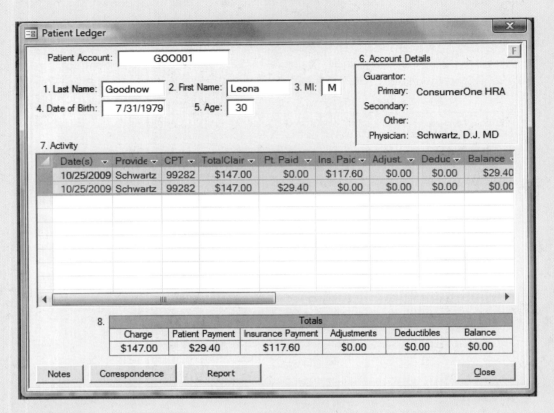

FIGURE 9-50

Delmar/Cengage Learning

STEP 4

When finished, close the Patient Ledger and Payment Posting windows. The Patient Selection window for posting payments should be available to select the next patient. If not, click on the *Posting Payments button* on the Main Menu.

CASE STUDY 9-G: STEARN, WILMA

STEP 1

Patient Stearn was in the neighborhood on 12/04/2009 and decided to stop in the office personally to make her payment. Select patient Stearn from the list to apply a payment.

STEP 2

Click to view the Patient Ledger. Note the amount due. The patient pays with cash. She gives $15.00 and receives $0.51 in change. She is also given a receipt for her payment. Post the cash payment of $13.83 to procedure 99213 and a payment of $0.66 to procedure 85014. Be sure to select *PATCASH* in Field 7 for each entry to properly indicate the type of payment. Check your screen with Figure 9-51 and Figure 9-52 before posting the payments.

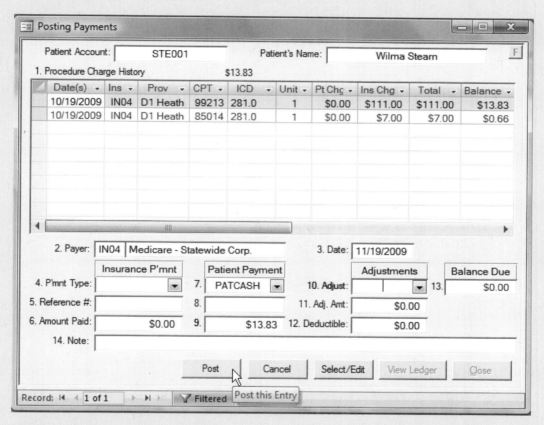

FIGURE 9-51

Delmar/Cengage Learning

Case Study 9-G Continues >>

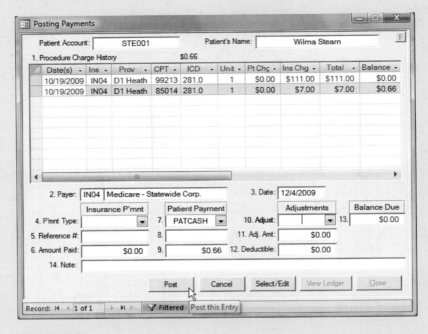

FIGURE 9-52

Delmar/Cengage Learning

STEP 3

View the Patient Ledger and check your work with Figure 9-53. When finished, close all open windows and return to the Main Menu.

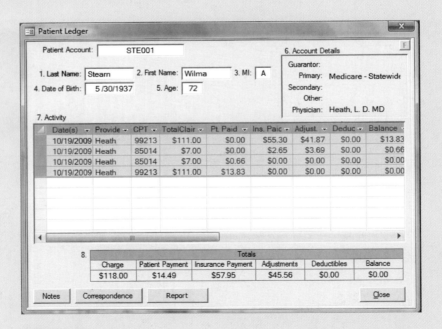

FIGURE 9-53

Delmar/Cengage Learning

CASE STUDY 9-H: YBARRA, ELANE

STEP 1

Refer to the personal check in Source Document 9-9 in the Source Document Appendix and inspect the check information. Select patient Ybarra from the Posting Payments area.

STEP 2

The patient has paid the remainder balance of $127.16. Post the payment to each date of service, and then check your work with Figure 9-54 through Figure 9–57 before posting each one. Continue to use 12/04/2009 as the date of posting.

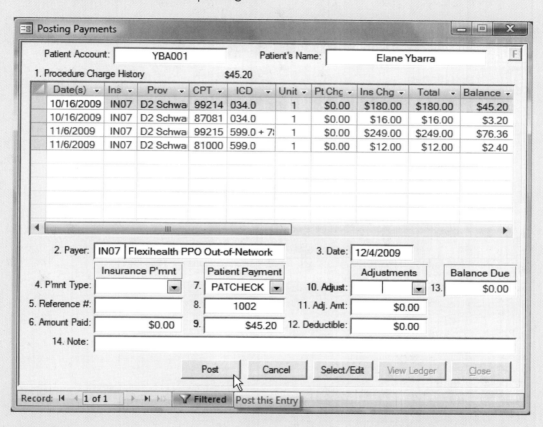

FIGURE 9-54

Delmar/Cengage Learning

Case Study 9-H Continues >>

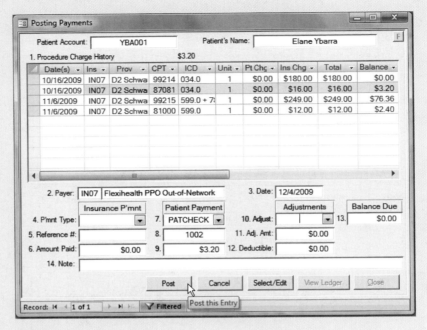

FIGURE 9-55

Delmar/Cengage Learning

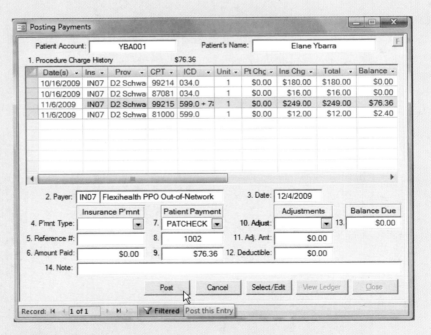

FIGURE 9-56

Delmar/Cengage Learning

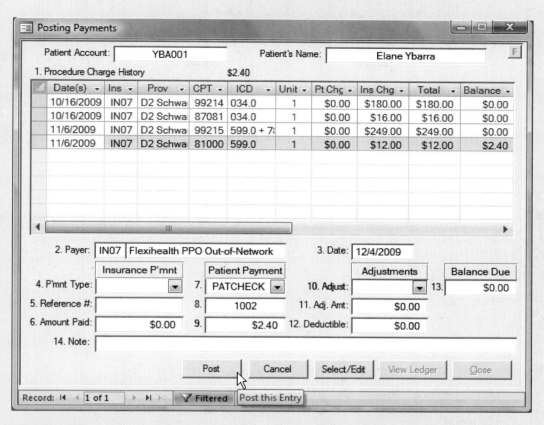

FIGURE 9-57

Delmar/Cengage Learning

Case Study 9-H Continues >>

STEP 3

When each payment posting has been completed, check the Patient Ledger with Figure 9-58.

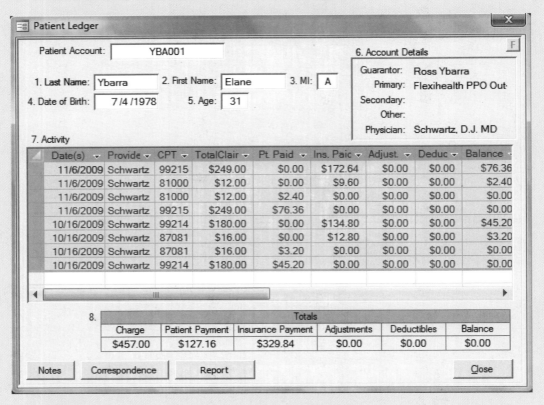

FIGURE 9-58

Delmar/Cengage Learning

STEP 4

When finished, close the Patient Ledger and Payment Posting windows. Return to the Main Menu of MOSS.

AGING PATIENT ACCOUNTS AND COLLECTIONS

Part of the patient billing procedure includes aging accounts. **Aging** refers to categorizing balances due according to the length of time they have been unpaid. These categories are divided into segments that average out to 30 days. In other words, an unpaid balance can be 30, 60, 90, or 120 (or more) days past due. Unpaid balances that are in the zero to 30-day category are not considered as past due, and are referred to as **current** accounts. Pursuing patients who are seriously delinquent with their payments is discussed later in this unit.

In the medical office, balances in the zero to 30-day category usually represent recent services, and are often pending insurance payment for patients with coverage. This is one of the factors that make aging accounts and billing patients tricky in the field of medicine. In any industry where claims are sent to insurance companies for partial or full reimbursement, a time lag exists. This time lag may cause certain balances to appear past due, when, in reality, the primary and/or secondary insurance is processing the claim. For patients with secondary insurance, a past-due balance could appear on an account for well past 30 to 45 days until that payment arrives.

Statements from medical offices often confuse patients, since the total balance due could reflect portions still pending from the insurance company. As you have learned, dunning messages that inform patients of the amount for which they are responsible to pay is a collections practice that can increase cash flow. However, for patients who are slow to pay, or consistently fail to pay, more effective collections techniques may be required beyond providing dunning messages on accounts.

THE COLLECTIONS PROCESS

As mentioned numerous times in this book, the best collections practices begin with financial counseling of new patients before service charges are incurred. A practice's brochure outlining payment policies, provider participation with health plans, and a specific contact person for financial matters helps avoid misunderstandings. Diligent collection of co-payments and other balances that are due at the time of service is the most effective collections technique for new and established patients. Additionally, having a timely and consistent schedule with regard to insurance billing, patient billing, and follow-up of payment promises plays a strong role in compliance.

The collections process, and when to take certain action, differs widely from office to office. Your employer will determine protocols for collections. For example, some offices initiate a phone call to the patient as soon as the account is 15 to 30 days past due. Other offices send a reminder on the patient's statement, or even a letter, before placing phone calls to patients to collect money. The tactics, time frames, and even specific letters and authorized payment arrangements, should be decided ahead of time, so that a plan of action is in place. Without this plan, there is little to no structure for successful collections.

Figure 9–59 provides guidelines for collections that fit most medical offices. Remember, prompt follow-up is the key. When a balance due remains unpaid beyond 15 days from the billed date, it probably will not be paid, unless further collections action is initiated.

WRITING COLLECTION LETTERS

Aside from dunning messages, most medical offices begin the collections process with a letter. The main purpose of any collection letter is to open a line of communication and offer assistance. Letters, early in the process, should not only encourage timely payment and ask for cooperation, but also maintain a sense of goodwill. In fact, initial collection letters are reminders to pay, more than anything else. They are generally viewed as less assertive than calling the patient, and more likely to be well received.

Carefully worded letters that take care not to appear overly assertive or unfair will deliver the best results. A patient should always be given the opportunity to pay within a reasonable amount of time. Using the physician as a participant in the collections process for both letter-writing and telephone collections is an excellent strategy for a better response.

As indicated in Figure 9-59, collection letters can be prepared for patients who do not pay on balances due within 15 days of a statement. The further past due a balance becomes, the more assertive the collections tactics become, both by letter and telephone. For larger balances, the collection letter should include an alternative for payment. This could be a reminder that major credit cards are accepted, or that a monthly payment arrangement can be set up directly with the office. Again, the

Time Past Due	Recommended Action
Time of service.	Payment and insurance policies are discussed with patient or guarantor.
Within 30 days after services are rendered.	First billing statement is sent; patients without insurance are reminded to pay. Patients with insurance are billed for applicable remainder balances, co-payments or deductibles.
Within 15 days of first billing statement.	Initiate collections for patients with balances due that have not responded to the first billing statement. A letter or telephone call is initiated.
60 days after services are rendered.	Second billing statement is sent, with a stronger reminder. All payments from insurance companies should have been received for patients with health plans.
Within 15 days of second billing statement.	A letter or telephone call is initiated. Offer payment arrangements; obtain commitment in writing with a schedule of when payments are due.
90 days after services are rendered.	Third billing statement is sent, with a strong reminder or warning. If needed, consult with manager or physician to plan next collections action.
Within 15 days of third billing statement.	A letter or telephone call is initiated. Another attempt to schedule payment arrangements is made. Notice is given of impending assignment to a collections agency or credit reporting system.
120 days after services are rendered.	Final collections action is initiated. Consult with the physician or office manager to apprise of which patients will be assigned to collections agency. A letter is prepared advising the patient of the action to be taken. If no further action is to be taken, the balance is adjusted as a bad debt and the patient account is flagged.

FIGURE 9-59

Collection guidelines. *Delmar/Cengage Learning*

objective is communication with the patient so that the medical office will be contacted and a solution worked out.

Study the sample collection letters found in Figure 9-60 and Figure 9-61. Which one is appropriate for use as an initial collection letter? Note the use of the physician in each letter as a participant of the collections process. How might this affect patient response to the letter? How does the first letter in Figure 9-60 compare in wording and message to the letter in Figure 9-61? It is clear that the choice of words, and even how sentences are structured, have an impact on what the letter projects to the reader. Next, study the letter in Figure 9-62. How does this letter compare to the others? At what stage of the collections process would you expect a delinquent patient to receive this letter?

Douglasville Medicine Associates
5076 Brand Blvd., Suite 401
Douglasville, NY 01234
Ph: (123) 456-7890
Fax: (123) 456-7891
Email: admin@dfma.com
Website: www.dfma.com

ERIC GORDON
485 Slate Dr.
Douglasville, NY 01234

Date: 05/23/20XX
Account No GOR001
Student No: Student1

Dear Mr. Gordon:

Our account manager has brought your current balance to my attention. Have you forgotten to send payment? In order to keep your account up to date, please remit $175.00 today. An envelope has been enclosed for your convenience.

If there is any reason a full payment cannot be made, a monthly payment can be arranged. I have instructed my staff to assist you in any way so that your obligation can be satisfied. I look forward to your cooperation with this matter.

Sincerely,

L.D. Heath, M.D. (or, administrative staff member signature)

FIGURE 9-60

Sample collection letter. *Delmar/Cengage Learning*

Douglasville Medicine Associates
5076 Brand Blvd., Suite 401
Douglasville, NY 01234
Ph: (123) 456-7890
Fax: (123) 456-7891
Email: admin@dfma.com
Website: www.dfma.com

ERIC GORDON
485 Slate Dr.
Douglasville, NY 01234

Date: 05/23/20XX
Account No GOR001
Student No: Student1

Dear Mr. Gordon:

Our account manager has privately discussed your current balance with me. We are concerned that you have not contacted our office regarding your balance. After reviewing your account, I ask that you call our office immediately for assistance. Our staff is ready to prepare a payment plan that will bring your account up to date and assist you with paying your obligation.

All patients that choose not to communicate with our staff or take advantage of payment arrangements will force us to no longer carry balances on our account and require payment at the time of service. Please avoid any alternative collection action by contacting us today. We look forward to your full cooperation.

Sincerely,

L.D. Heath, M.D. (or, administrative staff member signature)

FIGURE 9-61

Sample collection letter. *Delmar/Cengage Learning*

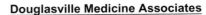

Douglasville Medicine Associates
5076 Brand Blvd., Suite 401
Douglasville, NY 01234
Ph: (123) 456-7890
Fax: (123) 456-7891
Email: admin@dfma.com
Website: www.dfma.com

ERIC GORDON
485 Slate Dr.
Douglasville, NY 01234

Date: 5/23/20XX
Account No: GOR001
Student No: Student1

Dear Mr. Gordon:

According to our records, the balance on your account remains unpaid. Our office has requested payment several times, and has offered alternate payment arrangements. Our requests appear to have been ignored.

I have instructed my account manager to withhold action on your account for the next five business days. Every effort will be made to answer your questions and provide you with a reasonable payment arrangement. If we do not receive a response, from you, alternative action will be taken to collect this obligation.

We hope you will avoid this action by contacting our office today to discuss your account and make arrangements.

Sincerely,

L.D. Heath, MD (or, administrative staff member signature)

FIGURE 9-62

Sample collection letter. *Delmar/Cengage Learning*

All collection letters should be addressed directly to the debtor, or guarantor, of record. The outside of the envelope cannot be marked with notices that state "delinquent" or "past due," or any other indication that the envelope content is a debt collection item.

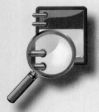

LET'S TRY IT! 9-9 WRITING COLLECTION LETTERS—BLAIR, DONALD

Objective: The reader prepares collection letters for patients who have overdue balances on their accounts, or other issues that require resolution.

STEP 1

Open the Patient Ledger for Donald Blair. He has an overdue balance of $1,832.00. His primary plan, Aetna, has determined, after further investigation, that patient Blair's fracture was a work-related injury and has notified the medical office that payment is denied. Aetna recommends that the patient notify his employer and a Workers' Comp claim be initiated. Using Figure 9-60 as a model, prepare a draft of a collection letter on note paper, dated January 4, 2010. Indicate why the claim was denied, and if not reported to the employer, the full amount is due from the patient.

STEP 2

At the bottom of the Patient Ledger screen, click on the *Correspondence button*. This opens an Output To window. Select a location for saving the letter (hard drive, flash drive, My Documents folder, etc.). Use the patient's last name and your last name for identification purposes, as shown in Figure 9-63.

T: Write down the name e folder where you saved ile so it can be retrieved in next steps.

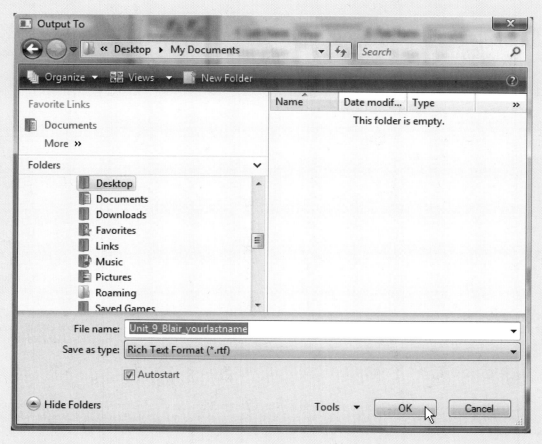

FIGURE 9-63

Delmar/Cengage Learning

STEP 3

Click on the *OK button*. The default word processing software installed on your computer opens the letterhead, ready to input the draft letter. If not, you may open your word processor (MS Word, WordPad, WordPerfect, etc.) and then find and open the file by navigating to the folder where it was saved. When displayed on the screen, the practice letterhead for Douglasville Medicine Associates is ready to use to type the letter. See Figure 9-64 for an example.

STEP 4

Change the date to January 4, 2010. Next, click on the sentence "*Type your message here*" and delete it. You are now ready to begin typing the letter to Donald Blair, using the draft that was previously prepared. Check your work with Figure 9-65. Your letter may be worded in a different manner, but the message and tone should be similar.

continues

Douglasville Medicine Associates
5076 Brand Blvd., Suite 401
Douglasville, NY 01234
Ph: (123) 456-7890
Fax: (123) 456-7891
Email: admin@dfma.com
Website: www.dfma.com

DONALD BLAIR
32 Hoover Blvd
Ridgeland, NY 27744

Date: 6/8/2010
Account No: BLA002
Student No: Student1

Dear Mr. Blair:

Type message here...

FIGURE 9-64

Delmar/Cengage Learning

Douglasville Medicine Associates
5076 Brand Blvd., Suite 401
Douglasville, NY 01234
Ph: (123) 456-7890
Fax: (123) 456-7891
Email: admin@dfma.com
Website: www.dfma.com

DONALD BLAIR
32 Hoover Blvd
Ridgeland, NY 27744

Date: 6/8/2010
Account No: BLA002
Student No: Student1

Dear Mr. Blair:

Our account manager has brought your current balance to my attention. Your insurance company, Aetna, has informed us that the services provided on 6/12/2009 were denied payment. After further investigation, they have determined that your injuries were work-related, and have advised that you notify your employer and initiate a Workers' Compensation claim.

Please contact your employer so that this claim can be paid. If it is not reported to the employer, you will be responsible for the full amount due. I have instructed my staff to assist you in any way so that your obligation can be satisfied. I look forward to your cooperation with this matter.

Sincerely,

L.D. Heath, M.D.

FIGURE 9-65

Delmar/Cengage Learning

STEP 5

Use Dr. Heath's signature block, as shown in Figure 9-65. Resave the letter, and then print it for your records, or turn it in to your instructor as directed.

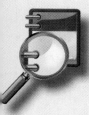

LET'S TRY IT! 9-10 WRITING COLLECTION LETTERS—CALDWELL, MEGAN

Objective: The reader prepares collection letters for patients who have overdue balances on their accounts, or other issues that require resolution.

STEP 1

Open the Patient Ledger for Megan Caldwell. She has an overdue balance of $20.00. This is a co-payment for an office visit that has been past due since December, 2008. Patient Caldwell has not responded to any previous collection letters or phone calls. The matter was brought to Dr. Schwartz's attention, and he has approved the patient being referred to the collections agency. However, he would like a letter sent to the patient for one last attempt to collect this small amount. He has suggested giving the patient five business days from the date of the letter to pay. Dr. Schwartz would like to include a sentence that mentions he hopes that this small balance will be paid soon and that no further action will be needed. Using Figure 9-62 as a model, prepare a draft of a collection letter on note paper, dated January 4, 2010.

STEP 2

T: Write down the name e folder where you saved ile so it can be retrieved in ext steps.

At the bottom of the Patient Ledger screen, click on the *Correspondence button*. This opens an Output To window. Select a location for saving the letter (hard drive, diskette, My Documents folder, etc.). Use the patient's last name and your last name for identification purposes, as shown in Figure 9-66.

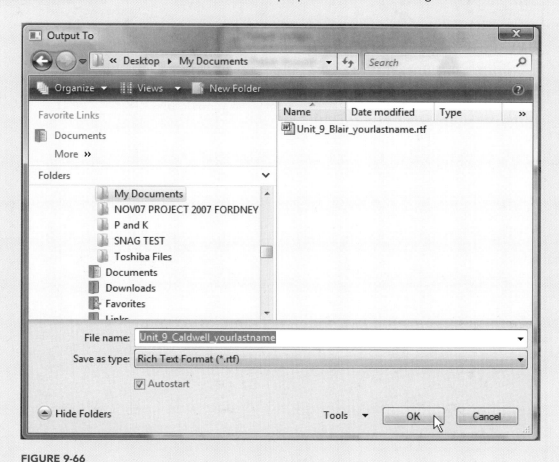

FIGURE 9-66

Delmar/Cengage Learning

continues

WRITING COLLECTION LETTERS—CALDWELL, MEGAN *continued*

STEP 3

Click on the *OK button*. The default word processing software installed on your computer opens the letterhead, ready to input the draft letter. If not, you may open your word processor (MS Word, WordPad, WordPerfect, etc.) and then find and open the file by navigating to the folder where it was saved. When displayed on the screen, the practice letterhead for Douglasville Medicine Associates is ready to use to type the letter.

STEP 4

Change the date to January 4, 2010. Next, click on the sentence "*Type your message here*" and delete it. You are now ready to begin typing the letter to Megan Caldwell, using the draft that was previously prepared. Check your work with Figure 9-67. Your letter may be worded in a different manner, but the message and tone should be similar.

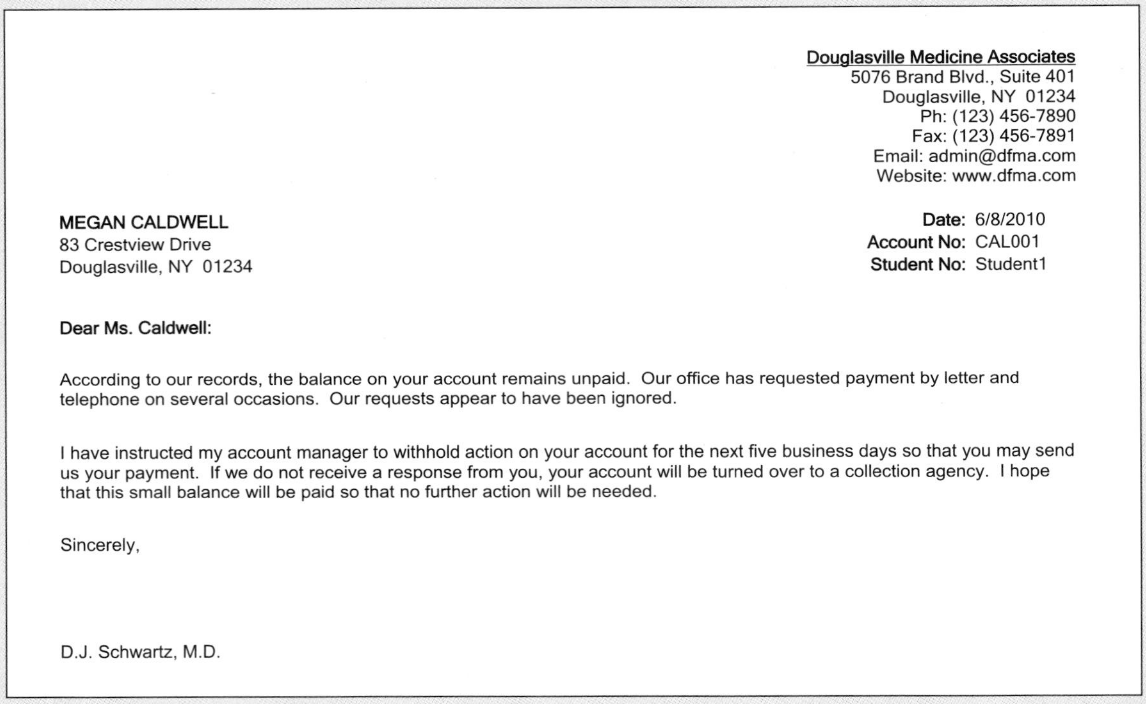

Douglasville Medicine Associates
5076 Brand Blvd., Suite 401
Douglasville, NY 01234
Ph: (123) 456-7890
Fax: (123) 456-7891
Email: admin@dfma.com
Website: www.dfma.com

MEGAN CALDWELL
83 Crestview Drive
Douglasville, NY 01234

Date: 6/8/2010
Account No: CAL001
Student No: Student1

Dear Ms. Caldwell:

According to our records, the balance on your account remains unpaid. Our office has requested payment by letter and telephone on several occasions. Our requests appear to have been ignored.

I have instructed my account manager to withhold action on your account for the next five business days so that you may send us your payment. If we do not receive a response from you, your account will be turned over to a collection agency. I hope that this small balance will be paid so that no further action will be needed.

Sincerely,

D.J. Schwartz, M.D.

FIGURE 9-67

Delmar/Cengage Learning

STEP 5

Use a signature block with Dr. D.J. Schwartz's name, as shown in Figure 9-67. Resave the letter, and then print it for your records, or turn it in to your instructor as directed.

DOS AND DON'TS OF TELEPHONE COLLECTIONS

Every business, including medical offices, that engages in the collection of debts must comply with state and federal regulations that concern collections. There are several guidelines that can be followed, especially when placing telephone calls for the purpose of collections. Some of the more common guidelines that adhere to most regulations are presented in the following list.

1. Calls should be placed only between 8 a.m. and 9 p.m. Calls at any other times, and even repeated calls, can be considered harassment.

2. Do not call the patient at work when it is known that personal calls cannot be accepted. If someone other than the patient answers the phone at the workplace, never reveal what the nature of the call is. Simply state your name and phone number where the patient should return the call.

3. Do not record conversations without the knowledge of the patient. This is considered an invasion of privacy.

4. Do not misrepresent yourself, such as posing as a collections agency, or engage in any other fraudulent activity. By contrast, a person cannot be threatened that his or her account will be turned over to a collections agency if there is no intent to do so. This is also considered misrepresentation.

5. For all telephone calls, be certain you are speaking to the appropriate person. Identify the person you are calling by using the full name for verification. Discussing a debt with any third party can be considered slander.

6. Do not use descriptive names that can be considered libel, such as calling a patient a "deadbeat" or a "delinquent." The patient should not be harassed verbally or threatened in any way.

In general, when calling patients for collections purposes, the collector should be respectful, nonassertive, and friendly during the conversation. This encourages a positive outcome and, ideally, a commitment to pay. After the initial greeting, the collector should state the purpose of the call. Again, no apologies are necessary; getting directly to the point, and securing a promise to pay, is the main objective.

For larger balances, the manager or physician should be consulted regarding an acceptable payment arrangement that can be offered to the patient. A monthly payment that will be due on a specific date each month makes tracking these payments easier. The debtor ideally should sign an agreement that clearly states the balance, amount of the monthly payment, and the dates on which those payments are expected. A notice should also be included on this document that outlines what the consequences are should the payment agreement not be followed. For example, a notice may read that an account may be considered delinquent and assigned to a collections agency if payment is more than five days late. It should also state that, if the patient anticipates the payment being late, he or she should call the office for assistance. See Figure 9-68 for an example of a written payment arrangement.

As with any collections activity, the details of the conversation should be documented. The Notes feature included with the Patient Ledger of MOSS is an ideal place for such notes. Follow the office policy of your employer if collection notes are to be kept in a specific location for reference purposes. If future follow-up is required, any staff member can review the notes and obtain information on what was discussed with the patient.

Douglasville Medicine Associates
5076 Brand Blvd., Suite 401
Douglasville, NY 01234
Ph: (123) 456-7890
Fax: (123) 456-7891
Email: admin@dfma.com
Website: www.dfma.com

PAYMENT ARRANGEMENT AGREEMENT   Date_____

I have been advised of the balance due on my account of $_____. I am in agreement that I am responsible for payment of this balance.

I agreement to pay the above balance as follows:

$_____ as the initial payment

$_____ due on the _____ of each month, until the balance is paid.

I understand that if any payment is more than five days past due as agreed above, my account will be considered delinquent. I will be responsible for any future collection costs if I default on this agreement.

I have read this arrangement and agree to the terms as stated.

_____ Date_____
Signature

_____
Printed Name

_____ Date_____
Authorized Signature for Practice

_____
Printed Name

FIGURE 9-68

A sample of a written payment agreement. *Delmar/Cengage Learning*

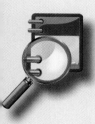

LET'S TRY IT! 9-11 ROLE-PLAY TELEPHONE COLLECTION CALLS

Objective: The reader practices a sample collections dialogue between a collector and a patient. Then, the details of the conversation are documented on the patient's record.

Collector: Hello, this is (your name) from Douglasville Medicine Associates. Am I speaking with Patty Practice?

Patient: Yes, this is Patty.

Collector: Good (morning, afternoon), Ms. Practice. My name is (your name). Dr. Heath has asked me to call you today to find out if there is a problem with your account. Over the past two months, our office has sent reminder notices regarding your balance. Ms. Practice, have you been receiving our statements?

Patient: I'm not sure.

Collector: Is your mailing address 123 Main Street in Douglasville?

Patient: Yes, it is. Apartment 116. How much do I owe?

Collector: Your current balance is $91.00.

Patient: I don't understand. I have insurance; shouldn't that be covered by my health plan?

Collector: Your health plan did not cover the procedure on October 28. The insurance company sent an explanation of the denial to you by mail. We received a copy of it at our office.

Patient: Well, I don't have that kind of money right now.

Collector: Ms. Practice, Dr. Heath and I have discussed your account in private. The doctor is willing to accept a monthly payment of $30.00 until this balance is paid. Would $30.00 create a financial hardship for you? (If the patient says it will create a hardship, ask what monthly or biweekly payment amount would be comfortable.)

Patient: I guess I could do that. Can you send me another bill?

Collector: Ms. Practice, our policy is to have all payment arrangements in writing. If you can send a payment within the next five business days for the first $30.00, we would be happy to set up a regular monthly due date for the remaining payments. Can I schedule an appointment for you to come to the office and set up your payment arrangement with our account manager?

The telephone call then can be concluded with the scheduling of a convenient appointment. Thank the patient, and say that you look forward to her cooperation with this matter. The patient should also be advised that her agreement to the payment arrangement will be made known to the doctor. It is best for the patient to be aware that the doctor has continued involvement in the collections process. This also may help strengthen the patient's commitment to pay.

Next, document the pertinent details of the telephone call. Since Patty Practice has an account, record the agreement that was made in the Notes section of the Patient Ledger as follows:

STEP 1

Click on the *drop-down menu* and select Patient Ledger, as shown in Figure 9-69. Select the account for Patty Practice to open her ledger for viewing.

continues

ROLE-PLAY TELEPHONE COLLECTION CALLS *continued*

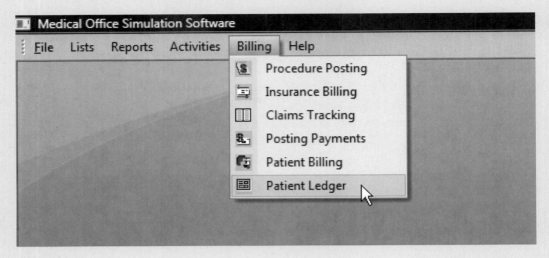

FIGURE 9-69

Delmar/Cengage Learning

STEP 2

Click on the *Notes button* located at the bottom left of the ledger screen, as shown in Figure 9-70. When the Notes window opens, click on the *Add button* in order to add a new note to the record.

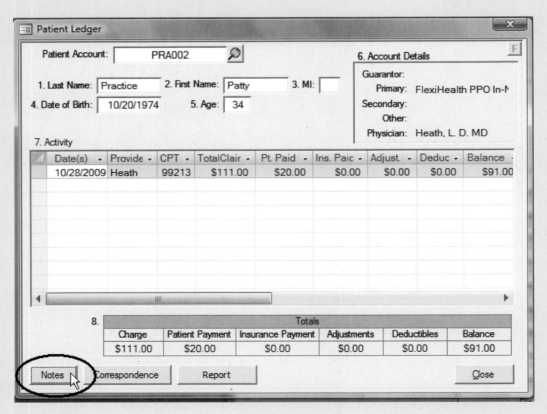

FIGURE 9-70

Delmar/Cengage Learning

STEP 3

Click inside the *Note box* and type the following: "12/31/2009. Spoke to patient on the telephone, verified address, discussed reason she has a $91.00 balance. Patient agreed to pay balance with 3 monthly payments of $30.00. Scheduled appointment on 01/06/2010 for her to sign an agreement." (Type your last name at the end of the note.) Compare your note to the example in Figure 9-71.

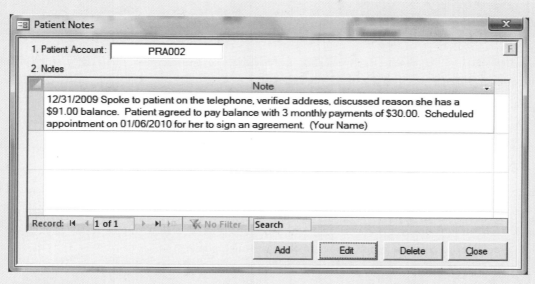

FIGURE 9-71

Delmar/Cengage Learning

It is obvious from the example dialogue shown above for Patty Practice that the collector must be prepared before placing collection calls. Knowing the balance due, how many reminders have been sent, why the money is owed, and knowledge of the health plan, assist in having an effective conversation. Anticipate every resistance and be ready with a solution. As mentioned earlier, all details of the collection call should be documented in the appropriate location for future reference and follow-up.

FINAL NOTES

The responsibilities of the administrative staff in a medical office go well beyond greeting patients and preparing insurance claims for billing. Long after insurance claims have been sent and payments received, effective follow-up of balances due from patients and secondary plans is essential. Collection of delinquent accounts becomes a separate challenge, requiring special skills not only in dealing with people, but also becoming savvy in pursuing insurance companies that are slow to pay. In the next unit, our attention will be turned to the tracking of, and following up on, insurance payments. Much like individual patients, many health plans have payment delays, denials, and suspended claims that require action at different levels. This is yet another component of the reimbursement process and, once again, software can assist in simplifying the work.

Whether a medical assistant decides to specialize in the art of collections and become a medical collector, or to use basic techniques as part of the billing tasks, the reimbursement cycle is not complete without patient billing and collections.

CHECK YOUR KNOWLEDGE

1. From the following list, select effective techniques for good communication when discussing financials with patients. Place a check in the blank provided.

_____ a. Practice good manners, with frequent use of "please" and "thank you."

_____ b. Maintain a professional demeanor.

_____ c. Advise the patient that accounts are assigned to a collections agency whenever payments are late.

_____ d. Greet patients and welcome them to the office before discussing financials.

_____ e. Discuss payment arrangements and hardship issues with patients while others are seated in the waiting room.

_____ f. If a patient's insurance has a low reimbursement rate, or is slow to pay, be sure to tell the patient in order to encourage him or her to change health plans.

_____ g. Use clear and specific language with a friendly tone.

_____ h. Remain calm and use tact when dealing with an angry patient.

2. An itemized bill that specifies the balance due and is sent to the patient on a monthly basis is called

a. a ledger.

b. a statement.

c. an explanation of benefits.

d. none of the above.

3. The most effective time of the month for patients to receive statements is

a. the first of the month.

b. the 1st and 15th of the month.

c. approximately five days before a payday.

d. five days after a payday.

4. The main purpose of any collection letter is

a. to threaten the patient into paying his or her bill.

b. to encourage payment, but maintain goodwill.

c. to open a line of communication and offer assistance.

d. to provide a reminder to pay.

e. b, c, and d above.

f. all of the above.

5. A technique for sending statements that spreads the flow of income through the month and divides patients into small billing groups is referred to as _____.

6. A note included on statements that explains balances, encourages payment, or warns of impending collections action is called a _____.

7. Today, a medical assistant has received 17 personal checks from patients that need to be posted. The checks have been batched together. In order to protect the checks from being cashed or improperly used by any other party, the checks are stamped with a(n) _____.

8. List some examples of how the results from various reports can be used in the medical office.

_____

_____

_____

9. List five main items that should be inspected on each personal check before accepting it as payment.

_____

_____

_____

10. Describe the action to be taken when a patient writes "paid in full" on the memo line of a personal check, yet the payment is less than the balance due on the account.

_____

_____

_____

11. When a patient has a primary and/or secondary insurance, explain why the balance due may appear delinquent even though the account is current (not late).

_____

_____

_____

12. How does a practice's information brochure or pamphlet help with payment collections from patients?

_____

_____

_____

13. List six important guidelines to use in order to properly place collection calls by telephone.

_____

_____

_____

14. Explain the importance of offering patients alternative methods of paying a balance.

_____

_____

_____

15. How does documenting collections activity (details of conversations or when letters are sent) assist the staff of a medical office?

_____

_____

_____

Posting Secondary Insurance Payments and Electronic RA Payments

OBJECTIVES

Upon completion of this unit, the reader should be able to:

- **Demonstrate posting payments from secondary insurance companies using MOSS**

- **Demonstrate posting payments based on an electronic Remittance Advice (RA) using MOSS**

In Unit 8, posting payments from insurance companies and applying those payments to patient accounts were discussed. The *Let's Try It!* exercises provided an opportunity to practice reading EOBs and RAs from insurance companies. EOBs helped to determine the amount of the payments, adjustments, and other data relevant to the fees charged for services. Many of the patients of the Douglasville Medicine Associates group practice have dual insurance. When the primary paid its portion of a claim, the secondary was billed for any remaining balances, and will pay according to the benefits of the plan.

An EOB or RA will also accompany payments received from secondary insurance plans. Like the EOBs from primary insurance, it is common for several patients to be included on one EOB, with one payment being applicable to several different patient accounts. It is helpful to review the Patient Ledger when an EOB and payment are received from a secondary plan. This allows review of payments already posted from the primary insurance, and any balances due. It may also be helpful to retrieve the EOB from the primary insurance and review details of the payments, adjustments, or amounts applied to deductibles. Comparing the Patient Ledger and the EOB from primary and secondary plans can help with understanding the entire payment cycle.

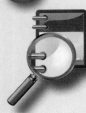

LET'S TRY IT! 10-1 POSTING SECONDARY INSURANCE PAYMENTS FROM CENTURY SENIORGAP

Objective: The reader posts payments from Century SeniorGap, a Medicare supplemental insurance plan, to patient accounts. The Patient Ledger and insurance EOB are referenced as needed to complete the task. The date of posting is 12/30/2009.

CASE STUDY 10-A: MUÑOZ, GERALDO

STEP 1

Start MOSS.

STEP 2

Refer to Source Document 10-1 in the Source Document Appendix, which shows an EOB from Century SeniorGap. Study the EOB and identify the patients and column headings. Click on the *Posting Payments button* on the Main Menu. Select patient Geraldo Muñoz from the list and click the *Apply Payment button.*

STEP 3

Next, click the *View Ledger button* and compare the EOB information to the ledger. The service dates, charges, Medicare payments, and balances should match up to details provided for patient Muñoz. When finished, close the ledger and return to the Posting Payments screen.

STEP 4

Since this is a payment made by the secondary insurance, you will need to select the plan with the locator bar on the bottom left of the screen. Click so that *record 2* is shown on the screen, indicated by Field 2 displaying Century SeniorGap. Check your screen with Figure 10-1 before proceeding.

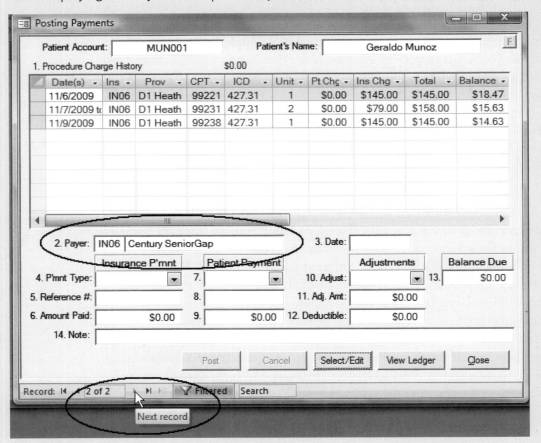

FIGURE 10-1

Delmar/Cengage Learning

STEP 5

Payments are posted in the same manner as learned in Unit 8. Select the *line entry* for service on 11/6/2009 in the top section by clicking on it, and then click on the *Select/Edit button*. This displays a balance of $18.27 in Field 13, as shown in Figure 10-2.

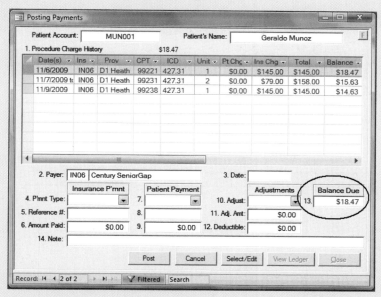

FIGURE 10-2

Delmar/Cengage Learning

NT: 12/30/2009

STEP 6

Enter the date of posting in Field 3. Next, tab to Field 4 and select Insurance Payment by dropping down the box. Enter the Century SeniorGap claim number, as shown on the EOB, in Field 5. Enter the payment of $14.80, as shown on the EOB, in Field 6. Upon pressing *Enter*, the amount due in Field 13 now displays zero. Check your screen with Figure 10-3.

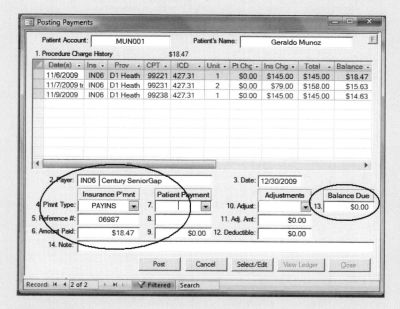

FIGURE 10-3

Delmar/Cengage Learning

Case Study 10-A Continues >>

STEP 7

Click on the *Post button* to apply the payment. View the ledger and check the Balance Due for the 11/06/2009 line entry. It should now read zero. See Figure 10-4.

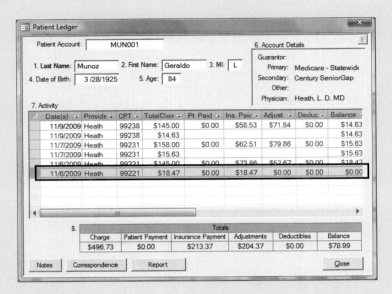

FIGURE 10-4

Delmar/Cengage Learning

STEP 8

Close the Patient Ledger screen. Repeat the instructions in previous Step 2 through Step 7 and post the payment for services on 11/07 through 11/08/09 shown on Source Document 10-1. Check your work with Figure 10-5 before clicking on the *Post button.*

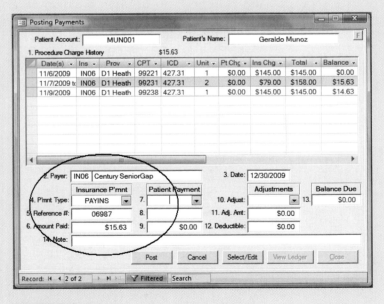

FIGURE 10-5

Delmar/Cengage Learning

STEP 9

Repeat the instructions in previous Step 2 through Step 7 and post the payment for services on 11/09/09 shown on Source Document 10-1. Check your work with Figure 10-6 before clicking on the *Post button.*

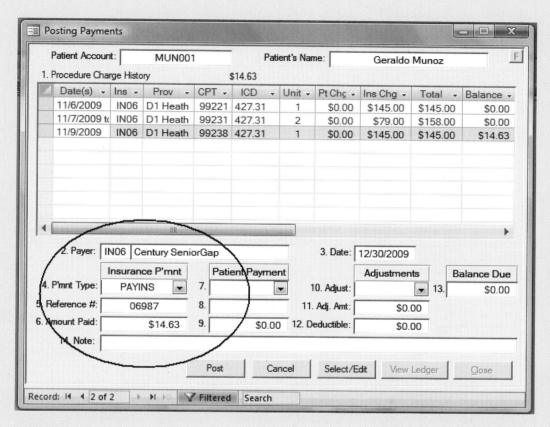

FIGURE 10-6

Delmar/Cengage Learning

Case Study 10-A Continues >>

Case Study 10-A Continued

STEP 10

When finished, check the Patient Ledger for patient Muñoz with Figure 10-7. All balance columns in Field 7 on the ledger should now read zero. The account is current, since both insurance plans have paid.

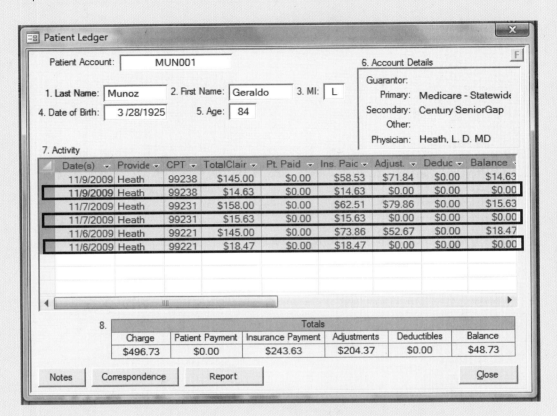

FIGURE 10-7

Delmar/Cengage Learning

STEP 11

Close all open windows and return to the Patient Selection list for posting payments.

CASE STUDY 10-B: TOMANAGA, MARIE

Continuing with the EOB from Century SeniorGap in Source Document 10-1, complete the following steps to post the payments for patient Tomanaga.

STEP 1

Start MOSS.

STEP 2

Study the EOB and identify the patients and column headings. Click on the *Posting Payments button* on the Main Menu. Select patient Marie Tomanaga from the list.

STEP 3

Next, click the *View Ledger button* and compare the EOB information to the ledger. The service dates, charges, Medicare payments, and balances should match up to details provided for patient Tomanaga. When finished, close the ledger and return to the Posting Payments screen.

STEP 4

Since this is a payment made by the secondary insurance, you will need to select the plan with the locator bar on the bottom left of the screen. Click so that *record 2* is shown on the screen, indicated by Field 2 displaying Century SeniorGap. Check your screen with Figure 10-8 before proceeding.

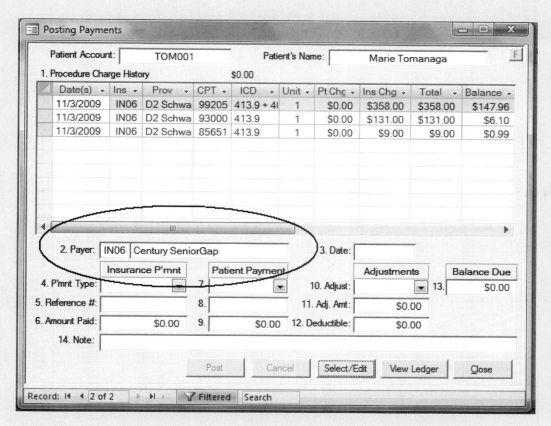

FIGURE 10-8

Delmar/Cengage Learning

Case Study 10-B Continues >>

Case Study 10-B Continued

STEP 5

Select the *line entry* for service on 11/3/2009, CPT 99205 in the top section by clicking on it, and then click on the *Select/Edit button*. This displays a balance of $147.96 in Field 13, as shown in Figure 10-9.

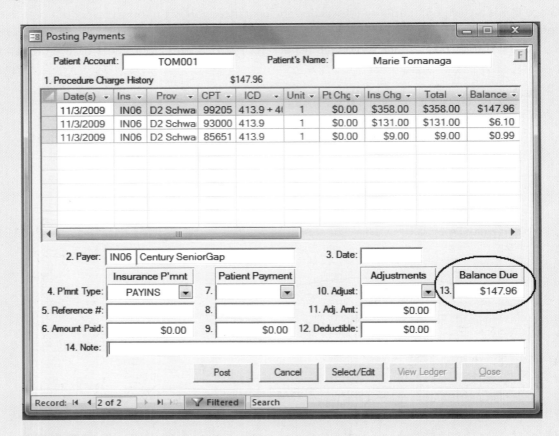

FIGURE 10-9

Delmar/Cengage Learning

NT: 12/30/2009

STEP 6

Enter the date of posting in Field 3. Next, tab to Field 4 and select Insurance Payment by dropping down the box. Enter the Century SeniorGap claim number, as shown on the EOB, in Field 5. Enter the payment of $147.96, as shown on the EOB, in Field 6. Upon pressing *Enter*, the amount due in Field 13 now displays zero. Check your screen with Figure 10-10.

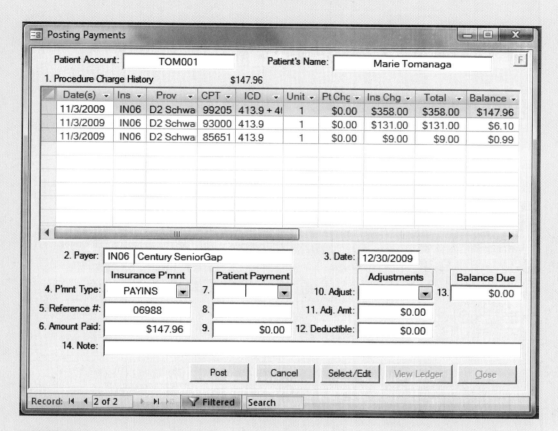

FIGURE 10-10

Delmar/Cengage Learning

Case Study 10-B Continues >>

Case Study 10-B Continued

STEP 7

Click on the *Post button* to apply the payment. View the ledger and check the Balance Due for the 11/03/2009 line entry for CPT 99205. It should now read zero. See Figure 10-11.

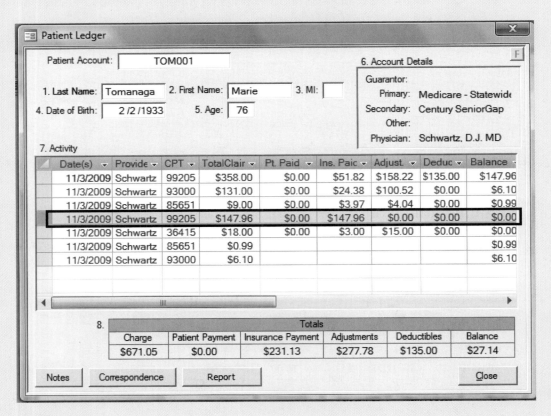

FIGURE 10-11

Delmar/Cengage Learning

STEP 8

Close the Patient Ledger screen. Repeat the instructions in previous Step 2 through Step 7 and post the payment for the next service on 11/03/2009, CPT 93000. Check your work with Figure 10-12 before clicking on the *Post button*.

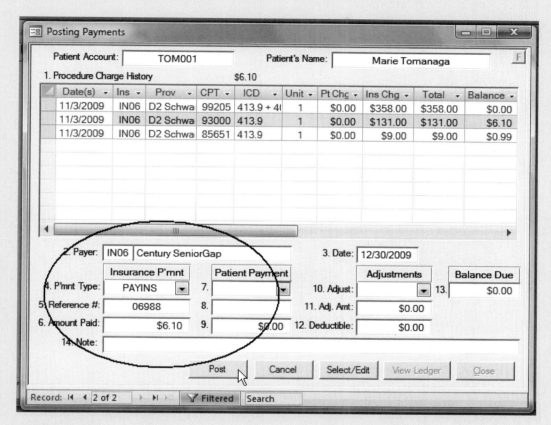

FIGURE 10-12

Delmar/Cengage Learning

Case Study 10-B Continues >>

STEP 9

Repeat the instructions in previous Step 2 through Step 7 and post the payment for the last service on 11/3/2009, CPT 85651 shown on Source Document 10-1. Check your work with Figure 10-13 before clicking on the *Post button*.

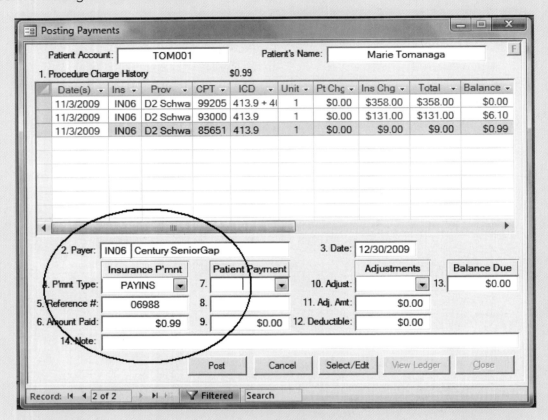

FIGURE 10-13

Delmar/Cengage Learning

STEP 10

When finished, check the Patient Ledger for patient Tomanaga with Figure 10-14. All balance columns in Field 7 on the ledger should now read zero. The account is current, since both insurance plans have paid.

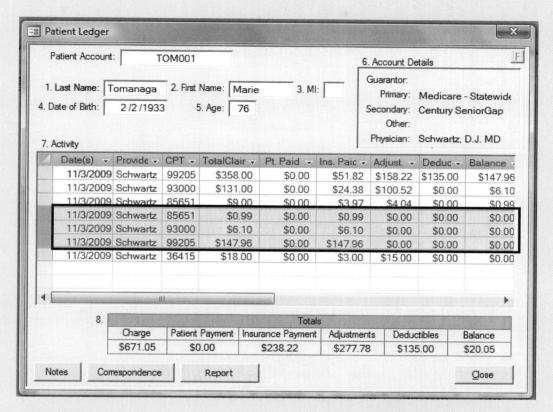

FIGURE 10-14

Delmar/Cengage Learning

STEP 11

Close all open windows and return to the Patient Selection list for posting payments.

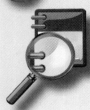

LET'S TRY IT! 10-2 POSTING SECONDARY INSURANCE PAYMENTS FROM MEDICAID

Objective: The reader posts payments from Medicaid as the secondary insurance to patient accounts. The Patient Ledger and insurance RA should be referenced as needed to complete the task. The date of posting is 12/30/2009.

CASE STUDY 10-C: BLANC, FRANCOIS
STEP 1
Start MOSS.

STEP 2
Refer to Source Document 10-2 in the Source Document Appendix, which shows an RA from Medicaid. Study the RA and identify the patients and column headings. Open the ledger for Francois Blanc, the first patient listed on the RA. Compare the ledger to the numbers on the RA regarding payments.

STEP 3
Click on the *Posting Payments button* on the Main Menu. Select patient Blanc from the list. Next, select the secondary insurance by using the locator bar on the bottom left of the screen. Click so that *record 2* is shown on the screen, indicated by Field 2 displaying Medicaid, as shown in Figure 10-15.

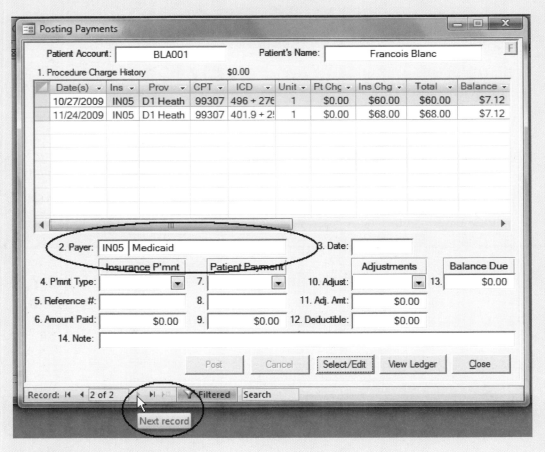

FIGURE 10-15

Delmar/Cengage Learning

STEP 4

In the top section, select the *line entry* for procedure 99307 on 10/27/2009 by clicking on it. Then, click on the *Select/Edit button.* This displays a balance of $7.12 in Field 13.

STEP 5

Post the payment as previously learned. Use the RA number, found in the top left corner, as the reference for Field 5. Check your work with Figure 10-16 before posting the payment.

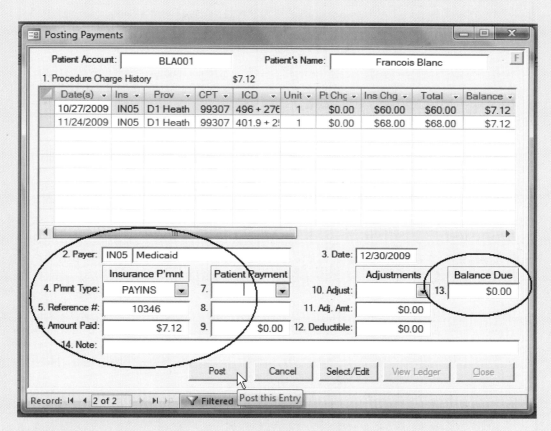

FIGURE 10-16

Delmar/Cengage Learning

Case Study 10-C Continues >>

STEP 6

Continuing with patient Blanc, post the next payment in the same manner for procedure 99307, done on 11/24/2009. Check your work with Figure 10-17 before posting the payment.

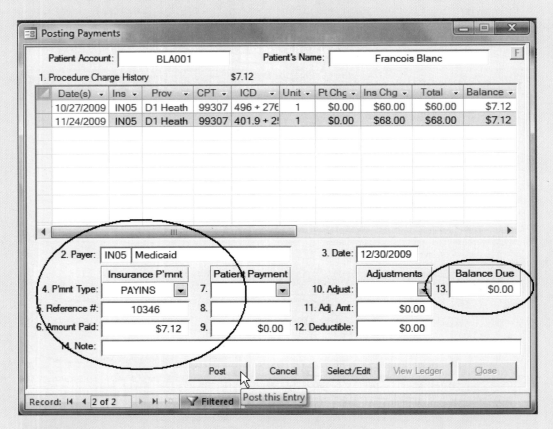

FIGURE 10-17

Delmar/Cengage Learning

STEP 7

When finished, compare the Patient Ledger for patient Blanc with Figure 10-18.

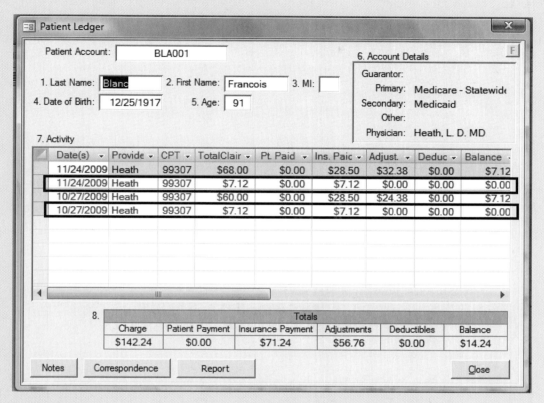

FIGURE 10-18

Delmar/Cengage Learning

STEP 8

Close all open windows and return to the Main Menu in MOSS.

CASE STUDY 10-D: CHANG, XAO

STEP 1

Refer to Source Document 10-2 in the Source Document Appendix, which shows an RA from Medicaid. Study the RA and identify the patients and column headings. Open the ledger for Xao Chang and compare the ledger to the numbers on the RA regarding payments.

STEP 2

Click on the *Posting Payments button* on the Main Menu. Select patient Chang from the list. Next, select the secondary insurance by using the locator bar on the bottom left of the screen. Click so that *record 2* is shown on the screen, indicated by Field 2 displaying Medicaid, as shown in Figure 10-19.

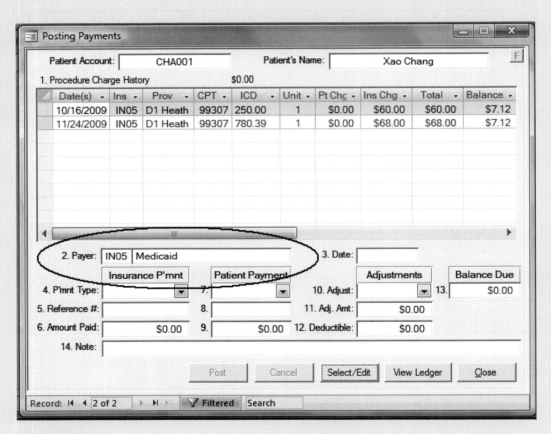

FIGURE 10-19

Delmar/Cengage Learning

STEP 3

In the top section, select the *line entry* for procedure 99307 on 10/16/2009 by clicking on it. Then, click on the *Select/Edit button*. This displays a balance of $7.12 in Field 13.

STEP 4

Post the payment as previously learned. Use the RA number, found in the top left corner, as the reference for Field 5. Check your work with Figure 10-20 before posting the payment.

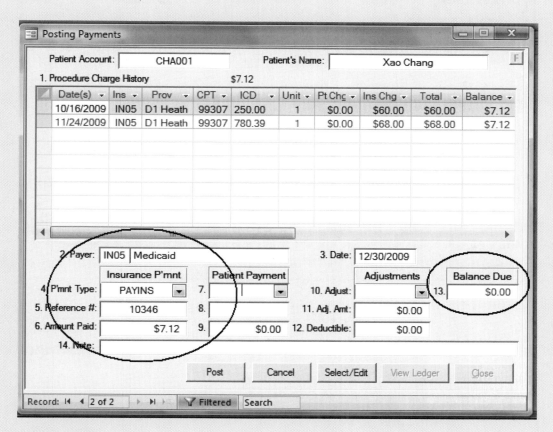

FIGURE 10-20

Delmar/Cengage Learning

Case Study 10-D Continues >>

STEP 5

Continuing with patient Chang, post the next payment in the same manner for procedure 99307, done on 11/24/2009. Check your work with Figure 10-21 before posting the payment.

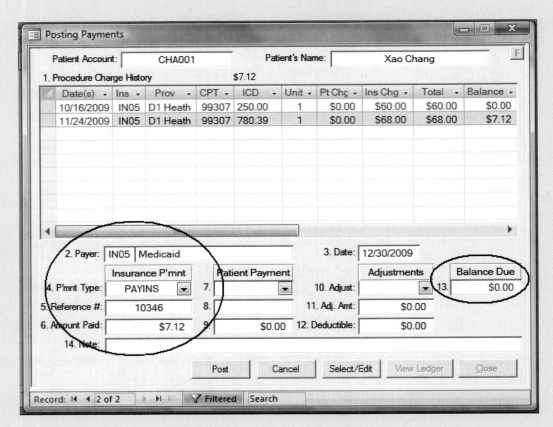

FIGURE 10-21

Delmar/Cengage Learning

STEP 6

When finished, compare the Patient Ledger for patient Chang with Figure 10-22.

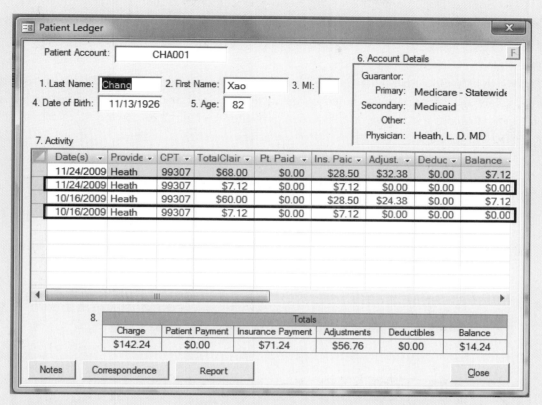

FIGURE 10-22

Delmar/Cengage Learning

STEP 7

Close all open windows and return to the Main Menu in MOSS.

CASE STUDY 10-E: PINKSTON, ANNA

STEP 1

Refer to Source Document 10-2 in the Source Document Appendix, which shows an RA from Medicaid. Study the RA and identify the patients and column headings. Open the ledger for Anna Pinkston and compare the ledger to the numbers on the RA regarding payments.

STEP 2

Click on the *Posting Payments button* on the Main Menu. Select patient Pinkston from the list. Next, select the secondary insurance by using the locator bar on the bottom left of the screen. Click so that *record 2* is shown on the screen, indicated by Field 2 displaying Medicaid, as shown in Figure 10-23.

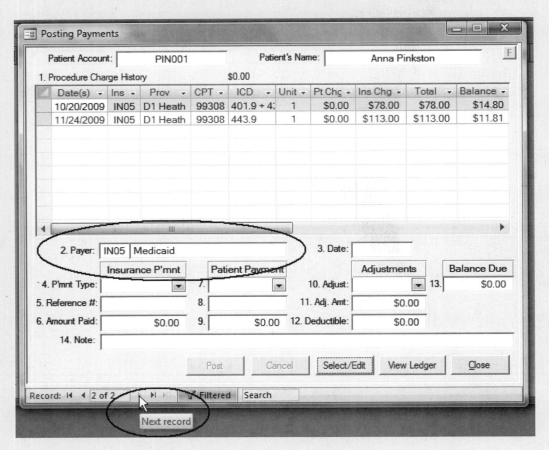

FIGURE 10-23

Delmar/Cengage Learning

STEP 3

In the top section, select the *line entry* for procedure 99308 on 10/20/2009 by clicking on it. Then, click on the *Select/Edit button*. This displays a balance of $14.80 in Field 13.

STEP 4

Post the payment as previously learned. Use the RA number, found in the top left corner, as the reference for Field 5. Check your work with Figure 10-24 before posting the payment.

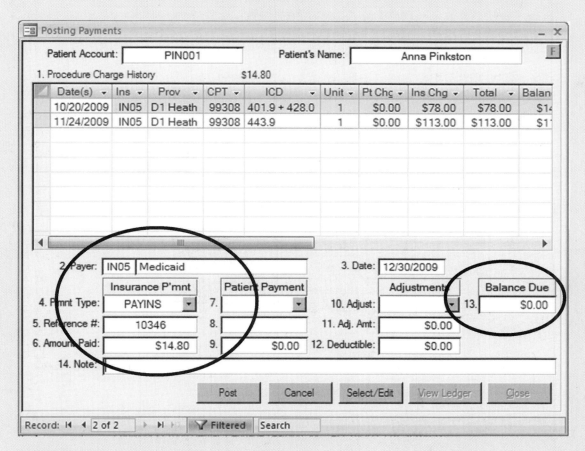

FIGURE 10-24

Delmar/Cengage Learning

Case Study 10-E Continues >>

STEP 5

Continuing with patient Pinkston, post the next payment in the same manner for procedure 99308, done on 11/24/2009. Check your work with Figure 10-25 before posting the payment.

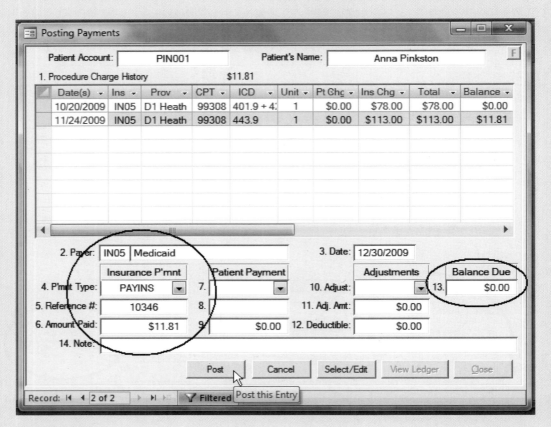

FIGURE 10-25

Delmar/Cengage Learning

STEP 6

When finished, compare the Patient Ledger for patient Pinkston with Figure 10-26.

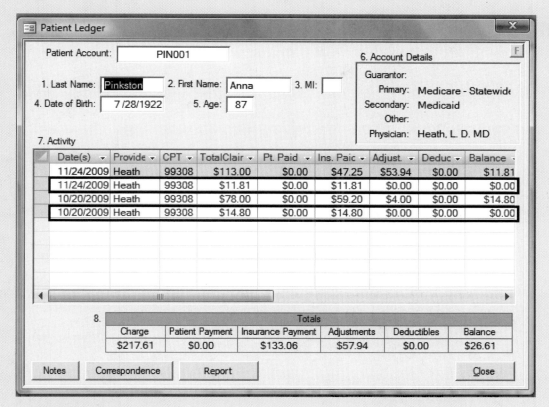

FIGURE 10-26

Delmar/Cengage Learning

STEP 7

Close all open windows and return to the Main Menu in MOSS.

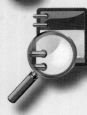

LET'S TRY IT! 10-3 POSTING SECONDARY INSURANCE PAYMENTS FROM MEDICARE

Objective: The reader posts payments from Medicare, as a secondary insurance, to the applicable patient accounts. The patient ledger and insurance RA should be referenced as needed to complete the task. The date of posting is 12/30/2009.

CASE STUDY 10-F: MANALY, RICHARD

STEP 1

Start MOSS.

STEP 2

Refer to Source Document 10-3 in the Source Document Appendix, which shows an RA from Medicare as secondary payer (MSP). Study the RA and identify the patients and column headings. Open the Patient Ledger for Richard Manaly, the first patient listed on the RA. Compare the ledger to the numbers on the RA regarding payments. Take note of the following guidelines:

A. The column headings are at the very top, going across, and correspond to the figures below, in bold. These look similar to the Medicare RAs used to post payments in Unit 8.

B. The line going across, starting with Name, includes the patient information. Notice the HIC number (Medicare ID number), ACNT number (account number at the medical office), and the internal control number (ICN), which is used as the reference in Field 5 for posting.

C. The explanation codes are located at the bottom of the RA. This helps you determine what the contractual write-off (CO) is, the primary insurance paid (OA-23), and the patient responsibility to pay (PR). The PROV-PD column provides the total paid to the provider by the primary insurance, and what Medicare pays as the secondary. For each patient on this RA, notice that Medicare has paid the co-insurance amount, which would have been the patient's responsibility if the patient had not had secondary coverage.

STEP 3

Close patient Manaly's ledger, then click on the *Posting Payments button* on the Main Menu. Select patient Manaly from the list. Next, select the secondary insurance by using the locator bar on the bottom left of the screen. Click so that *record 2* is shown on the screen, indicated by Field 2 displaying Medicare, as shown in Figure 10-27.

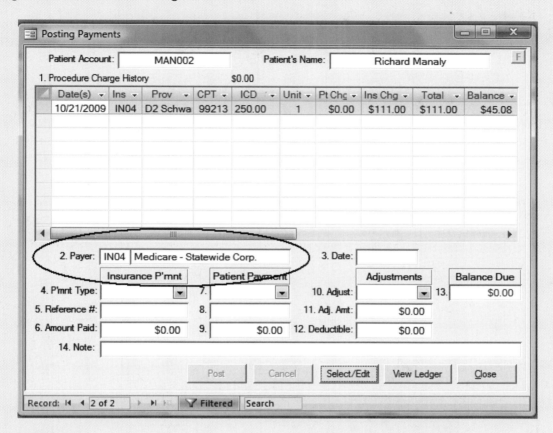

FIGURE 10-27

Delmar/Cengage Learning

Case Study 10-F Continues >>

STEP 4

In the top section, select the *line entry* for procedure 99213 on 10/21/2009 by clicking on it. Then, click on the *Select/Edit button*. This displays a balance of $45.08 in Field 13.

HINT: Use 12/30/2009 as the date of posting.

STEP 5

Post the payment of $16.48 as previously learned. Use the ICN number for patient Manaly as the reference for Field 5. Check your work with Figure 10-28 before clicking on the *Post button*.

NOTE: Medicare did not pay the $28.60 non-covered portion. The patient needs to pay this out-of-pocket expense since Dr. Schwartz is an out-of-network physician for FlexiHealth PPO.

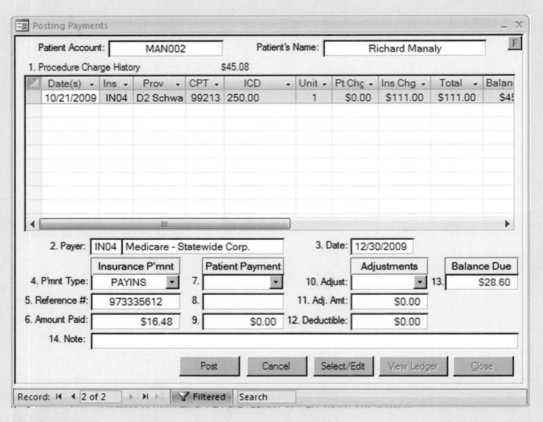

FIGURE 10-28

Delmar/Cengage Learning

STEP 6

When finished, compare the Patient Ledger to Figure 10-29. Close all open windows and return to the Patient Selection window for posting payments.

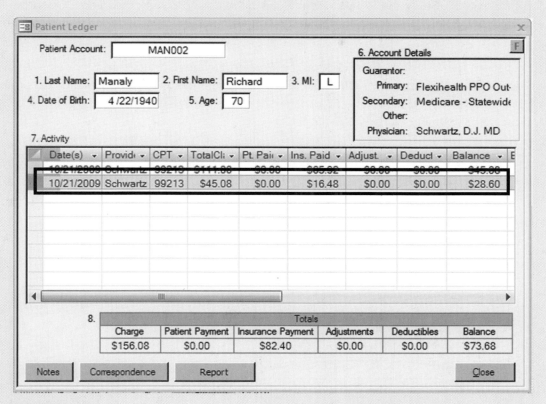

FIGURE 10-29

Delmar/Cengage Learning

CASE STUDY 10-G: RUHL, MARY

STEP 1

Refer to Source Document 10-3 in the Source Document Appendix, which shows an RA from Medicare as MSP. Study the RA and identify the patients and column headings. Open the Patient Ledger for Mary Ruhl, and compare the ledger to the numbers on the RA regarding payments

STEP 2

Close patient Ruhl's ledger, then click on the *Posting Payments button* on the Main Menu. Select patient Ruhl from the list. Next, select the secondary insurance by using the locator bar on the bottom left of the screen. Click so that *record 2* is shown on the screen, indicated by Field 2 displaying Medicare, as shown in Figure 10-30.

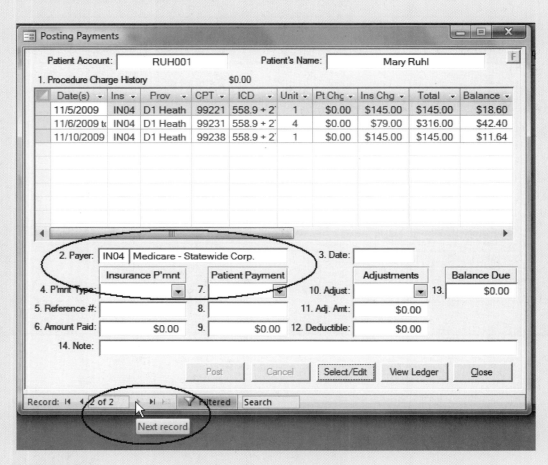

FIGURE 10-30

Delmar/Cengage Learning

STEP 3

In the top section, select the *line entry* for procedure 99221 on 11/05/2009 by clicking on it. Then, click on the *Select/Edit button*. This displays a balance of $18.60 in Field 13.

STEP 4

Post the payment of $18.60 as previously learned. Use the ICN number for patient Ruhl as the reference for Field 5. Check your work with Figure 10-31 before clicking on the *Post button*.

NT: Use 12/30/2009 as the te of posting.

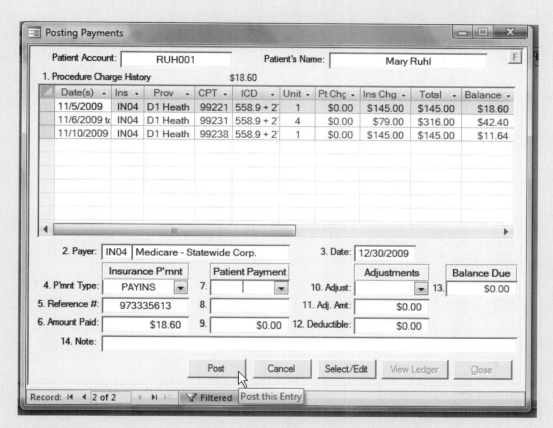

FIGURE 10-31

Delmar/Cengage Learning

Case Study 10-G Continues >>

STEP 5

In the top section, select the *line entry* for procedure 99231 on 11/06/2009 by clicking on it. Then, click on the *Select/Edit button*. This displays a balance of $42.40 in Field 13.

STEP 6

Post the payment of $42.40 as previously learned. Use the ICN number for patient Ruhl as the reference for Field 5. Check your work with Figure 10-32 before clicking on the *Post button*.

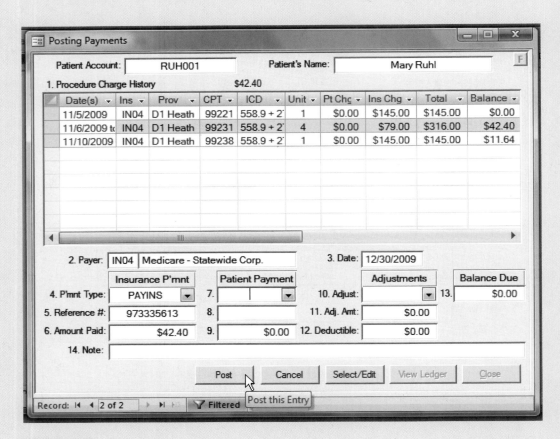

FIGURE 10-32

Delmar/Cengage Learning

STEP 7

In the top section, select the *line entry* for procedure 99238 on 11/10/2009 by clicking on it. Then, click on the *Select/Edit button*. This displays a balance of $11.64 in Field 13.

HINT: Use 12/30/2009 as the date of posting.

STEP 8

Post the payment of $11.64 as previously learned. Use the ICN number for patient Ruhl as the reference for Field 5. Check your work with Figure 10-33 before clicking on the *Post button*.

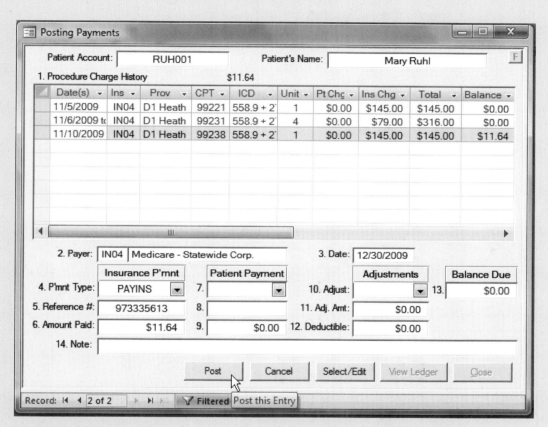

FIGURE 10-33

Delmar/Cengage Learning

Case Study 10-G Continues >>

Case Study 10-G Continued

STEP 9

When finished, compare the Patient Ledger to Figure 10-34.

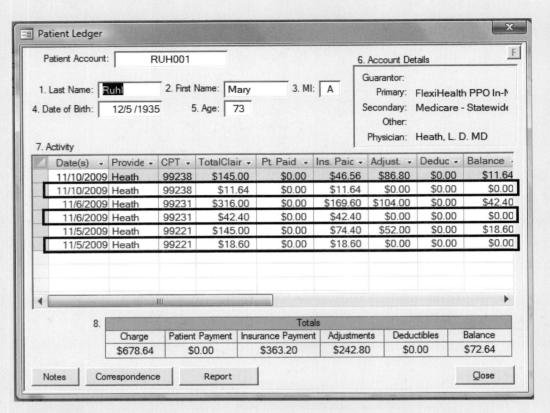

FIGURE 10-34

Delmar/Cengage Learning

STEP 10

Close all open windows and return to the Main Menu in MOSS.

LET'S TRY IT! 10-4 POSTING PAYMENTS FROM AN ELECTRONIC PAYMENT ADVICE FOR SIGNAL HMO PATIENTS

Objective: The reader posts payments received as shown on an electronic payment advice for patients with the Signal HMO health plan. The payment was electronically transferred to the bank account; however, each payment as it pertains to the individual account is applied.

PRINTING AN ELECTRONIC PAYMENT ADVICE

STEP 1

Start MOSS.

STEP 2

Click on the *Claims Tracking button* on the Main Menu, and then select Signal HMO from the list of insurance plans. See Figure 10-35.

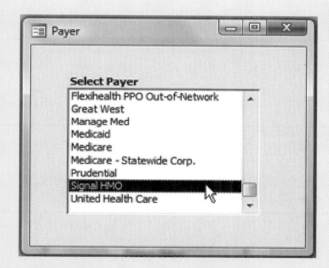

FIGURE 10-35

Delmar/Cengage Learning

continues

POSTING PAYMENTS FROM AN ELECTRONIC PAYMENT ADVICE FOR SIGNAL HMO PATIENTS *continued*

STEP 3

Enter the start date of 10/01/2009 and end date of 11/30/2009; click on *OK* after each entry. When finished, the Provider Payment Advice for Signal HMO will display (an example of the first page is shown in Figure 10-36).

PROVIDER PAYMENT ADVICE
Signal HMO
Student1

Patient Name   **KIMBERLY BEALS   (BEA001)**

Claim ID	DOS	Procedure	Charges	Allowed Amount	Patient Responsibility	Rejected Amount	Paid to Provider	Remarks
1000355	11/3/2009	36415	$18.00	$15.93	$0.00	$0.00	$15.93	A
1000354	11/3/2009	80053	$47.00	$41.60	$0.00	$0.00	$41.60	A
1000353	11/3/2009	99204	$283.00	$250.46	$10.00	$0.00	$240.46	A
Patient Totals			$348.00	$307.98	$10.00	$0.00	$297.98	

Patient Name   **David James   (JAM001)**

Claim ID	DOS	Procedure	Charges	Allowed Amount	Patient Responsibility	Rejected Amount	Paid to Provider	Remarks
1000361	11/9/2009	99213	$111.00	$98.24	$10.00	$0.00	$88.24	A
1000362	11/9/2009	86308	$17.00	$15.05	$0.00	$0.00	$15.05	A
Patient Totals			$128.00	$113.28	$10.00	$0.00	$103.28	

Patient Name   **MARTIN MONTNER   (MON001)**

Claim ID	DOS	Procedure	Charges	Allowed Amount	Patient Responsibility	Rejected Amount	Paid to Provider	Remarks
1000334	10/22/2009	87081	$16.00	$14.16	$0.00	$0.00	$14.16	A
1000333	10/22/2009	99204	$283.00	$250.46	$10.00	$0.00	$240.46	A
Patient Totals			$299.00	$264.62	$10.00	$0.00	$254.62	

FIGURE 10-36

Delmar/Cengage Learning

STEP 4

Print the Payment Advice by clicking on the *Print icon* on the top left of the screen, or see Source Document 10-4 in the Source Document Appendix. Review the information regarding charges, allowed amounts, patient responsibility, and amounts paid to the provider. Because the plan is an HMO, the patient is not responsible for any amount other than the co-payment or amounts that were rejected. For each patient listed below, calculate in the spaces below what the adjustment will be for each service provided.

BEALS

Code:	Charges:	Ins Paid:	Pt Paid:	Adjustment

JAMES

Code:	Charges:	Ins Paid:	Pt Paid:	Adjustment

MONTNER

Code:	Charges:	Ins Paid:	Pt Paid:	Adjustment

SHINN

Code:	Charges:	Ins Paid:	Pt Paid:	Adjustment

SYKES

Code:	Charges:	Ins Paid:	Pt Paid:	Adjustment

VILLANOVA

Code:	Charges:	Ins Paid:	Pt Paid:	Adjustment

Now, check your work before entering data into MOSS to be sure you have correctly interpreted the source documents.

continues

POSTING PAYMENTS FROM AN ELECTRONIC PAYMENT ADVICE FOR SIGNAL HMO PATIENTS *continued*

BEALS

Code:	Charges:	Ins Paid:	Pt Paid:	Adjustment
36415	$ 18.00	$ 15.93	0.00	$ 2.07
80053	$ 47.00	$ 41.60	0.00	$ 5.40
99204	$283.00	$240.46	$10.00	$32.54

JAMES

Code:	Charges:	Ins Paid:	Pt Paid:	Adjustment
99213	$111.00	$88.24	$10.00	$12.76
86308	$ 17.00	$15.05	$ 0.00	$ 1.95

MONTNER

Code:	Charges:	Ins Paid:	Pt Paid:	Adjustment
87081	$ 16.00	$ 14.16	$ 0.00	$ 1.84
99204	$283.00	$240.46	$10.00	$32.54

SHINN

Code:	Charges:	Ins Paid:	Pt Paid:	Adjustment
99213	$111.00	$ 88.24	$10.00	$12.76
85031	$ 11.00	$ 9.74	$ 0.00	$ 1.26
99214	$180.00	$149.30	$10.00	$20.70

SYKES

Code:	Charges:	Ins Paid:	Pt Paid:	Adjustment
99213	$111.00	$ 88.24	$10.00	$12.76
99214	$180.00	$149.30	$10.00	$20.70
36415	$ 18.00	$ 15.93	$ 0.00	$ 2.07
85031	$ 11.00	$ 9.74	$ 0.00	$ 1.26

VILLANOVA

Code:	Charges:	Ins Paid:	Pt Paid:	Adjustment
82947	$ 19.00	$ 16.82	$ 0.00	$ 2.18
99201	$130.00	$105.05	$10.00	$14.95

CASE STUDY 10-H: BEALS, KIMBERLY

STEP 1

Click on the *Posting Payments button* from the Main Menu and select patient Beals. As previously learned, post the payment for CPT 36415 on 11/03/2009. Use 11/30/2009 as the posting date, and the Claim ID in Field 5 as the reference number. Check your work with Figure 10-37 before clicking on the *Post button*.

NT: Claim ID numbers may fer on the reports. Use the e displayed on the report oduced by your software.

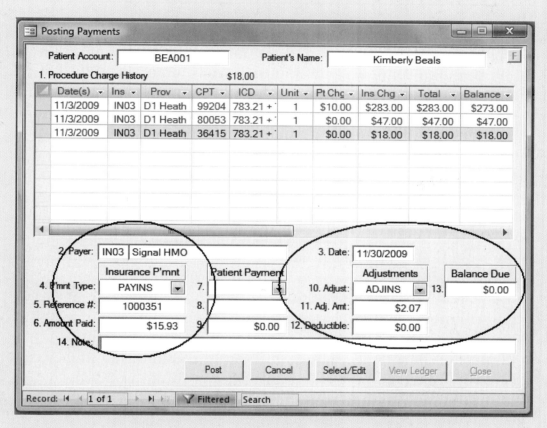

FIGURE 10-37

Delmar/Cengage Learning

Case Study 10-H Continues >>

STEP 2

Post the remaining two payments for procedures 80053 and 99204. Check your work with Figures 10-38 and 10-39 before clicking on the *Post button* for each payment.

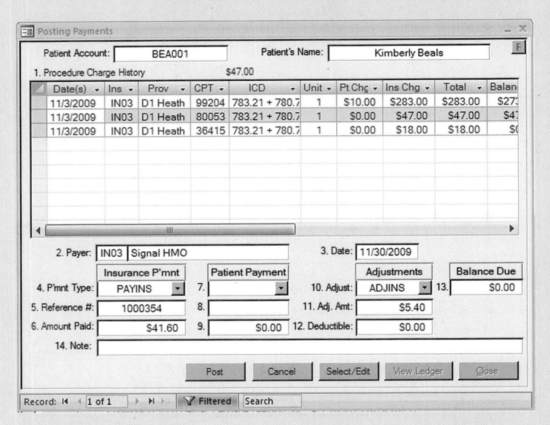

FIGURE 10-38

Delmar/Cengage Learning

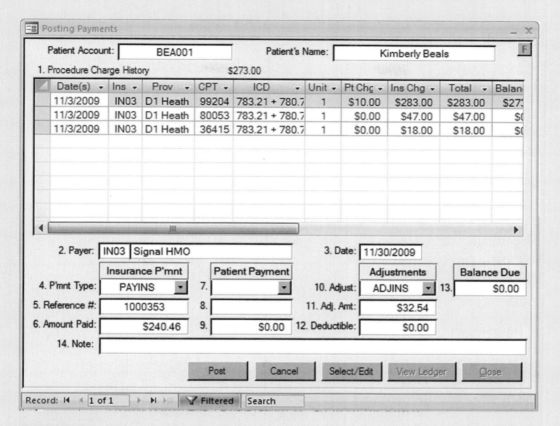

FIGURE 10-39

Delmar/Cengage Learning

STEP 3

View the Patient Ledger for patient Beals to check your work.

CASE STUDY 10-I: JAMES, DAVID

STEP 1

Select patient David James from the Posting Payment patient list.

STEP 2

As previously learned, post the payment as listed on the electronic Payment Advice for CPT 99213 on 11/09/2009. Use 11/30/2009 as the posting date, and the Claim ID in Field 5 as the reference number. Check your work with Figure 10-40 before clicking on the *Post button*.

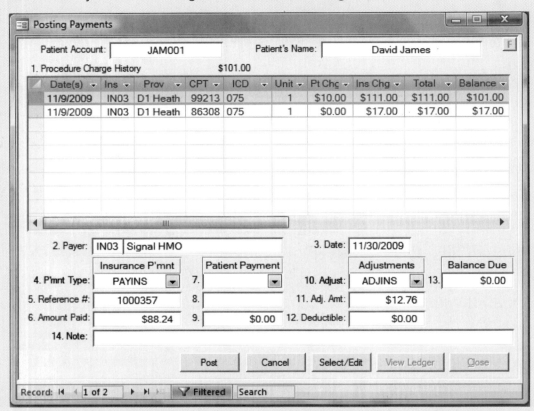

FIGURE 10-40

Delmar/Cengage Learning

STEP 3

Post the remaining payment for procedure 86308. Check your work with Figure 10-41 before clicking on the *Post button* for each payment.

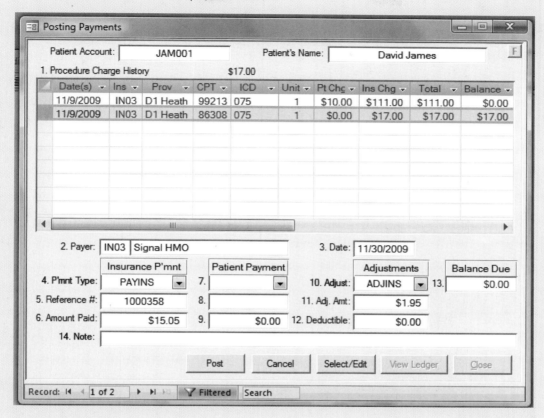

FIGURE 10-41

Delmar/Cengage Learning

Case Study 10-I Continues >>

STEP 4

View the Patient Ledger for patient James and check your work with Figure 10-42.

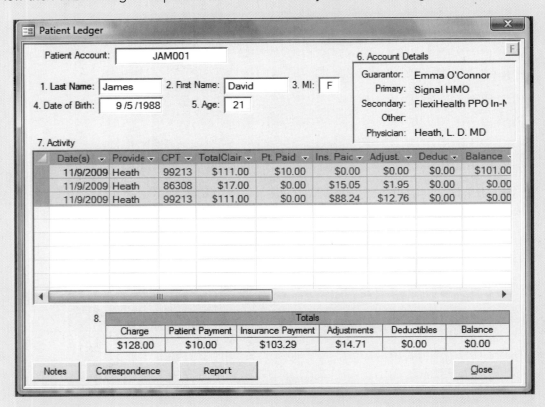

FIGURE 10-42

Delmar/Cengage Learning

STEP 5

Close all open windows and return to the Patient Selection screen for Posting Payments.

CASE STUDY 10-J: MONTNER, MARTIN

STEP 1

Select patient Martin Montner from the Posting Payments patient list.

STEP 2

As previously learned, post the payment as listed on the electronic Payment Advice for CPT 87081 on 10/22/2009. Use 11/30/2009 as the posting date, and the Claim ID in Field 5 as the reference number. Check your work with Figure 10-43 before clicking on the *Post button*.

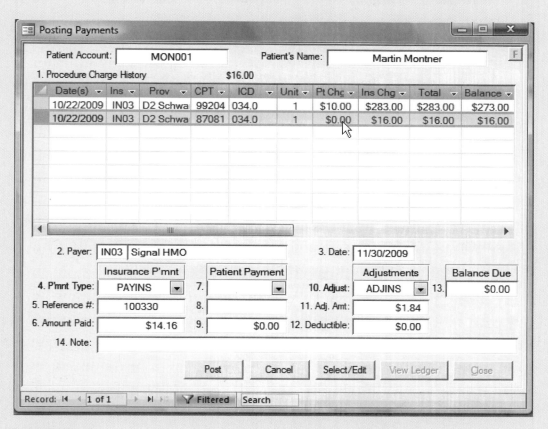

FIGURE 10-43

Delmar/Cengage Learning

Case Study 10-J Continues >>

STEP 3

Post the remaining payment for procedure 99204. Check your work with Figure 10-44 before clicking on the *Post button* for each payment.

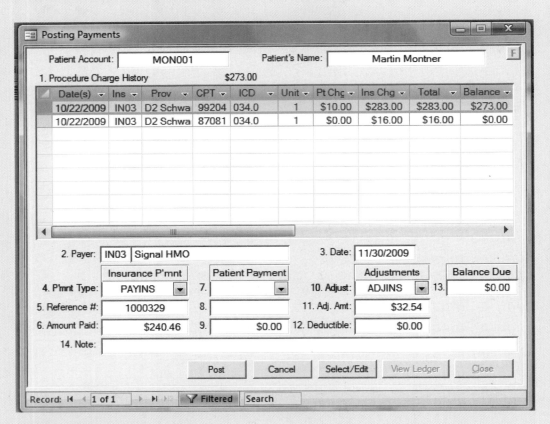

FIGURE 10-44

Delmar/Cengage Learning

STEP 4

View the Patient Ledger for patient Montner and check your work with Figure 10-45.

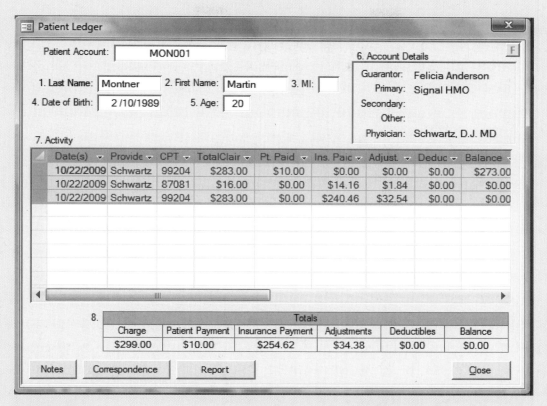

FIGURE 10-45

Delmar/Cengage Learning

STEP 5

Close all open windows and return to the Patient Selection screen for Posting Payments.

CASE STUDY 10-K: SHINN, ROBERT

STEP 1

Select patient Robert Shinn from the Posting Payments patient list.

STEP 2

As previously learned, post the payment as listed on the electronic Payment Advice for CPT 99213 on 10/30/2009. Use 11/30/2009 as the posting date, and the Claim ID in Field 5 as the reference number. Check your work with Figure 10-46 before clicking on the *Post button*.

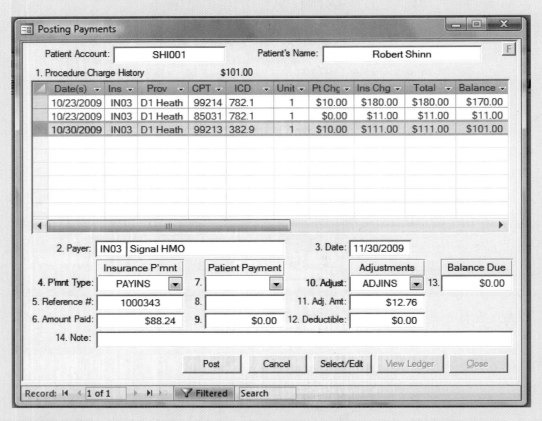

FIGURE 10-46

Delmar/Cengage Learning

STEP 3

Post the remaining payments for procedures 85031 and 99214. Check your work with Figures 10-47 and 10-48 before clicking on the *Post button* for each payment.

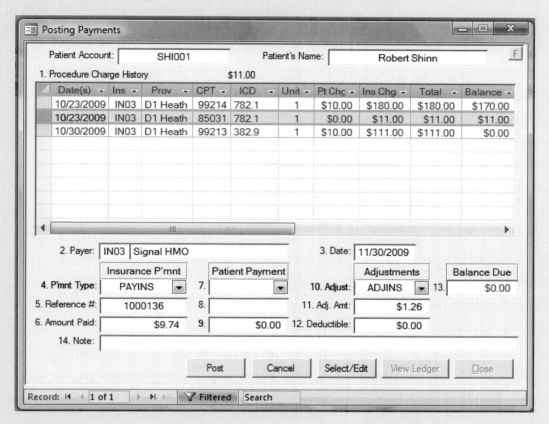

FIGURE 10-47

Delmar/Cengage Learning

Case Study 10-K Continues >>

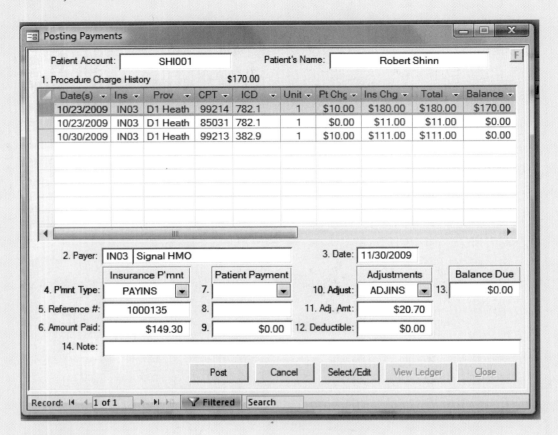

FIGURE 10-48

Delmar/Cengage Learning

STEP 4

View the Patient Ledger for patient Shinn and check your work with Figure 10-49.

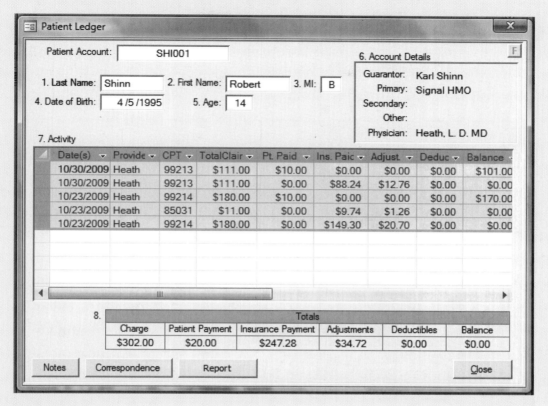

FIGURE 10-49

Delmar/Cengage Learning

STEP 5

Close all open windows and return to the Patient Selection screen for Posting Payments.

CASE STUDY 10-L: SYKES, EUGENE

STEP 1

Select patient Eugene Sykes from the Posting Payments patient list.

STEP 2

As previously learned, post the payment as listed on the electronic Payment Advice for CPT 99213 on 10/16/2009. Use 11/30/2009 as the posting date, and the Claim ID in Field 5 as the reference number. Check your work with Figure 10-50 before clicking on the *Post button*.

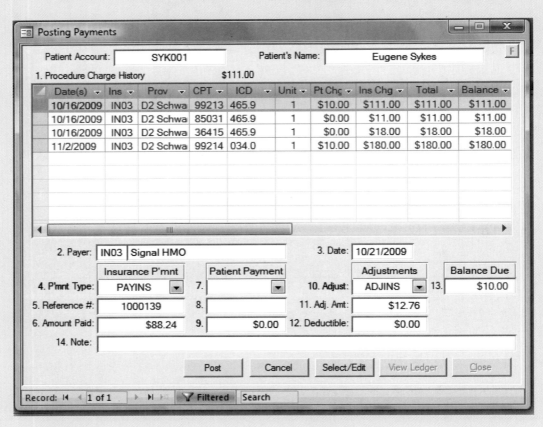

FIGURE 10-50

Delmar/Cengage Learning

STEP 3

Post the remaining payments for procedures 99214, 36415, and 85031. Check your work with Figure 10-51 to Figure 10-53 before clicking on the *Post button* for each payment.

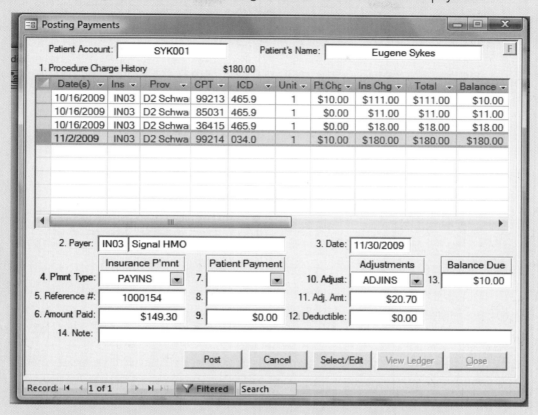

FIGURE 10-51

Delmar/Cengage Learning

Case Study 10-L Continues >>

Case Study 10-L Continued

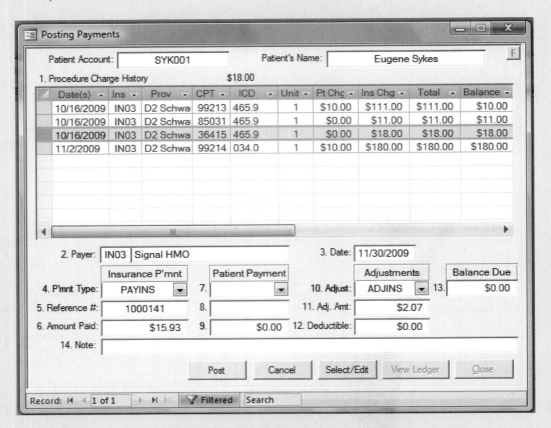

FIGURE 10-52

Delmar/Cengage Learning

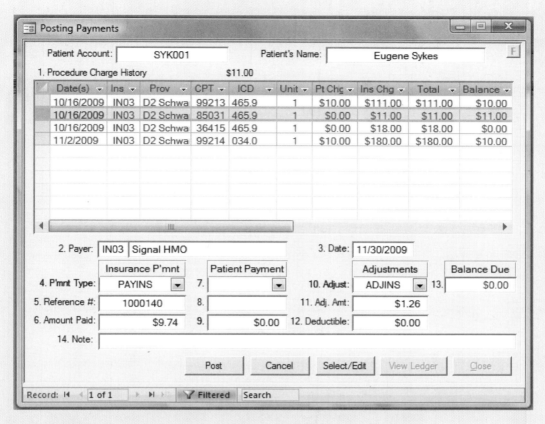

FIGURE 10-53

Delmar/Cengage Learning

Case Study 10-L Continues >>

STEP 4

View the Patient Ledger for Patient Sykes and check your work with Figure 10-54.

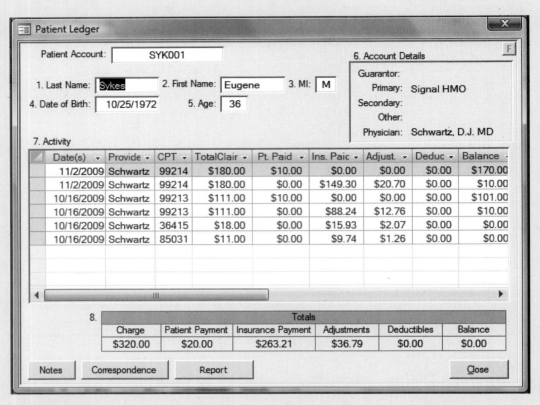

FIGURE 10-54

Delmar/Cengage Learning

STEP 5

Close all open windows and return to the Patient Selection screen for Posting Payments.

CASE STUDY 10-M: VILLANOVA, RICKY

STEP 1

Select patient Ricky Villanova from the Posting Payments patient list.

STEP 2

As previously learned, post the payment as listed on the electronic Payment Advice for CPT 82947 on 10/27/2009. Use 11/30/2009 as the posting date, and the Claim ID in Field 5 as the reference number. Check your work with Figure 10-55 before clicking on the *Post button*.

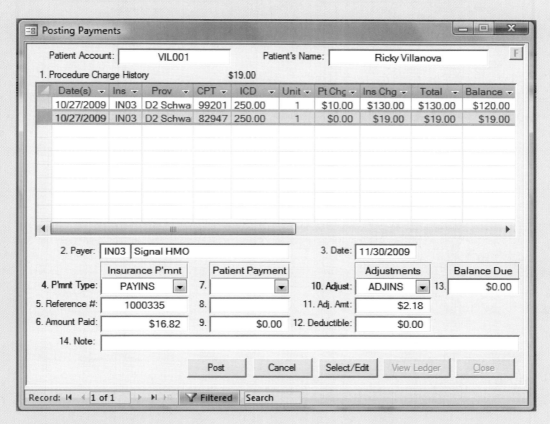

FIGURE 10-55

Delmar/Cengage Learning

Case Study 10-M Continues >>

STEP 3

Post the remaining payment for procedure 99201. Check your work with Figure 10-56 before clicking on the *Post button* for each payment.

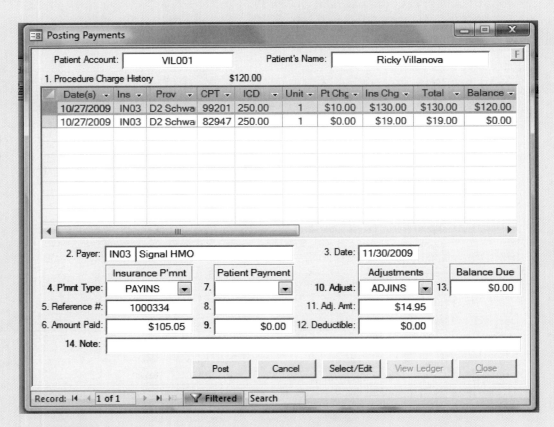

FIGURE 10-56

Delmar/Cengage Learning

STEP 4

View the Patient Ledger for Patient Villanova and check your work with Figure 10-57.

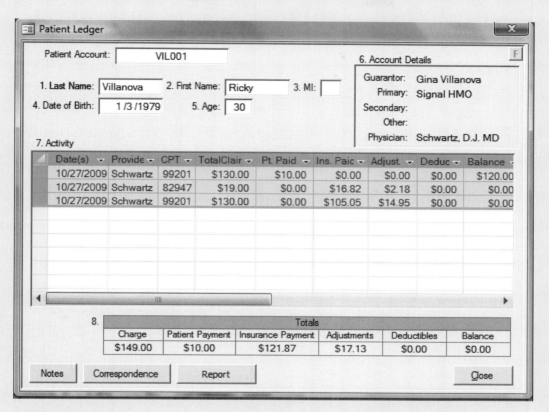

FIGURE 10-57

Delmar/Cengage Learning

STEP 5

Close all open windows and return to the Main Menu of MOSS.

FINAL NOTES

Once you have learned how to post payments by reading EOBs or RAs from primary insurance companies, and also to apply payments from patients to their accounts, the task of posting payments from other sources is familiar. Posting payments from secondary insurance plans is very similar to any other payment posted to the patient account. Reading the EOB or RA requires some initial analysis, but once the Patient Ledger and transactions are reviewed, it is relatively simple to pick out the balances, or even to identify problems with claims that will need further attention or follow-up. In the last unit of this book, you will learn how to identify problem claims, and then to follow up and track these claims to ensure the best possible, fair, and complete payments.

1. When posting payments from secondary insurance payers, explain why comparing the primary insurance EOB or RA and/or the patient ledger to the secondary EOB/RA is useful.

   _____

   _____

   _____

2. When posting a payment in MOSS from secondary insurance payers, it is important to identify and change the payer name in the posting screen. Explain your answer.

   a. True

   b. False

3. When all primary and secondary insurance payments, including adjustments, and patient payments have been posted to a patient account, the patient's balance due should be _____ for those services.

Insurance Claims Follow-up and Dispute Resolution

OBJECTIVES

Upon completion of this unit, the reader should be able to:

- **Discuss tracking of unpaid insurance claims and follow-up action required**

- **Identify types of problem insurance claims**

- **Explain the appeals process for unpaid or disputed Medicare claims and insurance claims in general**

- **Demonstrate the writing of an appeals letter to an insurance plan to dispute a reimbursement issue**

KEY TERMS

Appeal

Claims review

Denial

Lost claim

Pending claim

Suspended claim

One of the last components of the reimbursement process includes the tracking and follow-up of unpaid or problem claims from insurance companies. This is a form of collections, except in this case the insurance company, not an individual patient, has delayed or denied payment. Such claims need to be reviewed by the medical staff responsible for this task. Any necessary action needs to be taken swiftly, because time limits are often in effect. Whether the action involves rebilling the claim, providing documentation or reports, or disputing a payment decision by submitting a request for a formal review or appeal, such claims need to be pursued without delay.

It is important to remember that patients with dual insurance may have a longer time frame for waiting until a balance is completely paid. This is because the primary insurance must be billed and then must pay first before a secondary claim can be initiated. The secondary claim must be accompanied by a copy of the EOB or RA from the primary insurance. As discussed in an earlier unit, the only exception to this is when claims are automatically crossed over by the primary insurance. Accordingly, patients with dual insurance will have a longer wait time between payments, and should be carefully monitored before claims follow-up is initiated.

TRACKING AND FOLLOW-UP OF OUTSTANDING INSURANCE CLAIMS

The tracking and follow-up of insurance claims that have not been paid, or are outstanding, is one of the responsibilities of the administrative medical staff. If a payment amount is disputed, or if there is a disagreement regarding a payment denial, prompt and appropriate action must be taken to resolve the issue. Most insurance companies have limited time frames in which claim reviews or appeals must be initiated, before they are no longer allowed. Some are as short as 60 days, others a full year or more. Carefully tracking these problem claims is important so that opportunities to recover money are not lost.

Medical practice management software provides the capability to generate reports that assist in aging outstanding claims. These reports provide the first step in pinpointing potential problem claims that have not yet been paid. Some of these may just require rebilling; others will require more in-depth action.

As mentioned in Unit 8, paying careful attention to notes and messages from insurance carriers, provided on the EOBs and RAs, alerts the staff to claims that have been denied, or are suspended for further information or documentation. In addition, the reason for nonpayment, or even partial payment, is usually provided on the EOB. If these claims require more research and possible follow-up action or dispute, the time to separate them and take action is at the time the notice is received. In busy medical offices, handling EOBs containing problem claims that are allowed to go for several days or weeks before being addressed becomes an overwhelming task. Often, deadlines are missed and the money due is never challenged or recovered.

TYPES OF PROBLEM CLAIMS

There are different types of problem claims that the administrative staff needs to handle. Some of the more common types are listed here.

1. **Denials.** Also referred to as denied claims, **denials** are those claims that have not been paid, and a reason has been given. In fact, the law requires that insurance companies disclose to the policyholder why a claim has been denied. If the claim originated from the provider's office, it is customary for the provider to be notified as well, usually on the EOB. The reasons claims are denied can be numerous. These may include insurance guidelines were not being followed, or the services were incorrectly billed, or the services are excluded by the plan. Preauthorization may have been required and not obtained prior to the service being rendered. Some services are considered to be included, or "bundled," with other services, and are therefore denied for payment when billed separately. Each denial must be carefully studied and, if possible, corrections and resubmissions made so that payment can be received.

2. **Errors.** Some claims are denied because the medical office omitted or incorrectly submitted information on the claim. Errors made by the office are the main cause of denials, more than any other reason. Examples of such errors include incorrect policy numbers, not providing the insured's name and information, transposition of numbers, not confirming which insurance is the primary payer, incorrect dates of service, missing or invalid provider numbers, CPT and ICD coding errors, duplication of charges that have already been submitted, and missing referral information. Again, care and diligence on the part of the administrative staff can avoid the majority of these types of errors before claims are even processed. The best solution to reducing denied claims is to make certain that the billing procedures being followed are actually producing "clean" claims.

3. **Suspended or pending claims.** Suspended or pending claims are usually being reviewed. A claim in suspension might simply require more information from the provider, and until it is received, the claim is pending payment. In other instances, the claim may need to be reviewed by medical professionals who represent the insurance company. These reviews may be done to confirm medical necessity, investigate complicated claims, or for other reasons. After the additional information is received, or the claim is reviewed, a decision regarding whether it will be paid, denied, or the reimbursement reduced, will follow.

4. **Payments made to patients by the insurance company.** This does not happen as much as it used to in the days when indemnity plans were the most common type of coverage. However, on occasion, the reimbursement check for services may be sent directly to the patient instead of to the provider. This may be due to an error made by the insurance carrier, or because assignment of benefits was not properly signed and disclosed on the claim, showing that payment was to be made to the provider. In either case, when the patient has been paid in full, or even received a partial payment for services billed to the insurance company, it becomes a collections issue for the medical office. There are times that the medical office is not notified that payment has been made to the patient. By contacting the insurance company directly, it can be confirmed that the patient has received payment. The patient will then need to be notified and billed for the amount due. Further collections action, or even legal steps, may need to be taken if the patient refuses to pay the provider.

5. **Lost claims.** Lost claims are claims that the insurance company has no record of having received. Practice management software and clearinghouses have reduced the incidence of lost claims a great deal, especially by providing editing features and producing reports of claims that have been electronically transmitted. Paper claims are more likely to be lost, or insurance carriers can become backlogged. If a claim appears to be lost, usually after 30 to 45 days of inactivity without payment or notice of any kind, it is a good idea to trace the claim with the insurance company. This can be done either with a letter or by placing a phone call to the insurance company. If there is no record of the claim, it is appropriate to rebill it. Some offices provide the insurance company with a copy of the original claim and a letter stating the date of the original billing. However, if the original claim and the rebilled claim cross each other, expect one of the claims to be denied as a duplicate claim.

DISPUTING PAYMENT DECISIONS

If the administrative medical staff encounters claims that have been denied payment, or for which the payment has been reduced, the reasons surrounding these denials must be isolated and addressed. Otherwise, the same denial will happen repeatedly on the same type of claims in the future. This creates a vicious cycle of nonpayment that never gets corrected, which wastes valuable time and resources, not only for the provider and the office, but also for the patient.

All problem claims that stem from errors made by the medical office, or from misinterpretations of the health plan guidelines, require changes in procedure. The office manager and/or physician should be apprised of the problem, and an effort should be made by all responsible parties to take corrective action. Only when proper procedures are being followed as required by each health plan will the medical office be able to dispute problem claims and be successful with their resolution.

Once all internal problems with office procedures and billing protocols have been identified and corrected, claims that continue to be inadequately paid or denied should be pursued with the insurance company. This is done in the form of a request for review, or an appeal.

CLAIMS REVIEW AND APPEALS

Each health plan has its own process for disputing payment decisions. Almost all have time limits in which a review or appeal of a claim can be requested. Prompt action is essential. A **claims review**, or **appeal**, is a request for the claim to be reconsidered (reviewed) for payment, and to have the original decision appealed, or reversed. Some insurance companies separate these so that a request for review is first, and then the appeals process is the next step, if resolution is not reached.

How does one know what action to take when a claim is disputed? Each health plan supplies a provider manual, either in hard copy or available online, to the physicians or facilities that participate in their plan or have a contract with them. The manual outlines the plan details, billing requirements, and claims review process. The EOB often provides instructions for having a claim reviewed if the provider disagrees with the payment decision. It is not necessary to be a plan participant to request a claim review; however, the request needs to be made in writing.

For all written review requests, insurance companies require that the letter explain the reasons the payment decision is being disputed. Some insurance companies have special forms that need to be filled out and submitted. Providing a copy of the EOB, including supporting documentation or even references to the same or similar cases that have been paid in the past by the same insurance company, helps support the dispute. Figure 11-1 illustrates a generic form letter that can be used as a guide for composing letters to insurance companies requesting an appeal.

There is no guarantee that the request for review or appeal will be successful. However, if the reasons are valid, it is certainly worth the effort to pursue payment discrepancies. The most common reasons for requesting a claims review or appeal are denials that are not properly explained, and excessive reduction of the payment with improper or incorrect qualification by the insurance company. Complicated procedures that have been underpaid, despite unusual circumstances, special skills, or extended time involvement, should also be challenged.

The process may take much time, often months of waiting for a decision, and possibly periodic resubmission to the next level. However, the benefits often outweigh simply writing off the balance. Because of potential stall tactics, and the alleged practice of unwarranted claim denials by third-party payers, it would be a miserable loss of revenue for the billing staff not to pursue legitimate inquiries. It also gives the provider leverage for future claims if the appeal is won.

THE MEDICARE APPEALS PROCESS

A significant increase in audit activity by contractors for the Centers for Medicare & Medicaid Services (CMS) began in 2010 and is expected to continue. There is an overall intent to identify and recover payment errors. This increased activity has come about because of the transition of the hospital review function from CMS-contracted quality improvement organizations to CMS-contracted fiscal intermediaries (FI), as well as Medicare administrative contractors and other Medicare claims processors. CMS will soon introduce the permanent Medicare Recovery Audit Contractor (RAC) program.

The RAC program will focus on returning dollars to the Medicare trust funds from improper payments, and identifying underpayments that need to be repaid to providers. It has provided CMS with ways for detecting improper payments made in the past, and new tools for preventing future such payments. By 2010, CMS plans to have four RACs in place.

Douglasville Medicine Associates
5076 Brand Blvd., Suite 401
Douglasville, NY 01234
Ph: (123) 456-7890
Fax: (123) 456-7891
Email: admin@dfma.com
Website: www.dfma.com

December 10, 20XX

Insurance Carrier
Address
City, State, ZIP

ATTENTION: CLAIM APPEALS

Patient:
Insured:
ID number:
Group number:
Provider:
Claim Number:

To whom it may concern:

In reference to the above captioned claim, our office disagrees with the decision made regarding payment on this claim. Our records indicate that (followed by an explanation of the claim, and why there is a disagreement).

We have attached copies of the (procedure note, operative report, medical record, consultation, etc.), that supports the services billed on this claim. Therefore, we request that this claim be reviewed and expect prompt payment (or additional payment).

If you require further information, do not hesitate contacting me. Thank you in advance for your attention to this matter.

Sincerely,

Your Name
Your Title

FIGURE 11-1

A sample letter of appeal for use when disputing a payment made by an insurance carrier. *Delmar/Cengage Learning*

These changes will surely bring about an increase in audit activity that will most likely trigger increased denials of Medicare claims. This may result in Medicare providers having to make decisions about whether to go through the appeals process for these Medicare payment denials.

Medicare has very specific steps to follow for the appeals process. If a beneficiary or the Medicare provider is dissatisfied with the carrier's decision on a Part B claim, the law allows steps to be followed in order to appeal coverage or payment amount issues.

CMS implemented changes to the Medicare appeals process in 2005. The first level in the appeals process is called redetermination. A provider must submit a redetermination request in writing within 120 calendar days of receiving notice of initial determination (as shown on the Medicare RA—standard paper or electronic version). There is no minimum amount for which a request can be made at this level. A sample of form CMS 20027 used for this first step is shown in Figure 11-2.

DEPARTMENT OF HEALTH AND HUMAN SERVICES
CENTERS FOR MEDICARE & MEDICAID SERVICES

MEDICARE REDETERMINATION REQUEST FORM

1. Beneficiary's Name: ______________________________

2. Medicare Number: ______________________________

3. Description of Item or Service in Question: ______________________________

4. Date the Service or Item was Received: ______________________________

5. I do not agree with the determination of my claim. MY REASONS ARE:

____

____

____

6. Date of the initial determination notice ______________________________

(If you received your initial determination notice more than 120 days ago, include your reason for not making this request earlier.)

____

____

____

7. Additional Information Medicare Should Consider: ______________________________

____

____

____

8. Requester's Name: ______________________________

9. Requester's Relationship to the Beneficiary: ______________________________

10. Requester's Address: ______________________________

____

11. Requester's Telephone Number: ______________________________

12. Requester's Signature: ______________________________

13. Date Signed: ______________________________

14. ❑ I have evidence to submit. (Attach such evidence to this form.)
❑ I do not have evidence to submit.

NOTICE: Anyone who misrepresents or falsifies essential information requested by this form may upon conviction be subject to fine or imprisonment under Federal Law.

Form CMS-20027 (05/05) EF 05/2005

FIGURE 11-2

Medicare Redetermination Request Form. *Courtesy of the Centers for Medicare & Medicaid Services*

DEPARTMENT OF HEALTH AND HUMAN SERVICES
CENTERS FOR MEDICARE & MEDICAID SERVICES

MEDICARE RECONSIDERATION REQUEST FORM

1. Beneficiary's Name: _____

2. Medicare Number: _____

3. Description of Item or Service in Question: _____

4. Date the Service or Item was Received: _____

5. I do not agree with the determination of my claim. MY REASONS ARE:

   _____

   _____

   _____

6. Date of the redetermination notice _____
   (If you received your redetermination more than 180 days ago, include your reason for not making this request earlier.)

   _____

   _____

   _____

7. Additional Information Medicare Should Consider: _____

   _____

   _____

   _____

8. Requester's Name: _____

9. Requester's Relationship to the Beneficiary: _____

10. Requester's Address: _____

    _____

11. Requester's Telephone Number: _____

12. Requester's Signature: _____

13. Date Signed: _____

14. ❑ I have evidence to submit. (Attach such evidence to this form.)
    ❑ I do not have evidence to submit.

15. Name of the Medicare Contractor that Made the Redetermination: _____

NOTICE: Anyone who misrepresents or falsifies essential information requested by this form may upon conviction be subject to fine or imprisonment under Federal Law.

Form CMS-20033 (05/05) EF (05/2005)

FIGURE 11-3

Medicare Reconsideration Request Form. *Courtesy of the Centers for Medicare & Medicaid Services*

The second step in the appeals process is called reconsideration. A provider dissatisfied with a carrier's redetermination decision may file a request for reconsideration, to be conducted by a qualified independent carrier (QIC). The request must be filed within 180 calendar days of the date that the notice of an unfavorable redetermination was received. There is no minimum amount required to go to this step. When conducting its review, the QIC considers evidence and findings upon which the initial determination and redetermination were based, plus any additional evidence submitted by the parties, or that the QIC obtains on its own. If an initial determination involved a decision regarding the medical necessity of an item or service, the QIC's reconsideration must involve a panel of physicians or appropriate health care professionals, and must be based on clinical experience, the patient's medical records, and medical, technical, and scientific evidence on record. Where the claim involves physician services, the reviewing professional must be a physician; however, the physician reviewer need not be in the same specialty as the physician whose claims have been denied. A sample of form CMS 20033 used for this second step is shown in Figure 11-3. This step is the last opportunity that the provider will have to submit new evidence supporting the request for reconsideration.

The third step of the appeals process is the Administrative Law Judge (ALJ) hearing. To request an ALJ hearing, follow the instructions in the reconsideration letter received from the QIC. A provider who wants escalation to this next level must file the request within 60 days following receipt of the unfavorable QIC decision, and the provider must be seeking a minimum amount of $120.00 (as of 2009). ALJ hearings may be conducted by video-teleconference, if it is available; if not, the ALJ may conduct an in-person or a telephone hearing.

The ALJ must issue a decision within 90 calendar days of receipt of the request for a hearing and explain any unfavorable decisions. However, Medicare regulations have an array of authorized circumstances under which this deadline can be extended if necessary.

The fourth step of the appeals process is the Medicare Appeals Council (MAC). In order to file a request for a MAC review, refer to the ALJ instructions. A MAC review request must be filed within 60 days following receipt of the ALJ's decisions. The MAC currently operates under regulations issued by both the Department of Health and Human Services (HHS) and the Social Security Administration (SSA). If the council does not issue a decision on a provider-initiated review within 90 days, the provider may request escalation to the next step, which is filing with the federal district court.

Visit the following Web site which contains actual case studies of decisions made by MAC:

http://www.hhs.gov/dab/macdecision/

ASSERTIVE COLLECTIONS TACTICS FOR PRIVATE THIRD-PARTY PAYERS

Occasionally, despite the best efforts of the billing staff with tracking and following up claims, and with handling requests for review and appeal, some cases require more assertive action. Private third-party payers who appear abusive in their reimbursement practices and consistently reduce or deny payments without giving proper explanation, or who are simply unfair, may require other alternative ways to be approached. There are some specific actions that can be taken to pursue proper payment from insurance payers.

1. **Contact the payer directly.** If letters and forms are not producing results, calling the insurance carrier directly is the next option. It is important to always document the full name, phone number, and extension of each individual spoken to, including their title. Initially, a representative handles telephone inquiries. If any statements are made regarding the reason for denials or

reduced payments, request that these be made in writing and sent to the medical office. Complete notes should be taken regarding the details of each conversation, so that the information can be referred to during subsequent follow-up calls you may need to place.

If the information or results are not satisfactory, request to speak to the manager or supervisor, or, if necessary, take your issue to the next level: the president or chief executive officer (CEO). It should be clear to the payer that you will make a hard effort to find resolution.

2. **Soliciting help from the insured.** Sometimes, involving the insured (or patient) with matters related to reimbursement can be effective. The insured can directly contact the insurance company, either in writing or by telephone, and make an inquiry regarding reimbursement issues.

In cases where there is good reason to pursue an issue with the state insurance commissioner, a letter can be prepared on behalf of the patient. The state insurance commissioner has several responsibilities, including monitoring insurance companies to ensure protection for the policyholders, and ensuring that their interests are properly served. The state commissioner has authority to arbitrate cases, so sending a complaint to this resource might capture the attention of the payer. However, the complaint must originate from the insured. All information related to the dispute, including the health plan information, policyholder information, statement of the complaint, and all supporting claims and documentation should be included. Because of this, the medical office can assist the patient as needed to prepare his or her complaint. Once the complaint has been reviewed by the insured, it can be signed by him or her and sent by certified mail, return receipt requested.

3. **Involving the employer benefits department.** Many employers base their decision on staying with a particular health plan based not only on cost, but also on the satisfaction of their employees with the plan. The employer pays high premiums for coverage for a group of employees. In turn, the employer is the insurance company's client. If there are consistent problems with service, reimbursement, or other issues, employees can take their complaints to their employer benefits department. Intervention from the employer with the payer may yield favorable results. At the very least, it will indicate to the employer when dissatisfaction with a health plan becomes an issue with the employees.

LET'S TRY IT! 11-1 PREPARE A LETTER OF APPEAL TO SIGNAL HMO

Objective: The reader will prepare a letter of appeal to Signal HMO for patient Patty Practice, requesting a review of services rendered on 11/3/2009 for CPT 99204.

STEP 1
Start MOSS.

STEP 2
Review the electronic Payment Advice shown in Source Document 11-1 in the Source Document Appendix. Review the services and payments for all patients, carefully comparing CPT codes and payments. Are there discrepancies? What conclusions did you arrive at after re-evaluating the payments from the insurance plan? It appears that for CPT 99204, the amount allowed was reduced on patient Practice's service date compared to what was allowed for Montner. Patient Montner was allowed $234.53 more for the same service than patient Practice was. After reviewing both patient files, there is no valid reason found why this downgrading of the allowable took place, and the reason code is the same for both services (see the Remark column on the Payment Advice).

continues

PREPARE A LETTER OF APPEAL TO SIGNAL HMO *continued*

STEP 3

Using Figure 11-1 as a guide, prepare a draft of an appeals letter to Signal HMO, requesting a redetermination of service 99204 on 11/03/2009. Include the Claim ID number, date of service, and the patient name, as shown on the Payment Advice from Signal HMO. Indicate that a copy of the office notes, and a copy of the Payment Advice showing a higher allowable on the same service with another patient, have been enclosed with the letter. Use a signature block for yourself, and your title as "Administrative Medical Assistant." Be sure to include an enclosures line that indicates two documents are included with the letter.

STEP 4

Open the Patient Ledger for patient Practice and click on the *Correspondence button*. Save the letter file on the hard drive, or where indicated by your instructor. Use your last name, the patient's last name, and the words "appeals Signal HMO," as shown in Figure 11-4, as the file name.

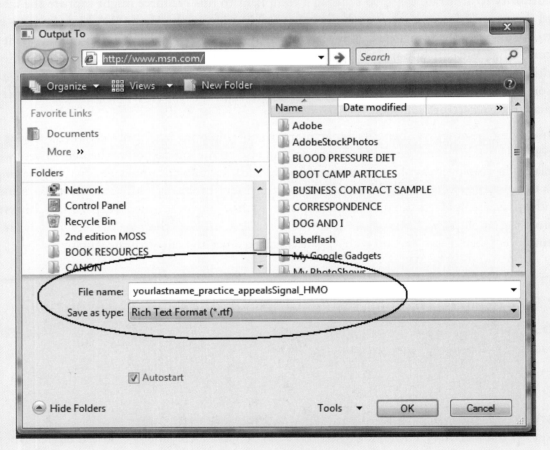

FIGURE 11-4

Delmar/Cengage Learning

STEP 5

When the practice letterhead opens, prepare the top section as shown in Figure 11-5. The address for Signal HMO was obtained from the Lists menu of insurance centers, as shown in Figure 11-6.

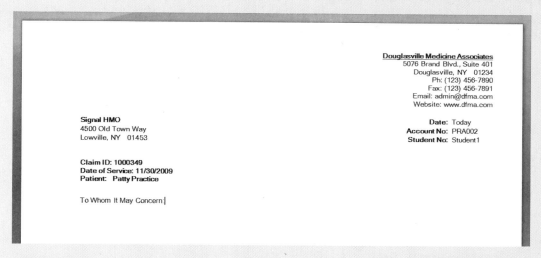

FIGURE 11-5

Delmar/Cengage Learning

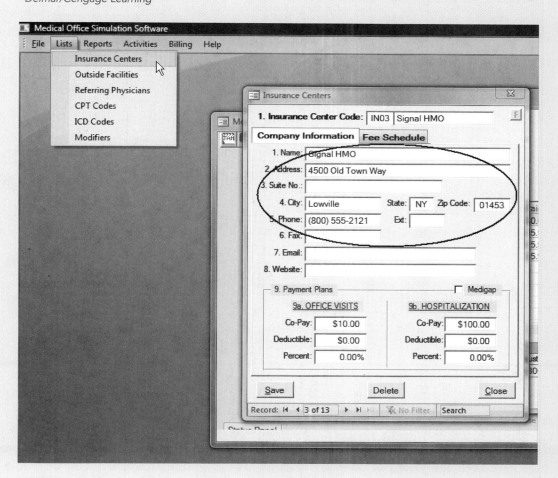

FIGURE 11-6

Delmar/Cengage Learning

continues

PREPARE A LETTER OF APPEAL TO SIGNAL HMO *continued*

STEP 6

Type the draft you prepared in Step 3 in the body of the letterhead for the practice. Compare your letter to the sample shown in Figure 11-7. Your letter might be worded somewhat differently, but the main ideas should have been communicated in a similar way.

Douglasville Medicine Associates
5076 Brand Blvd., Suite 401
Douglasville, NY 01234
Ph: (123) 456-7890
Fax: (123) 456-7891
Email: admin@dfma.com
Website: www.dfma.com

Signal HMO
4500 Old Town Way
Lowville, NY 01453

Date: Today
Account No: PRA002
Student No: Student1

Claim ID: 1000349
Date of Service: 11/3/2009
Patient: Patty Practice

To Whom It May Concern:

In reference to the above captioned claim, our office disagrees with the allowed amount for procedure 99204 on 11/3/2009. We have been allowed at a higher rate in the past, as indicated on a copy of a Payment Advice enclosed with this letter for date 10/22/2009. We have also enclosed a copy of the office notes for the services received by Patty Practice on 11/3/2009.

We request that the allowed amount be reviewed and a redetermination made so that payment can be corrected and the additional amount due sent to our office.

If you require further information, do not hesitate to contact me. Thank you in advance for your attention to this matter.

Sincerely,

Your Name
Administrative Medical Assistant

Enclosures: 2

FIGURE 11-7
Delmar/Cengage Learning

STEP 7

Click on *Save* when the letter is finished, and then print the letter for mailing, or turn it in to your instructor as directed.

STEP 8

Close all windows in MOSS and return to the Main Menu.

FINAL NOTES

Tracking and following up insurance claims are critical components of the reimbursement process. There have been allegations in the past regarding payers who intentionally delay or reduce payments, fully expecting the vast majority of medical offices will not question or pursue these claims.

Without question, it is of utmost importance that the administrative staff maintains the highest level of correct billing and coding practices. Eliminating any questionable aspect of a claim that increases its potential to become a problem claim, is a must. This begins with an excellent front-desk and billing staff at the medical office.

It is important to note that, in addition to pursuing health plans that consistently deny or reduce payments on legitimate claims, tracking payment patterns also assists in provider decisions. For instance, it is possible that participation with certain plans is of little benefit in the overall financial picture of the practice. By tracking payment patterns, time usage for pursuing payments and requesting reviews, and knowing the bottom line in dollars, your employer will be well equipped with information for making decisions regarding continuing participation with certain plans. Maintaining participation only with quality plans that have fair reimbursement practices on behalf of its policyholders fosters better patient relations and a solvent medical practice.

CHECK YOUR KNOWLEDGE

1. Explain why patients with dual insurance coverage may have a longer time frame for waiting until a balance is completely paid.

   _____

   _____

   _____

2. List and describe four common types of problem insurance claims in the medical office.

   _____

   _____

   _____

3. Discuss the importance of pursuing unpaid insurance claims promptly.

   _____

   _____

   _____

4. Explain why a suspended, or pending, claim should be researched before rebilling the claim.

   _____

   _____

   _____

5. Explain why problem claims that are caused by errors or improper billing procedures in the medical office have an effect on future claims.

   _____

   _____

   _____

6. How does the medical staff know which procedures to follow when an insurance claim needs to be disputed or reviewed for a particular insurance carrier?

_____

_____

_____

7. List and describe the steps involved in the Medicare appeals process.

_____

_____

_____

8. Describe ways a patient (or policyholder) can become involved in the process of disputing a payment decision made by his or her health plan.

_____

_____

_____

9. Describe how tracking payment patterns of insurance companies can assist the provider in making decisions regarding continuing participation with an insurance plan.

_____

_____

_____

Appendix
Source Documents

SOURCE DOCUMENT 5-1

Welcome To Our Office	NEW PATIENT INFORMATION	DATE _____

PLEASE PRINT

LAST NAME	FIRST NAME	MI	SSN		GENDER	MARITAL STATUS	DATE OF BIRTH
Montner	Martin		999-38-1672		Male	Single	2/10/89

ADDRESS	APT/UNIT	CITY	STATE	ZIP	HOME PH (123)	WORK PH ( ) EXT:
316 Slate Dr.		Douglasville	NY	01234	457-2166	

EMPLOYER/SCHOOL	EMPLOYER ADDRESS	CITY	STATE	ZIP
City Junior College	200 E. Midway Blvd.	Douglasville	NY	01234

REFERRING PHYSICIAN (LAST NAME, FIRST NAME)	ADDRESS	CITY	STATE	ZIP	PHONE

GUARANTOR – Person responsible for payment: ☐ self   ☐ spouse/other   ☒ parent   ☐ legal guardian If not "self", please complete the following:

LAST NAME	FIRST NAME	MI	SSN	GENDER	DATE OF BIRTH
Anderson	Felicia	S.	999-16-2133	Female	11/22/65

ADDRESS (IF DIFFERENT FROM PATIENT)	CITY	STATE	ZIP	HOME PH ( )	ALT. PHONE
Same					

EMPLOYER NAME	EMPLOYER ADDRESS	CITY STATE	ZIP	WORK PHONE EXT
Big Top Paper Warehouse	416 Industry Ln.	Douglasville	01235	123-555-6182

OTHER RESPONSIBLE PARTY:

LAST NAME	FIRST NAME	MI	SSN	GENDER	DATE OF BIRTH

ADDRESS (IF DIFFERENT FROM PATIENT)	CITY	STATE	ZIP	HOME PH ( )	ALT. PHONE

EMPLOYER NAME	EMPLOYER ADDRESS	CITY STATE	ZIP	WORK PHONE EXT

INSURANCE - PRIMARY

PLAN NAME	PATIENT RELATIONSHIP TO INSURED:
Signal HMO	☐ self ☐ spouse ☒ child ☐ other Full-time student

POLICYHOLDER INFORMATION

LAST NAME	FIRST NAME	MI	DATE OF BIRTH	ID#	POLICY #	GROUP #
Anderson	Felicia	S.	11/22/65	999162133-02		BTPW39

EMPLOYER NAME	PCP NAME, IF APPLICABLE:
Big Top Paper Warehouse	

INSURANCE - SECONDARY

PLAN NAME	PATIENT RELATIONSHIP TO INSURED: ☐ self ☐ spouse ☐ child ☐ other

POLICYHOLDER INFORMATION

LAST NAME	FIRST NAME	MI	DATE OF BIRTH	ID#	POLICY #	GROUP #

EMPLOYER NAME	PCP NAME, IF APPLICABLE:

ACCIDENT? ☐ YES ☐ NO IF YES, DATE OF INJURY	OCCUR AT WORK? ☐ YES ☐ NO	AUTO INVOLVED: ☐ YES ☐ NO	STATE

NAME OF ATTORNEY	PHONE NUMBER EXT.		

INSURANCE AUTHORIZATION AND ASSIGNMENT

Name of Policy Holder __Felicia Anderson_____   HIC Number _____

I request that payment of authorized Medicare/Other Insurance company benefits be made either to me or on my behalf to _____Dr. Schwartz_____
For any services furnished me by that party who accepts assignment/physician. Regulations pertaining to Medicare assignment of benefits apply.
I authorize the release of protected health information to the Social Security Administration and Centers for Medicare and Medicaid Services or its intermediaries or carriers any information needed for this or a related Medicare claim/other Insurance Company claim...(Section 11288 f the Social Security Act and if 31 U.S.C. Sections 3801-3812 provides penalties for withholding this information).

Signature _____*Felicia Anderson*_____   Date__10/21/09_____

Registration form for Martin Montner. *Used with permission. InHealth Record Systems, Inc. 5076 Winters Chapel Road, Atlanta, GA 30360, 800-477-7374.* http://www.inhealthrecords.com

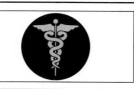

Signal HMO

PCP: Douglasville Medicine Associates
D.J. Schwartz, M.D.
(123)456-7890

Felicia S. Anderson   999162133   01
Martin Montner   Dependent   02

Copayment Schedule

PCP Office Visits $ 10.00
Specialists Visits $ 30.00
Emergency Room $ 100.00
Hospitalization   Authorization

Preauthorization 800-123-8877

Bank Code   E25/A10
361   Member Group Number: BTPW39   Type of Coverage

Insurance card for Martin Montner. *Delmar/Cengage Learning*

SOURCE DOCUMENT 5-3

Welcome To Our Office   NEW PATIENT INFORMATION   DATE _____

PLEASE PRINT

LAST NAME	FIRST NAME	MI	SSN		GENDER	MARITAL STATUS	DATE OF BIRTH
Adams	Minnie		999-57-1266		Female	Single	9/4/28

ADDRESS	APT/UNIT	CITY	STATE	ZIP	HOME PH (123)	WORK PH ( ) EXT:
1876 Slate Dr.	2B	Douglasville	NY	01234	457-3688	

EMPLOYER/SCHOOL	EMPLOYER ADDRESS	CITY	STATE	ZIP
Retired				

REFERRING PHYSICIAN (LAST NAME, FIRST NAME)	ADDRESS	CITY	STATE	ZIP	PHONE
Samantha Green	1600 Midway Ave #102	Douglasville	NY	01234	

GUARANTOR - Person responsible for payment: ☒ self   ☐ spouse/other   ☐ parent   ☐ legal guardian If not "self", please complete the following:

LAST NAME	FIRST NAME	MI	SSN		GENDER	DATE OF BIRTH

ADDRESS (IF DIFFERENT FROM PATIENT)	CITY	STATE	ZIP	HOME PH ( )	ALT. PHONE

EMPLOYER NAME	EMPLOYER ADDRESS	CITY	STATE	ZIP	WORK PHONE	EXT

OTHER RESPONSIBLE PARTY:

LAST NAME	FIRST NAME	MI	SSN		GENDER	DATE OF BIRTH	

ADDRESS (IF DIFFERENT FROM PATIENT)	CITY	STATE	ZIP	HOME PH ( )	ALT. PHONE

EMPLOYER NAME	EMPLOYER ADDRESS	CITY STATE	ZIP	WORK PHONE	EXT

INSURANCE - PRIMARY

PLAN NAME	PATIENT RELATIONSHIP TO INSURED:
Medicare	☒ self ☐ spouse ☐ child ☐ other

POLICYHOLDER INFORMATION

LAST NAME	FIRST NAME	MI	DATE OF BIRTH	ID#	POLICY #	GROUP #
Adams	Minnie		9/4/28	999571266A		

EMPLOYER NAME	PCP NAME, IF APPLICABLE:

INSURANCE - SECONDARY

PLAN NAME	PATIENT RELATIONSHIP TO INSURED: ☐ self ☐ spouse ☐ child ☐ other

POLICYHOLDER INFORMATION

LAST NAME	FIRST NAME	MI	DATE OF BIRTH	ID#	POLICY #	GROUP #

EMPLOYER NAME	PCP NAME, IF APPLICABLE:

ACCIDENT? ☐ YES ☒ NO IF YES, DATE OF INJURY	OCCUR AT WORK? ☐ YES ☒ NO	AUTO INVOLVED: ☐ YES ☒ NO	STATE
NAME OF ATTORNEY	PHONE NUMBER EXT.		

INSURANCE AUTHORIZATION AND ASSIGNMENT

Name of Policy Holder __Minnie Adams__   HIC Number _____

I request that payment of authorized Medicare/Other Insurance company benefits be made either to me or on my behalf to __Dr. Heath__
For any services furnished me by that party who accepts assignment/physician. Regulations pertaining to Medicare assignment of benefits apply.
I authorize the release of protected health information to the Social Security Administration and Centers for Medicare and Medicaid Services or its intermediaries or carriers any information needed for this or a related Medicare claim/other Insurance Company claim...(Section 11288 f the Social Security Act and if 31 U.S.C. Sections 3801-3812 provides penalties for withholding this information).

Signature __Minnie Adams__   Date __10/28/09__

MEDICARE		HEALTH INSURANCE
HEALTH CARE FINANCING ADMINISTRATION		

NAME OF BENEFICIARY
Minnie Adams

MEDICARE CLAIM NUMBER   SEX
999571266A   Female

IS ENTITLED TO

HOSPIAL   (PART A)

MEDICAL   (PART B)

SIGN ➜
HERE _____ *Minnie Adams* _____

Insurance card for Minnie Adams. *Delmar/Cengage Learning*

SOURCE DOCUMENT 5-5

Welcome To Our Office

NEW PATIENT INFORMATION DATE _____

PLEASE PRINT

LAST NAME	FIRST NAME	MI	SSN		GENDER	MARITAL STATUS	DATE OF BIRTH
Corbett	Melissa	A.	999-52-3168		Female	Single	6/16/97

ADDRESS	APT/UNIT	CITY	STATE	ZIP	HOME PH (123)	WORK PH ( ) EXT:
1230 Granite St.	4A	Douglasville	NY	01234	457-2133	

EMPLOYER/SCHOOL	EMPLOYER ADDRESS	CITY	STATE	ZIP
Clear Lake Middle School				

REFERRING PHYSICIAN (LAST NAME, FIRST NAME)	ADDRESS	CITY	STATE	ZIP	PHONE

GUARANTOR - Person responsible for payment: ☐ self ☐ spouse/other ☒ parent ☐ legal guardian _If not "self", please complete the following:_

LAST NAME	FIRST NAME	MI	SSN		GENDER	DATE OF BIRTH
Corbett	Daniel	M.	999-30-1255		Male	6/14/73

ADDRESS (IF DIFFERENT FROM PATIENT)	CITY	STATE	ZIP	HOME PH ( )	ALT. PHONE
Same					

EMPLOYER NAME	EMPLOYER ADDRESS	CITY STATE	ZIP	WORK PHONE EXT
Banterfield Hobby	9211 Midway Blvd.	Douglasville	01234	123-528-3110

OTHER RESPONSIBLE PARTY:

LAST NAME	FIRST NAME	MI	SSN	GENDER	DATE OF BIRTH	
Corbett	Janice	S.	999-30-1232	Female	3/31/73	Mother

ADDRESS (IF DIFFERENT FROM PATIENT)	CITY	STATE	ZIP	HOME PH ( )	ALT. PHONE
Same					

EMPLOYER NAME	EMPLOYER ADDRESS	CITY STATE	ZIP	WORK PHONE EXT
Homemaker				

INSURANCE - PRIMARY

PLAN NAME	PATIENT RELATIONSHIP TO INSURED:
Flexihealth PPO	☐ self ☐ spouse ☒ child ☐ other

POLICYHOLDER INFORMATION

LAST NAME	FIRST NAME	MI	DATE OF BIRTH	ID#	POLICY #	GROUP #
Corbett	Daniel	M.	6/14/73	999301255-04		BH225

EMPLOYER NAME	PCP NAME, IF APPLICABLE:
Banterfield Hobby	

INSURANCE - SECONDARY

PLAN NAME	PATIENT RELATIONSHIP TO INSURED: ☐ self ☐ spouse ☐ child ☐ other

POLICYHOLDER INFORMATION

LAST NAME	FIRST NAME	MI	DATE OF BIRTH	ID#	POLICY #	GROUP #

EMPLOYER NAME	PCP NAME, IF APPLICABLE:

ACCIDENT? ☐ YES ☒ NO IF YES, DATE OF INJURY	OCCUR AT WORK? ☐ YES ☒ NO	AUTO INVOLVED: ☐ YES ☒ NO	STATE
NAME OF ATTORNEY	PHONE NUMBER EXT.		

INSURANCE AUTHORIZATION AND ASSIGNMENT

Name of Policy Holder ____Daniel Corbett_____ HIC Number _____

I request that payment of authorized Medicare/Other Insurance company benefits be made either to me or on my behalf to ____Dr. Heath_____

For any services furnished me by that party who accepts assignment/physician. Regulations pertaining to Medicare assignment of benefits apply.

I authorize the release of protected health information to the Social Security Administration and Centers for Medicare and Medicaid Services or its intermediaries or carriers any information needed for this or a related Medicare claim/other Insurance Company claim...(Section 11288 f the Social Security Act and if 31 U.S.C. Sections 3801-3812 provides penalties for withholding this information).

Signature ____Daniel Corbett_____ Date____10/29/09_____

Registration form for Melissa Corbett. *Used with permission. InHealth Record Systems, Inc. 5076 Winters Chapel Road, Atlanta, GA 30360, 800-477-7374. http://www.inhealthrecords.com*

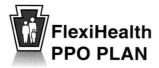

**FlexiHealth
PPO PLAN**

Insurer 81564

Your Health First SM

Insured:	Corbett, Daniel M.	999301255-01
Employer:	Banterfield Hobby	Network 45A-2
Group:	BH225	

Family Plan

Corbett, Janice S.	999301255-02
Corbett, Mira A.	999301255-03
Corbett, Melissa A.	999301255-04

Physician Co-pay: $20.00
Hospital Services: $400.00 Annual family deductible.
Surgery & Hospitalization: Requires preauthorization 800-123-3654

Insurance card for Melissa Corbett. *Delmar/Cengage Learning*

SOURCE DOCUMENT 5-7

Welcome To Our Office   NEW PATIENT INFORMATION   DATE _____

PLEASE PRINT

LAST NAME	FIRST NAME	MI	SSN		GENDER	MARITAL STATUS	DATE OF BIRTH
Zuhl	Rodney	A.	999-61-9213		Male	Single	12/21/84

ADDRESS	APT/UNIT	CITY	STATE	ZIP	HOME PH (123)	WORK PH ( ) EXT:
62 Pebble Trail	15	Douglasville	NY	01234	457-4448	

EMPLOYER/SCHOOL	EMPLOYER ADDRESS	CITY	STATE	ZIP
Unemployed				

REFERRING PHYSICIAN (LAST NAME, FIRST NAME)	ADDRESS	CITY	STATE	ZIP	PHONE

GUARANTOR - Person responsible for payment: ☒ self   ☐ spouse/other   ☐ parent   ☐ legal guardian <u>If not "self", please complete the following:</u>

LAST NAME	FIRST NAME	MI	SSN		GENDER	DATE OF BIRTH

ADDRESS (IF DIFFERENT FROM PATIENT)	CITY	STATE	ZIP	HOME PH ( )	ALT. PHONE

EMPLOYER NAME	EMPLOYER ADDRESS	CITY	STATE	ZIP	WORK PHONE EXT

OTHER RESPONSIBLE PARTY:

LAST NAME	FIRST NAME	MI	SSN		GENDER	DATE OF BIRTH	

ADDRESS (IF DIFFERENT FROM PATIENT)	CITY	STATE	ZIP	HOME PH ( )	ALT. PHONE

EMPLOYER NAME	EMPLOYER ADDRESS	CITY STATE	ZIP	WORK PHONE EXT

INSURANCE - PRIMARY

PLAN NAME	PATIENT RELATIONSHIP TO INSURED:
Self pay	☐ self ☐ spouse ☐ child ☐ other

POLICYHOLDER INFORMATION

LAST NAME	FIRST NAME	MI	DATE OF BIRTH	ID#	POLICY #	GROUP #

EMPLOYER NAME	PCP NAME, IF APPLICABLE:

INSURANCE - SECONDARY

PLAN NAME	PATIENT RELATIONSHIP TO INSURED: ☐ self ☐ spouse ☐ child ☐ other

POLICYHOLDER INFORMATION

LAST NAME	FIRST NAME	MI	DATE OF BIRTH	ID#	POLICY #	GROUP #

EMPLOYER NAME	PCP NAME, IF APPLICABLE:

ACCIDENT? ☐ YES ☐ NO IF YES, DATE OF INJURY	OCCUR AT WORK? ☐ YES ☐ NO	AUTO INVOLVED: ☐ YES ☐ NO	STATE

NAME OF ATTORNEY	PHONE NUMBER EXT.

INSURANCE AUTHORIZATION AND ASSIGNMENT

Name of Policy Holder _____ HIC Number _____
I request that payment of authorized Medicare/Other Insurance company benefits be made either to me or on my behalf to _____
For any services furnished me by that party who accepts assignment/physician. Regulations pertaining to Medicare assignment of benefits apply.
I authorize the release of protected health information to the Social Security Administration and Centers for Medicare and Medicaid Services or its intermediaries or carriers any information needed for this or a related Medicare claim/other Insurance Company claim...(Section 11288 f the Social Security Act and if 31 U.S.C. Sections 3801-3812 provides penalties for withholding this information).

Signature *Rodney Zuhl* _____   Date 10/30/2009 _____

SOURCE DOCUMENT 5-8

Welcome To Our Office
PLEASE PRINT

NEW PATIENT INFORMATION

DATE _____

LAST NAME	FIRST NAME	MI	SSN		GENDER	MARITAL STATUS	DATE OF BIRTH
Tomanaga	Marie		999-21-3166		Female	Married	2/2/33

ADDRESS	APT/UNIT	CITY	STATE	ZIP	HOME PH (123)	WORK PH ( ) EXT:
2301 Marbie Way		Douglasville	NY	01234	457-2110	

EMPLOYER/SCHOOL	EMPLOYER ADDRESS	CITY	STATE	ZIP
Retired				

REFERRING PHYSICIAN (LAST NAME, FIRST NAME)	ADDRESS	CITY	STATE	ZIP	PHONE

GUARANTOR - Person responsible for payment: ☒ self ☐ spouse/other ☐ parent ☐ legal guardian If not "self", please complete the following:

LAST NAME	FIRST NAME	MI	SSN	GENDER	DATE OF BIRTH

ADDRESS (IF DIFFERENT FROM PATIENT)	CITY	STATE	ZIP	HOME PH ( )	ALT. PHONE

EMPLOYER NAME	EMPLOYER ADDRESS	CITY	STATE	ZIP	WORK PHONE	EXT

OTHER RESPONSIBLE PARTY:

LAST NAME	FIRST NAME	MI	SSN	GENDER	DATE OF BIRTH
Tomanaga	Walter		999-52-1133	Male	2/20/28

ADDRESS (IF DIFFERENT FROM PATIENT)	CITY	STATE	ZIP	HOME PH ( )	ALT. PHONE
Same					

EMPLOYER NAME	EMPLOYER ADDRESS	CITY STATE	ZIP	WORK PHONE	EXT
Retired					

INSURANCE - PRIMARY

PLAN NAME	PATIENT RELATIONSHIP TO INSURED:
Medicare	☒ self ☐ spouse ☐ child ☐ other

POLICYHOLDER INFORMATION

LAST NAME	FIRST NAME	MI	DATE OF BIRTH	ID#	POLICY #	GROUP #
Tomanaga	Marie		2/2/33	999213166A		

EMPLOYER NAME	PCP NAME, IF APPLICABLE:

INSURANCE - SECONDARY

PLAN NAME	PATIENT RELATIONSHIP TO INSURED:
Century SeniorGap	☒ self ☐ spouse ☐ child ☐ other

POLICYHOLDER INFORMATION

LAST NAME	FIRST NAME	MI	DATE OF BIRTH	ID#	POLICY #	GROUP #
Tomanaga	Marie		2/2/33	999213166		MG612

EMPLOYER NAME	PCP NAME, IF APPLICABLE:

ACCIDENT? ☐ YES ☒ NO IF YES, DATE OF INJURY	OCCUR AT WORK? ☒ YES ☐ NO	AUTO INVOLVED: ☐ YES ☒ NO	STATE

NAME OF ATTORNEY	PHONE NUMBER	EXT.

INSURANCE AUTHORIZATION AND ASSIGNMENT

Name of Policy Holder Marie Tomanaga _____ HIC Number _____

I request that payment of authorized Medicare/Other Insurance company benefits be made either to me or on my behalf to Dr. Schwartz

For any services furnished me by that party who accepts assignment/physician. Regulations pertaining to Medicare assignment of benefits apply.

I authorize the release of protected health information to the Social Security Administration and Centers for Medicare and Medicaid Services or its intermediaries or carriers any information needed for this or a related Medicare claim/other Insurance Company claim...(Section 11288 f the Social Security Act and if 31 U.S.C. Sections 3801-3812 provides penalties for withholding this information).

Signature *Marie Tomanaga* _____ Date 11/3/09 _____

Registration form for Marie Tomanaga. *Used with permission. InHealth Record Systems, Inc. 5076 Winters Chapel Road, Atlanta, GA 30360, 800-477-7374. http://www.inhealthrecords.com*

MEDICARE		HEALTH INSURANCE

HEALTH CARE FINANCING ADMINISTRATION

NAME OF BENEFICIARY
Marie Tomanaga

MEDICARE CLAIM NUMBER   SEX
999213166A   Female

IS ENTITLED TO

HOSPITAL   (PART A)

MEDICAL   (PART B)

SIGN ➜
HERE   _Marie Tomanaga_____

Century
SeniorGap

Medigap Plan J - Region 23-5

Insured: Marie Tomanaga   999213166
Medigap Number: MG612

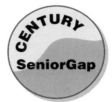

Insurer: CentSG   02CENT/09/TTGAP

Insurance cards for Marie Tomanaga. *Delmar/Cengage Learning*

SOURCE DOCUMENT 5-10

Welcome To Our Office
PLEASE PRINT

NEW PATIENT INFORMATION

DATE _____

LAST NAME	FIRST NAME	MI	SSN		GENDER	MARITAL STATUS	DATE OF BIRTH
Villanova	Ricky		999-32-1106		Male	Married	1/3/79

ADDRESS	APT/UNIT	CITY	STATE	ZIP	HOME PH (123)	WORK PH ( ) EXT:
8123 Slate Ct.	15	Douglasville	NY	01234	457-6122	Same

EMPLOYER/SCHOOL	EMPLOYER ADDRESS	CITY	STATE	ZIP
Self employed	8123 Slate Ct.	Douglasville	NY	01234

REFERRING PHYSICIAN (LAST NAME, FIRST NAME)	ADDRESS	CITY	STATE	ZIP	PHONE
Joseph Reed					

GUARANTOR - Person responsible for payment: ☐ self ☒ spouse/other ☐ parent ☐ legal guardian If not "self", please complete the following:

LAST NAME	FIRST NAME	MI	SSN	GENDER	DATE OF BIRTH
Villanova	Gina	M.	999-61-9923	Female	6/30/82

ADDRESS (IF DIFFERENT FROM PATIENT)	CITY	STATE	ZIP	HOME PH ( )	ALT. PHONE
Same					

EMPLOYER NAME	EMPLOYER ADDRESS	CITY	STATE	ZIP	WORK PHONE EXT
Morgan Associates	385 Granite St.	Douglasville		01235	123-528-1996

OTHER RESPONSIBLE PARTY:

LAST NAME	FIRST NAME	MI	SSN	GENDER	DATE OF BIRTH	

ADDRESS (IF DIFFERENT FROM PATIENT)	CITY	STATE	ZIP	HOME PH ( )	ALT. PHONE

EMPLOYER NAME	EMPLOYER ADDRESS	CITY STATE	ZIP	WORK PHONE EXT

INSURANCE - PRIMARY

PLAN NAME	PATIENT RELATIONSHIP TO INSURED:
Signal HMO	☐ self ☒ spouse ☐ child ☐ other

POLICYHOLDER INFORMATION

LAST NAME	FIRST NAME	MI	DATE OF BIRTH	ID#	POLICY #	GROUP #
Villanova	Gina	M.	6/30/82	999619923-02		MA8991

EMPLOYER NAME	PCP NAME, IF APPLICABLE:
Morgan Associates	

INSURANCE - SECONDARY

PLAN NAME	PATIENT RELATIONSHIP TO INSURED: ☐ self ☐ spouse ☐ child ☐ other
None	

POLICYHOLDER INFORMATION

LAST NAME	FIRST NAME	MI	DATE OF BIRTH	ID#	POLICY #	GROUP #

EMPLOYER NAME	PCP NAME, IF APPLICABLE:

ACCIDENT? ☐ YES ☐ NO IF YES, DATE OF INJURY	OCCUR AT WORK? ☐ YES ☐ NO	AUTO INVOLVED: ☐ YES ☐ NO	STATE

NAME OF ATTORNEY	PHONE NUMBER EXT.		

INSURANCE AUTHORIZATION AND ASSIGNMENT

Name of Policy Holder ___Gina Villanova_____ HIC Number _____

I request that payment of authorized Medicare/Other Insurance company benefits be made either to me or on my behalf to _Dr. Schwartz_____
For any services furnished me by that party who accepts assignment/physician. Regulations pertaining to Medicare assignment of benefits apply.
I authorize the release of protected health information to the Social Security Administration and Centers for Medicare and Medicaid Services or its intermediaries or carriers any information needed for this or a related Medicare claim/other Insurance Company claim...(Section 11288 f the Social Security Act and if 31 U.S.C. Sections 3801-3812 provides penalties for withholding this information).

Signature ___Gina Villanova_____ Date___10/27/09_____

Registration form for Ricky Villanova. *Used with permission. InHealth Record Systems, Inc. 5076 Winters Chapel Road, Atlanta, GA 30360, 800-477-7374. http://www.inhealthrecords.com*

SOURCE DOCUMENT 5-11

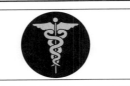

Signal **HMO**

PCP: Douglasville Medicine Associates
D.J. Schwartz, M.D.
(123)456-7890

Gina Villanova   999619923   01
Ricky Villanova   Dependent   02

Copayment Schedule

PCP Office Visits	$ 10.00
Specialists Visits	$ 30.00
Emergency Room	$ 100.00
Hospitalization	Authorization

Preauthorization 800-123-8877

Bank Code
361   Member Group Number: MA8991

E25/A10
Type of Coverage

Insurance card for Ricky Villanova. *Delmar/Cengage Learning*

SOURCE DOCUMENT 5-12

Welcome To Our Office
PLEASE PRINT

NEW PATIENT INFORMATION

DATE _____

LAST NAME	FIRST NAME	MI	SSN		GENDER	MARITAL STATUS	DATE OF BIRTH
Pradhan	Kabin		999-56-9844		Male	Single	12/2/51

ADDRESS	APT/UNIT	CITY	STATE	ZIP	HOME PH (123	WORK PH (123) EXT:
2213 Boulder Ct.		Douglasville	NY	01234	457-2189	528-9772

EMPLOYER/SCHOOL	EMPLOYER ADDRESS	CITY	STATE	ZIP
Allcity Mortgage Co.	2158 Midway Blvd.	Douglasville	NY	01235

REFERRING PHYSICIAN (LAST NAME, FIRST NAME)	ADDRESS	CITY	STATE	ZIP	PHONE

GUARANTOR - Person responsible for payment: ☒ self ☐ spouse/other ☐ parent ☐ legal guardian If not "self", please complete the following:

LAST NAME	FIRST NAME	MI	SSN		GENDER	DATE OF BIRTH

ADDRESS (IF DIFFERENT FROM PATIENT)	CITY	STATE	ZIP	HOME PH ( )	ALT. PHONE

EMPLOYER NAME	EMPLOYER ADDRESS	CITY	STATE	ZIP	WORK PHONE	EXT

OTHER RESPONSIBLE PARTY:

LAST NAME	FIRST NAME	MI	SSN		GENDER	DATE OF BIRTH	

ADDRESS (IF DIFFERENT FROM PATIENT)	CITY	STATE	ZIP	HOME PH ( )	ALT. PHONE

EMPLOYER NAME	EMPLOYER ADDRESS	CITY STATE	ZIP	WORK PHONE	EXT

INSURANCE – PRIMARY

PLAN NAME	PATIENT RELATIONSHIP TO INSURED:
ConsumerOne HRA	☒ self ☐ spouse ☐ child ☐ other

POLICYHOLDER INFORMATION

LAST NAME	FIRST NAME	MI	DATE OF BIRTH	ID#	POLICY #	GROUP #
Pradhan	Kabin		12/2/51	999569844		ACM0211

EMPLOYER NAME	PCP NAME, IF APPLICABLE:

INSURANCE – SECONDARY

PLAN NAME	PATIENT RELATIONSHIP TO INSURED: ☐ self ☐ spouse ☐ child ☐ other

POLICYHOLDER INFORMATION

LAST NAME	FIRST NAME	MI	DATE OF BIRTH	ID#	POLICY #	GROUP #

EMPLOYER NAME	PCP NAME, IF APPLICABLE:

ACCIDENT? ☐ YES ☒ NO IF YES, DATE OF INJURY	OCCUR AT WORK? ☐ YES ☒ NO	AUTO INVOLVED: ☐ YES ☒ NO	STATE

NAME OF ATTORNEY	PHONE NUMBER EXT.

INSURANCE AUTHORIZATION AND ASSIGNMENT

Name of Policy Holder ___Kabin Pradhan___ HIC Number _____

I request that payment of authorized Medicare/Other Insurance company benefits be made either to me or on my behalf to _Dr. Schwartz_
For any services furnished me by that party who accepts assignment/physician. Regulations pertaining to Medicare assignment of benefits apply.
I authorize the release of protected health information to the Social Security Administration and Centers for Medicare and Medicaid Services or its intermediaries or carriers any information needed for this or a related Medicare claim/other Insurance Company claim...(Section 11288 f the Social Security Act and if 31 U.S.C. Sections 3801-3812 provides penalties for withholding this information).

Signature ___Kabin Pradhan___ Date ___11/03/09___

Registration form for Kabin Pradhan. *Used with permission. InHealth Record Systems, Inc. 5076 Winters Chapel Road, Atlanta, GA 30360, 800-477-7374. http://www.inhealthrecords.com*

SOURCE DOCUMENT 5-13

Consumer **ONE**

Benefits Card
Health Reimbursement Arrangement

Participant: Pradhan, Kabin
ID Number: 999569844
Employer Group: ACM0211

Preventative Care: 100%
EPA – Call 800-123-8253
Level 3 - 80/20

In-Network Preferred

Plan Code GP123123

Insurance card for Kabin Pradhan. *Delmar/Cengage Learning*

SOURCE DOCUMENT 5-14

Welcome To Our Office
PLEASE PRINT

NEW PATIENT INFORMATION

DATE _____

LAST NAME	FIRST NAME	MI	SSN		GENDER	MARITAL STATUS	DATE OF BIRTH
Beals	Kimberly	L.	999-22-9899		Female	Single	10/20/69

ADDRESS		APT/UNIT	CITY	STATE	ZIP	HOME PH (123)	WORK PH (123) EXT:
5526 Gravel Way			Douglasville	NY	01234	457-3210	528-1132

EMPLOYER/SCHOOL	EMPLOYER ADDRESS		CITY	STATE	ZIP
Clear Lake Elementary	5899 Pebble Trail		Douglasville	NY	01234

REFERRING PHYSICIAN (LAST NAME, FIRST NAME)	ADDRESS	CITY	STATE	ZIP	PHONE

GUARANTOR - Person responsible for payment: ☒ self ☐ spouse/other ☐ parent ☐ legal guardian If not "self", please complete the following:

LAST NAME	FIRST NAME	MI	SSN		GENDER	DATE OF BIRTH

ADDRESS (IF DIFFERENT FROM PATIENT)	CITY	STATE	ZIP	HOME PH ( )	ALT. PHONE

EMPLOYER NAME	EMPLOYER ADDRESS	CITY	STATE	ZIP	WORK PHONE	EXT

OTHER RESPONSIBLE PARTY:

LAST NAME	FIRST NAME	MI	SSN		GENDER	DATE OF BIRTH

ADDRESS (IF DIFFERENT FROM PATIENT)	CITY	STATE	ZIP	HOME PH ( )	ALT. PHONE

EMPLOYER NAME	EMPLOYER ADDRESS	CITY STATE	ZIP	WORK PHONE	EXT

INSURANCE - PRIMARY

PLAN NAME	PATIENT RELATIONSHIP TO INSURED:
Signal HMO	☒ self ☐ spouse ☐ child ☐ other

POLICYHOLDER INFORMATION

LAST NAME	FIRST NAME	MI	DATE OF BIRTH	ID#	POLICY #	GROUP #
Beals	Kimberly	L.	10/20/69	999229899-00		CLE5610

EMPLOYER NAME	PCP NAME, IF APPLICABLE:
Clear Lake Elementary	

INSURANCE - SECONDARY

PLAN NAME	PATIENT RELATIONSHIP TO INSURED: ☐ self ☐ spouse ☐ child ☐ other

POLICYHOLDER INFORMATION

LAST NAME	FIRST NAME	MI	DATE OF BIRTH	ID#	POLICY #	GROUP #

EMPLOYER NAME	PCP NAME, IF APPLICABLE:

ACCIDENT? ☐ YES ☒ NO IF YES, DATE OF INJURY	OCCUR AT WORK? ☐ YES ☒ NO	AUTO INVOLVED: ☐ YES ☒ NO	STATE

NAME OF ATTORNEY	PHONE NUMBER EXT.

INSURANCE AUTHORIZATION AND ASSIGNMENT

Name of Policy Holder Kimberly L. Beals _____ HIC Number _____

I request that payment of authorized Medicare/Other Insurance company benefits be made either to me or on my behalf to Dr. Heath
For any services furnished me by that party who accepts assignment/physician. Regulations pertaining to Medicare assignment of benefits apply.
I authorize the release of protected health information to the Social Security Administration and Centers for Medicare and Medicaid Services or its intermediaries or carriers any information needed for this or a related Medicare claim/other Insurance Company claim...(Section 11288 f the Social Security Act and if 31 U.S.C. Sections 3801-3812 provides penalties for withholding this information).

Signature _____ Kimberly Beals _____   Date___ 11/03/09 _____

Registration form for Kimberly Beals. *Used with permission. InHealth Record Systems, Inc. 5076 Winters Chapel Road, Atlanta, GA 30360, 800-477-7374. http://www.inhealthrecords.com*

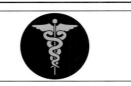

Signal HMO

PCP: Douglasville Medicine Associates
L.D. Heath, M.D.
(123)456-7890

Kimberly Beals   999229899   00

Copayment Schedule

PCP Office Visits $ 10.00
Specialists Visits $ 30.00
Emergency Room $ 100.00
Hospitalization   Authorization

Preauthorization 800-123-8877

Bank Code
  361   Member Group Number: CLE5610

E25/A10
Type of Coverage

Insurance card for Kimberly Beals. *Delmar/Cengage Learning*

SOURCE DOCUMENT 5-16

Welcome To Our Office
PLEASE PRINT

NEW PATIENT INFORMATION

DATE _____

LAST NAME	FIRST NAME	MI	SSN		GENDER	MARITAL STATUS	DATE OF BIRTH
Kinzler	Linda		999-63-4521		Female	Single	2/27/83

ADDRESS	APT/UNIT	CITY	STATE	ZIP	HOME PH (123)	WORK PH ( ) EXT:
913 Boulder Parkway		Douglasville	NY	01234	457-5688	

EMPLOYER/SCHOOL	EMPLOYER ADDRESS	CITY	STATE	ZIP
Unemployed				

REFERRING PHYSICIAN (LAST NAME, FIRST NAME)	ADDRESS	CITY	STATE	ZIP	PHONE

GUARANTOR - Person responsible for payment: ☐ self ☒ spouse/other ☐ parent ☐ legal guardian If not "self", please complete the following:

LAST NAME	FIRST NAME	MI	SSN		GENDER	DATE OF BIRTH
Wade	Jennifer	A.	999-12-5813		Female	5/5/82

ADDRESS (IF DIFFERENT FROM PATIENT)	CITY	STATE	ZIP	HOME PH ( )	ALT. PHONE
Same					

EMPLOYER NAME	EMPLOYER ADDRESS	CITY STATE	ZIP	WORK PHONE EXT
Tech Consultants, Inc.	321B Industry Lane	Douglasville	01235	123-528-5166

OTHER RESPONSIBLE PARTY:

LAST NAME	FIRST NAME	MI	SSN	GENDER	DATE OF BIRTH	

ADDRESS (IF DIFFERENT FROM PATIENT)	CITY	STATE	ZIP	HOME PH ( )	ALT. PHONE

EMPLOYER NAME	EMPLOYER ADDRESS	CITY STATE	ZIP	WORK PHONE EXT

INSURANCE - PRIMARY

PLAN NAME	PATIENT RELATIONSHIP TO INSURED:
Flexihealth PPO	☐ self ☐ spouse ☐ child ☒ other

POLICYHOLDER INFORMATION

LAST NAME	FIRST NAME	MI	DATE OF BIRTH	ID#	POLICY #	GROUP #
Wade	Jennifer	A.	5/5/82	999125813-02		TC1015

EMPLOYER NAME	PCP NAME, IF APPLICABLE:		
Tech Consultants, Inc.			

INSURANCE - SECONDARY

PLAN NAME	PATIENT RELATIONSHIP TO INSURED: ☐ self ☐ spouse ☐ child ☐ other

POLICYHOLDER INFORMATION

LAST NAME	FIRST NAME	MI	DATE OF BIRTH	ID#	POLICY #	GROUP #

EMPLOYER NAME	PCP NAME, IF APPLICABLE:		

ACCIDENT? ☐ YES ☐ NO IF YES, DATE OF INJURY	OCCUR AT WORK? ☐ YES ☐ NO	AUTO INVOLVED: ☐ YES ☐ NO	STATE

NAME OF ATTORNEY	PHONE NUMBER EXT.	

INSURANCE AUTHORIZATION AND ASSIGNMENT

Name of Policy Holder _Jennifer Wade_____ HIC Number _____

I request that payment of authorized Medicare/Other Insurance company benefits be made either to me or on my behalf to _Dr. Heath_____

For any services furnished me by that party who accepts assignment/physician. Regulations pertaining to Medicare assignment of benefits apply. I authorize the release of protected health information to the Social Security Administration and Centers for Medicare and Medicaid Services or its intermediaries or carriers any information needed for this or a related Medicare claim/other Insurance Company claim...(Section 11288 f the Social Security Act and if 31 U.S.C. Sections 3801-3812 provides penalties for withholding this information).

Signature _____ _Jennifer Wade_____ Date_ 11/09/09 _____

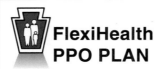

**FlexiHealth
PPO PLAN**

Insurer 81564

Your Health First ᔆᴹ

Insured:	Wade, Jennifer 999125813-01
Employer:	Tech Consultants, Inc.
Group:	TCI015

Family/Spousal/Partner Premier Plan

Additional Insured:
Kinzler, Linda   999125813-02

Physician Co-pay: $20.00
Hospital Services: $400.00 Annual family deductible.
Surgery & Hospitalization: Requires preauthorization 800-123-7426

Insurance card for Linda Kinzler. *Delmar/Cengage Learning*

SOURCE DOCUMENT 5-18

Community General Hospital									RECORD OF ADMISSION	

PATIENT NAME		ROOM NO.	HOSP. NO.	ADDRESS LINE - 1			ADDRESS LINE - 2	
Tate, Jason		410B		8812 Marble Way			APT. 103	

AGE	BIRTHDATE	SEX	BIRTHPLACE	CITY	STATE	ZIP CODE	COUNTRY CODE
	3-5-67	M	St. Petersburg, FL	Douglasville	NY	01235	22

SSAN	NATIONALITY	CIVIL ST.	MILITARY	RELIGION		CHURCH	PATIENT TELEPHONE
999561133				UNK			(123)457-2216

SPOUSE INFORMATION

NAME OF HUSBAND OR NAME OF WIFE	SPOUSE BIRTHPLACE	SPOUSE EMPLOYER NAME

SPOUSE ADDRESS	SPOUSE EMPLOYER ADDRESS

NAME OF FATHER	BIRTHPLACE	NAME OF MOTHER	BIRTHPLACE

NOTIFY IN CASE OF EMERGENCY

NAME	RELATIONSHIP	ADDRESS	TELEPHONE
Wittek, Jeanne	Girlfriend	UNK	(123)427-5721

PATIENT EMPLOYER NAME	EMPLOYER ADDRESS	EMPLOYER TELEPHONE	GUARANTOR OCCUPATION
Hi-Lo Concrete	1120 Industry Lane, Douglasville	(123)522-6899	Construction

GUARANTOR NAME	GUARANTOR TELEPHONE	HOSPITALIZATION INSURANCE
Self		Flexihealth PPO In-Network

GUARANTOR ADDRESS - 1	CITY	ID Number: 999561133 Group: HLC321

GUARANTOR ADDRESS - 2	STATE	ZIP CODE	DATE	TIME	PLACE	EVENT	INJURY DUE TO ACCID.

ADMITTING PHYSICIAN	CONSULTING PHYSICIAN	ADMITTING SERVICE	SMOKER	ADMITTING DIAGNOSIS				
Heath	Lambert	Medicine	Yes	Peptic Ulcer				

ALLERGIES	DATE LAST ADM.	PREV. ADM. NO.	ADMISSION DATE	TIME OF ADMISSION	INITIALS	DISCHARGE DATE
Sulfa						

FINANCIAL CLASS	MEDICAL RECORDS NUMBER	ADMISSION CODE	HOME 1	SHORT TERM HOSPITAL 2	SKILLED NURSING FACILITY 3	INTERMEDIATE CARE FACILITY 4	OTHER 5	LEFT AMA 7	EXPIRED 20	TIME
	6082145									

PRINCIPAL DIAGNOSIS: 536.9   ADVANCE DIRECTIVE =   CODE

SECONDARY DIAGNOSIS: 780.6, 311

Preauthorization

obtained

#22136900

PRINCIPAL OPERATION/DATE:

SECONDARY OPERATIONS:

Consultation With _____ *Jeanette Lambert, M.D. Gastroenterology* _____

Results: ☐ Recovered ☒ Improved ☐ Not Improved ☐ Not Treated ☐ Diagnosis Only ☐ Died ☐ Released Against Advice

Cause of Death _____ Autopsy: ☐ Yes ☐ No

I have examined and approved this complete medical on _____ 20 _____

Signed _____ Attending Physician

ADMISSION - SUMMARY SHEET

Face sheet for Jason Tate. *Delmar/Cengage Learning*

SOURCE DOCUMENT 5-19

New York County Hospital								RECORD OF ADMISSION	

New York County Hospital — **RECORD OF ADMISSION**

PATIENT NAME			ROOM NO.	HOSP. NO.	ADDRESS LINE - 1			ADDRESS LINE - 2	
Munoz, Geraldo L.			211B		1287 Boulder Ct.				

AGE	BIRTHDATE	SEX	BIRTHPLACE	CITY	STATE	ZIP CODE	COUNTRY CODE
	3-28-25	M	Dominican Republic	Douglasville	NY	01234	22

SSAN	NATIONALITY	CIVIL ST.	MILITARY	RELIGION	CHURCH		PATIENT TELEPHONE
999832166			NO	Cath			(123)457-0018

SPOUSE INFORMATION	NAME OF HUSBAND OR NAME OF WIFE	SPOUSE BIRTHPLACE	SPOUSE EMPLOYER NAME
	SPOUSE ADDRESS		SPOUSE EMPLOYER ADDRESS

	NAME OF FATHER	BIRTHPLACE	NAME OF MOTHER	BIRTHPLACE
	Munoz, Jose Maria	Dominican Republic	Munoz, Lisy	Dominican Republic

NOTIFY IN CASE OF EMERGENCY	NAME	RELATIONSHIP	ADDRESS	TELEPHONE
	Anzalone, Elisa	Sister	5611 Whitestone Dr. Douglasville	(123)427-6133

PATIENT EMPLOYER NAME	EMPLOYER ADDRESS	EMPLOYER TELEPHONE	GUARANTOR OCCUPATION
Retired			

GUARANTOR NAME	GUARANTOR TELEPHONE	HOSPITALIZATION INSURANCE
Self		Medicare Statewide Corp 999832166A
GUARANTOR ADDRESS - 1	CITY	Century SeniorGap 999832166 MG5121

GUARANTOR ADDRESS - 2	STATE	ZIP CODE	DATE	TIME	PLACE	EVENT	INJURY DUE TO ACCID.

ADMITTING PHYSICIAN	CONSULTING PHYSICIAN	ADMITTING SERVICE	SMOKER	ADMITTING DIAGNOSIS
Heath	Romanov	Medicine	Yes	Atrial Fibrillation

ALLERGIES	DATE LAST ADM.	PREV. ADM. NO.	ADMISSION DATE	TIME OF ADMISSION	INITIALS	DISCHARGE DATE
NKA						

FINANCIAL CLASS	MEDICAL RECORDS NUMBER	ADMISSION CODE	HOME 1	SHORT TERM HOSPITAL 2	SKILLED NURSING FACILITY 3	INTERMEDIATE CARE FACILITY 4	OTHER 5	LEFT AMA 7	EXPIRED 20	TIME
	3116110									

PRINCIPAL DIAGNOSIS: 427.31   ADVANCE DIRECTIVE =   CODE

SECONDARY DIAGNOSIS: None

PRINCIPAL OPERATION/DATE: N/A

SECONDARY OPERATIONS:

Consultation With _____ *Yuri Romanov, M.D. Cardiology* _____

Results: ☐ Recovered   ☐ Improved   ☐ Not Improved   ☐ Not Treated   ☒ Diagnosis Only   ☐ Died   ☐ Released Against Advice

Cause of Death _____   Autopsy: ☐ Yes   ☐ No

I have examined and approved this complete medical on _____ 20 _____

Signed _____ Attending Physician

ADMISSION - SUMMARY SHEET

Face sheet for Geraldo Munoz. *Delmar/Cengage Learning*

SOURCE DOCUMENT 5-20

New York County Hospital

RECORD OF ADMISSION

PATIENT NAME			ROOM NO.	HOSP. NO.		ADDRESS LINE - 1				ADDRESS LINE - 2	
Ruhl, Mary A.			209A			1233 Gravel Way					

AGE	BIRTHDATE	SEX	BIRTHPLACE		CITY		STATE	ZIP CODE		COUNTRY CODE	
	12-5-35	F	Douglasville, NY		Douglasville		NY	01234		22	

SSAN	NATIONALITY	CIVIL ST.	MILITARY	RELIGION			CHURCH		PATIENT TELEPHONE	
999526778			NO	BAP					(123)457-2133	

SPOUSE INFORMATION

NAME OF HUSBAND OR NAME OF WIFE	SPOUSE BIRTHPLACE	SPOUSE EMPLOYER NAME
Ruhl, Robert M.	Toronto, Canada	Banterfield Hobby

SPOUSE ADDRESS	SPOUSE EMPLOYER ADDRESS
1233 Gravel Way Douglasville, NY	9211 Midway Blvd., Douglasville

NAME OF FATHER	BIRTHPLACE	NAME OF MOTHER	BIRTHPLACE

NOTIFY IN CASE OF EMERGENCY

NAME	RELATIONSHIP	ADDRESS	TELEPHONE
Ruhl, Robert M.	Spouse		(123)457-2133

PATIENT EMPLOYER NAME	EMPLOYER ADDRESS	EMPLOYER TELEPHONE	GUARANTOR OCCUPATION
Retired			Sales clerk

GUARANTOR NAME	GUARANTOR TELEPHONE	HOSPITALIZATION INSURANCE
Ruhl, Robert M.		1. Flexihealth PPO 999321168-02 Group BH225

GUARANTOR ADDRESS - 1	CITY	
		2. Medicare Statewide Corp 999321168B

GUARANTOR ADDRESS - 2	STATE	ZIP CODE	DATE	TIME	PLACE	EVENT	INJURY DUE TO ACCID.

ADMITTING PHYSICIAN	CONSULTING PHYSICIAN	ADMITTING SERVICE	SMOKER	ADMITTING DIAGNOSIS	
Heath		Medicine	No	Gastroenteritis	

ALLERGIES	DATE LAST ADM.	PREV. ADM. NO.	ADMISSION DATE	TIME OF ADMISSION	INITIALS	DISCHARGE DATE

FINANCIAL CLASS	MEDICAL RECORDS NUMBER	ADMISSION CODE	HOME	SHORT TERM HOSPITAL	SKILLED NURSING FACILITY	INTERMEDIATE CARE FACILITY	OTHER	LEFT AMA	EXPIRED	TIME
	3115321		1	2	3	4	5	7	20	

PRINCIPAL DIAGNOSIS: 558.9

ADVANCE DIRECTIVE =   **CODE**

SECONDARY DIAGNOSIS: 276.5, 780.6

Preauthorization

obtained

#22136950

PRINCIPAL OPERATION/DATE: N/A

SECONDARY OPERATIONS:

Consultation With _____

Results: ☐ Recovered   ☐ Improved   ☐ Not Improved   ☐ Not Treated   ☐ Diagnosis Only   ☐ Died   ☐ Released Against Advice

Cause of Death _____ Autopsy: ☐ Yes   ☐ No

I have examined and approved this complete medical on_____ 20 _____

Signed _____ Attending Physician

ADMISSION - SUMMARY SHEET

Face sheet for Mary Ruhl. *Delmar/Cengage Learning*

SOURCE DOCUMENT 5-21

New York County Hospital   RECORD OF ADMISSION

PATIENT NAME	ROOM NO.	HOSP. NO.	ADDRESS LINE - 1			ADDRESS LINE - 2	
Mallory, Christina	201C		516 Ridgeway Rd.				

AGE	BIRTHDATE	SEX	BIRTHPLACE		CITY	STATE	ZIP CODE	COUNTRY CODE
	2-20-1990	F	Chicago, IL		Douglasville	NY	01234	22

SSAN	NATIONALITY	CIVIL ST.	MILITARY	RELIGION	CHURCH	PATIENT TELEPHONE
999561134			NO	LUTH		(123)457-2321

SPOUSE INFORMATION	NAME OF HUSBAND OR NAME OF WIFE	SPOUSE BIRTHPLACE	SPOUSE EMPLOYER NAME
	SPOUSE ADDRESS		SPOUSE EMPLOYER ADDRESS

NOTIFY IN CASE OF EMERGENCY	NAME OF FATHER	BIRTHPLACE	NAME OF MOTHER	BIRTHPLACE
	Mallory, Michael	UNK	Brendon, Louise	UNK

	NAME	RELATIONSHIP	ADDRESS	TELEPHONE
	Mallory, Michael	Father		(123)427-6110

PATIENT EMPLOYER NAME	EMPLOYER ADDRESS	EMPLOYER TELEPHONE	GUARANTOR OCCUPATION
Student-Full time	Central University		Plumber

GUARANTOR NAME	GUARANTOR TELEPHONE	HOSPITALIZATION INSURANCE
Mallory, Michael		Flexihealth PPO Group: PP2891

GUARANTOR ADDRESS - 1	CITY	
		Mallory, Michael 999510226-B2

GUARANTOR ADDRESS - 2	STATE	ZIP CODE	DATE	TIME	PLACE	EVENT	INJURY DUE TO ACCID.

ADMITTING PHYSICIAN	CONSULTING PHYSICIAN	ADMITTING SERVICE	SMOKER	ADMITTING DIAGNOSIS
Heath	Johnson	Medicine	No	Drug reaction, post antibiotic therapy

ALLERGIES			DATE LAST ADM.	PREV. ADM. NO.	ADMISSION DATE	TIME OF ADMISSION	INITIALS	DISCHARGE DATE
NKA								

FINANCIAL CLASS	MEDICAL RECORDS NUMBER	ADMISSION CODE	HOME	SHORT TERM HOSPITAL	SKILLED NURSING FACILITY	INTERMEDIATE CARE FACILITY	OTHER	LEFT AMA	EXPIRED	TIME
	3118986		1	2	3	4	5	7	20	

PRINCIPAL DIAGNOSIS:
995.2   ADVANCE DIRECTIVE =   CODE

SECONDARY DIAGNOSIS:
708.9, 780.79   Preauthorization

                                                 obtained

                                                 #22139631

PRINCIPAL OPERATION/DATE:
N/A

SECONDARY OPERATIONS:

Consultation With _____ *Randall Johnson, M.D. Immunology* _____

Results: ☐ Recovered ☐ Improved ☐ Not Improved ☐ Not Treated ☐ Diagnosis Only ☐ Died ☐ Released Against Advice

Cause of Death _____ Autopsy: ☐ Yes ☐ No

I have examined and approved this complete medical on _____ 20 ____

Signed _____ Attending Physician

ADMISSION - SUMMARY SHEET

Face sheet for Christina Mallory. *Delmar/Cengage Learning*

SOURCE DOCUMENT 5-22

Community General Hospital

EMERGENCY ROOM • OUTPATIENT RECORD

PATIENT NUMBER	TYPE	PATIENT NAME		AGE	BIRTHDATE	SEX	M/S	DATE OF SERVICE	TIME	CLERK INIT.
6086515		Goodnow, Leona M			7-31-79	F	M			

ADDRESS - LINE 1	ADDRESS - LINE 2	CITY	STATE	ZIP CODE	TELEPHONE
321 White Stone Dr.		Douglasville	NY	01234	(123)457-1113

PATIENT SSAN	NOTIFY IN CASE OF EMERGENCY - NAME	RELATIONSHIP	ADDRESS	TELEPHONE
999910156	Goodnow, Thomas L.	Spouse	321 White Stone Dr.	(123)457-1113

INSURANCE COMPANY	CONTRACT OR GROUP NUMBER	DATE	PLACE	A C C I D E N T
ConsumerOne HRA 999151189-02	Group TRG01			
Thomas Goodnow		TIME	EVENT	

GUARANTOR NAME	GUARANTOR ADDRESS	CITY	STATE	ZIP CODE	GUAR. TELEPHONE	G U A R A N T O R
Goodnow, Thomas	Same					

GUARANTOR EMPLOYER	GUARANTOR OCCUPATION	GUAR. EMPL. ADDRESS	GUAR. EMPL. TELEPHONE
The Rockwell Group	Investor	650 Midway Blvd., Douglasville	(123)528-3511

PREV. SERVICE	PREV. SERV. DATE	IF MINOR - PARENT NAME	MED. REC. #	ATTENDING/2ND PHYSICIAN
			6086515	Schwartz

	X -RAY	LAB	RESP TH.	PHY TH.	EKG	I.V.	DRUGS	SUPPLIES	OTHER	M.D.	E.R. RM	TOTOAL DUE

AUTHORIZATION FOR TREATMENT, GARANTEE OF PAYMENT, ASSIGNMENT OF INSURANCE BENEFITS

1. The undersigned has been informed of the emergency treatment considered necessary for the above named patient, and that treatment and procedures will be performed by physicians, members of house staff and employees of the hospital. Authorization is hereby granted for such treatment and procedures. The undersigned has read the above authorization and understands the same and certifies that no guarantee or assurance has been made as to the results that may be obtained.
2. The undersigned agrees to pay for services rendered by Hospital upon release of patient.
3. I/we hereby assign any hospital benefits, sick benefits, injury benefics due to a liability of a Third party, payable by any party, for the above patient, to Hospital unless I pay the account in full upon release of patient.
4. I/we hereby authorize the "Administrator of Hospital" to furnish from its records any information requested by the before mentioned insurance companies in connection with the above assignment. I do hereby appoint the "Controller" of Hospital as my lawful attorney to endorse for me any checks made payable to me for benefits or claims collected under the above assignment and to apply any credit balance to any other account I may owe said hospital.

DATE	TIME	SIGNED PATIENT	Leona Goodnow	SIGNED GUARANTOR	Thomas Goodnow

CHIEF COMLAINT (If accident state How, When, and Where)
Difficulty breathing, chest tightness

Leona Goodnow

TEMP.	PULSE	RESP.	B/P	ALLERGIES	MEDICATIONS - HOME	E.R. - PHYSICIAN	TET. TOX.
98²	112	28	130/88	NKA	Albuterol, Accolate	Schwartz	

NURSES NOTES:

c/o shortness of breath, wet cough, chest tightness Hx: Asthma aggravated by exposure to

cats and dander.

NURSES'S SIGNATURE (RN or LNP)
G. Jones, RN

LAB DATA (including X-Rays, EKGs, etc.)

PHYSICIAN"S REPORT

25 yo WF, WD, WN presents c difficulty breathing. States she was visiting a friend with several cats. Exposure to fur and

dander x 4 hrs. Started to feel chest tightness, developed wet cough, states "lots of phlegm" in chest and throat. Exam

reveals rales/rhonchi, upper lungs. Marked wheezing on expiration. Pt. states chest feels tight and painful on inspiration.

Impression: Moderate respiratory distress

Hx asthma and bronchitis

DIAGNOSIS: Asthmatic bronchitis 493.90

TREATMENT:
Nebulizer/albuterol treatment, relief within 20 mins.

CONDITION ON DISC		
IMP	STABLE	EXPIRED

INSTRUCTIONS TO PATIENT:

1. Albuterol Inhaler puffs qid x 2 days, then prn

2. Maintain Accolate dose

3. Start Symbicort 220 mcg two puffs hs – f/up in 1 WK @ office

FOLLOW-UP WITH
Schwartz M.D.

Leona Goodnow

DJ Schwartz M.D.

PATIEN'S SIGNATURE ON DISCHARGE BY SIGNING HERE I CERTIFY THAT I UNDERSTAND THE FOLLOWW-UP INSTRUCTIONS RECIEVED BY ME IN WRITING, WHICH ARE EXPLAINED TO ME.	DATE - TIME OF DISC.	PHYSICIAN'S SIGNATURE

Emergency outpatient record for Leona Goodnow. *Delmar/Cengage Learning*

SOURCE DOCUMENT 6-1

PLEASE RETURN THIS FORM TO RECEPTIONIST	NAME Manaly, Richard

2332

PLACE OF SERVICE:
(X) OFFICE
( ) NEW YORK COUNTY HOSPITAL
( ) COMMUNITY GENERAL HOSPITAL
( ) RETIREMENT INN NURSING HOME
( ) _____

DATE OF SERVICE 10/21/09

A. OFFICE VISITS - New Patient

Code	History	Exam	Dec.	Time	
99201	Prob. Foc.	Prob. Foc.	Straight	10 min.	_____
99202	Ex. Prob. Foc.	Ex. Prob. Foc.	Straight	20 min.	_____
99203	Detail	Detail	Low	30 min.	_____
99204	Comp.	Comp.	Mod.	45 min.	_____
99205	Comp.	Comp.	High	60 min.	_____

B. OFFICE VISIT - Established Patient

Code	History	Exam	Dec.	Time	
99211	Minimal	Minimal	Minimal	5 min.	_____
99212	Prob. Foc.	Prob. Foc.	Straight	10min.	_____
X 99213	Ex. Prob. Foc.	Ex. Prob. Foc.	Low	15 min.	1
99214	Detail	Detail	Mod.	25 min.	_____
99215	Comp.	Comp.	High	40 min.	_____

C. HOSPITAL CARE   Dx Units

1. Initial Hospital Care (30 min)	____ ___	99221	_____
2. Subsequent Care	____ ___	99231	_____
3. Critical Care (30-74 min)	____ ___	99291	_____
4. each additional 30 min.	____ ___	99292	_____
5. Discharge Services	____ ___	99238	_____
6. Emergency Room	____ ___	99282	_____

D. NURSING HOME CARE   Dx Units

Initial Care - New Pt.

1. Expanded	____ ___	99322	_____
2. Detailed	____ ___	99323	_____

Subsequent Care - Estab. Pt.

3. Problem Focused	____ ___	99307	_____
4. Expanded	____ ___	99308	_____
5. Detailed	____ ___	99309	_____
5. Comprehensive	____ ___	99310	_____

E. PROCEDURES

1. Arthrocentesis, Small Jt.	____	20600	_____
2. Colonoscopy	____	45378	_____
3. EKG w/interpretation	____	93000	_____
4. X-Ray Chest, PA/LAT	____	71020	_____

F. LAB

1. Blood Sugar	____	82947	_____
2. CBC w/differential	____	85031	_____
3. Cholesterol	____	82465	_____
4. Comprehensive Metabolic Panel	____	80053	_____
5. ESR	____	85651	_____
6. Hematocrit	____	85014	_____
7. Mono Screen	____	86308	_____
8. Pap Smear	____	88150	_____
9. Potassium	____	84132	_____
10. Preg. Test, Quantitative	____	84702	_____
11. Routine Venipuncture	____	36415	_____

F. Cont'd   Dx Units

12. Strep Screen	____	87081	_____
13. UA, Routine w/Micro	____	81000	_____
14. UA, Routine w/o Micro	____	81002	_____
15. Uric Acid	____	84550	_____
16. VDRL	____	86592	_____
17. Wet Prep	____	82710	_____
18. _____	____	____	_____

G. INJECTIONS

1. Influenza Virus Vaccine	____	90658	_____
2. Pneumoccocal Vaccine	____	90772	_____
3. Tetanus Toxoids	____	90703	_____
4. Therapeutic Subcut/IM	____	90732	_____
5. Vaccine Administration	____	90471	_____
6. Vaccine - each additional	____	90472	_____

H. MISCELLANEOUS

1. _____ ____ _____
2. _____ ____ _____

AMOUNT PAID $ 0

Mark diagnosis with (1=Primary, 2=Secondary, 3=Tertiary)	DIAGNOSIS NOT LISTED BELOW _____

DIAGNOSIS	ICD-9-CM 1, 2, 3	DIAGNOSIS	ICD-9-CM 1, 2, 3	DIAGNOSIS	ICD-9-CM 1, 2, 3
Abdominal Pain	789.0	Dehydration	276.51	Otitis Media, Acute NOS	382.9
Allergic Rhinitis, Unspec.	477.9	Depression, NOS	311	Peptic Ulcer Disease	536.9
Angina Pectoris, Unspec.	413.9	Diabetes Mellitus, Type II Controlled	250.00 1	Peripheral Vascular Disease NOS	443.9
Anemia, Iron Deficiency, Unspec.	280.9	Diabetes Mellitus, Type II Controlled	250.02	Pharyngitis, Acute	462
Anemia, NOS	285.9	Drug Reaction, NOS	995.29	Pneumonia, Organism Unspec.	486
Anemia, Pernicious	281.0	Dysuria	788.1	Prostatitis, NOS	601.9
Asthma w/ Exacerbation	493.92	Eczema, NOS	692.2	PVC	427.69
Asthmatic Bronchitis, Unspec.	493.90	Edema	782.3	Rash, Non Specific	782.1
Atrial Fibrillation	427.31	Fever, Unknown Origin	780.6	Seizure Disorder NOS	780.39
Atypical Chest Pain, Unspec.	786.59	Gastritis, Acute w/o Hemorrhage	535.00	Serous Otitis Media, Chronic, Unspec.	381.10
Bronchiolitis, due to RSV	466.11	Gastroenteritis, NOS	558.9	Sinusitis, Acute NOS	461.9
Bronchitis, Acute	466.0	Gastroesophageal Reflux	530.81	Tonsillitis, Acute	463.
Bronchitis, NOS	490	Hepatitis A, Infectious	070.1	Upper Respiratory Infection, Acute NOS	465.9
Cardiac Arrest	427.5	Hypercholesterolemia, Pure	272.0	Urinary Tract Infection, Unspec.	599.0
Cardiopulmonary Disease, Chronic, Unspec.	416.9	Hypertension, Unspec.	401.9	Urticaria, Unspec.	708.9
Cellulitis, NOS	682.9	Hypoglycemia NOS	251.2	Vertigo, NOS	780.4
Congestive Heart Failure, Unspec.	428.0	Hypokalemia	276.8	Viral Infection NOS	079.99
Contact Dermatitis NOS	692.9	Impetigo	684	Weakness, Generalized	780.79
COPD NOS	496	Lymphadenitis, Unspec.	289.3	Weight Loss, Abnormal	783.21
CVA, Acute, NOS	434.91	Mononucleosis	075		
CVA, Old or Healed	438.9	Myocardial Infarction, Acute, NOS	410.9		
Degenerative Arthritis		Organic Brain Syndrome	310.9		
(Specify Site) _____	715.9	Otitis Externa, Acute NOS	380.10		

ABN: I UNDERSTAND THAT MEDICARE PROBABLY WILL NOT COVER THE SERVICES LISTED BELOW

A. _____ B. _____ C. _____

Date _____   Patient Signature _____

Doctor's Signature *D.J. Schwartz*

RETURN: _____ Days 3 Weeks _____ Months _____

REF# 122949 SB (05.07.09)   TO REORDER CALL INHEALTH RECORD SYSTEMS 800-477-7374

DOUGLASVILLE MEDICINE ASSOCIATES
5076 BRAND BLVD., SUITE 401
DOUGLASVILLE, NY 01234
PHONE No. (123) 456-7890

❏ L.D. HEATH, M.D.   ☒ D.J. SCHWARTZ, M.D.
NPI# 9995010111   NPI# 9995020212
EIN# 00-1234560

SOURCE DOCUMENT 6-2

PLEASE RETURN THIS FORM TO RECEPTIONIST

NAME Montner, Martin

2333

PLACE OF SERVICE:	(X) OFFICE	( ) NEW YORK COUNTY HOSPITAL	( ) RETIREMENT INN NURSING HOME	
	( ) COMMUNITY GENERAL HOSPITAL	( ) _____		**DATE OF SERVICE** 10/22/09

A. OFFICE VISITS - New Patient

Code	History	Exam	Dec.	Time	
___ 99201	Prob. Foc.	Prob. Foc.	Straight	10 min.	___
___ 99202	Ex. Prob. Foc.	Ex. Prob. Foc.	Straight	20 min.	___
___ 99203	Detail	Detail	Low	30 min.	___
X 99204	Comp.	Comp.	Mod.	45 min.	034.0
___ 99205	Comp.	Comp.	High	60 min.	___

B. OFFICE VISIT - Established Patient

Code	History	Exam	Dec.	Time	
___ 99211	Minimal	Minimal	Minimal	5 min.	___
___ 99212	Prob. Foc.	Prob. Foc.	Straight	10 min.	___
___ 99213	Ex. Prob. Foc.	Ex. Prob. Foc.	Low	15 min.	___
___ 99214	Detail	Detail	Mod.	25 min.	___
___ 99215	Comp.	Comp.	High	40 min.	___

C. HOSPITAL CARE   Dx Units

1. Initial Hospital Care (30 min) ___ ___ 99221 ___
2. Subsequent Care ___ ___ 99231 ___
3. Critical Care (30-74 min) ___ ___ 99291 ___
4. each additional 30 min. ___ ___ 99292 ___
5. Discharge Services ___ ___ 99238 ___
6. Emergency Room ___ ___ 99282 ___

D. NURSING HOME CARE

	Dx	Units
Initial Care - New Pt.		
1. Expanded	___	99322
2. Detailed	___	99323
Subsequent Care - Estab. Pt.		
3. Problem Focused	___	99307
4. Expanded	___	99308
5. Detailed	___	99309
5. Comprehensive	___	99310

E. PROCEDURES

1. Arthrocentesis, Small Jt. ___ 20600 ___
2. Colonoscopy ___ 45378 ___
3. EKG w/interpretation ___ 93000 ___
4. X-Ray Chest, PA/LAT ___ 71020 ___

F. LAB

1. Blood Sugar ___ 82947 ___
2. CBC w/differential ___ 85031 ___
3. Cholesterol ___ 82465 ___
4. Comprehensive Metabolic Panel ___ 80053 ___
5. ESR ___ 85651 ___
6. Hematocrit ___ 85014 ___
7. Mono Screen ___ 86308 ___
8. Pap Smear ___ 88150 ___
9. Potassium ___ 84132 ___
10. Preg. Test, Quantitative ___ 84702 ___
11. Routine Venipuncture ___ 36415 ___

F. Cont'd   Dx   Units

		Dx		Units
12. Strep Screen	034.0	87081	1
13. UA, Routine w/Micro	___	81000	___
14. UA, Routine w/o Micro	___	81002	___
15. Uric Acid	___	84550	___
16. VDRL	___	86592	___
17. Wet Prep	___	82710	___
18. _____	___		___

G. INJECTIONS

1. Influenza Virus Vaccine ___ 90658 ___
2. Pneumoccocal Vaccine ___ 90772 ___
3. Tetanus Toxoids ___ 90703 ___
4. Therapeutic Subcut/IM ___ 90732 ___
5. Vaccine Administration ___ 90471 ___
6. Vaccine - each additional ___ 90472 ___

H. MISCELLANEOUS

1. _____ ___
2. _____ ___

AMOUNT PAID $ 10.00

Mark diagnosis with
(1=Primary, 2=Secondary, 3=Tertiary)

DIAGNOSIS NOT LISTED BELOW ___ 034.0 Strep Throat

DIAGNOSIS	ICD-9-CM 1, 2, 3	DIAGNOSIS	ICD-9-CM 1, 2, 3	DIAGNOSIS	ICD-9-CM 1, 2, 3
Abdominal Pain	789.0 ___	Dehydration	276.51 ___	Otitis Media, Acute NOS	382.9 ___
Allergic Rhinitis, Unspec.	477.9 ___	Depression, NOS	311 ___	Peptic Ulcer Disease	536.9 ___
Angina Pectoris, Unspec.	413.9 ___	Diabetes Mellitus, Type II Controlled	250.00 ___	Peripheral Vascular Disease NOS	443.9 ___
Anemia, Iron Deficiency, Unspec.	280.9 ___	Diabetes Mellitus, Type II Controlled	250.02 ___	Pharyngitis, Acute	462 ___
Anemia, NOS	285.9 ___	Drug Reaction, NOS	995.29 ___	Pneumonia, Organism Unspec.	486 ___
Anemia, Pernicious	281.0 ___	Dysuria	788.1 ___	Prostatitis, NOS	601.9 ___
Asthma w/ Exacerbation	493.92 ___	Eczema, NOS	692.2 ___	PVC	427.69 ___
Asthmatic Bronchitis, Unspec.	493.90 ___	Edema	782.3 ___	Rash, Non Specific	782.1 ___
Atrial Fibrillation	427.31 ___	Fever, Unknown Origin	780.6 ___	Seizure Disorder NOS	780.39 ___
Atypical Chest Pain, Unspec.	786.59 ___	Gastritis, Acute w/o Hemorrhage	535.00 ___	Serous Otitis Media, Chronic, Unspec.	381.10 ___
Bronchiolitis, due to RSV	466.11 ___	Gastroenteritis, NOS	558.9 ___	Sinusitis, Acute NOS	461.9 ___
Bronchitis, Acute	466.0 ___	Gastroesophageal Reflux	530.81 ___	Tonsillitis, Acute	463. ___
Bronchitis, NOS	490 ___	Hepatitis A, Infectious	070.1 ___	Upper Respiratory Infection, Acute NOS	465.9 ___
Cardiac Arrest	427.5 ___	Hypercholesterolemia, Pure	272.0 ___	Urinary Tract Infection, Unspec.	599.0 ___
Cardiopulmonary Disease, Chronic, Unspec.	416.9 ___	Hypertension, Unspec.	401.9 ___	Urticaria, Unspec.	708.9 ___
Cellulitis, NOS	682.9 ___	Hypoglycemia NOS	251.2 ___	Vertigo, NOS	780.4 ___
Congestive Heart Failure, Unspec.	428.0 ___	Hypokalemia	276.8 ___	Viral Infection NOS	079.99 ___
Contact Dermatitis NOS	692.9 ___	Impetigo	684 ___	Weakness, Generalized	780.79 ___
COPD NOS	496 ___	Lymphadenitis, Unspec.	289.3 ___	Weight Loss, Abnormal	783.21 ___
CVA, Acute, NOS	434.91 ___	Mononucleosis	075 ___		
CVA, Old or Healed	438.9 ___	Myocardial Infarction, Acute, NOS	410.9 ___		
Degenerative Arthritis (Specify Site)	715.9 ___	Organic Brain Syndrome	310.9 ___		
		Otitis Externa, Acute NOS	380.10 ___		

ABN: I UNDERSTAND THAT MEDICARE PROBABLY WILL NOT COVER THE SERVICES LISTED BELOW

A. _____ B. _____ C. _____

Patient

Date _____ Signature _____

Doctor's Signature D.J. Schwartz

RETURN: 5-7 Days ___ Weeks ___ Months ___

DOUGLASVILLE MEDICINE ASSOCIATES
5076 BRAND BLVD., SUITE 401
DOUGLASVILLE, NY 01234
PHONE No. (123) 456-7890

❑ L.D. HEATH, M.D.   ☒ D.J. SCHWARTZ, M.D.
NPI# 9995010111   NPI# 9995020212
EIN# 00-1234560

REF# 122949 SB (05.07.09)   TO REORDER CALL INHEALTH RECORD SYSTEMS 800-477-7374

Superbill for Martin Montner. *Used with permission. InHealth Record Systems, Inc. 5076 Winters Chapel Road, Atlanta, GA 30360, 800-477-7374. http://www.inhealthrecords.com*

SOURCE DOCUMENT 6-3

PLEASE RETURN THIS FORM TO RECEPTIONIST	NAME *Conway, John*
	2334

PLACE OF SERVICE:
(X) OFFICE   ( ) RETIREMENT INN NURSING HOME
( ) NEW YORK COUNTY HOSPITAL
( ) COMMUNITY GENERAL HOSPITAL   ( ) _____

DATE OF SERVICE *10/23/09*

A. OFFICE VISITS - New Patient

Code	History	Exam	Dec.	Time	
___ 99201	Prob. Foc.	Prob. Foc.	Straight	10 min.	_____
___ 99202	Ex. Prob. Foc.	Ex. Prob. Foc.	Straight	20 min.	_____
___ 99203	Detail	Detail	Low	30 min.	_____
___ 99204	Comp.	Comp.	Mod.	45 min.	_____
___ 99205	Comp.	Comp.	High	60 min.	_____

B. OFFICE VISIT - Established Patient

Code	History	Exam	Dec.	Time	
___ 99211	Minimal	Minimal		5 min.	_____
___ 99212	Prob. Foc.	Prob. Foc.	Straight	10min.	_____
___ 99213	Ex. Prob. Foc.	Ex. Prob. Foc.	Low	15 min.	_____
X 99214	Detail	Detail	Mod.	25 min.	*1,2*
___ 99215	Comp.	Comp.	High	40 min.	_____

C. HOSPITAL CARE

	Dx	Units	
1. Initial Hospital Care (30 min)	___ ___	99221	_____
2. Subsequent Care	___ ___	99231	_____
3. Critical Care (30-74 min)	___ ___	99291	_____
4. each additional 30 min.	___ ___	99292	_____
5. Discharge Services	___ ___	99238	_____
6. Emergency Room	___ ___	99282	_____

D. NURSING HOME CARE

	Dx	Units	
Initial Care - New Pt.			
1. Expanded	___	99322	_____
2. Detailed	___	99323	_____
Subsequent Care - Estab. Pt.			
3. Problem Focused	___	99307	_____
4. Expanded	___	99308	_____
5. Detailed	___	99309	_____
5. Comprehensive	___	99310	_____

E. PROCEDURES

1. Arthrocentesis, Small Jt. ____	20600	_____
2. Colonoscopy	45378	_____
3. EKG w/interpretation ____	93000	_____
4. X-Ray Chest, PA/LAT ____	71020	_____

F. LAB

1. Blood Sugar	___	82947	_____
2. CBC w/differential	*2*	85031	X
3. Cholesterol		82465	_____
4. Comprehensive Metabolic Panel	___	80053	_____
5. ESR	___	85651	_____
6. Hematocrit	___	85014	_____
7. Mono Screen	___	86308	_____
8. Pap Smear	___	88150	_____
9. Potassium	___	84132	_____
10. Preg. Test, Quantitative	___	84702	_____
11. Routine Venipuncture	___	36415	_____

F. Cont'd

		Dx	Units	
12. Strep Screen		____	87081	_____
13. UA, Routine w/Micro		____	81000	_____
14. UA, Routine w/o Micro		____	81002	_____
15. Uric Acid		____	84550	_____
16. VDRL		____	86592	_____
17. Wet Prep		____	82710	_____
18.				

G. INJECTIONS

1. Influenza Virus Vaccine	____	90658	_____
2. Pneumoccocal Vaccine	____	90772	_____
3. Tetanus Toxoids	____	90703	_____
4. Therapeutic Subcut/IM	____	90732	_____
5. Vaccine Administration	____	90471	_____
6. Vaccine - each additional	____	90472	_____

H. MISCELLANEOUS

1. _____ ____ _____
2. _____ ____ _____

AMOUNT PAID $ *0*

Mark diagnosis with (1=Primary, 2=Secondary, 3=Tertiary)

DIAGNOSIS NOT LISTED BELOW _____

DIAGNOSIS	ICD-9-CM 1, 2, 3	DIAGNOSIS	ICD-9-CM 1, 2, 3	DIAGNOSIS	ICD-9-CM 1, 2, 3
Abdominal Pain	789.00 *1*	Dehydration	276.51 ___	Otitis Media, Acute NOS	382.9 ___
Allergic Rhinitis, Unspec.	477.9 ___	Depression, NOS	311 ___	Peptic Ulcer Disease	536.9 ___
Angina Pectoris, Unspec.	413.9 ___	Diabetes Mellitus, Type II Controlled	250.00 ___	Peripheral Vascular Disease NOS	443.9 ___
Anemia, Iron Deficiency, Unspec.	280.9 ___	Diabetes Mellitus, Type II Controlled	250.02 ___	Pharyngitis, Acute	462 ___
Anemia, NOS	285.9 ___	Drug Reaction, NOS	995.29 ___	Pneumonia, Organism Unspec.	486 ___
Anemia, Pernicious	281.0 ___	Dysuria	788.1 ___	Prostatitis, NOS	601.9 ___
Asthma w/ Exacerbation	493.92 ___	Eczema, NOS	692.2 ___	PVC	427.69 ___
Asthmatic Bronchitis, Unspec.	493.90 ___	Edema	782.3 ___	Rash, Non Specific	782.1 ___
Atrial Fibrillation	427.31 ___	Fever, Unknown Origin	780.6 *2*	Seizure Disorder NOS	780.39 ___
Atypical Chest Pain, Unspec.	786.59 ___	Gastritis, Acute w/o Hemorrhage	535.00 ___	Serous Otitis Media, Chronic, Unspec.	381.10 ___
Bronchiolitis, due to RSV	466.11 ___	Gastroenteritis, NOS	558.9 ___	Sinusitis, Acute NOS	461.9 ___
Bronchitis, Acute	466.0 ___	Gastroesophageal Reflux	530.81 ___	Tonsillitis, Acute	463. ___
Bronchitis, NOS	490 ___	Hepatitis A, Infectious	070.1 ___	Upper Respiratory Infection, Acute NOS	465.9 ___
Cardiac Arrest	427.5 ___	Hypercholesterolemia, Pure	272.0 ___	Urinary Tract Infection, Unspec.	599.0 ___
Cardiopulmonary Disease, Chronic, Unspec.	416.9 ___	Hypertension, Unspec.	401.9 ___	Urticaria, Unspec.	708.9 ___
Cellulitis, NOS	682.9 ___	Hypoglycemia NOS	251.2 ___	Vertigo, NOS	780.4 ___
Congestive Heart Failure, Unspec.	428.0 ___	Hypokalemia	276.8 ___	Viral Infection NOS	079.99 ___
Contact Dermatitis NOS	692.9 ___	Impetigo	684 ___	Weakness, Generalized	780.79 ___
COPD NOS	496 ___	Lymphadenitis, Unspec.	289.3 ___	Weight Loss, Abnormal	783.21 ___
CVA, Acute, NOS	434.91 ___	Mononucleosis	075 ___		
CVA, Old or Healed	438.9 ___	Myocardial Infarction, Acute, NOS	410.9 ___		
Degenerative Arthritis (Specify Site)	715.9 ___	Organic Brain Syndrome	310.9 ___		
		Otitis Externa, Acute NOS	380.10 ___		

ABN: I UNDERSTAND THAT MEDICARE PROBABLY WILL NOT COVER THE SERVICES LISTED BELOW

A. _____ B. _____ C. _____
                             Patient

Date _____ Signature _____

Doctor's Signature *LD Heath*

RETURN: *3* Days _____ Weeks _____ Months

DOUGLASVILLE MEDICINE ASSOCIATES
5076 BRAND BLVD., SUITE 401
DOUGLASVILLE, NY 01234
PHONE No. (123) 456-7890

☒ L.D. HEATH, M.D.   ❑ D.J. SCHWARTZ, M.D.
NPI# 9995010111   NPI# 9995020212
EIN# 00-1234560

REF# 122949 SB (05.07.09)   TO REORDER CALL INHEALTH RECORD SYSTEMS 800-477-7374

Superbill for John Conway. *Used with permission. InHealth Record Systems, Inc. 5076 Winters Chapel Road, Atlanta, GA 30360, 800-477-7374. http://www.inhealthrecords.com*

SOURCE DOCUMENT 6-4

PLEASE RETURN THIS FORM TO RECEPTIONIST	NAME Shektar, Paula

2335

PLACE OF SERVICE:
(X) OFFICE
( ) NEW YORK COUNTY HOSPITAL
( ) COMMUNITY GENERAL HOSPITAL
( ) RETIREMENT INN NURSING HOME
( ) _____

DATE OF SERVICE 10/23/09

A. OFFICE VISITS - New Patient

Code	History	Exam	Dec.	Time	
___ 99201	Prob. Foc.	Prob. Foc.	Straight	10 min.	_____
___ 99202	Ex. Prob. Foc.	Ex. Prob. Foc.	Straight	20 min.	_____
___ 99203	Detail	Detail	Low	30 min.	_____
___ 99204	Comp.	Comp.	Mod.	45 min.	_____
___ 99205	Comp.	Comp.	High	60 min.	_____

B. OFFICE VISIT - Established Patient

Code	History	Exam	Dec.	Time	
___ 99211	Minimal	Minimal	Minimal	5 min.	_____
___ 99212	Prob. Foc.	Prob. Foc.	Straight	10min.	_____
___ 99213	Ex. Prob. Foc.	Ex. Prob. Foc.	Low	15 min.	_____
X 99214	Detail	Detail	Mod.	25 min.	1
___ 99215	Comp.	Comp.	High	40 min.	_____

C. HOSPITAL CARE   Dx Units

1. Initial Hospital Care (30 min) ____ ___ 99221 _____
2. Subsequent Care ____ ___ 99231 _____
3. Critical Care (30-74 min) ____ ___ 99291 _____
4. each additional 30 min. ____ ___ 99292 _____
5. Discharge Services ____ ___ 99238 _____
6. Emergency Room ____ ___ 99282 _____

D. NURSING HOME CARE
                                        Dx Units

Initial Care - New Pt.
1. Expanded ____ 99322 _____
2. Detailed ____ 99323 _____

Subsequent Care - Estab. Pt.
3. Problem Focused ____ 99307 _____
4. Expanded ____ 99308 _____
5. Detailed ____ 99309 _____
5. Comprehensive ____ 99310 _____

E. PROCEDURES
1. Arthrocentesis, Small Jt. ____ 20600 _____
2. Colonoscopy ____ 45378 _____
3. EKG w/interpretation ____ 93000 _____
4. X-Ray Chest, PA/LAT ____ 71020 _____

F. LAB
1. Blood Sugar ____ 82947 _____
2. CBC w/differential ____ 85031 _____
3. Cholesterol ____ 82465 _____
4. Comprehensive Metabolic Panel ____ 80053 _____
5. ESR ____ 85651 _____
6. Hematocrit ____ 85014 _____
7. Mono Screen ____ 86308 _____
8. Pap Smear ____ 88150 _____
9. Potassium ____ 84132 _____
10. Preg. Test, Quantitative ____ 84702 _____
11. Routine Venipuncture ____ 36415 _____

F. Cont'd   Dx Units
12. Strep Screen ____ 87081 _____
13. UA, Routine w/Micro ____ 81000 _____
14. UA, Routine w/o Micro ____ 81002 _____
15. Uric Acid ____ 84550 _____
16. VDRL ____ 86592 _____
17. Wet Prep ____ 82710 _____
18. _____ ____ ____ _____

G. INJECTIONS
1. Influenza Virus Vaccine ____ 90658 _____
2. Pneumoccocal Vaccine ____ 90772 _____
3. Tetanus Toxoids ____ 90703 _____
4. Therapeutic Subcut/IM ____ 90732 _____
5. Vaccine Administration ____ 90471 _____
6. Vaccine - each additional ____ 90472 _____

H. MISCELLANEOUS
1. _____ ____ _____
2. _____ ____ _____

AMOUNT PAID $ _____

Mark diagnosis with (1=Primary, 2=Secondary, 3=Tertiary)	DIAGNOSIS NOT LISTED BELOW _____

DIAGNOSIS	ICD-9-CM 1, 2, 3	DIAGNOSIS	ICD-9-CM 1, 2, 3	DIAGNOSIS	ICD-9-CM 1, 2, 3
Abdominal Pain	789.0	Dehydration	276.51	Otitis Media, Acute NOS	382.9
Allergic Rhinitis, Unspec.	477.9	Depression, NOS	311	Peptic Ulcer Disease	536.9
Angina Pectoris, Unspec.	413.9	Diabetes Mellitus, Type II Controlled	250.00	Peripheral Vascular Disease NOS	443.9
Anemia, Iron Deficiency, Unspec.	280.9	Diabetes Mellitus, Type II Controlled	250.02	Pharyngitis, Acute	462
Anemia, NOS	285.9	Drug Reaction, NOS	995.29	Pneumonia, Organism Unspec.	486
Anemia, Pernicious	281.0	Dysuria	788.1	Prostatitis, NOS	601.9
Asthma w/ Exacerbation	493.92	Eczema, NOS	692.2	PVC	427.69
Asthmatic Bronchitis, Unspec.	493.90	Edema	782.3	Rash, Non Specific	782.1
Atrial Fibrillation	427.31	Fever, Unknown Origin	780.6	Seizure Disorder NOS	780.39
Atypical Chest Pain, Unspec.	786.59	Gastritis, Acute w/o Hemorrhage	535.00	Serous Otitis Media, Chronic, Unspec.	381.10
Bronchiolitis, due to RSV	466.11	Gastroenteritis, NOS	558.9	Sinusitis, Acute NOS	461.9
Bronchitis, Acute	466.0	Gastroesophageal Reflux	530.81	Tonsillitis, Acute	463.
Bronchitis, NOS	490	Hepatitis A, Infectious	070.1	Upper Respiratory Infection, Acute NOS	465.9
Cardiac Arrest	427.5	Hypercholesterolemia, Pure	272.0	Urinary Tract Infection, Unspec.	599.0
Cardiopulmonary Disease, Chronic, Unspec.	416.9	Hypertension, Unspec.	401.9	Urticaria, Unspec.	708.9
Cellulitis, NOS	682.9	Hypoglycemia NOS	251.2	Vertigo, NOS	780.4
Congestive Heart Failure, Unspec.	428.0 1	Hypokalemia	276.8	Viral Infection NOS	079.99
Contact Dermatitis NOS	692.9	Impetigo	684	Weakness, Generalized	780.79
COPD NOS	496	Lymphadenitis, Unspec.	289.3	Weight Loss, Abnormal	783.21
CVA, Acute, NOS	434.91	Mononucleosis	075		
CVA, Old or Healed	438.9	Myocardial Infarction, Acute, NOS	410.9		
Degenerative Arthritis		Organic Brain Syndrome	310.9		
(Specify Site) _____	715.9	Otitis Externa, Acute NOS	380.10		

ABN: I UNDERSTAND THAT MEDICARE PROBABLY WILL NOT COVER THE SERVICES LISTED BELOW

A. _____ B. _____ C. _____

                Patient
Date _____ Signature _____

Doctor's
Signature   *D.J. Schwartz*

RETURN: _____ Days _____ Weeks   1   Months _____

DOUGLASVILLE MEDICINE ASSOCIATES
5076 BRAND BLVD., SUITE 401
DOUGLASVILLE, NY 01234
PHONE No. (123) 456-7890
☐ L.D. HEATH, M.D.   ☒ D.J. SCHWARTZ, M.D.
NPI# 9995010111   NPI# 9995020212
EIN# 00-1234560

REF# 122949 SB (05.07.09)   TO REORDER CALL INHEALTH RECORD SYSTEMS 800-477-7374

Superbill for Paula Shektar. Used with permission. InHealth Record Systems, Inc. 5076 Winters Chapel Road, Atlanta, GA 30360, 800-477-7374. http://www.inhealthrecords.com

SOURCE DOCUMENT 6-5

<table>
<tr><td colspan="2">**PLEASE RETURN THIS FORM TO RECEPTIONIST**</td><td>NAME Villanova, Ricky</td></tr>
</table>

2336

PLACE OF SERVICE:
(X) OFFICE
( ) NEW YORK COUNTY HOSPITAL
( ) COMMUNITY GENERAL HOSPITAL
( ) RETIREMENT INN NURSING HOME
( ) _____

DATE OF SERVICE 10/27/09

A. OFFICE VISITS - New Patient

	Code	History	Exam	Dec.	Time	
X	99201	Prob. Foc.	Prob. Foc.	Straight	10 min.	1
	99202	Ex. Prob. Foc.	Ex. Prob. Foc.	Straight	20 min.	
	99203	Detail	Detail	Low	30 min.	
	99204	Comp.	Comp.	Mod.	45 min.	
	99205	Comp.	Comp.	High	60 min.	

B. OFFICE VISIT - Established Patient

Code	History	Exam	Dec.	Time	
99211	Minimal	Minimal	Minimal	5 min.	
99212	Prob. Foc.	Prob. Foc.	Straight	10min.	
99213	Ex. Prob. Foc.	Ex. Prob. Foc.	Low	15 min.	
99214	Detail	Detail	Mod.	25 min.	
99215	Comp.	Comp.	High	40 min.	

C. HOSPITAL CARE   Dx Units

1.	Initial Hospital Care (30 min)		99221	
2.	Subsequent Care		99231	
3.	Critical Care (30-74 min)		99291	
4.	each additional 30 min.		99292	
5.	Discharge Services		99238	
6.	Emergency Room		99282	

D. NURSING HOME CARE   Dx   Units

Initial Care - New Pt.

1.	Expanded		99322
2.	Detailed		99323

Subsequent Care - Estab. Pt.

3.	Problem Focused		99307
4.	Expanded		99308
5.	Detailed		99309
5.	Comprehensive		99310

E. PROCEDURES

1.	Arthrocentesis, Small Jt.		20600
2.	Colonoscopy		45378
3.	EKG w/interpretation		93000
4.	X-Ray Chest, PA/LAT		71020

F. LAB

1.	Blood Sugar	1	82947	X
2.	CBC w/differential		85031	
3.	Cholesterol		82465	
4.	Comprehensive Metabolic Panel		80053	
5.	ESR		85651	
6.	Hematocrit		85014	
7.	Mono Screen		86308	
8.	Pap Smear		88150	
9.	Potassium		84132	
10.	Preg. Test, Quantitative		84702	
11.	Routine Venipuncture		36415	

F. Cont'd   Dx   Units

12.	Strep Screen		87081
13.	UA, Routine w/Micro		81000
14.	UA, Routine w/o Micro		81002
15.	Uric Acid		84550
16.	VDRL		86592
17.	Wet Prep		82710
18.	_____		_____

G. INJECTIONS

1.	Influenza Virus Vaccine		90658
2.	Pneumoccocal Vaccine		90772
3.	Tetanus Toxoids		90703
4.	Therapeutic Subcut/IM		90732
5.	Vaccine Administration		90471
6.	Vaccine - each additional		90472

H. MISCELLANEOUS

1. _____
2. _____

AMOUNT PAID $ 10.00

Mark diagnosis with (1=Primary, 2=Secondary, 3=Tertiary)

DIAGNOSIS NOT LISTED BELOW _____

DIAGNOSIS	ICD-9-CM 1, 2, 3	DIAGNOSIS	ICD-9-CM 1, 2, 3	DIAGNOSIS	ICD-9-CM 1, 2, 3
Abdominal Pain	789.0	Dehydration	276.51	Otitis Media, Acute NOS	382.9
Allergic Rhinitis, Unspec.	477.9	Depression, NOS	311	Peptic Ulcer Disease	536.9
Angina Pectoris, Unspec.	413.9	Diabetes Mellitus, Type II Controlled	250.00 1	Peripheral Vascular Disease NOS	443.9
Anemia, Iron Deficiency, Unspec.	280.9	Diabetes Mellitus, Type II Controlled	250.02	Pharyngitis, Acute	462
Anemia, NOS	285.9	Drug Reaction, NOS	995.29	Pneumonia, Organism Unspec.	486
Anemia, Pernicious	281.0	Dysuria	788.1	Prostatitis, NOS	601.9
Asthma w/ Exacerbation	493.92	Eczema, NOS	692.2	PVC	427.69
Asthmatic Bronchitis, Unspec.	493.90	Edema	782.3	Rash, Non Specific	782.1
Atrial Fibrillation	427.31	Fever, Unknown Origin	780.6	Seizure Disorder NOS	780.39
Atypical Chest Pain, Unspec.	786.59	Gastritis, Acute w/o Hemorrhage	535.00	Serous Otitis Media, Chronic, Unspec.	381.10
Bronchiolitis, due to RSV	466.11	Gastroenteritis, NOS	558.9	Sinusitis, Acute NOS	461.9
Bronchitis, Acute	466.0	Gastroesophageal Reflux	530.81	Tonsillitis, Acute	463.
Bronchitis, NOS	490	Hepatitis A, Infectious	070.1	Upper Respiratory Infection, Acute NOS	465.9
Cardiac Arrest	427.5	Hypercholesterolemia, Pure	272.0	Urinary Tract Infection, Unspec.	599.0
Cardiopulmonary Disease, Chronic, Unspec.	416.9	Hypertension, Unspec.	401.9	Urticaria, Unspec.	708.9
Cellulitis, NOS	682.9	Hypoglycemia NOS	251.2	Vertigo, NOS	780.4
Congestive Heart Failure, Unspec.	428.0	Hypokalemia	276.8	Viral Infection NOS	079.99
Contact Dermatitis NOS	692.9	Impetigo	684	Weakness, Generalized	780.79
COPD NOS	496	Lymphadenitis, Unspec.	289.3	Weight Loss, Abnormal	783.21
CVA, Acute, NOS	434.91	Mononucleosis	075		
CVA, Old or Healed	438.9	Myocardial Infarction, Acute, NOS	410.9		
Degenerative Arthritis		Organic Brain Syndrome	310.9		
(Specify Site)	715.9	Otitis Externa, Acute NOS	380.10		

ABN: I UNDERSTAND THAT MEDICARE PROBABLY WILL NOT COVER THE SERVICES LISTED BELOW

A. _____ B. _____ C. _____
Patient

Date _____ Signature _____

Doctor's Signature   D.J. Schwartz

RETURN: _____ Days _____ Weeks 1 Months _____

REF# 122949 SB (05.07.09)   TO REORDER CALL INHEALTH RECORD SYSTEMS 800-477-7374

DOUGLASVILLE MEDICINE ASSOCIATES
5076 BRAND BLVD., SUITE 401
DOUGLASVILLE, NY 01234
PHONE No. (123) 456-7890
❏ L.D. HEATH, M.D.   ☒ D.J. SCHWARTZ, M.D.
NPI# 9995010111   NPI# 9995020212
EIN# 00-1234560

Superbill for Ricky Villanova. Used with permission. InHealth Record Systems, Inc. 5076 Winters Chapel Road, Atlanta, GA 30360, 800-477-7374. http://www.inhealthrecords.com

SOURCE DOCUMENT 6-6

PLEASE RETURN THIS FORM TO RECEPTIONIST

NAME   Adams, Minnie

2337

PLACE OF SERVICE:
(X) OFFICE
( ) NEW YORK COUNTY HOSPITAL
( ) COMMUNITY GENERAL HOSPITAL
( ) RETIREMENT INN NURSING HOME
( ) _____

DATE OF SERVICE   10/28/09

A. OFFICE VISITS - New Patient

Code	History	Exam	Dec.	Time	
___ 99201	Prob. Foc.	Prob. Foc.	Straight	10 min.	
___ 99202	Ex. Prob. Foc.	Ex. Prob. Foc.	Straight	20 min.	___
X 99203	Detail	Detail	Low	30 min.	1
___ 99204	Comp.	Comp.	Mod.	45 min.	
___ 99205	Comp.	Comp.	High	60 min.	

B. OFFICE VISIT - Established Patient

Code	History	Exam	Dec.	Time	
___ 99211	Minimal	Minimal	Minimal	5 min.	
___ 99212	Prob. Foc.	Prob. Foc.	Straight	10 min.	
___ 99213	Ex. Prob. Foc.	Ex. Prob. Foc.	Low	15 min.	
___ 99214	Detail	Detail	Mod.	25 min.	
___ 99215	Comp.	Comp.	High	40 min.	

C. HOSPITAL CARE   Dx Units

1. Initial Hospital Care (30 min) ___ ___ 99221 ___
2. Subsequent Care ___ ___ 99231 ___
3. Critical Care (30-74 min) ___ ___ 99291 ___
4. each additional 30 min. ___ ___ 99292 ___
5. Discharge Services ___ ___ 99238 ___
6. Emergency Room ___ ___ 99282 ___

D. NURSING HOME CARE   Dx Units

Initial Care - New Pt.
1. Expanded ___ ___ 99322 ___
2. Detailed ___ ___ 99323 ___

Subsequent Care - Estab. Pt.
3. Problem Focused ___ ___ 99307 ___
4. Expanded ___ ___ 99308 ___
5. Detailed ___ ___ 99309 ___
5. Comprehensive ___ ___ 99310 ___

E. PROCEDURES

1. Arthrocentesis, Small Jt. ___ 20600
2. Colonoscopy ___ 45378
3. EKG w/interpretation ___ 93000
4. X-Ray Chest, PA/LAT ___ 71020

F. LAB

1. Blood Sugar ___ 82947 ___
2. CBC w/differential ___ 85031 ___
3. Cholesterol ___ 82465 ___
4. Comprehensive Metabolic Panel 1 80053 X ___
5. ESR ___ 85651 ___
6. Hematocrit ___ 85014 ___
7. Mono Screen ___ 86308 ___
8. Pap Smear ___ 88150 ___
9. Potassium ___ 84132 ___
10. Preg. Test, Quantitative ___ 84702 ___
11. Routine Venipuncture 1 36415 X

F. Cont'd   Dx Units

12. Strep Screen ___ 87081 ___
13. UA, Routine w/Micro ___ 81000 ___
14. UA, Routine w/o Micro ___ 81002 ___
15. Uric Acid ___ 84550 ___
16. VDRL ___ 86592 ___
17. Wet Prep ___ 82710 ___
18. ___ ___ ___

G. INJECTIONS

1. Influenza Virus Vaccine ___ 90658 ___
2. Pneumoccocal Vaccine ___ 90772 ___
3. Tetanus Toxoids ___ 90703 ___
4. Therapeutic Subcut/IM ___ 90732 ___
5. Vaccine Administration ___ 90471 ___
6. Vaccine - each additional ___ 90472 ___

H. MISCELLANEOUS

1. _____ ___
2. _____ ___

AMOUNT PAID $ _____

Mark diagnosis with
(1=Primary, 2=Secondary, 3=Tertiary)

DIAGNOSIS NOT LISTED BELOW _____

DIAGNOSIS	ICD-9-CM 1, 2, 3	DIAGNOSIS	ICD-9-CM 1, 2, 3	DIAGNOSIS	ICD-9-CM 1, 2, 3
Abdominal Pain	789.0 ___	Dehydration	276.51 ___	Otitis Media, Acute NOS	382.9 ___
Allergic Rhinitis, Unspec.	477.9 ___	Depression, NOS	311 ___	Peptic Ulcer Disease	536.9 ___
Angina Pectoris, Unspec.	413.9 ___	Diabetes Mellitus, Type II Controlled	250.00 ___	Peripheral Vascular Disease NOS	443.9 ___
Anemia, Iron Deficiency, Unspec.	280.9 ___	Diabetes Mellitus, Type II Controlled	250.02 ___	Pharyngitis, Acute	462 ___
Anemia, NOS	285.9 ___	Drug Reaction, NOS	995.29 ___	Pneumonia, Organism Unspec.	486 ___
Anemia, Pernicious	281.0 ___	Dysuria	788.1 ___	Prostatitis, NOS	601.9 ___
Asthma w/ Exacerbation	493.92 ___	Eczema, NOS	692.2 ___	PVC	427.69 ___
Asthmatic Bronchitis, Unspec.	493.90 ___	Edema	782.3 ___	Rash, Non Specific	782.1 ___
Atrial Fibrillation	427.31 ___	Fever, Unknown Origin	780.6 ___	Seizure Disorder NOS	780.39 ___
Atypical Chest Pain, Unspec.	786.59 ___	Gastritis, Acute w/o Hemorrhage	535.00 ___	Serous Otitis Media, Chronic, Unspec.	381.10 ___
Bronchiolitis, due to RSV	466.11 ___	Gastroenteritis, NOS	558.9 ___	Sinusitis, Acute NOS	461.9 ___
Bronchitis, Acute	466.0 ___	Gastroesophageal Reflux	530.81 ___	Tonsillitis, Acute	463. ___
Bronchitis, NOS	490 ___	Hepatitis A, Infectious	070.1 ___	Upper Respiratory Infection, Acute NOS	465.9 ___
Cardiac Arrest	427.5 ___	Hypercholesterolemia, Pure	272.0 ___	Urinary Tract Infection, Unspec.	599.0 ___
Cardiopulmonary Disease, Chronic, Unspec.	416.9 ___	Hypertension, Unspec.	401.9 ___	Urticaria, Unspec.	708.9 ___
Cellulitis, NOS	682.9 ___	Hypoglycemia NOS	251.2 ___	Vertigo, NOS	780.4 ___
Congestive Heart Failure, Unspec.	428.0 ___	Hypokalemia	276.8 ___	Viral Infection NOS	079.99 ___
Contact Dermatitis NOS	692.9 ___	Impetigo	684 ___	Weakness, Generalized	780.79 ___
COPD NOS	496 ___	Lymphadenitis, Unspec.	289.3 ___	Weight Loss, Abnormal	783.21 ___
CVA, Acute, NOS	434.91 ___	Mononucleosis	075 ___		
CVA, Old or Healed	438.9 1	Myocardial Infarction, Acute, NOS	410.9 ___		
Degenerative Arthritis		Organic Brain Syndrome	310.9 ___		
(Specify Site)	715.9 ___	Otitis Externa, Acute NOS	380.10 ___		

ABN: I UNDERSTAND THAT MEDICARE PROBABLY WILL NOT COVER THE SERVICES LISTED BELOW

A. _____ B. _____ C. _____
                     Patient
Date _____   Signature _____

Doctor's Signature   LD Heath

RETURN: _____ Days _____ Weeks   PRN   Months

REF# 122949 SB (05.07.09)   TO REORDER CALL INHEALTH RECORD SYSTEMS 800-477-7374

DOUGLASVILLE MEDICINE ASSOCIATES
5076 BRAND BLVD., SUITE 401
DOUGLASVILLE, NY 01234
PHONE No. (123) 456-7890
(X) L.D. HEATH, M.D.   ( ) D.J. SCHWARTZ, M.D.
NPI# 9995010111   NPI# 9995020212
EIN# 00-1234560

SOURCE DOCUMENT 6-7

PLEASE RETURN THIS FORM TO RECEPTIONIST	NAME Worthington, Cynthia

2339

PLACE OF SERVICE:
(X) OFFICE
( ) NEW YORK COUNTY HOSPITAL
( ) COMMUNITY GENERAL HOSPITAL
( ) RETIREMENT INN NURSING HOME
( ) _____

DATE OF SERVICE __10/30/09__

A. OFFICE VISITS - New Patient

Code	History	Exam	Dec.	Time	
___ 99201	Prob. Foc.	Prob. Foc.	Straight	10 min.	_____
___ 99202	Ex. Prob. Foc.	Ex. Prob. Foc.	Straight	20 min.	_____
___ 99203	Detail	Detail	Low	30 min.	_____
___ 99204	Comp.	Comp.	Mod.	45 min.	_____
___ 99205	Comp.	Comp.	High	60 min.	_____

B. OFFICE VISIT - Established Patient

Code	History	Exam	Dec.	Time	
___ 99211	Minimal	Minimal		5 min.	_____
___ 99212	Prob. Foc.	Prob. Foc.	Straight	10 min.	_____
X 99213	Ex. Prob. Foc.	Ex. Prob. Foc.	Low	15 min.	1
___ 99214	Detail	Detail	Mod.	25 min.	_____
___ 99215	Comp.	Comp.	High	40 min.	_____

C. HOSPITAL CARE

		Dx	Units	
1.	Initial Hospital Care (30 min)	____	99221	_____
2.	Subsequent Care	____	99231	_____
3.	Critical Care (30-74 min)	____	99291	_____
4.	each additional 30 min.	____	99292	_____
5.	Discharge Services	____	99238	_____
6.	Emergency Room	____	99282	_____

D. NURSING HOME CARE

		Dx	Units	
Initial Care - New Pt.				
1.	Expanded	____	99322	_____
2.	Detailed	____	99323	_____
Subsequent Care - Estab. Pt.				
3.	Problem Focused	____	99307	_____
4.	Expanded	____	99308	_____
5.	Detailed	____	99309	_____
5.	Comprehensive	____	99310	_____

E. PROCEDURES

1.	Arthrocentesis, Small Jt.	____	20600
2.	Colonoscopy	____	45378
3.	EKG w/interpretation	____	93000
4.	X-Ray Chest, PA/LAT	____	71020

F. LAB

1.	Blood Sugar	____	82947
2.	CBC w/differential	____	85031
3.	Cholesterol	____	82465
4.	Comprehensive Metabolic Panel	____	80053
5.	ESR	____	85651
6.	Hematocrit	____	85014
7.	Mono Screen	____	86308
8.	Pap Smear	____	88150
9.	Potassium	____	84132
10.	Preg. Test, Quantitative	____	84702
11.	Routine Venipuncture	____	36415

F. Cont'd

			Dx	Units	
12.	Strep Screen	____		87081	_____
13.	UA, Routine w/Micro	____		81000	_____
14.	UA, Routine w/o Micro	____		81002	_____
15.	Uric Acid	____		84550	_____
16.	VDRL	____		86592	_____
17.	Wet Prep	____		82710	_____
18.	_____	____		____	_____

G. INJECTIONS

1.	Influenza Virus Vaccine	____	90658
2.	Pneumoccocal Vaccine	____	90772
3.	Tetanus Toxoids	____	90703
4.	Therapeutic Subcut/IM	____	90732
5.	Vaccine Administration	____	90471
6.	Vaccine - each additional	____	90472

H. MISCELLANEOUS

1. _____ ____ _____
2. _____ ____ _____

AMOUNT PAID $ __20.00__

Mark diagnosis with (1=Primary, 2=Secondary, 3=Tertiary)	DIAGNOSIS NOT LISTED BELOW _____

DIAGNOSIS	ICD-9-CM 1, 2, 3	DIAGNOSIS	ICD-9-CM 1, 2, 3	DIAGNOSIS	ICD-9-CM 1, 2, 3
Abdominal Pain	789.0 ___	Dehydration	276.51 ___	Otitis Media, Acute NOS	382.9 ___
Allergic Rhinitis, Unspec.	477.9 ___	Depression, NOS	311 ___	Peptic Ulcer Disease	536.9 ___
Angina Pectoris, Unspec.	413.9 ___	Diabetes Mellitus, Type II Controlled	250.00 ___	Peripheral Vascular Disease NOS	443.9 ___
Anemia, Iron Deficiency, Unspec.	280.9 ___	Diabetes Mellitus, Type II Controlled	250.02 ___	Pharyngitis, Acute	462 ___
Anemia, NOS	285.9 ___	Drug Reaction, NOS	995.29 ___	Pneumonia, Organism Unspec.	486 ___
Anemia, Pernicious	281.0 ___	Dysuria	788.1 ___	Prostatitis, NOS	601.9 ___
Asthma w/ Exacerbation	493.92 ___	Eczema, NOS	692.2 ___	PVC	427.69 ___
Asthmatic Bronchitis, Unspec.	493.90 ___	Edema	782.3 ___	Rash, Non Specific	782.1 _1_
Atrial Fibrillation	427.31 ___	Fever, Unknown Origin	780.6 ___	Seizure Disorder NOS	780.39 ___
Atypical Chest Pain, Unspec.	786.59 ___	Gastritis, Acute w/o Hemorrhage	535.00 ___	Serous Otitis Media, Chronic, Unspec.	381.10 ___
Bronchiolitis, due to RSV	466.11 ___	Gastroenteritis, NOS	558.9 ___	Sinusitis, Acute NOS	461.9 ___
Bronchitis, Acute	466.0 ___	Gastroesophageal Reflux	530.81 ___	Tonsillitis, Acute	463. ___
Bronchitis, NOS	490 ___	Hepatitis A, Infectious	070.1 ___	Upper Respiratory Infection, Acute NOS	465.9 ___
Cardiac Arrest	427.5 ___	Hypercholesterolemia, Pure	272.0 ___	Urinary Tract Infection, Unspec.	599.0 ___
Cardiopulmonary Disease, Chronic, Unspec.	416.9 ___	Hypertension, Unspec.	401.9 ___	Urticaria, Unspec.	708.9 ___
Cellulitis, NOS	682.9 ___	Hypoglycemia NOS	251.2 ___	Vertigo, NOS	780.4 ___
Congestive Heart Failure, Unspec.	428.0 ___	Hypokalemia	276.8 ___	Viral Infection NOS	079.99 ___
Contact Dermatitis NOS	692.9 ___	Impetigo	684 ___	Weakness, Generalized	780.79 ___
COPD NOS	496 ___	Lymphadenitis, Unspec.	289.3 ___	Weight Loss, Abnormal	783.21 ___
CVA, Acute, NOS	434.91 ___	Mononucleosis	075 ___		
CVA, Old or Healed	438.9 ___	Myocardial Infarction, Acute, NOS	410.9 ___		
Degenerative Arthritis		Organic Brain Syndrome	310.9 ___		
(Specify Site)	715.9 ___	Otitis Externa, Acute NOS	380.10 ___		

ABN: I UNDERSTAND THAT MEDICARE PROBABLY WILL NOT COVER THE SERVICES LISTED BELOW

A. _____ B. _____ C. _____
Patient
Date _____ Signature _____

Doctor's Signature __LD Heath__

RETURN: _____ Days __1__ Weeks _____ Months _____

DOUGLASVILLE MEDICINE ASSOCIATES
5076 BRAND BLVD., SUITE 401
DOUGLASVILLE, NY 01234
PHONE No. (123) 456-7890
(X) L.D. HEATH, M.D.   ( ) D.J. SCHWARTZ, M.D.
NPI# 9995010111   NPI# 9995020212
EIN# 00-1234560

REF# 122949 SB (05.07.09)   TO REORDER CALL INHEALTH RECORD SYSTEMS 800-477-7374

SOURCE DOCUMENT 6-8

PLEASE RETURN THIS FORM TO RECEPTIONIST	NAME Zuhl, Rodney

2340

	(X) OFFICE	( ) RETIREMENT INN NURSING HOME
PLACE OF	( ) NEW YORK COUNTY HOSPITAL	
SERVICE:	( ) COMMUNITY GENERAL HOSPITAL	( ) _____ **DATE OF SERVICE** 10/30/09

A. OFFICE VISITS - New Patient

	Code	History	Exam	Dec.	Time	
____	99201	Prob. Foc.	Prob. Foc.	Straight	10 min.	____
____	99202	Ex. Prob. Foc.	Ex. Prob. Foc.	Straight	20 min.	____
X	99203	Detail	Detail	Low	30 min.	1
____	99204	Comp.	Comp.	Mod.	45 min.	____
____	99205	Comp.	Comp.	High	60 min.	____

B. OFFICE VISIT - Established Patient

	Code	History	Exam	Dec.	Time	
____	99211	Minimal	Minimal	Minimal	5 min.	____
____	99212	Prob. Foc.	Prob. Foc.	Straight	10min.	____
____	99213	Ex. Prob. Foc.	Ex. Prob. Foc.	Low	15 min.	____
____	99214	Detail	Detail	Mod.	25 min.	____
____	99215	Comp.	Comp.	High	40 min.	____

C. HOSPITAL CARE   Dx Units

1.	Initial Hospital Care (30 min)	____ ____	99221	____
2.	Subsequent Care	____ ____	99231	____
3.	Critical Care (30-74 min)	____ ____	99291	____
4.	each additional 30 min.	____ ____	99292	____
5.	Discharge Services	____ ____	99238	____
6.	Emergency Room	____ ____	99282	____

D. NURSING HOME CARE   Dx Units

Initial Care - New Pt.

1.	Expanded	____ ___	99322	____
2.	Detailed	____ ___	99323	____

Subsequent Care - Estab. Pt.

3.	Problem Focused	____ ___	99307	____
4.	Expanded	____ ___	99308	____
5.	Detailed	____ ___	99309	____
5.	Comprehensive	____ ___	99310	____

E. PROCEDURES

1.	Arthrocentesis, Small Jt.	____	20600	____
2.	Colonoscopy	____	45378	____
3.	EKG w/interpretation	____	93000	____
4.	X-Ray Chest, PA/LAT	____	71020	____

F. LAB

1.	Blood Sugar	____	82947	____
2.	CBC w/differential	____	85031	____
3.	Cholesterol	____	82465	____
4.	Comprehensive Metabolic Panel	____	80053	____
5.	ESR	____	85651	____
6.	Hematocrit	____	85014	____
7.	Mono Screen	____	86308	____
8.	Pap Smear	____	88150	____
9.	Potassium	____	84132	____
10.	Preg. Test, Quantitative	____	84702	____
11.	Routine Venipuncture	____	36415	____

F. Cont'd   Dx Units

12.	Strep Screen	____	87081	____
13.	UA, Routine w/Micro	1	81000	X
14.	UA, Routine w/o Micro	____	81002	____
15.	Uric Acid	____	84550	____
16.	VDRL	1	86592	X
17.	Wet Prep	____	82710	____
18.	_____	____	____	____

G. INJECTIONS

1.	Influenza Virus Vaccine	____	90658	____
2.	Pneumoccocal Vaccine	____	90772	____
3.	Tetanus Toxoids	____	90703	____
4.	Therapeutic Subcut/IM	____	90732	____
5.	Vaccine Administration	____	90471	____
6.	Vaccine - each additional	____	90472	____

H. MISCELLANEOUS

1. _____ ____ ____
2. _____ ____ ____

AMOUNT PAID $ 200.70

Mark diagnosis with (1=Primary, 2=Secondary, 3=Tertiary)

DIAGNOSIS NOT LISTED _____ BELOW _____

DIAGNOSIS	ICD-9-CM 1, 2, 3	DIAGNOSIS	ICD-9-CM 1, 2, 3	DIAGNOSIS	ICD-9-CM 1, 2, 3
Abdominal Pain	789.0_	Dehydration	276.51	Otitis Media, Acute NOS	382.9
Allergic Rhinitis, Unspec.	477.9	Depression, NOS	311	Peptic Ulcer Disease	536.9
Angina Pectoris, Unspec.	413.9	Diabetes Mellitus, Type II Controlled	250.00	Peripheral Vascular Disease NOS	443.9
Anemia, Iron Deficiency, Unspec.	280.9	Diabetes Mellitus, Type II Controlled	250.02	Pharyngitis, Acute	462
Anemia, NOS	285.9	Drug Reaction, NOS	995.29	Pneumonia, Organism Unspec.	486
Anemia, Pernicious	281.0	Dysuria	788.1 1	Prostatitis, NOS	601.9
Asthma w/ Exacerbation	493.92	Eczema, NOS	692.2	PVC	427.69
Asthmatic Bronchitis, Unspec.	493.90	Edema	782.3	Rash, Non Specific	782.1
Atrial Fibrillation	427.31	Fever, Unknown Origin	780.6	Seizure Disorder NOS	780.39
Atypical Chest Pain, Unspec.	786.59	Gastritis, Acute w/o Hemorrhage	535.00	Serous Otitis Media, Chronic, Unspec.	381.10
Bronchiolitis, due to RSV	466.11	Gastroenteritis, NOS	558.9	Sinusitis, Acute NOS	461.9
Bronchitis, Acute	466.0	Gastroesophageal Reflux	530.81	Tonsillitis, Acute	463.
Bronchitis, NOS	490	Hepatitis A, Infectious	070.1	Upper Respiratory Infection, Acute NOS	465.9
Cardiac Arrest	427.5	Hypercholesterolemia, Pure	272.0	Urinary Tract Infection, Unspec.	599.0
Cardiopulmonary Disease, Chronic, Unspec.	416.9	Hypertension, Unspec.	401.9	Urticaria, Unspec.	708.9
Cellulitis, NOS	682.9	Hypoglycemia NOS	251.2	Vertigo, NOS	780.4
Congestive Heart Failure, Unspec.	428.0	Hypokalemia	276.8	Viral Infection NOS	079.99
Contact Dermatitis NOS	692.9	Impetigo	684	Weakness, Generalized	780.79
COPD NOS	496	Lymphadenitis, Unspec.	289.3	Weight Loss, Abnormal	783.21
CVA, Acute, NOS	434.91	Mononucleosis	075		
CVA, Old or Healed	438.9	Myocardial Infarction, Acute, NOS	410.9		
Degenerative Arthritis		Organic Brain Syndrome	310.9		
(Specify Site) _____	715.9	Otitis Externa, Acute NOS	380.10		

ABN: I UNDERSTAND THAT MEDICARE PROBABLY WILL NOT COVER THE SERVICES LISTED BELOW

A. _____ B. _____ C. _____
Patient

Date _____ Signature _____

Doctor's Signature _D J Schwartz_

RETURN: 5 Days _____ Weeks _____ Months _____

REF# 122949 SB (05.07.09)   TO REORDER CALL INHEALTH RECORD SYSTEMS 800-477-7374

DOUGLASVILLE MEDICINE ASSOCIATES
5076 BRAND BLVD., SUITE 401
DOUGLASVILLE, NY 01234
PHONE No. (123) 456-7890
☐ L.D. HEATH, M.D.   ☒ D.J. SCHWARTZ, M.D.
NPI# 9995010111   NPI# 9995020212
EIN# 00-1234560

SOURCE DOCUMENT 6-9

PLEASE RETURN THIS FORM TO RECEPTIONIST

NAME Shinn, Robert

2341

PLACE OF SERVICE:
(X) OFFICE
( ) NEW YORK COUNTY HOSPITAL
( ) COMMUNITY GENERAL HOSPITAL
( ) RETIREMENT INN NURSING HOME
( ) _____

DATE OF SERVICE 10/30/09

A. OFFICE VISITS - New Patient

Code	History	Exam	Dec.	Time	
____ 99201	Prob. Foc.	Prob. Foc.	Straight	10 min.	_____
____ 99202	Ex. Prob. Foc.	Ex. Prob. Foc.	Straight	20 min.	_____
____ 99203	Detail	Detail	Low	30 min.	_____
____ 99204	Comp.	Comp.	Mod.	45 min.	_____
____ 99205	Comp.	Comp.	High	60 min.	_____

B. OFFICE VISIT - Established Patient

Code	History	Exam	Dec.	Time	
____ 99211	Minimal	Minimal	Minimal	5 min.	_____
____ 99212	Prob. Foc.	Prob. Foc.	Straight	10min.	_____
X 99213	Ex. Prob. Foc.	Ex. Prob. Foc.	Low	15 min.	I
____ 99214	Detail	Detail	Mod.	25 min.	_____
____ 99215	Comp.	Comp.	High	40 min.	_____

C. HOSPITAL CARE

		Dx	Units	
1.	Initial Hospital Care (30 min)	____	___ 99221	_____
2.	Subsequent Care	____	___ 99231	_____
3.	Critical Care (30-74 min)	____	___ 99291	_____
4.	each additional 30 min.	____	___ 99292	_____
5.	Discharge Services	____	___ 99238	_____
6.	Emergency Room	____	___ 99282	_____

D. NURSING HOME CARE

		Dx	Units	
Initial Care - New Pt.				
1.	Expanded	____	___ 99322	_____
2.	Detailed	____	___ 99323	_____
Subsequent Care - Estab. Pt.				
3.	Problem Focused	____	___ 99307	_____
4.	Expanded	____	___ 99308	_____
5.	Detailed	____	___ 99309	_____
5.	Comprehensive	____	___ 99310	_____

E. PROCEDURES

1.	Arthrocentesis, Small Jt.	____	20600 _____
2.	Colonoscopy	____	45378 _____
3.	EKG w/interpretation	____	93000 _____
4.	X-Ray Chest, PA/LAT	____	71020 _____

F. LAB

1.	Blood Sugar	____	82947 _____
2.	CBC w/differential	____	85031 _____
3.	Cholesterol	____	82465 _____
4.	Comprehensive Metabolic Panel	____	80053 _____
5.	ESR	____	85651 _____
6.	Hematocrit	____	85014 _____
7.	Mono Screen	____	86308 _____
8.	Pap Smear	____	88150 _____
9.	Potassium	____	84132 _____
10.	Preg. Test, Quantitative	____	84702 _____
11.	Routine Venipuncture	____	36415 _____

F. Cont'd

		Dx	Units	
12.	Strep Screen	____	87081	_____
13.	UA, Routine w/Micro	____	81000	_____
14.	UA, Routine w/o Micro	____	81002	_____
15.	Uric Acid	____	84550	_____
16.	VDRL	____	86592	_____
17.	Wet Prep	____	82710	_____
18.	_____	____	____	_____

G. INJECTIONS

1.	Influenza Virus Vaccine	____	90658 _____
2.	Pneumoccoccal Vaccine	____	90772 _____
3.	Tetanus Toxoids	____	90703 _____
4.	Therapeutic Subcut/IM	____	90732 _____
5.	Vaccine Administration	____	90471 _____
6.	Vaccine - each additional	____	90472 _____

H. MISCELLANEOUS

1. _____ ____ _____
2. _____ ____ _____

AMOUNT PAID $ 10.00

Mark diagnosis with
(1=Primary, 2=Secondary, 3=Tertiary)

DIAGNOSIS
NOT LISTED _____
BELOW _____

DIAGNOSIS	ICD-9-CM 1, 2, 3	DIAGNOSIS	ICD-9-CM 1, 2, 3	DIAGNOSIS	ICD-9-CM 1, 2, 3
Abdominal Pain	789.0	Dehydration	276.51	Otitis Media, Acute NOS	382.9 I
Allergic Rhinitis, Unspec.	477.9	Depression, NOS	311	Peptic Ulcer Disease	536.9
Angina Pectoris, Unspec.	413.9	Diabetes Mellitus, Type II Controlled	250.00	Peripheral Vascular Disease NOS	443.9
Anemia, Iron Deficiency, Unspec.	280.9	Diabetes Mellitus, Type II Controlled	250.02	Pharyngitis, Acute	462
Anemia, NOS	285.9	Drug Reaction, NOS	995.29	Pneumonia, Organism Unspec.	486
Anemia, Pernicious	281.0	Dysuria	788.1	Prostatitis, NOS	601.9
Asthma w/ Exacerbation	493.92	Eczema, NOS	692.2	PVC	427.69
Asthmatic Bronchitis, Unspec.	493.90	Edema	782.3	Rash, Non Specific	782.1
Atrial Fibrillation	427.31	Fever, Unknown Origin	780.6	Seizure Disorder NOS	780.39
Atypical Chest Pain, Unspec.	786.59	Gastritis, Acute w/o Hemorrhage	535.00	Serous Otitis Media, Chronic, Unspec.	381.10
Bronchiolitis, due to RSV	466.11	Gastroenteritis, NOS	558.9	Sinusitis, Acute NOS	461.9
Bronchitis, Acute	466.0	Gastroesophageal Reflux	530.81	Tonsillitis, Acute	463.
Bronchitis, NOS	490	Hepatitis A, Infectious	070.1	Upper Respiratory Infection, Acute NOS	465.9
Cardiac Arrest	427.5	Hypercholesterolemia, Pure	272.0	Urinary Tract Infection, Unspec.	599.0
Cardiopulmonary Disease, Chronic, Unspec.	416.9	Hypertension, Unspec.	401.9	Urticaria, Unspec.	708.9
Cellulitis, NOS	682.9	Hypoglycemia NOS	251.2	Vertigo, NOS	780.4
Congestive Heart Failure, Unspec.	428.0	Hypokalemia	276.8	Viral Infection NOS	079.99
Contact Dermatitis NOS	692.9	Impetigo	684	Weakness, Generalized	780.79
COPD NOS	496	Lymphadenitis, Unspec.	289.3	Weight Loss, Abnormal	783.21
CVA, Acute, NOS	434.91	Mononucleosis	075		
CVA, Old or Healed	438.9	Myocardial Infarction, Acute, NOS	410.9		
Degenerative Arthritis		Organic Brain Syndrome	310.9		
(Specify Site) ___	715.9	Otitis Externa, Acute NOS	380.10		

ABN: I UNDERSTAND THAT MEDICARE PROBABLY WILL NOT COVER THE SERVICES LISTED BELOW

A._____ B._____ C._____

Patient

Date _____ Signature _____

Doctor's Signature ___ L D Heath ___

RETURN:_____ Days 1 Weeks _____ Months _____

DOUGLASVILLE MEDICINE ASSOCIATES
5076 BRAND BLVD., SUITE 401
DOUGLASVILLE, NY 01234
PHONE No. (123) 456-7890
(X) L.D. HEATH, M.D.   ( ) D.J. SCHWARTZ, M.D.
NPI# 9995010111   NPI# 9995020212
EIN# 00-1234560

REF# 122949 SB (05.07.09)   TO REORDER CALL INHEALTH RECORD SYSTEMS 800-477-7374

Superbill for Robert Shinn. *Used with permission. InHealth Record Systems, Inc. 5076 Winters Chapel Road, Atlanta, GA 30360, 800-477-7374. http://www.inhealthrecords.com*

SOURCE DOCUMENT 6-10

PLEASE RETURN THIS FORM TO RECEPTIONIST

NAME Pradhan, Kabin

2342

PLACE OF SERVICE:
(X) OFFICE
( ) NEW YORK COUNTY HOSPITAL
( ) COMMUNITY GENERAL HOSPITAL
( ) RETIREMENT INN NURSING HOME
( ) _____

DATE OF SERVICE 11/03/09

A. OFFICE VISITS - New Patient

	Code	History	Exam	Dec.	Time	
X	99201	Prob. Foc.	Prob. Foc.	Straight	10 min.	I
	99202	Ex. Prob. Foc.	Ex. Prob. Foc.	Straight	20 min.	
	99203	Detail	Detail	Low	30 min.	
	99204	Comp.	Comp.	Mod.	45 min.	
	99205	Comp.	Comp.	High	60 min.	

B. OFFICE VISIT - Established Patient

Code	History	Exam	Dec.	Time	
99211	Minimal	Minimal	Minimal	5 min.	
99212	Prob. Foc.	Prob. Foc.	Straight	10min.	
99213	Ex. Prob. Foc.	Ex. Prob. Foc.	Low	15 min.	
99214	Detail	Detail	Mod.	25 min.	
99215	Comp.	Comp.	High	40 min.	

C. HOSPITAL CARE   Dx Units

1.	Initial Hospital Care (30 min)	___ ___	99221	___
2.	Subsequent Care	___ ___	99231	___
3.	Critical Care (30-74 min)	___ ___	99291	___
4.	each additional 30 min.	___ ___	99292	___
5.	Discharge Services	___ ___	99238	___
6.	Emergency Room	___ ___	99282	___

D. NURSING HOME CARE

Dx Units

Initial Care - New Pt.

1.	Expanded	___	99322 ___
2.	Detailed	___	99323 ___

Subsequent Care - Estab. Pt.

3.	Problem Focused	___	99307 ___
4.	Expanded	___	99308 ___
5.	Detailed	___	99309 ___
5.	Comprehensive	___	99310 ___

E. PROCEDURES

1.	Arthrocentesis, Small Jt.	___	20600 ___
2.	Colonoscopy		45378 ___
3.	EKG w/interpretation	___	93000 ___
4.	X-Ray Chest, PA/LAT	___	71020 ___

F. LAB

1.	Blood Sugar	___	82947 ___
2.	CBC w/differential	___	85031 ___
3.	Cholesterol	___	82465 ___
4.	Comprehensive Metabolic Panel	___	80053 ___
5.	ESR	___	85651 ___
6.	Hematocrit	___	85014 ___
7.	Mono Screen	___	86308 ___
8.	Pap Smear	___	88150 ___
9.	Potassium	___	84132 ___
10.	Preg. Test, Quantitative	___	84702 ___
11.	Routine Venipuncture	___	36415 ___

F. Cont'd

Dx Units

12.	Strep Screen	___	87081 ___
13.	UA, Routine w/Micro	___	81000 ___
14.	UA, Routine w/o Micro	___	81002 ___
15.	Uric Acid	___	84550 ___
16.	VDRL	___	86592 ___
17.	Wet Prep	___	82710 ___
18.	_____	___	___

G. INJECTIONS

1.	Influenza Virus Vaccine	___	90658 ___
2.	Pneumoccocal Vaccine	___	90772 ___
3.	Tetanus Toxoids	___	90703 ___
4.	Therapeutic Subcut/IM	___	90732 ___
5.	Vaccine Administration	___	90471 ___
6.	Vaccine - each additional	___	90472 ___

H. MISCELLANEOUS

1. _____ ___
2. _____ ___

AMOUNT PAID $ ___ Ø

Mark diagnosis with (1=Primary, 2=Secondary, 3=Tertiary)

DIAGNOSIS NOT LISTED BELOW _____

DIAGNOSIS	ICD-9-CM 1, 2, 3	DIAGNOSIS	ICD-9-CM 1, 2, 3	DIAGNOSIS	ICD-9-CM 1, 2, 3
Abdominal Pain	789.0 ___	Dehydration	276.51 ___	Otitis Media, Acute NOS	382.9 ___
Allergic Rhinitis, Unspec.	477.9 ___	Depression, NOS	311 ___	Peptic Ulcer Disease	536.9 ___
Angina Pectoris, Unspec.	413.9 ___	Diabetes Mellitus, Type II Controlled	250.00 ___	Peripheral Vascular Disease NOS	443.9 ___
Anemia, Iron Deficiency, Unspec.	280.9 ___	Diabetes Mellitus, Type II Controlled	250.02 ___	Pharyngitis, Acute	462 ___
Anemia, NOS	285.9 ___	Drug Reaction, NOS	995.29 ___	Pneumonia, Organism Unspec.	486 ___
Anemia, Pernicious	281.0 ___	Dysuria	788.1 ___	Prostatitis, NOS	601.9 ___
Asthma w/ Exacerbation	493.92 ___	Eczema, NOS	692.2 ___	PVC	427.69 ___
Asthmatic Bronchitis, Unspec.	493.90 ___	Edema	782.3 ___	Rash, Non Specific	782.1 ___
Atrial Fibrillation	427.31 ___	Fever, Unknown Origin	780.6 ___	Seizure Disorder NOS	780.39 ___
Atypical Chest Pain, Unspec.	786.59 ___	Gastritis, Acute w/o Hemorrhage	535.00 ___	Serous Otitis Media, Chronic, Unspec.	381.10 ___
Bronchiolitis, due to RSV	466.11 ___	Gastroenteritis, NOS	558.9 ___	Sinusitis, Acute NOS	461.9 ___
Bronchitis, Acute	466.0 ___	Gastroesophageal Reflux	530.81 I	Tonsillitis, Acute	463. ___
Bronchitis, NOS	490 ___	Hepatitis A, Infectious	070.1 ___	Upper Respiratory Infection, Acute NOS	465.9 ___
Cardiac Arrest	427.5 ___	Hypercholesterolemia, Pure	272.0 ___	Urinary Tract Infection, Unspec.	599.0 ___
Cardiopulmonary Disease, Chronic, Unspec.	416.9 ___	Hypertension, Unspec.	401.9 ___	Urticaria, Unspec.	708.9 ___
Cellulitis, NOS	682.9 ___	Hypoglycemia NOS	251.2 ___	Vertigo, NOS	780.4 ___
Congestive Heart Failure, Unspec.	428.0 ___	Hypokalemia	276.8 ___	Viral Infection NOS	079.99 ___
Contact Dermatitis NOS	692.9 ___	Impetigo	684 ___	Weakness, Generalized	780.79 ___
COPD NOS	496 ___	Lymphadenitis, Unspec.	289.3 ___	Weight Loss, Abnormal	783.21 ___
CVA, Acute, NOS	434.91 ___	Mononucleosis	075 ___		
CVA, Old or Healed	438.9 ___	Myocardial Infarction, Acute, NOS	410.9 ___		
Degenerative Arthritis		Organic Brain Syndrome	310.9 ___		
(Specify Site)	715.9 ___	Otitis Externa, Acute NOS	380.10 ___		

ABN: I UNDERSTAND THAT MEDICARE PROBABLY WILL NOT COVER THE SERVICES LISTED BELOW

A. _____ B. _____ C. _____

Patient

Date _____ Signature _____

Doctor's Signature _D J Schwartz_

RETURN: _____ Days _____ Weeks __1__ Months

DOUGLASVILLE MEDICINE ASSOCIATES
5076 BRAND BLVD., SUITE 401
DOUGLASVILLE, NY 01234
PHONE No. (123) 456-7890
❑ L.D. HEATH, M.D.   ☒ D.J. SCHWARTZ, M.D.
NPI# 9995010111   NPI# 9995020212
EIN# 00-1234560

REF# 122949 SB (05.07.09)   TO REORDER CALL INHEALTH RECORD SYSTEMS 800-477-7374

SOURCE DOCUMENT 6-11

PLEASE RETURN THIS FORM TO RECEPTIONIST

NAME Tomanaga, Marie

2343

PLACE OF SERVICE:
(X) OFFICE
( ) NEW YORK COUNTY HOSPITAL
( ) COMMUNITY GENERAL HOSPITAL
( ) RETIREMENT INN NURSING HOME
( ) _____

DATE OF SERVICE 11/03/09

A. OFFICE VISITS - New Patient

Code	History	Exam	Dec.	Time	
99201	Prob. Foc.	Prob. Foc.	Straight	10 min.	
99202	Ex. Prob. Foc.	Ex. Prob. Foc.	Straight	20 min.	
99203	Detail	Detail	Low	30 min.	
99204	Comp.	Comp.	Mod.	45 min.	
X 99205	Comp.	Comp.	High	60 min.	1, 2

B. OFFICE VISIT - Established Patient

Code	History	Exam	Dec.	Time	
99211	Minimal	Minimal	Minimal	5 min.	
99212	Prob. Foc.	Prob. Foc.	Straight	10min.	
99213	Ex. Prob. Foc.	Ex. Prob. Foc.	Low	15 min.	
99214	Detail	Detail	Mod.	25 min.	
99215	Comp.	Comp.	High	40 min.	

C. HOSPITAL CARE

		Dx	Units	
1.	Initial Hospital Care (30 min)		99221	
2.	Subsequent Care		99231	
3.	Critical Care (30-74 min)		99291	
4.	each additional 30 min.		99292	
5.	Discharge Services		99238	
6.	Emergency Room		99282	

D. NURSING HOME CARE

		Dx	Units
	Initial Care - New Pt.		
1.	Expanded		99322
2.	Detailed		99323
	Subsequent Care - Estab. Pt.		
3.	Problem Focused		99307
4.	Expanded		99308
5.	Detailed		99309
5.	Comprehensive		99310

E. PROCEDURES

		Dx	Units	
1.	Arthrocentesis, Small Jt.		20600	
2.	Colonoscopy		45378	
3.	EKG w/interpretation	1	93000	X
4.	X-Ray Chest, PA/LAT		71020	

F. LAB

		Dx	Units	
1.	Blood Sugar		82947	
2.	CBC w/differential		85031	
3.	Cholesterol		82465	
4.	Comprehensive Metabolic Panel		80053	
5.	ESR	1	85651	X
6.	Hematocrit		85014	
7.	Mono Screen		86308	
8.	Pap Smear		88150	
9.	Potassium		84132	
10.	Preg. Test, Quantitative		84702	
11.	Routine Venipuncture	1	36415	X

F. Cont'd

		Dx	Units	
12.	Strep Screen		87081	
13.	UA, Routine w/Micro		81000	
14.	UA, Routine w/o Micro		81002	
15.	Uric Acid		84550	
16.	VDRL		86592	
17.	Wet Prep		82710	
18.	_____		____	

G. INJECTIONS

1.	Influenza Virus Vaccine		90658	
2.	Pneumococcal Vaccine		90772	
3.	Tetanus Toxoids		90703	
4.	Therapeutic Subcut/IM		90732	
5.	Vaccine Administration		90471	
6.	Vaccine - each additional		90472	

H. MISCELLANEOUS

1. _____ ____
2. _____ ____

AMOUNT PAID $ ____Ø____

Mark diagnosis with
(1=Primary, 2=Secondary, 3=Tertiary)

DIAGNOSIS NOT LISTED BELOW _____

DIAGNOSIS	ICD-9-CM	1, 2, 3	DIAGNOSIS	ICD-9-CM	1, 2, 3	DIAGNOSIS	ICD-9-CM	1, 2, 3
Abdominal Pain	789.0		Dehydration	276.51		Otitis Media, Acute NOS	382.9	
Allergic Rhinitis, Unspec.	477.9		Depression, NOS	311		Peptic Ulcer Disease	536.9	
Angina Pectoris, Unspec.	413.9	1	Diabetes Mellitus, Type II Controlled	250.00		Peripheral Vascular Disease NOS	443.9	
Anemia, Iron Deficiency, Unspec.	280.9		Diabetes Mellitus, Type II Controlled	250.02		Pharyngitis, Acute	462	
Anemia, NOS	285.9		Drug Reaction, NOS	995.29		Pneumonia, Organism Unspec.	486	
Anemia, Pernicious	281.0		Dysuria	788.1		Prostatitis, NOS	601.9	
Asthma w/ Exacerbation	493.92		Eczema, NOS	692.2		PVC	427.69	
Asthmatic Bronchitis, Unspec.	493.90		Edema	782.3		Rash, Non Specific	782.1	
Atrial Fibrillation	427.31		Fever, Unknown Origin	780.6		Seizure Disorder NOS	780.39	
Atypical Chest Pain, Unspec.	786.59		Gastritis, Acute w/o Hemorrhage	535.00		Serous Otitis Media, Chronic, Unspec.	381.10	
Bronchiolitis, due to RSV	466.11		Gastroenteritis, NOS	558.9		Sinusitis, Acute NOS	461.9	
Bronchitis, Acute	466.0		Gastroesophageal Reflux	530.81		Tonsillitis, Acute	463.	
Bronchitis, NOS	490		Hepatitis A, Infectious	070.1		Upper Respiratory Infection, Acute NOS	465.9	
Cardiac Arrest	427.5		Hypercholesterolemia, Pure	272.0		Urinary Tract Infection, Unspec.	599.0	
Cardiopulmonary Disease, Chronic, Unspec.	416.9		Hypertension, Unspec.	401.9	2	Urticaria, Unspec.	708.9	
Cellulitis, NOS	682.9		Hypoglycemia NOS	251.2		Vertigo, NOS	780.4	
Congestive Heart Failure, Unspec.	428.0		Hypokalemia	276.8		Viral Infection NOS	079.99	
Contact Dermatitis NOS	692.9		Impetigo	684		Weakness, Generalized	780.79	
COPD NOS	496		Lymphadenitis, Unspec.	289.3		Weight Loss, Abnormal	783.21	
CVA, Acute, NOS	434.91		Mononucleosis	075				
CVA, Old or Healed	438.9		Myocardial Infarction, Acute, NOS	410.9				
Degenerative Arthritis			Organic Brain Syndrome	310.9				
(Specify Site)	715.9		Otitis Externa, Acute NOS	380.10				

ABN: I UNDERSTAND THAT MEDICARE PROBABLY WILL NOT COVER THE SERVICES LISTED BELOW

A. _____ B. _____ C. _____

Patient

Date _____ Signature _____

Doctor's Signature _D J Schwartz_

RETURN: _____ Days 3 Weeks _____ Months _____

REF# 122949 SB (05.07.09) TO REORDER CALL INHEALTH RECORD SYSTEMS 800-477-7374

DOUGLASVILLE MEDICINE ASSOCIATES
5076 BRAND BLVD., SUITE 401
DOUGLASVILLE, NY 01234
PHONE No. (123) 456-7890
☐ L.D. HEATH, M.D.   ☒ D.J. SCHWARTZ, M.D.
NPI# 9995010111   NPI# 9995020212
EIN# 00-1234560

Superbill for Marie Tomanaga. *Used with permission. InHealth Record Systems, Inc. 5076 Winters Chapel Road, Atlanta, GA 30360, 800-477-7374. http://www.inhealthrecords.com*

SOURCE DOCUMENT 6-12

PLEASE RETURN THIS FORM TO RECEPTIONIST

NAME   Beals, Kimberly

2344

PLACE OF SERVICE:
(X) OFFICE
( ) NEW YORK COUNTY HOSPITAL
( ) COMMUNITY GENERAL HOSPITAL
( ) RETIREMENT INN NURSING HOME
( ) _____

DATE OF SERVICE   11/03/09

A. OFFICE VISITS - New Patient

	Code	History	Exam	Dec.	Time	
	99201	Prob. Foc.	Prob. Foc.	Straight	10 min.	
	99202	Ex. Prob. Foc.	Ex. Prob. Foc.	Straight	20 min.	
	99203	Detail	Detail	Low	30 min.	
X	99204	Comp.	Comp.	Mod.	45 min.	1, 2
	99205	Comp.	Comp.	High	60 min.	

B. OFFICE VISIT - Established Patient

Code	History	Exam	Dec.	Time
99211	Minimal	Minimal	Minimal	5 min.
99212	Prob. Foc.	Prob. Foc.	Straight	10 min.
99213	Ex. Prob. Foc.	Ex. Prob. Foc.	Low	15 min.
99214	Detail	Detail	Mod.	25 min.
99215	Comp.	Comp.	High	40 min.

C. HOSPITAL CARE   Dx Units

1. Initial Hospital Care (30 min) ____ ____ 99221 _____
2. Subsequent Care ____ ____ 99231 _____
3. Critical Care (30-74 min) ____ ____ 99291 _____
4. each additional 30 min. ____ ____ 99292 _____
5. Discharge Services ____ ____ 99238 _____
6. Emergency Room ____ ____ 99282 _____

D. NURSING HOME CARE   Dx Units

Initial Care - New Pt.
1. Expanded ____ ____ 99322
2. Detailed ____ ____ 99323

Subsequent Care - Estab. Pt.
3. Problem Focused ____ ____ 99307 _____
4. Expanded ____ ____ 99308 _____
5. Detailed ____ ____ 99309 _____
5. Comprehensive ____ ____ 99310 _____

E. PROCEDURES

1. Arthrocentesis, Small Jt. ____ 20600
2. Colonoscopy ____ 45378
3. EKG w/interpretation ____ 93000
4. X-Ray Chest, PA/LAT ____ 71020

F. LAB

1. Blood Sugar ____ 82947 _____
2. CBC w/differential ____ 85031 _____
3. Cholesterol ____ 82465 _____
4. Comprehensive Metabolic Panel 1, 2 80053 X _____
5. ESR ____ 85651 _____
6. Hematocrit ____ 85014 _____
7. Mono Screen ____ 86308 _____
8. Pap Smear ____ 88150 _____
9. Potassium ____ 84132 _____
10. Preg. Test, Quantitative ____ 84702 _____
11. Routine Venipuncture 1, 2 36415 X

F. Cont'd   Dx Units

12. Strep Screen ____ 87081 _____
13. UA, Routine w/Micro ____ 81000 _____
14. UA, Routine w/o Micro ____ 81002 _____
15. Uric Acid ____ 84550 _____
16. VDRL ____ 86592 _____
17. Wet Prep ____ 82710 _____
18. _____ ____ ____ _____

G. INJECTIONS

1. Influenza Virus Vaccine ____ 90658 _____
2. Pneumoccocal Vaccine ____ 90772 _____
3. Tetanus Toxoids ____ 90703 _____
4. Therapeutic Subcut/IM ____ 90732 _____
5. Vaccine Administration ____ 90471 _____
6. Vaccine - each additional ____ 90472 _____

H. MISCELLANEOUS

1. _____ ____ ____
2. _____ ____ ____

AMOUNT PAID $ 10.00

Mark diagnosis with
(1=Primary, 2=Secondary, 3=Tertiary)

DIAGNOSIS NOT LISTED _____
BELOW _____

DIAGNOSIS	ICD-9-CM	1, 2, 3	DIAGNOSIS	ICD-9-CM	1, 2, 3	DIAGNOSIS	ICD-9-CM	1, 2, 3
Abdominal Pain	789.0		Dehydration	276.51		Otitis Media, Acute NOS	382.9	
Allergic Rhinitis, Unspec.	477.9		Depression, NOS	311		Peptic Ulcer Disease	536.9	
Angina Pectoris, Unspec.	413.9		Diabetes Mellitus, Type II Controlled	250.00		Peripheral Vascular Disease NOS	443.9	
Anemia, Iron Deficiency, Unspec.	280.9		Diabetes Mellitus, Type II Controlled	250.02		Pharyngitis, Acute	462	
Anemia, NOS	285.9		Drug Reaction, NOS	995.29		Pneumonia, Organism Unspec.	486	
Anemia, Pernicious	281.0		Dysuria	788.1		Prostatitis, NOS	601.9	
Asthma w/ Exacerbation	493.92		Eczema, NOS	692.2		PVC	427.69	
Asthmatic Bronchitis, Unspec.	493.90		Edema	782.3		Rash, Non Specific	782.1	
Atrial Fibrillation	427.31		Fever, Unknown Origin	780.6		Seizure Disorder NOS	780.39	
Atypical Chest Pain, Unspec.	786.59		Gastritis, Acute w/o Hemorrhage	535.00		Serous Otitis Media, Chronic, Unspec.	381.10	
Bronchiolitis, due to RSV	466.11		Gastroenteritis, NOS	558.9		Sinusitis, Acute NOS	461.9	
Bronchitis, Acute	466.0		Gastroesophageal Reflux	530.81		Tonsillitis, Acute	463.	
Bronchitis, NOS	490		Hepatitis A, Infectious	070.1		Upper Respiratory Infection, Acute NOS	465.9	
Cardiac Arrest	427.5		Hypercholesterolemia, Pure	272.0		Urinary Tract Infection, Unspec.	599.0	
Cardiopulmonary Disease, Chronic, Unspec.	416.9		Hypertension, Unspec.	401.9		Urticaria, Unspec.	708.9	
Cellulitis, NOS	682.9		Hypoglycemia NOS	251.2		Vertigo, NOS	780.4	
Congestive Heart Failure, Unspec.	428.0		Hypokalemia	276.8		Viral Infection NOS	079.99	
Contact Dermatitis NOS	692.9		Impetigo	684		Weakness, Generalized	780.79	2
COPD NOS	496		Lymphadenitis, Unspec.	289.3		Weight Loss, Abnormal	783.21	1
CVA, Acute, NOS	434.91		Mononucleosis	075				
CVA, Old or Healed	438.9		Myocardial Infarction, Acute, NOS	410.9				
Degenerative Arthritis			Organic Brain Syndrome	310.9				
(Specify Site)	715.9		Otitis Externa, Acute NOS	380.10				

ABN: I UNDERSTAND THAT MEDICARE PROBABLY WILL NOT COVER THE SERVICES LISTED BELOW

A. _____ B. _____ C. _____

Patient

Date _____ Signature _____

Doctor's Signature   L D Heath

RETURN: _____ Days   2   Weeks _____ Months _____

REF# 122949 SB (05.07.09)   TO REORDER CALL INHEALTH RECORD SYSTEMS 800-477-7374

DOUGLASVILLE MEDICINE ASSOCIATES
5076 BRAND BLVD., SUITE 401
DOUGLASVILLE, NY 01234
PHONE No. (123) 456-7890
☒ L.D. HEATH, M.D.   ☐ D.J. SCHWARTZ, M.D.
NPI# 9995010111   NPI# 9995020212
EIN# 00-1234560

Superbill for Kimberly Beals. *Used with permission. InHealth Record Systems, Inc. 5076 Winters Chapel Road, Atlanta, GA 30360, 800-477-7374. http://www.inhealthrecords.com*

SOURCE DOCUMENT 6-13

PLEASE RETURN THIS FORM TO RECEPTIONIST

NAME *Gordon, Eric*

2345

PLACE OF SERVICE:
(X) OFFICE
( ) NEW YORK COUNTY HOSPITAL
( ) COMMUNITY GENERAL HOSPITAL
( ) RETIREMENT INN NURSING HOME
( ) _____

DATE OF SERVICE 11/05/09

A. OFFICE VISITS - New Patient

Code	History	Exam	Dec.	Time	
___ 99201	Prob. Foc.	Prob. Foc.	Straight	10 min.	___
___ 99202	Ex. Prob. Foc.	Ex. Prob. Foc.	Straight	20 min.	___
___ 99203	Detail	Detail	Low	30 min.	___
___ 99204	Comp.	Comp.	Mod.	45 min.	___
___ 99205	Comp.	Comp.	High	60 min.	___

B. OFFICE VISIT - Established Patient

Code	History	Exam	Dec.	Time	
___ 99211	Minimal	Minimal	Minimal	5 min.	___
___ 99212	Prob. Foc.	Prob. Foc.	Straight	10 min.	___
X 99213	Ex. Prob. Foc.	Ex. Prob. Foc.	Low	15 min.	1
___ 99214	Detail	Detail	Mod.	25 min.	___
___ 99215	Comp.	Comp.	High	40 min.	___

C. HOSPITAL CARE Dx Units

1. Initial Hospital Care (30 min) ___ ___ 99221 ___
2. Subsequent Care ___ ___ 99231 ___
3. Critical Care (30-74 min) ___ ___ 99291 ___
4. each additional 30 min. ___ ___ 99292 ___
5. Discharge Services ___ ___ 99238 ___
6. Emergency Room ___ ___ 99282 ___

D. NURSING HOME CARE Dx Units

Initial Care - New Pt.
1. Expanded ___ ___ 99322 ___
2. Detailed ___ ___ 99323 ___

Subsequent Care - Estab. Pt.
3. Problem Focused ___ ___ 99307 ___
4. Expanded ___ ___ 99308 ___
5. Detailed ___ ___ 99309 ___
5. Comprehensive ___ ___ 99310 ___

E. PROCEDURES

1. Arthrocentesis, Small Jt. ___ 20600 ___
2. Colonoscopy ___ 45378 ___
3. EKG w/interpretation ___ 93000 ___
4. X-Ray Chest, PA/LAT ___ 71020 ___

F. LAB

1. Blood Sugar ___ 82947 ___
2. CBC w/differential ___ 85031 ___
3. Cholesterol ___ 82465 ___
4. Comprehensive Metabolic Panel ___ 80053 ___
5. ESR ___ 85651 ___
6. Hematocrit ___ 85014 ___
7. Mono Screen ___ 86308 ___
8. Pap Smear ___ 88150 ___
9. Potassium ___ 84132 ___
10. Preg. Test, Quantitative ___ 84702 ___
11. Routine Venipuncture ___ 36415 ___

F. Cont'd Dx Units

12. Strep Screen ___ 87081 ___
13. UA, Routine w/Micro ___ 81000 ___
14. UA, Routine w/o Micro ___ 81002 ___
15. Uric Acid ___ 84550 ___
16. VDRL ___ 86592 ___
17. Wet Prep ___ 82710 ___
18. ___ ___ ___

G. INJECTIONS

1. Influenza Virus Vaccine ___ 90658 ___
2. Pneumococcal Vaccine ___ 90772 ___
3. Tetanus Toxoids ___ 90703 ___
4. Therapeutic Subcut/IM ___ 90732 ___
5. Vaccine Administration ___ 90471 ___
6. Vaccine - each additional ___ 90472 ___

H. MISCELLANEOUS

1. _____ ___ ___
2. _____ ___ ___

AMOUNT PAID $ ___ 0 ___

Mark diagnosis with
(1=Primary, 2=Secondary, 3=Tertiary)

DIAGNOSIS NOT LISTED BELOW _____

DIAGNOSIS	ICD-9-CM 1, 2, 3	DIAGNOSIS	ICD-9-CM 1, 2, 3	DIAGNOSIS	ICD-9-CM 1, 2, 3
Abdominal Pain	789.0 ___	Dehydration	276.51 ___	Otitis Media, Acute NOS	382.9 ___
Allergic Rhinitis, Unspec.	477.9 ___	Depression, NOS	311 ___	Peptic Ulcer Disease	536.9 ___
Angina Pectoris, Unspec.	413.9 ___	Diabetes Mellitus, Type II Controlled	250.00 ___	Peripheral Vascular Disease NOS	443.9 ___
Anemia, Iron Deficiency, Unspec.	280.9 ___	Diabetes Mellitus, Type II Controlled	250.02 ___	Pharyngitis, Acute	462 ___
Anemia, NOS	285.9 ___	Drug Reaction, NOS	995.29 ___	Pneumonia, Organism Unspec.	486 ___
Anemia, Pernicious	281.0 ___	Dysuria	788.1 ___	Prostatitis, NOS	601.9 ___
Asthma w/ Exacerbation	493.92 ___	Eczema, NOS	692.2 ___	PVC	427.69 ___
Asthmatic Bronchitis, Unspec.	493.90 ___	Edema	782.3 ___	Rash, Non Specific	782.1 ___
Atrial Fibrillation	427.31 ___	Fever, Unknown Origin	780.6 ___	Seizure Disorder NOS	780.39 ___
Atypical Chest Pain, Unspec.	786.59 ___	Gastritis, Acute w/o Hemorrhage	535.00 ___	Serous Otitis Media, Chronic, Unspec.	381.10 ___
Bronchiolitis, due to RSV	466.11 ___	Gastroenteritis, NOS	558.9 ___	Sinusitis, Acute NOS	461.9 ___
Bronchitis, Acute	466.0 ___	Gastroesophageal Reflux	530.81 _1_	Tonsillitis, Acute	463. ___
Bronchitis, NOS	490 ___	Hepatitis A, Infectious	070.1 ___	Upper Respiratory Infection, Acute NOS	465.9 ___
Cardiac Arrest	427.5 ___	Hypercholesterolemia, Pure	272.0 ___	Urinary Tract Infection, Unspec.	599.0 ___
Cardiopulmonary Disease, Chronic, Unspec.	416.9 ___	Hypertension, Unspec.	401.9 ___	Urticaria, Unspec.	708.9 ___
Cellulitis, NOS	682.9 ___	Hypoglycemia NOS	251.2 ___	Vertigo, NOS	780.4 ___
Congestive Heart Failure, Unspec.	428.0 ___	Hypokalemia	276.8 ___	Viral Infection NOS	079.99 ___
Contact Dermatitis NOS	692.9 ___	Impetigo	684 ___	Weakness, Generalized	780.79 ___
COPD NOS	496 ___	Lymphadenitis, Unspec.	289.3 ___	Weight Loss, Abnormal	783.21 ___
CVA, Acute, NOS	434.91 ___	Mononucleosis	075 ___		
CVA, Old or Healed	438.9 ___	Myocardial Infarction, Acute, NOS	410.9 ___		
Degenerative Arthritis (Specify Site)	715.9 ___	Organic Brain Syndrome	310.9 ___		
		Otitis Externa, Acute NOS	380.10 ___		

ABN: I UNDERSTAND THAT MEDICARE PROBABLY WILL NOT COVER THE SERVICES LISTED BELOW

A. _____ B. _____ C. _____

Patient

Date _____ Signature _____

Doctor's Signature *D J Schwartz*

RETURN: _____ Days _____ Weeks PRN Months _____

DOUGLASVILLE MEDICINE ASSOCIATES
5076 BRAND BLVD., SUITE 401
DOUGLASVILLE, NY 01234
PHONE No. (123) 456-7890
☐ L.D. HEATH, M.D.   ☒ D.J. SCHWARTZ, M.D.
NPI# 9995010111   NPI# 9995020212
EIN# 00-1234560

Superbill for Eric Gordon. *Used with permission. InHealth Record Systems, Inc. 5076 Winters Chapel Road, Atlanta, GA 30360, 800-477-7374. http://www.inhealthrecords.com*

SOURCE DOCUMENT 6-14

PLEASE RETURN THIS FORM TO RECEPTIONIST	NAME Ybarra, Elane
	2346

PLACE OF SERVICE:
(X) OFFICE   ( ) RETIREMENT INN NURSING HOME
( ) NEW YORK COUNTY HOSPITAL
( ) COMMUNITY GENERAL HOSPITAL   ( ) _____   **DATE OF SERVICE** 11/06/09

A. OFFICE VISITS - New Patient

Code	History	Exam	Dec.	Time	
99201	Prob. Foc.	Prob. Foc.	Straight	10 min.	___
99202	Ex. Prob. Foc.	Ex. Prob. Foc.	Straight	20 min.	___
99203	Detail	Detail	Low	30 min.	___
99204	Comp.	Comp.	Mod.	45 min.	___
99205	Comp.	Comp.	High	60 min.	___

B. OFFICE VISIT - Established Patient

Code	History	Exam	Dec.	Time	
99211	Minimal	Minimal	Minimal	5 min.	___
99212	Prob. Foc.	Prob. Foc.	Straight	10min.	___
99213	Ex. Prob. Foc.	Ex. Prob. Foc.	Low	15 min.	___
99214	Detail	Detail	Mod.	25 min.	___
X 99215	Comp.	Comp.	High	40 min.	1, 2

C. HOSPITAL CARE   Dx Units

1.	Initial Hospital Care (30 min) ___ ___	99221	___
2.	Subsequent Care ___ ___	99231	___
3.	Critical Care (30-74 min) ___ ___	99291	___
4.	each additional 30 min. ___	99292	___
5.	Discharge Services ___ ___	99238	___
6.	Emergency Room ___ ___	99282	___

D. NURSING HOME CARE   Dx Units

Initial Care - New Pt.
1.	Expanded	___	99322 ___
2.	Detailed	___	99323 ___

Subsequent Care - Estab. Pt.
3.	Problem Focused	___	99307 ___
4.	Expanded	___	99308 ___
5.	Detailed	___	99309 ___
5.	Comprehensive	___	99310 ___

E. PROCEDURES

1.	Arthrocentesis, Small Jt.	___	20600
2.	Colonoscopy	___	45378
3.	EKG w/interpretation	___	93000
4.	X-Ray Chest, PA/LAT	___	71020

F. LAB

1.	Blood Sugar	___	82947 ___
2.	CBC w/differential	___	85031 ___
3.	Cholesterol	___	82465 ___
4.	Comprehensive Metabolic Panel	___	80053 ___
5.	ESR	___	85651 ___
6.	Hematocrit	___	85014 ___
7.	Mono Screen	___	86308 ___
8.	Pap Smear	___	88150 ___
9.	Potassium	___	84132 ___
10.	Preg. Test, Quantitative	___	84702 ___
11.	Routine Venipuncture	___	36415 ___

F. Cont'd   Dx Units

12.	Strep Screen	87081	___
13.	UA, Routine w/Micro	81000	1 X
14.	UA, Routine w/o Micro	81002	___
15.	Uric Acid	84550	___
16.	VDRL	86592	___
17.	Wet Prep	82710	___
18.	_____	___	___

G. INJECTIONS

1.	Influenza Virus Vaccine	90658	___
2.	Pneumococcal Vaccine	90772	___
3.	Tetanus Toxoids	90703	___
4.	Therapeutic Subcut/IM	90732	___
5.	Vaccine Administration	90471	___
6.	Vaccine - each additional	90472	___

H. MISCELLANEOUS
1. _____ ___ ___
2. _____ ___ ___

AMOUNT PAID $ Ø

Mark diagnosis with (1=Primary, 2=Secondary, 3=Tertiary)	DIAGNOSIS NOT LISTED BELOW _____

DIAGNOSIS	ICD-9-CM 1, 2, 3	DIAGNOSIS	ICD-9-CM 1, 2, 3	DIAGNOSIS	ICD-9-CM 1, 2, 3
Abdominal Pain	789.0	Dehydration	276.51	Otitis Media, Acute NOS	382.9
Allergic Rhinitis, Unspec.	477.9	Depression, NOS	311	Peptic Ulcer Disease	536.9
Angina Pectoris, Unspec.	413.9	Diabetes Mellitus, Type II Controlled	250.00	Peripheral Vascular Disease NOS	443.9
Anemia, Iron Deficiency, Unspec.	280.9	Diabetes Mellitus, Type II Controlled	250.02	Pharyngitis, Acute	462
Anemia, NOS	285.9	Drug Reaction, NOS	995.29	Pneumonia, Organism Unspec.	486
Anemia, Pernicious	281.0	Dysuria	788.1	Prostatitis, NOS	601.9
Asthma w/ Exacerbation	493.92	Eczema, NOS	692.2	PVC	427.69
Asthmatic Bronchitis, Unspec.	493.90	Edema	782.3	Rash, Non Specific	782.1
Atrial Fibrillation	427.31	Fever, Unknown Origin	780.6	Seizure Disorder NOS	780.39
Atypical Chest Pain, Unspec.	786.59	Gastritis, Acute w/o Hemorrhage	535.00	Serous Otitis Media, Chronic, Unspec.	381.10
Bronchiolitis, due to RSV	466.11	Gastroenteritis, NOS	558.9	Sinusitis, Acute NOS	461.9
Bronchitis, Acute	466.0	Gastroesophageal Reflux	530.81	Tonsillitis, Acute	463.
Bronchitis, NOS	490	Hepatitis A, Infectious	070.1	Upper Respiratory Infection, Acute NOS	465.9
Cardiac Arrest	427.5	Hypercholesterolemia, Pure	272.0	Urinary Tract Infection, Unspec.	599.0 1
Cardiopulmonary Disease, Chronic, Unspec.	416.9	Hypertension, Unspec.	401.9	Urticaria, Unspec.	708.9
Cellulitis, NOS	682.9	Hypoglycemia NOS	251.2	Vertigo, NOS	780.4
Congestive Heart Failure, Unspec.	428.0	Hypokalemia	276.8	Viral Infection NOS	079.99
Contact Dermatitis NOS	692.9	Impetigo	684	Weakness, Generalized	780.79 2
COPD NOS	496	Lymphadenitis, Unspec.	289.3	Weight Loss, Abnormal	783.21
CVA, Acute, NOS	434.91	Mononucleosis	075		
CVA, Old or Healed	438.9	Myocardial Infarction, Acute, NOS	410.9		
Degenerative Arthritis (Specify Site)	715.9	Organic Brain Syndrome	310.9		
		Otitis Externa, Acute NOS	380.10		

ABN: I UNDERSTAND THAT MEDICARE PROBABLY WILL NOT COVER THE SERVICES LISTED BELOW

A. _____ B. _____ C. _____
Patient
Date _____ Signature _____

Doctor's Signature *D J Schwartz*

RETURN: _____ Days 1 Weeks _____ Months _____

REF# 122949 SB (05.07.09) TO REORDER CALL INHEALTH RECORD SYSTEMS 800-477-7374

DOUGLASVILLE MEDICINE ASSOCIATES
5076 BRAND BLVD., SUITE 401
DOUGLASVILLE, NY 01234
PHONE No. (123) 456-7890
☐ L.D. HEATH, M.D.   ☒ D.J. SCHWARTZ, M.D.
NPI# 9995010111   NPI# 9995020212
EIN# 00-1234560

SOURCE DOCUMENT 6-15

PLEASE RETURN THIS FORM TO RECEPTIONIST

NAME Kinzler, Linda

2347

PLACE OF SERVICE:
(X) OFFICE
( ) NEW YORK COUNTY HOSPITAL
( ) COMMUNITY GENERAL HOSPITAL
( ) RETIREMENT INN NURSING HOME
( ) _____

DATE OF SERVICE 11/09/09

A. OFFICE VISITS - New Patient

Code	History	Exam	Dec.	Time	
99201	Prob. Foc.	Prob. Foc.	Straight	10 min.	
99202	Ex. Prob. Foc.	Ex. Prob. Foc.	Straight	20 min.	
X 99203	Detail	Detail	Low	30 min.	
99204	Comp.	Comp.	Mod.	45 min.	
99205	Comp.	Comp.	High	60 min.	

B. OFFICE VISIT - Established Patient

Code	History	Exam	Dec.	Time	
99211	Minimal	Minimal	Minimal	5 min.	
99212	Prob. Foc.	Prob. Foc.	Straight	10min.	
99213	Ex. Prob. Foc.	Ex. Prob. Foc.	Low	15 min.	
99214	Detail	Detail	Mod.	25 min.	
99215	Comp.	Comp.	High	40 min.	

C. HOSPITAL CARE Dx Units

1. Initial Hospital Care (30 min) _____ _____ 99221 _____
2. Subsequent Care _____ _____ 99231 _____
3. Critical Care (30-74 min) _____ _____ 99291 _____
4. each additional 30 min. _____ _____ 99292 _____
5. Discharge Services _____ _____ 99238 _____
6. Emergency Room _____ _____ 99282 _____

D. NURSING HOME CARE Dx Units

Initial Care - New Pt.
1. Expanded _____ _____ 99322
2. Detailed _____ _____ 99323

Subsequent Care - Estab. Pt.
3. Problem Focused _____ _____ 99307
4. Expanded _____ _____ 99308
5. Detailed _____ _____ 99309
5. Comprehensive _____ _____ 99310

E. PROCEDURES

1. Arthrocentesis, Small Jt. _____ 20600
2. Colonoscopy _____ 45378
3. EKG w/interpretation _____ 93000
4. X-Ray Chest, PA/LAT _____ 71020

F. LAB

1. Blood Sugar _____ 82947 _____
2. CBC w/differential _____ 85031 _____
3. Cholesterol _____ 82465 _____
4. Comprehensive Metabolic Panel _____ 80053 _____
5. ESR _____ 85651 _____
6. Hematocrit _____ 85014 _____
7. Mono Screen _____ 86308 _____
8. Pap Smear _____ 88150 _____
9. Potassium _____ 84132 _____
10. Preg. Test, Quantitative _____ 84702 _____
11. Routine Venipuncture _____ 36415 _____

F. Cont'd Dx Units

12. Strep Screen _____ 87081 _____
13. UA, Routine w/Micro _____ 81000 _____
14. UA, Routine w/o Micro _____ 81002 _____
15. Uric Acid _____ 84550 _____
16. VDRL _____ 86592 _____
17. Wet Prep _____ 82710 _____
18. _____ _____ _____

G. INJECTIONS

1. Influenza Virus Vaccine 1 90658 X
2. Pneumoccocal Vaccine _____ 90772 _____
3. Tetanus Toxoids _____ 90703 _____
4. Therapeutic Subcut/IM _____ 90732 _____
5. Vaccine Administration _____ 90471 _____
6. Vaccine - each additional _____ 90472 _____

H. MISCELLANEOUS

1. _____ _____ _____
2. _____ _____ _____

AMOUNT PAID $ 42.00

Mark diagnosis with (1=Primary, 2=Secondary, 3=Tertiary)	DIAGNOSIS NOT LISTED BELOW _____

DIAGNOSIS	ICD-9-CM 1, 2, 3	DIAGNOSIS	ICD-9-CM 1, 2, 3	DIAGNOSIS	ICD-9-CM 1, 2, 3
Abdominal Pain	789.0	Dehydration	276.51	Otitis Media, Acute NOS	382.9
Allergic Rhinitis, Unspec.	477.9	Depression, NOS	311	Peptic Ulcer Disease	536.9
Angina Pectoris, Unspec.	413.9	Diabetes Mellitus, Type II Controlled	250.00	Peripheral Vascular Disease NOS	443.9
Anemia, Iron Deficiency, Unspec.	280.9	Diabetes Mellitus, Type II Controlled	250.02	Pharyngitis, Acute	462
Anemia, NOS	285.9	Drug Reaction, NOS	995.29	Pneumonia, Organism Unspec.	486
Anemia, Pernicious	281.0	Dysuria	788.1	Prostatitis, NOS	601.9
Asthma w/ Exacerbation	493.92	Eczema, NOS	692.2	PVC	427.69
Asthmatic Bronchitis, Unspec.	493.90 1	Edema	782.3	Rash, Non Specific	782.1
Atrial Fibrillation	427.31	Fever, Unknown Origin	780.6	Seizure Disorder NOS	780.39
Atypical Chest Pain, Unspec.	786.59	Gastritis, Acute w/o Hemorrhage	535.00	Serous Otitis Media, Chronic, Unspec.	381.10
Bronchiolitis, due to RSV	466.11	Gastroenteritis, NOS	558.9	Sinusitis, Acute NOS	461.9
Bronchitis, Acute	466.0	Gastroesophageal Reflux	530.81	Tonsillitis, Acute	463.
Bronchitis, NOS	490	Hepatitis A, Infectious	070.1	Upper Respiratory Infection, Acute NOS	465.9
Cardiac Arrest	427.5	Hypercholesterolemia, Pure	272.0	Urinary Tract Infection, Unspec.	599.0
Cardiopulmonary Disease, Chronic, Unspec.	416.9	Hypertension, Unspec.	401.9	Urticaria, Unspec.	708.9
Cellulitis, NOS	682.9	Hypoglycemia NOS	251.2	Vertigo, NOS	780.4
Congestive Heart Failure, Unspec.	428.0	Hypokalemia	276.8	Viral Infection NOS	079.99
Contact Dermatitis NOS	692.9	Impetigo	684	Weakness, Generalized	780.79
COPD NOS	496	Lymphadenitis, Unspec.	289.3	Weight Loss, Abnormal	783.21
CVA, Acute, NOS	434.91	Mononucleosis	075		
CVA, Old or Healed	438.9	Myocardial Infarction, Acute, NOS	410.9		
Degenerative Arthritis		Organic Brain Syndrome	310.9		
(Specify Site)	715.9	Otitis Externa, Acute NOS	380.10		

ABN: I UNDERSTAND THAT MEDICARE PROBABLY WILL NOT COVER THE SERVICES LISTED BELOW

A. _____ B. _____ C. _____

Patient Signature _____

Date _____

Doctor's Signature L D Heath

RETURN: _____ Days _____ Weeks PRN _____ Months

REF# 122949 SB (05.07.09) TO REORDER CALL INHEALTH RECORD SYSTEMS 800-477-7374

DOUGLASVILLE MEDICINE ASSOCIATES
5076 BRAND BLVD., SUITE 401
DOUGLASVILLE, NY 01234
PHONE No. (123) 456-7890
☒ L.D. HEATH, M.D. ☐ D.J. SCHWARTZ, M.D.
NPI# 9995010111 NPI# 9995020212
EIN# 00-1234560

Superbill for Linda Kinzler. *Used with permission. InHealth Record Systems, Inc. 5076 Winters Chapel Road, Atlanta, GA 30360, 800-477-7374. http://www.inhealthrecords.com*

SOURCE DOCUMENT 6-16

PLEASE RETURN THIS FORM TO RECEPTIONIST	NAME James, David
	2348

PLACE OF SERVICE:
(X) OFFICE
( ) NEW YORK COUNTY HOSPITAL
( ) COMMUNITY GENERAL HOSPITAL
( ) RETIREMENT INN NURSING HOME
( ) _____

DATE OF SERVICE 11/09/09

A. OFFICE VISITS - New Patient

Code	History	Exam	Dec.	Time	
___ 99201	Prob. Foc.	Prob. Foc.	Straight	10 min.	_____
___ 99202	Ex. Prob. Foc.	Ex. Prob. Foc.	Straight	20 min.	_____
___ 99203	Detail	Detail	Low	30 min.	_____
___ 99204	Comp.	Comp.	Mod.	45 min.	_____
___ 99205	Comp.	Comp.	High	60 min.	_____

B. OFFICE VISIT - Established Patient

Code	History	Exam	Dec.	Time	
___ 99211	Minimal	Minimal	Minimal	5 min.	_____
___ 99212	Prob. Foc.	Prob. Foc.	Straight	10min.	_____
X 99213	Ex. Prob. Foc.	Ex. Prob. Foc.	Low	15 min.	1
___ 99214	Detail	Detail	Mod.	25 min.	_____
___ 99215	Comp.	Comp.	High	40 min.	_____

C. HOSPITAL CARE   Dx Units

1. Initial Hospital Care (30 min)	___ ___	99221	_____
2. Subsequent Care	___ ___	99231	_____
3. Critical Care (30-74 min)	___ ___	99291	_____
4. each additional 30 min.	___ ___	99292	_____
5. Discharge Services	___ ___	99238	_____
6. Emergency Room	___ ___	99282	_____

D. NURSING HOME CARE   Dx Units

Initial Care - New Pt.

1. Expanded	___	99322	_____
2. Detailed	___	99323	_____

Subsequent Care - Estab. Pt.

3. Problem Focused	___	99307	_____
4. Expanded	___	99308	_____
5. Detailed	___	99309	_____
5. Comprehensive	___	99310	_____

E. PROCEDURES

1. Arthrocentesis, Small Jt.	___	20600
2. Colonoscopy	___	45378
3. EKG w/interpretation	___	93000
4. X-Ray Chest, PA/LAT	___	71020

F. LAB

1. Blood Sugar	___	82947	_____
2. CBC w/differential	___	85031	_____
3. Cholesterol	___	82465	_____
4. Comprehensive Metabolic Panel	___	80053	_____
5. ESR	___	85651	_____
6. Hematocrit	___	85014	_____
7. Mono Screen	1	86308	X
8. Pap Smear	___	88150	_____
9. Potassium	___	84132	_____
10. Preg. Test, Quantitative	___	84702	_____
11. Routine Venipuncture	___	36415	_____

F. Cont'd   Dx Units

12. Strep Screen	___	87081	_____
13. UA, Routine w/Micro	___	81000	_____
14. UA, Routine w/o Micro	___	81002	_____
15. Uric Acid	___	84550	_____
16. VDRL	___	86592	_____
17. Wet Prep	___	82710	_____
18. _____	___	_____	_____

G. INJECTIONS

1. Influenza Virus Vaccine	___	90658	_____
2. Pneumoccocal Vaccine	___	90772	_____
3. Tetanus Toxoids	___	90703	_____
4. Therapeutic Subcut/IM	___	90732	_____
5. Vaccine Administration	___	90471	_____
6. Vaccine - each additional	___	90472	_____

H. MISCELLANEOUS

1. _____ ___ _____
2. _____ ___ _____

AMOUNT PAID $ 10.00

Mark diagnosis with
(1=Primary, 2=Secondary, 3=Tertiary)

DIAGNOSIS NOT LISTED BELOW _____

DIAGNOSIS	ICD-9-CM 1, 2, 3	DIAGNOSIS	ICD-9-CM 1, 2, 3	DIAGNOSIS	ICD-9-CM 1, 2, 3
Abdominal Pain	789.0	Dehydration	276.51	Otitis Media, Acute NOS	382.9
Allergic Rhinitis, Unspec.	477.9	Depression, NOS	311	Peptic Ulcer Disease	536.9
Angina Pectoris, Unspec.	413.9	Diabetes Mellitus, Type II Controlled	250.00	Peripheral Vascular Disease NOS	443.9
Anemia, Iron Deficiency, Unspec.	280.9	Diabetes Mellitus, Type II Controlled	250.02	Pharyngitis, Acute	462
Anemia, NOS	285.9	Drug Reaction, NOS	995.29	Pneumonia, Organism Unspec.	486
Anemia, Pernicious	281.0	Dysuria	788.1	Prostatitis, NOS	601.9
Asthma w/ Exacerbation	493.92	Eczema, NOS	692.2	PVC	427.69
Asthmatic Bronchitis, Unspec.	493.90	Edema	782.3	Rash, Non Specific	782.1
Atrial Fibrillation	427.31	Fever, Unknown Origin	780.6	Seizure Disorder NOS	780.39
Atypical Chest Pain, Unspec.	786.59	Gastritis, Acute w/o Hemorrhage	535.00	Serous Otitis Media, Chronic, Unspec.	381.10
Bronchiolitis, due to RSV	466.11	Gastroenteritis, NOS	558.9	Sinusitis, Acute NOS	461.9
Bronchitis, Acute	466.0	Gastroesophageal Reflux	530.81	Tonsillitis, Acute	463.
Bronchitis, NOS	490	Hepatitis A, Infectious	070.1	Upper Respiratory Infection, Acute NOS	465.9
Cardiac Arrest	427.5	Hypercholesterolemia, Pure	272.0	Urinary Tract Infection, Unspec.	599.0
Cardiopulmonary Disease, Chronic, Unspec.	416.9	Hypertension, Unspec.	401.9	Urticaria, Unspec.	708.9
Cellulitis, NOS	682.9	Hypoglycemia NOS	251.2	Vertigo, NOS	780.4
Congestive Heart Failure, Unspec.	428.0	Hypokalemia	276.8	Viral Infection NOS	079.99
Contact Dermatitis NOS	692.9	Impetigo	684	Weakness, Generalized	780.79
COPD NOS	496	Lymphadenitis, Unspec.	289.3	Weight Loss, Abnormal	783.21
CVA, Acute, NOS	434.91	Mononucleosis	075 1		
CVA, Old or Healed	438.9	Myocardial Infarction, Acute, NOS	410.9		
Degenerative Arthritis (Specify Site)	715.9	Organic Brain Syndrome	310.9		
		Otitis Externa, Acute NOS	380.10		

ABN: I UNDERSTAND THAT MEDICARE PROBABLY WILL NOT COVER THE SERVICES LISTED BELOW

A. _____ B. _____ C. _____

Patient

Date _____ Signature _____

Doctor's Signature _L D Heath_

RETURN: _____ Days 2 Weeks _____ Months

REF# 122949 SB (05.07.09)   TO REORDER CALL INHEALTH RECORD SYSTEMS 800-477-7374

DOUGLASVILLE MEDICINE ASSOCIATES
5076 BRAND BLVD., SUITE 401
DOUGLASVILLE, NY 01234
PHONE No. (123) 456-7890
☒ L.D. HEATH, M.D.   ❏ D.J. SCHWARTZ, M.D.
NPI# 9995010111   NPI# 9995020212
EIN# 00-1234560

SOURCE DOCUMENT 6-17

Outside Services LOG
Drs. Heath and Schwartz

Ref. Number	Date(s) of Service	Patient Name	Facility Physician	Procedures Authorization #	Diagnosis (Primary/Secondary/ Tertiary)
001	11/24/2009	Blanc, Francois	Retirement Inn Nursing Home, Dr. Heath	Est. Pt. Problem Focused	Hypertension DM - Type II Uncontrolled
002	11/24/2009	Chang, Xao	Retirement Inn Nursing Home Dr. Heath	Est. Pt. Problem Focused	Seizure disorder
003	11/24/2009	Pinkston, Anna	Retirement Inn Nursing Home Dr. Heath	Est. Pt. Expanded	Peripheral Vascular Insufficiency
004	11/03/2009	Tate, Jason	Community General Hospital Dr. Heath	Initial hospital care (patient admitted) Auth # 2213690	Peptic Ulcer, fever of unknown origin, depression
004	11/04/2009	Tate, Jason	Community General Hospital Dr. Heath	Subsequent hospital care (inpatient)	Peptic Ulcer, fever of unknown origin, depression
004	11/05/2009	Tate, Jason	Community General Hospital Dr. Heath	Discharge services	Peptic Ulcer, fever of unknown origin, depression
005	11/06/2009	Munoz, Geraldo	New York County Hospital Dr. Heath	Initial hospital care (patient admitted)	Atrial fibrillation
005	11/07/2009 to 11/08/2009	Munoz, Geraldo	New York County Hospital Dr. Heath	Subsequent hospital care (inpatient)	Atrial fibrillation
005	11/09/2009	Munoz, Geraldo	New York County Hospital Dr. Heath	Discharge services	Atrial fibrillation

Outside Services LOG
Drs. Heath and Schwartz

Ref. Number	Date(s) of Service	Patient Name	Facility Physician	Procedures Authorization #	Diagnosis (Primary/Secondary/Tertiary)
006	11/05/2009	Ruhl, Mary	New York County Hospital Dr. Heath	Detailed hospital care (patient admitted) Auth # 22136950	Gastroenteritis, dehydration, fever of unknown origin
006	11/06/2009 to 11/09/2009	Ruhl, Mary	New York County Hospital Dr. Heath	Subsequent care	Gastroenteritis, dehydration, fever of unknown origin
006	11/10/2009	Ruhl, Mary	New York County Hospital Dr. Heath	Discharge service	Gastroenteritis, dehydration, fever of unknown origin
007	11/14/2009	Mallory, Christina	New York County Hospital Dr. Heath	Initial hospital care (admitted overnight for observation) Auth # 22136931	Drug reaction, post antibiotic therapy
007	11/15/2009	Mallory, Christina	New York County Hospital Dr. Heath	Discharge service	Drug reaction, post antibiotic therapy. Patient stable.
008	10/25/2009	Goodnow, Leona	Community General Hospital Dr. Schwartz	Emergency Room service (no admission, stable)	Asthma, exacerbation

Outside Services Log for Drs. Heath and Schwartz. *Delmar/Cengage Learning*

SOURCE DOCUMENT 8-1

```
Medicare Remittance Advice (MOSS Sample)
--------------------------------------------------------------------
11-30-2009 MEDICARE CLAIMS SUBMITTED FOR L.D. Heath, MD 999501
--------------------------------------------------------------------

ADAMS,  MINNIE              BILLED  ALLOWED DEDUCT    COINS  PROV-PD  MC-ADJUSTMEN
   HIC  999571266A          ASG Y   ICN  973332011
   ACNT ADA001
1028    102809  11  99203  200.00  106.99  0         21.40   85.59    93.01
1028    102809  11  80053   47.00   14.77  0          0.00   14.77    32.23
1028    102809  11  36415   18.00    3.00  0          0.00    3.00    15.00
            CLAIM TOTALS:  265.00  124.76  0         21.40  103.36   140.24


BLANC,  FRANCOIS            BILLED  ALLOWED DEDUCT    COINS  PROV-PD  MC-ADJUSTMEN
   HIC  999135611A          ASG Y   ICN     973332012
   ACNT BLA001
1027    102709  31  99307   60.00  35.62   0          7.12   28.50    24.38
1124    112409  32  99307   68.00  35.62   0          7.12   28.50    32.38
            CLAIM TOTALS:  128.00  71.24   0         14.24   57.00    56.76
CLAIM INFORMATION FORWARDED TO: MEDICAID


CHANG,  XAO                 BILLED  ALLOWED DEDUCT    COINS  PROV-PD  MC-ADJUSTMEN
   HIC  999321156A          ASG Y   ICN     973332013
ACNT CHA001
1016    101609  31  99307   60.00  35.62   0          7.12   28.50    24.38
1124    112409  32  99307   68.00  35.62   0          7.12   28.50    32.38
            CLAIM TOTALS:  128.00  71.24   0         14.24   57.00    56.76
CLAIM INFORMATION FORWARDED TO:  MEDICAID

TOTAL PAID TO PROVIDER: $217.36
```

Medicare Remittance Advice for Patients Adams, Blanc, and Chang. *Delmar/Cengage Learning*

SOURCE DOCUMENT 8-2

```
Medicare Remittance Advice (MOSS Sample)
11-30-2009 MEDICARE CLAIMS SUBMITTED FOR L.D. Heath, MD 999501
```

		BILLED	ALLOWED	DEDUCT	COINS	PROV-PD	MC-ADJUSTMENT

RAMIREZ, MANUEL
HIC   999512136A
ACNT RAM001

		BILLED	ALLOWED	DEDUCT	COINS	PROV-PD	MC-ADJUSTMENT
			ASG Y	ICN 973332020			
1030	11 99215	249.00	140.31	0.00	28.06	112.25	108.69
1030	11 45378	1518.00	451.54	0.00	90.30	361.24	1066.46
CLAIM TOTALS:		1767.00	591.85	0.00	118.36	473.49	1175.15

MUNOZ, GERALDO
HIC   999832166A
ACNT MUN001

		BILLED	ALLOWED	DEDUCT	COINS	PROV-PD	MC-ADJUSTMENT
			ASG Y	ICN 973332021			
1106	21 99221	145.00	92.33	0.00	18.47	73.86	52.67
1107	21 99231	158.00	78.14	0.00	15.63	62.51	79.86
1109	21 99238	145.00	73.16	0.00	14.63	58.53	71.84
CLAIM TOTALS:		448.00	243.63	0.00	48.73	194.90	204.37

PINKSTON, ANNA
HIC   999210132D
ACNT PIN001

		BILLED	ALLOWED	DEDUCT	COINS	PROV-PD	MC-ADJUSTMENT
			ASG Y	ICN 973332022			
1020	31 99308	78.00	74.00	0.00	14.80	59.20	4.00
1124	31 99308	113.00	59.06	0.00	11.81	47.25	53.94
CLAIM TOTALS:		191.00	133.06	0.00	26.61	106.45	57.94

CLAIM INFORMATION FORWARDED TO: MEDICAID

TOTAL PAID TO PROVIDER: $774.84

Medicare Remittance Advice for Patients Ramirez, Munoz, and Pinkston. *Delmar/Cengage Learning*

SOURCE DOCUMENT 8-3

```
Medicare Remittance Advice (MOSS Sample)
```

11-30-2009 MEDICARE CLAIMS SUBMITTED FOR L.D. Heath, MD 999501

MANGANO, VITO
HIC 999213899A ICN 973332030
ACNT ADA001

				BILLED ASG Y	ALLOWED	DEDUCT	COINS	PROV-PD	MC-ADJUSTMENT
1027	102709	11	99214	180.00	104.46	75.00	5.89	23.57	75.54
1027	102709	11	81000	12.00	4.43	0	0.89	3.54	7.57
1027	102709	11	36415	18.00	3.00	0	0.00	3.00	15.00
		CLAIM TOTALS:		210.00	111.89	75.00	6.78	30.11	98.11

TOTAL PAID TO PROVIDER: $30.11

11-30-2009 MEDICARE CLAIMS SUBMITTED FOR D.J. SCHWARTZ, MD 999502

TOMANAGA, MARIE
HIC 999131666A ICN 973332043
ACNT TOM001

				BILLED ASG Y	ALLOWED	DEDUCT	COINS	PROV-PD	MC-ADJUSTMENT
1103	110309	11	99205	358.00	199.78	135.00	12.96	51.82	158.22
1103	110309	11	93000	131.00	30.48	0.00	6.10	24.38	100.52
1103	110309	11	85651	9.00	4.96	0.00	0.99	3.97	4.04
1103	110309	11	36415	18.00	3.00	0.00	0.00	3.00	15.00
		CLAIM TOTALS:		516.00	238.22	135.00	20.05	83.17	277.78

TOTAL PAID TO PROVIDER: $83.17

Medicare Remittance Advice for Patients Mangano and Tomanaga. *Delmar/Cengage Learning*

SOURCE DOCUMENT 8-4

Explanation of Medical Benefits   **FlexiHealth PPO Plan**

Insured Name	Insured/Patient ID	Patient Name	Page 1
KRAMER, STANLEY	**999811169-01**	**KRAMER, STANLEY**	**11/30/2009**

Provider Name: **D.J. SCHWARTZ, MD - Out-of-Network Provider**
Reference Number: 987997

Service Date	Type of Service	Charge(s) Submitted	Not Covered or Discount	Amount Covered	Patient Co-payment Co-insurance Deductible	Covered Balance	Plan Liability	See Note
10/27/2009	99221 Initial Hosp Care	$145.00	52.00	93.00	93.00 Deductible	0.00	0.00	A, B
10/28/2009 to 10/29/2009	99231 Hosp Subsequent Care	$158.00	48.00	110.00	110.00 Deductible	0.00	0.00	A, B
10/30/2009	99212 Est. Pat/Level 2	$ 80.00	5.80	74.20	74.20 Deductible	0.00	0.00	A, B
					Total Paid: $0.00			

Notes on Benefit Determination:

A - This expense has been applied to plan deductible or co-pay.
B - Patient is responsible for non-covered amounts for Out-of-Network providers.

Flexihealth PPO Plan Explanation of Medical Benefits, Patient Kramer.

SOURCE DOCUMENT 8-5

Explanation of Medical Benefits   **FlexiHealth PPO Plan**

Insured Name	Insured/Patient ID	Patient Name	Page 1
WADE, JENNIFER	999125813-02	KINZLER, LINDA	11/30/2009

Service Date	Type of Service	Charge(s) Submitted	Not Covered or Discount	Amount Covered	Patient Co-payment Co-insurance Deductible	Covered Balance	Plan Liability	See Note
Provider Name: L.D. HEATH MD – In-Network Provider								
Reference Number: 987236								
11/09/2009	99203 New Pat/Level 3	$200.00	$20.00	$180.00	$20.00 co-pay	$160.00	$160.00	A
11/09/2009	90658 Flu Vaccination	$ 22.00	$22.00	$ 0.00	$ 0.00	$ 0.00	$ 0.00	B
						Total Paid:	**$160.00**	

Notes on Benefit Determination:

A - Preferred provider discount. Patient is not required to pay this amount.

B - Plan exclusion, patient responsibility.

Flexihealth PPO Plan Explanation of Medical Benefits, Patient Kinzler.

SOURCE DOCUMENT 8-6

Explanation of Medical Benefits   **FlexiHealth PPO Plan**

Insured Name	Insured/Patient ID	Patient Name		Page 1
MALLORY, MICHAEL	**999510226-B2**	**MALLORY, CHRISTINA**		**11/30/2009**

Service Date	Type of Service	Charge(s) Submitted	Not Covered or Discount	Amount Covered	Patient Co-payment Co-insurance Deductible	Covered Balance	Plan Liability	See Note
	Provider Name: **L.D. Heath, MD – In-Network Provider**							
	Reference Number: 987522							
11/14/2009	99221 Initial Hosp Care	$145.00	$ 52.00	$93.00	$18.60 co-ins	$74.40	$74.40	A
11/15/2009	99238 Hosp Discharge	$145.00	$ 86.80	$58.20	$11.64 co-ins	$46.56	$46.56	A
							Total Paid: $119.96	

Insured Name	Insured/Patient ID	Patient Name		
MANALY, RICHARD	**999236189**	**MANALY, RICHARD**		

	Provider Name: **D.J. Schwartz MD – Out-of-Network Provider**							
	Reference Number: 987523							
10/21/2009	99213 Est. Pat/Level 3	$111.00	$ 28.60	$82.40	$16.48 co-ins	$65.92	$65.92	B
							Total Paid: $65.92	

Insured Name	Insured/Patient ID	Patient Name		
RUHL, ROBERT	**999321168-02**	**RUHL, MARY**		

	Provider Name: **L.D. Heath, MD – In-Network Provider**							
	Reference Number: 987524							
11/05/2009	99221 Initial Hosp Care	$145.00	$ 52.00	$93.00	$18.60 co-ins	$74.40	$74.40	A
11/06/2009 to	99231 Hosp Subsequent Care	$316.00	$104.00	$212.00	$42.40 co-ins	$169.60	$ 169.60	A
11/09/2009								
11/10/2009	99238 Hosp Discharge	$145.00	$ 86.80	$58.20	$11.64 co-ins	$46.56	$46.56	A
							Total Paid: $290.56	

Notes on Benefit Determination:

A - Preferred provider discount. Patient is not required to pay this amount.

B - Patient is responsible for non-covered amounts for Out-of-Network providers.

Flexihealth PPO Plan Explanation of Medical Benefits, Patients Mallory, Manaly, and Ruhl.

Explanation of Medical Benefits   **FlexiHealth PPO Plan**

Insured Name	Insured/Patient ID	Patient Name
WORTHINGTON, CYNTHIA	999215992	WORTHINGTON, CYNTHIA

Provider Name: **L.D. Heath, MD – In-Network Provider**
Reference Number: 987556

Service Date	Type of Service	Charge(s) Submitted	Not Covered or Discount	Amount Covered	Patient Co-payment Co-insurance Deductible	Covered Balance	Plan Liability	See Note
10/30/2009	99213 Est. Pat/Level 3	$ 111.00	$ 28.60	$ 82.40	$ 20.00 co-pay	$ 62.40	$ 62.40	A
							Total Paid: $62.40	

Insured Name	Insured/Patient ID	Patient Name
YBARRA, ROSS	999113287	YBARRA, ELANE

Provider Name: **D.J. Schwartz MD – Out-of-Network Provider**
Reference Number: 987557

Service Date	Type of Service	Charge(s) Submitted	Not Covered or Discount	Amount Covered	Patient Co-payment Co-insurance Deductible	Covered Balance	Plan Liability	See Note
10/16/2009	99214 Est. Pat/Level 4	$ 180.00	$ 11.50	$ 168.50	$ 33.70 co-ins	$ 134.80	$ 134.80	B
10/16/2009	87081 Strep Screen	$ 16.00	$ 0.00	$ 16.00	$ 3.20 co-ins	$ 12.80	$ 12.80	B
11/06/2009	99215 Est. Pat/Level 5	$ 249.00	$ 33.20	$ 215.80	$ 43.16 co-ins	$ 172.64	$ 172.64	B
11/06/2009	81000 UA w/micro	$ 12.00	$ 0.00	$ 12.00	$ 2.40 co-ins	$ 9.60	$ 9.60	B
							Total Paid: $329.84	

Insured Name	Insured/Patient ID	Patient Name
TATE, JASON	999561133	TATE, JASON

Provider Name: **L.D. Heath, MD – In-Network Provider**
Reference Number: 987558

Service Date	Type of Service	Charge(s) Submitted	Not Covered or Discount	Amount Covered	Patient Co-payment Co-insurance Deductible	Covered Balance	Plan Liability	See Note
11/03/2009	99221 Hosp Admission	$ 145.00	$ 52.00	$ 93.00	$ 18.60 co-ins	$ 74.40	$ 74.40	A
11/04/2009	99231 Hosp Subsequentc Care	$ 79.00	$ 26.00	$ 53.00	$ 10.60 co-ins	$ 42.40	$ 42.40	A
11/05/2009	99238 Hosp Discharge	$ 145.00	$ 86.80	$ 58.20	$ 11.64 co-ins	$ 46.56	$ 46.56	A
							Total Paid: $163.36	

Notes on Benefit Determination:

Flexihealth PPO Plan Explanation of Medical Benefits, Patients Worthington, Ybarra, and Tate.

SOURCE DOCUMENT 8-8

Service Detail – ConsumerONE HRA

Date(s) of Service	Amount Charged	Amount Allowed	Amount Disallowed	Level One	Level Two	Level Three	Preventative Care	Patient Responsibility	Benefit Paid by HRA	*Remark Codes
Patient: John Conway			Claim #: 32155400		**Provider:**	HEATH	Douglasville Medicine Associates			
102309	$ 180.00	$ 168.70	$ 11.30	$ 168.70	0.00	0.00	0.00	$ 0.00	$ 168.70	001
102309	$ 11.00	$ 11.00	$ 0.00	$ 11.00	0.00	0.00	0.00	$ 0.00	$ 11.00	001
Patient: Leona Goodnow			Claim #: 32155401		**Provider:**	SCHWARTZ	Douglasville Medicine Associates			
102509	$ 147.00	$ 147.00	$ 0.00	$ 0.00	0.00	$ 147.00	0.00	$ 29.40	$ 117.60	003
Patient: Eric Gordon			Claim #: 32155402		**Provider:**	SCHWARTZ	Douglasville Medicine Associates			
102209	$ 180.00	$ 168.70	$ 11.30	$ 0.00	$ 168.70	0.00	0.00	$ 168.70	$ 0.00	001, 002
110509	$ 111.00	$ 88.00	$ 23.00	$ 0.00	$ 88.00	0.00	0.00	$ 88.00	$ 0.00	001, 002
Patient: Kabin Pradhan			Claim #: 32155403		**Provider:**	SCHWARTZ	Douglasville Medicine Associates			
110309	$ 130.00	$ 124.60	$ 5.40	$ 124.60	$ 0.00	0.00	0.00	$ 0.00	$ 124.60	001
TOTALS	$ 759.00	$ 708.00	$ 51.00	$ 304.30	$ 256.70	$ 147.00	0.00	$ 286.10	$ 421.90	*

*Remark Codes:

001 Level One EPA – Disallowed amount is an in-network provider write-off.

002 Level Two – Patient out-of-pocket responsibility up to $500.00; EPA exhausted

003 Level Three – In-Network 80/20 HRA reimbursement agreement.

ConsumerONE HRA Service Detail.

SOURCE DOCUMENT 9-1

Minnie Adams
1876 Slate Dr.
Douglasville, NY 01234

9-5678/1234   **55683**

DATE ___11/30/2009___

PAY TO THE
ORDER OF___Douglasville Medicine Assoc.___ | $ **21.40**

Twenty-one dollars 40/100 ------------------------------ DOLLARS

Memo___Oct 28, 2009___   *Minnie Adams*

⑈123456780⑈ 123⑈456⑈7⑈

Check from Minnie Adams. *Delmar/Cengage Learning*

SOURCE DOCUMENT 9-2

Eric Gordon
485 Slate Dr.
Douglasville, NY 01234

9-5678/1234   **998**

DATE ___12/1/2009___

PAY TO THE
ORDER OF___Dr. Schwartz___ | $ **256.70**

Two hundred fifty six 70/100 ----------------- DOLLARS

Memo___Deductibles___   *Eric Gordon*

⑈123456780⑈ 123⑈456⑈7⑈

Check from Eric Gordon. *Delmar/Cengage Learning*

SOURCE DOCUMENT 9-3

Stanley Kramer
58682 Pebble Trail
Douglasville, NY 01234

9-5678/1234   **1130**

DATE ___12/1/2009___

PAY TO THE
ORDER OF___Dr. Schwartz___ | $ **383.00**

Three hundred and eighty-three 00/100 ---------- DOLLARS

Memo___Acct: KRA001___   *Stanley Kramer*

⑈123456780⑈ 123⑈456⑈7⑈

Check from Stanley Kramer. *Delmar/Cengage Learning*

SOURCE DOCUMENT 9-4

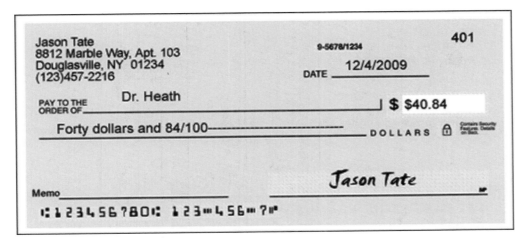

Michael Mallory
516 Ridgeway Rd.
Douglasville, NY 01234
(123)4572321

9-5678/1234

8552

DATE 12/01/2009

PAY TO THE ORDER OF **Douglasville Med Assoc** $ 30.24

Thirty dollars and 24 cents --------------------- DOLLARS

Memo **Account MAL001**   *Michael Mallory*

⑆123456780⑆ 123⑈456⑈7⑉

Check from Michael Mallory. *Delmar/Cengage Learning*

SOURCE DOCUMENT 9-5

Vito or Teresa Mangano
8123 Slate Court, Apt. 31
Douglasville, NY 01234

9-5678/1234

117

DATE 11/30/2009

PAY TO THE ORDER OF **Doctor Heath** $ 81.78

Eighty-one dollars and 78/100--------------- DOLLARS

Memo   *Vito Mangano*

⑆123456780⑆ 123⑈456⑈7⑉

Check from Vita Mangano. *Delmar/Cengage Learning*

SOURCE DOCUMENT 9-6

Jason Tate
8812 Marble Way, Apt. 103
Douglasville, NY 01234
(123)457-2216

9-5678/1234

401

DATE 12/4/2009

PAY TO THE ORDER OF **Dr. Heath** $ $40.84

Forty dollars and 84/100----------------------- DOLLARS

Memo   *Jason Tate*

⑆123456780⑆ 123⑈456⑈7⑉

Check from Jason Tate. *Delmar/Cengage Learning*

SOURCE DOCUMENT 9-7

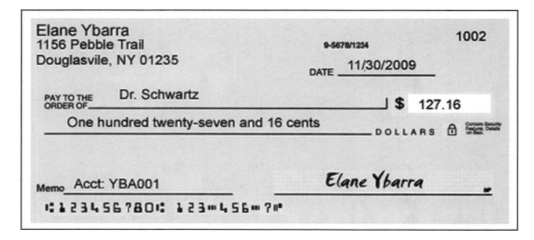

Cynthia Worthington
5857 Granite St.
Douglasville, NY 01235

3645

9-5678/1234

DATE 11/30/2009

PAY TO THE ORDER OF Douglasville Medicine Associates $ 20.00

Exactly twenty DOLLARS

Memo Co-payment 10/27/09

Cindy Worthington

⑆123456780⑆ 123⑉456⑉7⑊

Check from Cynthia Worthington. *Delmar/Cengage Learning*

SOURCE DOCUMENT 9-8

Thomas Goodnow
Leona Goodnow
321 White Stone Dr.
Douglasville, NY 01234

203

9-5678/1234

DATE 12/1/2009

PAY TO THE ORDER OF Douglasville Medicine Associates $ 29.40

Twenty-nine and 40/100 ----------------------------------- DOLLARS

Memo

Thomas Goodnow

⑆123456780⑆ 123⑉456⑉7⑊

Check from Thomas Goodnow. *Delmar/Cengage Learning*

SOURCE DOCUMENT 9-9

Elane Ybarra
1156 Pebble Trail
Douglasville, NY 01235

1002

9-5678/1234

DATE 11/30/2009

PAY TO THE ORDER OF Dr. Schwartz $ 127.16

One hundred twenty-seven and 16 cents DOLLARS

Memo Acct: YBA001

Elane Ybarra

⑆123456780⑆ 123⑉456⑉7⑊

Check from Elane Ybarra. *Delmar/Cengage Learning*

SOURCE DOCUMENT 10-1

Century SeniorGap
4500 Old Town Way
Lowville, NY 01453

December 21, 2009
Check Number: 1055458795666

Medigap Explanation of Benefits

Patient Name	Provider	Service Dates From	To	Provider Charged Amt	Medicare Allowed Amt	Medicare Paid Amt	Deductible	SeniorGap Paid
Munoz, Geraldo	Heath	1106	110609	145.00	92.33	73.86	0.00	18.47
999832166A	Heath	1107	110809	158.00	78.14	62.51	0.00	15.63
	Heath	1109	110909	145.00	73.16	58.53	0.00	14.63
SeniorGap Claim Number: 06987								
Tomanaga, Marie	Schwartz	1103	110309	358.00	199.78	51.82	135.00	147.96
999213166A	Schwartz	1103	110309	131.00	30.48	24.38	0.00	6.10
	Schwartz	1103	110309	9.00	4.96	3.97	0.00	0.99
	Schwartz	1103	110309	18.00	3.00	3.00	0.00	0.00
SeniorGap Claim Number: 06988						Check Total:		204.68

Medigap Explanation of Benefits. *Delmar/Cengage Learning*

SOURCE DOCUMENT 10-2

STATE DEPARTMENT OF MEDICAID SERVICES
MEDICAID MANAGEMENT INFORMATION SYSTEM
REMITTANCE ADVICE

AS OF 12162009

RA NUMBER 10346

CLAIM TYPE: MBS

Provider Name: LD HEATH
Provider ID: 890012

* PAID CLAIMS *

RECIPIENT IDENTIFICATION NAME	NUMBER	CLAIM QTY	SERVICE DATES FROM	THRU	BILLED CHARGES	DEDUCTIBLE AMOUNT	COINSURANCE AMOUNT	PMT AMT
BLANC, F	9991335611							
PROC: 99307		1	10/27/2009	10/27/2009	60.00	0.00	7.12	7.12
PROC: 99307		1	11/24/2009	11/24/2009	68.00	0.00	7.12	7.12
MEDICARE APPROVED AMT:					128.00			
MEDICARE PAID AMT:					57.00			
MEDICARE PAID DATE:12/16/2009								
CHANG, X	999321156							
PROC: 99307		1	10/16/2009	10/16/2009	60.00	0.00	7.12	7.12
PROC: 99307		1	11/24/2004	11/24/2009	68.00	0.00	7.12	7.12
MEDICARE APPROVED AMT:					128.00			
MEDICARE PAID AMT:					57.00			
MEDICARE PAID DATE:12/16/2009								
PINKSTON, A	999210132							
PROC: 99308		1	10/20/2009	10/20/2009	78.00	0.00	14.80	14.80
PROC: 99308		1	11/24/2009	11/24/2009	113.00	0.00	11.81	11.81
MEDICARE APPROVED AMT:					191.00			
MEDICARE PAID AMT:					106.45			
MEDICARE PAID DATE:11/25/2009								
CLAIMS PAID ON THIS RA:	6		TOTAL BILLED:		55.09		TOTAL PAID:	55.09

Remittance Advice from the State Department Medicaid Services. *Delmar/Cengage Learning*

SOURCE DOCUMENT 10-3

MSP PROVIDER REMITTANCE ADVICE   12/16/2009

PROV	SERV	DATE	POS	NOS	PROC	BILLED	ALLOWED	DEDUCT	COINS	GRP/RC	AMT	PROV PD
NAME MANALY, RICHARD			HIC	999236189A	ACNT	MAN002	ICN	973335612	ASG	N		
SCHWARTZ	1021	102109	11	1	99213	111.00	82.40	0.00	16.48	OA	28.60	28.60
999502										OA-23	65.92	65.92
										PR	16.48	16.48
PT RESP	0.00	CLAIM TOTALS				111.00		NET PAID	16.48			
NAME RUHL, MARY			HIC	999321168B	ACNT	RUH001	ICN	973335613	ASG	Y		
HEATH	1105	110509	21	1	99221	145.00	126.40	0.00	18.60	CO	18.60	18.60
999502										OA-23	74.40	74.40
										PR	18.60	18.60
HEATH	1106	110909	21	4	99231	316.00	212.00	0.00	42.40	CO	104.00	104.00
999502										OA-23	169.60	169.60
										PR	42.40	42.40
HEATH	1110	111009	21	1	99238	145.00	58.20	0.00	11.64	CO	86.80	86.80
999502										OA-23	46.56	46.56
										PR	11.64	11.64
PT RESP	0.00	CLAIM TOTALS				606.00		NET PAID	72.64			

GRP/RC

CO – Contractual obligation, the patient may not be billed for this amount

OA – Other Adjustment

OA-23: Amount primary insurance paid, claim reduced as part of COB

PR – Patient responsibility

SOURCE DOCUMENT 10-4

PROVIDER PAYMENT ADVICE
Signal HMO
Student1

Patient Name Kimberly Beals (BEA001)

Claim ID	DOS	Procedure	Charges	Allowed Amount	Patient Responsibility	Rejected Amount	Paid to Provider	Remarks
1000351	11/3/2009	36415	$18.00	$15.93	$0.00	$0.00	$15.93	A
1000350	11/3/2009	80053	$47.00	$41.60	$0.00	$0.00	$41.60	A
1000349	11/3/2009	99204	$283.00	$250.46	$10.00	$0.00	$240.46	A
Patient Totals			$348.00	$307.98	$10.00	$0.00	$297.98	

Patient Name David James (JAM001)

Claim ID	DOS	Procedure	Charges	Allowed Amount	Patient Responsibility	Rejected Amount	Paid to Provider	Remarks
1000357	11/9/2009	99213	$111.00	$98.24	$10.00	$0.00	$88.24	A
1000358	11/9/2009	86308	$17.00	$15.05	$0.00	$0.00	$15.05	A
Patient Totals			$128.00	$113.28	$10.00	$0.00	$103.28	

Patient Name Martin Montner (MON001)

Claim ID	DOS	Procedure	Charges	Allowed Amount	Patient Responsibility	Rejected Amount	Paid to Provider	Remarks
1000330	10/22/2009	87081	$16.00	$14.16	$0.00	$0.00	$14.16	A
1000329	10/22/2009	99204	$283.00	$250.46	$10.00	$0.00	$240.46	A
Patient Totals			$299.00	$264.62	$10.00	$0.00	$254.62	

PROVIDER PAYMENT ADVICE
Signal HMO
Student1

Patient Name Robert Shinn (SHI001)

Claim ID	DOS	Procedure	Charges	Allowed Amount	Patient Responsibility	Rejected Amount	Paid to Provider	Remarks
1000343	10/30/2009	99213	$111.00	$98.24	$10.00	$0.00	$88.24	A
1000136	10/23/2009	85031	$11.00	$9.74	$0.00	$0.00	$9.74	A
1000135	10/23/2009	99214	$180.00	$159.30	$10.00	$0.00	$149.30	A
Patient Totals			$302.00	$267.28	$20.00	$0.00	$247.28	

Patient Name Eugene Sykes (SYK001)

Claim ID	DOS	Procedure	Charges	Allowed Amount	Patient Responsibility	Rejected Amount	Paid to Provider	Remarks
1000139	10/16/2009	99213	$111.00	$98.24	$10.00	$0.00	$88.24	A
1000154	11/2/2009	99214	$180.00	$159.30	$10.00	$0.00	$149.30	A
1000141	10/16/2009	36415	$18.00	$15.93	$0.00	$0.00	$15.93	A
1000140	10/16/2009	85031	$11.00	$9.74	$0.00	$0.00	$9.74	A
Patient Totals			$320.00	$283.21	$20.00	$0.00	$263.21	

Patient Name Ricky Villanova (VIL001)

Claim ID	DOS	Procedure	Charges	Allowed Amount	Patient Responsibility	Rejected Amount	Paid to Provider	Remarks
1000335	10/27/2009	82947	$19.00	$16.82	$0.00	$0.00	$16.82	A
1000334	10/27/2009	99201	$130.00	$115.05	$10.00	$0.00	$105.05	A
Patient Totals			$149.00	$131.87	$10.00	$0.00	$121.87	

Provider Payment Advice from Signal HMO. *Delmar/Cengage Learning*

SOURCE DOCUMENT 11-1

PROVIDER PAYMENT ADVICE
Signal HMO
Student1

Patient Name Patty Practice (PRA002)

Claim ID	DOS	Procedure	Charges	Allowed Amount	Patient Responsibility	Rejected Amount	Paid to Provider	Remarks
1000351	11/3/2009	36415	$18.00	$15.93	$0.00	$0.00	$15.93	A
1000350	11/3/2009	80053	$47.00	$15.93	$0.00	$0.00	$15.93	A
1000349	11/3/2009	99204	$283.00	$15.93	$10.00	$0.00	$5.93	A
Patient Totals			$348.00	$47.79	$10.00	$0.00	$37.79	

Patient Name David James (JAM001)

Claim ID	DOS	Procedure	Charges	Allowed Amount	Patient Responsibility	Rejected Amount	Paid to Provider	Remarks
1000357	11/9/2009	99213	$111.00	$98.24	$10.00	$0.00	$88.24	A
1000358	11/9/2009	86308	$17.00	$15.05	$0.00	$0.00	$15.05	A
Patient Totals			$128.00	$113.28	$10.00	$0.00	$103.28	

Patient Name Martin Montner (MON001)

Claim ID	DOS	Procedure	Charges	Allowed Amount	Patient Responsibility	Rejected Amount	Paid to Provider	Remarks
1000330	10/22/2009	87081	$16.00	$14.16	$0.00	$0.00	$14.16	A
1000329	10/22/2009	99204	$283.00	$250.46	$10.00	$0.00	$240.46	A
Patient Totals			$299.00	$264.62	$10.00	$0.00	$254.62	

Provider Payment Advice from Signal HMO. *Delmar/Cengage Learning*

Glossary

Accepting assignment—when the physician or supplier agrees to accept the approved amount as full fee.

Active window—the vivid-colored title bar that is currently in use.

Adjustment—an amount taken away from (or added to) the balance of an account.

Aging—refers to categorizing balances due according to the length of time they have been unpaid.

Ambulatory surgical center—provides a facility where surgery, medical procedures, and skilled rehabilitation services are performed, and patients leave the center to return home the same day.

Ancillary office—an additional location that is part of the same practice or business entity.

Appeal—also called a claims review, is a request for the claim to be reconsidered (reviewed) for payment, and to have the original decision appealed, or reversed.

Application window—contains the actual software program.

Applications software—software that allows the computer user to perform specific tasks or work.

Appointment reminder card—a card that contains information for the next appointment, including day, date, and time.

Appointment scheduling system—a system that handles most of the tasks associated with patient visits to the office.

Arrowheads—indicators to the right or at the bottom of menu selections that designate more selections, or sub-menus, are available.

Arrows—indicators to the right or at the bottom of menu selections that designate more selections (or that a submenu) are available.

Attending physician—the doctor who has primary responsibility for the treatment and care of the patient.

Back office—also referred to as the clinical area, or that part of the office where health care professionals examine patients.

Bill pay system—a service that allows users to manage and pay bills online through a secure website; funds are typically taken directly from a bank account.

Billing cycle—refers to the time that elapses between regular statements being mailed to patients.

Birthday rule—an informal procedure used by insurers to help determine which health plan pays first when children are dependents on more than one health plan.

Black circles—indicators that menu options are selected or *on*.

Block billing—using a range of dates when the same CPT code applies to each of the consecutive dates.

Booting—refers to the computer using a special start-up program to load the operating system into memory when starting the computer.

Browser—a special window, such as Internet Explorer, used to search sites on the Internet.

Business associate agreement—allows covered entities to share PHI with business associates by assuring that the information will be appropriately safeguarded.

Cable modem—a device that enables high-speed Internet access using cable television wires instead of telephone lines.

Cancellation—a patient who had an appointment but called the office to either reschedule or opted not to visit the office.

Cancelled check—a check that has already been paid to the payee and processed by a financial institution.

Capitation—a special reimbursement method common to managed care in which the physician is reimbursed on a per patient rate plus co-payment, rather than a fee schedule for each medical procedure performed.

CD burner—a drive that can write (record) data onto a blank CD.

CD-R (Compact Disk-Recordable)—this type of CD allows data to be recorded or copied onto it.

CD-ROM (Compact Disk-Read Only Memory *or* **CD)**—the computer can use and transfer data from the CD but cannot erase from or add data to it.

Centers for Medicare & Medicaid Services (CMS)—serves the needs of Medicare and Medicaid beneficiaries.

Central processing unit (CPU)—the brain of the personal computer without which the computer cannot run programs, perform calculations, or direct instructions to other parts of the computer.

Charges—fees for procedures performed.

Checkmarks—indicators that show menu options are selected or *on*.

Claims review—also called an appeal, is a request for the claim to be reconsidered (reviewed) for payment, and to have the original decision appealed, or reversed.

Closed panel HMO—also known as a staff model; a plan that contracts with physicians to provide services exclusively to their members.

CMS–1500—the claim form approved by the Centers for Medicare & Medicaid Services (CMS) and used by the Medicare program for submitting claims from physicians and suppliers; also accepted by the majority of insurance carriers whenever paper claims need to be submitted.

COB—see Coordination of benefits.

Co-insurance—the percentage of cost the primary insurance company will not pay.

Command buttons—buttons used, when clicked, to execute a function, such as *Save*, *Close*, *Cancel*, and *OK*.

Consultation—when another physician renders an opinion and advice regarding a patient's diagnosis and treatment.

Consumer-driven health plans—new products now visible in the medical insurance marketplace that give medical consumers more choices and control over spending by having access to funds reserved for health care.

Coordination of benefits (COB)—means benefits are paid such that no more than 100 percent of usual, customary, and reasonable (UCR) expenses are covered under the combined benefits of all plans; applies when a patient is covered by more than one plan.

Co-payment—a fixed payment at each office visit for which the patient is responsible.

Covered entities—users protected under the HIPAA privacy rules.

CPT-4—see Current Procedural Terminology codes.

CPU—see Central processing unit.

Current accounts—unpaid balances that are in the zero to 30-day category.

Current Procedural Terminology codes (CPT-4)—codes that identify procedures performed for patients.

Cyclic billing—a method of splitting overall patient accounts into smaller segments that are billed according to specific designators at different times during the month.

Data—information.

Data processing—the input, processing, and output cycle of a computer.

Database management programs—software programs that enable information to be stored, modified, and retrieved.

Dedicated server—a server that performs only the specific tasks it was set up to do.

Deductible—an out-of-pocket expense the patient must pay before the insurance company will pay on covered services.

Demographic information—basic information regarding the patient that includes address, phone number, date of birth, gender, marital status, employer, school, etc.

Denial—also referred to as denied claims, are those that have not been paid, and a reason has been given.

Desktop—a graphical interface provided by Windows that allows users to manage resources visually.

Dialog boxes—special windows that appear on the screen when more information or settings are required from the user, before a command can be executed.

Digital camera—an input device, used to convert pictures into digital files.

Digital file—data in a format that can be recognized and used by the computer.

Disk—a round plate on which information, or data, can be recorded.

Document window—the window that displays the document created or opened within a program.

Double click—See Single/double click.

Dragging—also known as grabbing; holding down the left mouse button, and moving an item from one location on the computer screen to another.

Drive—a machine that is usually part of the computer system that reads data from a disk.

Drop-down box—a list that displays choices when clicked.

Dropping—letting go of the left mouse button so that the item that was dragged is left in its new location on the screen.

DSL (Digital subscriber line)—high-speed access to the Internet using existing copper wires used for telephone service in the home or office without interfering with voice services.

Dun—a demand for payment.

Dunning message—a short collection note that appears on a patient's bill.

DVD (Digital versatile disk)—similar to a CD, but based on a different technology; can hold five to ten times more data than a CD.

EHR— Electronic Health Records integrate all elements of a patient's health history, which may include medications, lab work, x-rays, scans, EKGs, medical diagnoses, and more as digital documentation.

Electronic payment and statement (EPS) system—will transfer payments made on claims directly to the medical provider's financial institution by way of a clearinghouse.

Encounter form—also known as a superbill, a charge ticket, or visit/fee slip, contains all of the information insurance companies require in order to consider a claim for payment.

EOB—see Explanation of benefits.

EPS—See Electronic payment and statement (EPS) system.

Established patient—an individual who has received professional services from a physician within the past three years, or from another physician of the same specialty who belongs to the same group practice.

Exclusion—a service not covered by a health insurance plan.

Explanation of benefits (EOB)—shows the dates of service for a particular patient, which codes were considered for payment, and the physician or facility that rendered the services.

Face sheet—also known as the admission form, admitting sheet, data form, or patient information form; a common document in medical facilities that contains demographic information on the patient.

Fee schedule—much like a price list, allows the fee to be charged according to the costs assigned by the patient's insurance provider.

File maintenance system—a utility area of the program that contains common information used by various systems within the software.

Firewall—software residing on a computer that is configured with rules that allow certain traffic, programs, and other network requests to move to and from the computers connected to the server; helps protect from viruses, malicious attacks, or unauthorized access or use of certain areas or programs within the network.

Fiscal intermediary—also referred to as the Medicare carrier; insurance carriers who manage funds and make payments on behalf of the beneficiary.

Flagging—marking a file, indicating special action is required.

Floppy diskette—a disk that stores data, similar to the hard drive, except it is portable and holds less information.

Front office—also referred to as the administrative area; the hub of the medical facility.

FSA—see Health flexible spending account.

Grabbing—clicking on an object on the computer screen with the mouse and holding on to it in order to drag it to another location on the screen.

Group model HMO—resembles the closed panel model but, in this case, the HMO has an exclusive contract with a medical group practice.

Group plan—a single medical plan that provides coverage for a group of people.

Guarantor—the person responsible for paying medical expenses; often included on the registration form.

Hard copy—paper documents produced by the printer.

Hard drive—the disk that resides inside the computer and stores all file data and software programs.

Hardware—the physical parts of a computer.

Health flexible spending account (FSA)—provides a means for employees to put aside money for medical expenses that otherwise might not be reimbursed.

Health insurance claim number (HIC)—refers to the patient's Medicare number.

Health Insurance Portability and Accountability Act (HIPAA)—a bill that provides guidelines for the protection of patient health information.

Health reimbursement arrangement (HRA)—an arrangement between employer and insured that provides funds for health care expenses.

Health unit coordinators—individuals who manage the administrative tasks of the nurse's station.

HIC—see Health insurance claim number.

HIPAA—see Health Insurance Portability and Accountability Act.

Hospital—a facility that provides 24-hour care to patients with the highest level of medical need.

Hot keys—keyboard selections for accessing menu options without using the mouse.

Hot-swapped—removing one device from and plugging a different device into the same slot with smooth transition from one to the other.

HRA—see Health reimbursement arrangement.

ICD-9—see International Classification of Diseases.

Increment box—also called a spinner, looks like a text box with a special button on the right that contains a small arrowhead pointing up and another one pointing down; typically found where choices involving size or quantity (number) are involved.

Indemnity plan—sometimes called traditional or commercial insurance; patients have few restrictions but more responsibility.

Independent practice association—see Open panel HMO.

Individual plan—a medical insurance plan purchased directly by the policyholder from an insurance company or through an agent.

In-network benefits—services received from authorized providers.

Inpatient—a patient who stays in the hospital for more than 24 hours.

Input—adding information; common input devices include the keyboard and the mouse.

Insurance billing system—designed to prepare claims that will be sent to insurance companies in order to receive payment for services rendered by medical providers.

Insurance card—issued by the insurance company, containing information about the policyholder.

Insurance verification—contacting the insurance company, either by telephone or by using online resources on the computer, in order to verify that the patient is indeed eligible to receive benefits.

Interface—the activity of programs communicating and functioning with each other.

International Classification of Diseases (ICD-9)—a set of codes used to identify patients' diagnoses.

Internet—a global network that connects millions of computers, enabling the exchange of data, news, and other information.

Internet Explorer—a special window that displays Web pages on the Internet for viewing.

LAN—see Local area network.

Large group health plan—a plan provided by an employer with more than 100 employees.

Liability insurance—coverage that protects against claims based on negligence, inappropriate action, or inaction which results in injury to someone or damage to property.

Limiting charge—The cap on the amount that can be charged above Medicare's approved amount by a Medicare NON-PAR provider that does not accept assignment on a claim.

Local area network—the most common type of network for computers that are located in the same building.

Lost claim—the insurance company has no record of having received the claim.

Mainframes—large, powerful computers capable of supporting hundreds or thousands of users simultaneously.

Major medical—covers expenses for catastrophic illness or accidents that go beyond what is covered by basic insurance or funds available in arrangement agreements.

Managed care—a system of health plans that attempts to control costs by limiting access to health care and focusing on preventative medicine.

Medicaid—also known as Title XIX; a federal/state entitlement program that provides medical assistance for families and individuals with low incomes and resources.

Medical savings account (MSA)—a combination of a high-deductible insurance plan with a savings account.

Medicare + Choice HMOs—function like any other HMO; the beneficiary has a PCP who manages care and must authorize special services or referrals to specialists.

Medicare + Choice plan (M+C)—also known as Medicare part C; provides all coverage available with original Medicare and may even offer additional services not covered by original Medicare.

Medicare + Choice PPOs—plans that offer a network of providers from which the beneficiary may choose without consulting his or her PCP.

Medicare Part A—covers inpatient hospital, skilled nursing facility, home health, and hospice care.

Medicare Part B—covers professional services that are reasonable and medically necessary.

Medigap—coverage that helps pay for the deductible and co-insurance and other "gaps" in coverage in the Medicare plan.

Microprocessor—also known as the central processing unit (CPU); the brain of the personal computer without which the computer cannot run programs, perform calculations, or direct instructions to other parts of the computer.

Modem—a device that translates digital information from the computer into analog signals used by telephones, and vice versa; literally *modulate-dem*odulate.

MSA—see Medical savings account.

National provider identification (NPI)—a 10-character number developed to eventually replace the PIN numbers for all insurances, including Medicare UPIN numbers.

Network—computers that are interconnected, or linked, so that information can be exchanged between them for many users.

Network HMO—see Open panel HMO.

New patient—an individual who has not received services from the physician, or an associate physician of the same group with the same specialty, within the past three years.

Node—see Workstation.

No-fault—insurance that pays for health care services resulting from injury to the patient, or for damage to property, regardless of who is at fault for causing the accident.

No-show—a patient with a scheduled appointment who simply does not show up and did not call the office to advise that he or she would not be coming.

Nursing home—an entity that provides nursing care and rehabilitation services to people with illnesses, injuries, or functional disabilities; most facilities serve the elderly, but some provide services to younger individuals with special needs.

Office hours—the time when the ongoing responsibilities of office management are completed.

Online—when connections between computers (workstations-to-servers or workstations-to-workstations) are made via Internet connectivity.

Open panel HMO—also known as a Network HMO and an independent practice association (IPA); includes physicians who provide services to enrollees of the plan in their own offices.

Operating system (OS)—the system that allows software and devices to function, and gives the user a way to communicate with the computer.

Output—anything that comes out of a computer, including information.

Parallel port—a 25-pin socket, most popular for plugging in the printer.

Participating physician—a physician who has agreed to treat specific patient populations and has negotiated for reimbursement under a contract with an insurance company.

Patient billing system—uses claims sent to insurance companies, along with payments received and posted, to generate statements.

Patient hours—those times during the workday that are dedicated to patient visits in the clinical back office.

Protection and Affordable Care Act—includes a large number of health-related provisions that will be put into effect over the next several years, estimated to be in full effect by 2018. These provisions include expanding Medicaid eligibility, providing incentives for businesses to provide health care benefits to their employees, additional support for medical research, and eliminating pre-existing condition exclusions, among others.

Patient registration system—allows the user to input information about each patient in the practice.

PCP—see Primary care physician.

Pending claim—also called a suspended claim, is one that is usually being reviewed.

Peripherals—hardware devices connected to the computer.

Personal computer (PC)—a desktop computer dedicated to the use of one individual.

PHI—see Protected health information.

Plug-and-play (PnP)—hardware that is automatically configured by the computer during installation.

Pointer—an on-screen, mouse-driven character, usually an arrow, that is used to perform grabbing, dragging, dropping, and clicking tasks by the mouse.

Posting payments system—applies the payment to the patient's account.

Primary care physician (PCP)—the physician who decides when the patient can see a specialist or receive special services and procedures; most PCPs practice general medicine and include family physicians and internists.

Primary insurance—the first insurance company that is billed for patient services.

Private fee-for-service plans (PFFS)—these plans are much like indemnity plans, and, in fact, are similar to original Medicare; however, these private plans determine the amount providers will be reimbursed.

Procedure posting—the process of entering procedure charges.

Procedure posting system—applies fees to the patient's account along with other information relevant to the encounter between patient and physician.

Processing—the performance of arithmetical and logical operations so that data can be productively used or manipulated by a computer.

Progress notes—handwritten or typed notes provided by the physician to document the details of a patient's visit.

Prompt—a special window with a message for the user.

Protected health information (PHI)—health information that can be individually identified in any form: orally, on paper, or electronically.

Provider identification numbers (PIN)—issued by health insurance companies to identify providers and verify credentials properly.

Provider sponsored organizations (PSOs)—either a single provider or a group of affiliated providers who render services to the beneficiary.

RAM—See Random Access Memory.

Random access memory (RAM)—the actual memory of the computer that temporarily holds currently opened software programs and files while they are in use by the computer.

Recall postcards—also known as tickler files; reminder systems designed to monitor distant follow-up appointments and provide a mailer that can be sent to patients approximately one to two months before an appointment should be scheduled.

Reference sheet—shows all patients scheduled for an office visit.

Referral—the actual transfer of a patient to a new physician, for partial or complete care, for a specific medical problem.

Registration form—also called a patient information data sheet; filled out by the person, or guardian of the person, to be treated by the physician.

Remittance advice (RA)—also known as an EOB; information regarding claims that were sent, either electronically or on paper claim forms, and that now are documented and returned to the medical office by the insurance carrier.

Report generation system—retrieves and organizes the data from various parts of the practice management software program into useful information or reports.

Restrictive endorsements—information that identifies the party who cashes a check and indicates that it is to be used "for deposit only;" used whenever a patient pays with a check, money order, or cashier's check.

Scanner—an input device, used to convert pictures or text into digital files.

Scroll bars—bars situated on the computer screen used to move blocks of text up and down or from left to right in a window.

Serial port—a simple port that can be identified by its 9-pin socket.

Server—a computer that is accessible to other computers in a network, usually on a smaller scale than mainframes.

Shared server—provides access to software, disk drives, and other areas to the users connected to them.

Shortcut keys—keyboard selections for accessing menu options without using the mouse.

Silicon chip—a small wafer of semiconductor material composed of electrical components that are responsible for all functions that run the computer; contained in the microprocessor.

Single/double click—a function of the mouse that allows the computer to select, open, or execute a command.

Skilled nursing facility (SNF)—for patients who need 24-hour nursing supervision in order to ensure their medical, psychological, and social needs are met.

SNF—see Skilled Nursing Facility.

Social Services—provides patient assistance in a number of areas, including information regarding financial resources to fit individual needs and eligibility.

Software program—specific instructions the computer follows that cause it to behave in a certain manner.

Source documents—documentation used as reference by the medical office staff.

Spreadsheet programs—software programs that allow information, mostly numbers, to be used in rows and columns; mathematical formulas can be applied to numbers for various uses and results.

Staff model—see Closed panel HMO.

Stand-alone unit—a computer that is not part of a network; all information is stored and used from that computer unit only.

Statement—an itemized bill that specifies the balance due on a patient's account.

Superbill—also known as an encounter form, a charge ticket, or visit/fee slip; contains all of the information insurance companies require in order to consider a claim for payment.

Suspended claim—also called a pending claim, is one that is usually being reviewed.

Systems software—the operating system (OS) that enables the computer to communicate between its various components.

Text box—an area to enter text or numbers in a software program.

Tickler files—also known as recall postcards; reminder systems designed to monitor distant follow-up appointments and provide a mailer that can be sent to patients approximately one to two months before an appointment should be scheduled.

Title bar—the bar along the top of a window that displays the name of the program or document on the left side of the bar.

Toolbar—a collection of buttons that can be clicked to activate the most common commands of a software program.

UCR—see Usual, customary and reasonable rate.

Underlined letters—indicators, or menu options, of shortcut features that can be used with the keyboard.

Unique provider identification number (UPIN)—a six-position, alphanumeric identifier that is assigned to all Medicare physicians, medical groups, and non-physician practitioners.

USB (Universal serial bus)—a universal port designed to standardize peripheral connectivity.

USB flash memory drive—sometimes called a jump drive; serves as additional storage, allowing files to be copied to and from the drive with up to 300 times the capacity of a floppy disk.

Usual, customary, and reasonable rate—also known as the UCR; calculated as part of an indemnity plan as the basis on which to make payment to the provider.

Walk-in patient—a person who comes to the office without an appointment.

Ward—a division of a hospital that contains rooms used for the temporary accommodation of patients.

WiFi—also called 802.11b; allows users with notebook computers and personal digital assistant (PDA) devices to wirelessly connect to networks, and through that, the Internet.

Windows Explorer—an application used to browse a PC for files and folders.

Word processing programs—software programs that allow the use of text for producing documents such as correspondence, reports, medical notes, and journal manuscripts.

Workers' compensation—insurance that employers are required to carry for employees who may get sick or injured on the job.

Work-in patient—a patient who calls the day before, or, on the same day that an appointment is needed.

Workstation—also called a node; a computer that is networked to the server.

Index

IMPORTANT! READ CAREFULLY: This End User License Agreement ("Agreement") sets forth the conditions by which Cengage Learning will make electronic access to the Cengage Learning-owned licensed content and associated media, software, documentation, printed materials, and electronic documentation contained in this package and/or made available to you via this product (the "Licensed Content"), available to you (the "End User"). BY CLICKING THE "I ACCEPT" BUTTON AND/OR OPENING THIS PACKAGE, YOU ACKNOWLEDGE THAT YOU HAVE READ ALL OF THE TERMS AND CONDITIONS, AND THAT YOU AGREE TO BE BOUND BY ITS TERMS, CONDITIONS, AND ALL APPLICABLE LAWS AND REGULATIONS GOVERNING THE USE OF THE LICENSED CONTENT.

1.0 SCOPE OF LICENSE

1.1 *Licensed Content.* The Licensed Content may contain portions of modifiable content ("Modifiable Content") and content which may not be modified or otherwise altered by the End User ("Non-Modifiable Content"). For purposes of this Agreement, Modifiable Content and Non-Modifiable Content may be collectively referred to herein as the "Licensed Content." All Licensed Content shall be considered Non-Modifiable Content, unless such Licensed Content is presented to the End User in a modifiable format and it is clearly indicated that modification of the Licensed Content is permitted.

1.2 Subject to the End User's compliance with the terms and conditions of this Agreement, Cengage Learning hereby grants the End User, a nontransferable, nonexclusive, limited right to access and view a single copy of the Licensed Content on a single personal computer system for noncommercial, internal, personal use only, and, to the extent that End User adopts the associated textbook for use in connection with a course, the limited right to provide, distribute, and display the Modifiable Content to course students who purchase the textbook, for use in connection with the course only. The End User shall not (i) reproduce, copy, modify (except in the case of Modifiable Content), distribute, display, transfer, sublicense, prepare derivative work(s) based on, sell, exchange, barter or transfer, rent, lease, loan, resell, or in any other manner exploit the Licensed Content; (ii) remove, obscure, or alter any notice of Cengage Learning's intellectual property rights present on or in the Licensed Content, including, but not limited to, copyright, trademark, and/or patent notices; or (iii) disassemble, decompile, translate, reverse engineer, or otherwise reduce the Licensed Content. Cengage reserves the right to use a hardware lock device, license administration software, and/or a license authorization key to control access or password protection technology to the Licensed Content. The End User may not take any steps to avoid or defeat the purpose of such measures. Use of the Licensed Content without the relevant required lock device or authorization key is prohibited. UNDER NO CIRCUMSTANCES MAY NON-SALEABLE ITEMS PROVIDED TO YOU BY CENGAGE (INCLUDING, WITHOUT LIMITATION, ANNOTATED INSTRUCTOR'S EDITIONS, SOLUTIONS MANUALS, INSTRUCTOR RESOURCES MATERIALS AND/OR TEST MATERIALS) BE SOLD, AUCTIONED, LICENSED OR OTHERWISE REDISTRIBUTED BY THE END USER.

2.0 TERMINATION

2.1 Cengage Learning may at any time (without prejudice to its other rights or remedies) immediately terminate this Agreement and/or suspend access to some or all of the Licensed Content, in the event that the End User does not comply with any of the terms and conditions of this Agreement. In the event of such termination by Cengage Learning, the End User shall immediately return any and all copies of the Licensed Content to Cengage Learning.

3.0 PROPRIETARY RIGHTS

3.1 The End User acknowledges that Cengage Learning owns all rights, title and interest, including, but not limited to all copyright rights therein, in and to the Licensed Content, and that the End User shall not take any action inconsistent with such ownership. The Licensed Content is protected by U.S., Canadian and other applicable copyright laws and by international treaties, including the Berne Convention and the Universal Copyright Convention. Nothing contained in this Agreement shall be construed as granting the End User any ownership rights in or to the Licensed Content.

3.2 Cengage Learning reserves the right at any time to withdraw from the Licensed Content any item or part of an item for which it no longer retains the right to publish, or which it has reasonable grounds to believe infringes copyright or is defamatory, unlawful, or otherwise objectionable.

4.0 PROTECTION AND SECURITY

4.1 The End User shall use its best efforts and take all reasonable steps to safeguard its copy of the Licensed Content to ensure that no unauthorized reproduction, publication, disclosure, modification, or distribution of the Licensed Content, in whole or in part, is made. To the extent that the End User becomes aware of any such unauthorized use of the Licensed Content, the End User shall immediately notify Cengage Learning. Notification of such violations may be made by sending an e-mail to infringement@cengage.com.

5.0 MISUSE OF THE LICENSED PRODUCT

5.1 In the event that the End User uses the Licensed Content in violation of this Agreement, Cengage Learning shall have the option of electing liquidated damages, which shall include all profits generated by the End User's use of the Licensed Content plus interest computed at the maximum rate permitted by law and all legal fees and other expenses incurred by Cengage Learning in enforcing its rights, plus penalties.

6.0 FEDERAL GOVERNMENT CLIENTS

6.1 Except as expressly authorized by Cengage Learning, Federal Government clients obtain only the rights specified in this Agreement and no other rights. The Government acknowledges that (i) all software and related documentation incorporated in the Licensed Content is existing commercial computer software within the meaning of FAR 27.405(b)(2); and (2) all other data delivered in whatever form, is limited rights data within the meaning of FAR 27.401. The restrictions in this section are acceptable as consistent with the Government's need for software and other data under this Agreement.

7.0 DISCLAIMER OF WARRANTIES AND LIABILITIES

7.1 Although Cengage Learning believes the Licensed Content to be reliable, Cengage Learning does not guarantee or warrant (i) any information or materials contained in or produced by the Licensed Content, (ii) the accuracy, completeness or reliability of the Licensed Content, or (iii) that the Licensed Content is free from errors or other material defects. THE LICENSED PRODUCT IS PROVIDED "AS IS," WITHOUT ANY WARRANTY OF ANY KIND AND CENGAGE LEARNING DISCLAIMS ANY AND ALL WARRANTIES, EXPRESSED OR IMPLIED, INCLUDING, WITHOUT LIMITATION, WARRANTIES OF MERCHANTABILITY OR FITNESS FOR A PARTICULAR PURPOSE. IN NO EVENT SHALL CENGAGE LEARNING BE LIABLE FOR: INDIRECT, SPECIAL, PUNITIVE OR CONSEQUENTIAL DAMAGES INCLUDING FOR LOST PROFITS, LOST DATA, OR OTHERWISE. IN NO EVENT SHALL CENGAGE LEARNING'S AGGREGATE LIABILITY HEREUNDER, WHETHER ARISING IN CONTRACT, TORT, STRICT LIABILITY OR OTHERWISE, EXCEED THE AMOUNT OF FEES PAID BY THE END USER HEREUNDER FOR THE LICENSE OF THE LICENSED CONTENT.

8.0 GENERAL

8.1 *Entire Agreement.* This Agreement shall constitute the entire Agreement between the Parties and supercedes all prior Agreements and understandings oral or written relating to the subject matter hereof.

8.2 *Enhancements/Modifications of Licensed Content.* From time to time, and in Cengage Learning's sole discretion, Cengage Learning may advise the End User of updates, upgrades, enhancements and/or improvements to the Licensed Content, and may permit the End User to access and use, subject to the terms and conditions of this Agreement, such modifications, upon payment of prices as may be established by Cengage Learning.

8.3 *No Export.* The End User shall use the Licensed Content solely in the United States and shall not transfer or export, directly or indirectly, the Licensed Content outside the United States.

8.4 *Severability.* If any provision of this Agreement is invalid, illegal, or unenforceable under any applicable statute or rule of law, the provision shall be deemed omitted to the extent that it is invalid, illegal, or unenforceable. In such a case, the remainder of the Agreement shall be construed in a manner as to give greatest effect to the original intention of the parties hereto.

8.5 *Waiver.* The waiver of any right or failure of either party to exercise in any respect any right provided in this Agreement in any instance shall not be deemed to be a waiver of such right in the future or a waiver of any other right under this Agreement.

8.6 *Choice of Law/Venue.* This Agreement shall be interpreted, construed, and governed by and in accordance with the laws of the State of New York, applicable to contracts executed and to be wholly preformed therein, without regard to its principles governing conflicts of law. Each party agrees that any proceeding arising out of or relating to this Agreement or the breach or threatened breach of this Agreement may be commenced and prosecuted in a court in the State and County of New York. Each party consents and submits to the nonexclusive personal jurisdiction of any court in the State and County of New York in respect of any such proceeding.

8.7 *Acknowledgment.* By opening this package and/or by accessing the Licensed Content on this Web site, THE END USER ACKNOWLEDGES THAT IT HAS READ THIS AGREEMENT, UNDERSTANDS IT, AND AGREES TO BE BOUND BY ITS TERMS AND CONDITIONS. IF YOU DO NOT ACCEPT THESE TERMS AND CONDITIONS, YOU MUST NOT ACCESS THE LICENSED CONTENT AND RETURN THE LICENSED PRODUCT TO CENGAGE LEARNING (WITHIN 30 CALENDAR DAYS OF THE END USER'S PURCHASE) WITH PROOF OF PAYMENT ACCEPTABLE TO CENGAGE LEARNING, FOR A CREDIT OR A REFUND. Should the End User have any questions/comments regarding this Agreement, please contact Cengage Learning at Delmar.help@cengage.com.

MOSS 2.0 SYSTEM REQUIREMENTS:

- Processor: minimum required by operating system
- Memory: minimum required by operating system
- Operating System: Microsoft Windows XP® with Service Pack 2, Windows Vista®
- 75 MB free hard drive space
- 800 × 600 monitor display
- Recommended: MS Access (MS Access Runtime supplied on disk)

Microsoft®, Windows®, Windows XP®, and Windows Vista® are trademarks of the Microsoft Corporation.

MOSS 2.0 SINGLE USER INSTALLATION INSTRUCTIONS:

1. Close all open programs and documents.
2. Place the MOSS 2.0 CD into your CD-ROM drive.
3. MOSS 2.0 should begin setup automatically. Follow the on-screen prompts to install MOSS and Microsoft Access Runtime:
   - Click "Next"
   - Click "I Accept" the terms of the license agreement
   - Click "Next"
   - Click the button next to "TYPICAL" as the setup type
   - Click "Install"
4. If MOSS does not begin setup automatically, follow these instructions:
   - Double click on My Computer.
   - Double click the Control Panel icon.
   - Utilize the Add/Remove Programs feature (for specific instructions on how to use, please reference the User Manual for your Operating System).
   - Click the Install button, and follow the prompts as indicated in Step 3.
5. When you finish installing MOSS, it will be accessible through the Start menu: *Start > Programs > MOSS 2.0*